The ESC Textbook of
Thrombosis

European Society of Cardiology publications portfolio

The ESC Textbook of Cardiovascular Medicine (Third Edition)
Edited by A. John Camm, Thomas F. Lüscher, Gerald Maurer and Patrick W. Serruys

The ESC Textbook of Preventive Cardiology
Edited by Stephan Gielen, Guy De Backer, Massimo Piepoli, and David Wood

The EHRA Book of Pacemaker, ICD, and CRT Troubleshooting: *Case-based learning with multiple choice questions*
Edited by Haran Burri, Carsten Israel, and Jean-Claude Deharo

The EACVI Echo Handbook
Edited by Patrizio Lancellotti and Bernard Cosyns

The ESC Handbook of Preventive Cardiology: *Putting prevention into practice*
Edited by Catriona Jennings, Ian Graham, and Stephan Gielen

The EACVI Textbook of Echocardiography (Second edition)
Edited by Patrizio Lancellotti, José Luis Zamorano, Gilbert Habib, and Luigi Badano

The EHRA Book of Interventional Electrophysiology: *Case-based learning with multiple choice questions*
Edited by Hein Heidbuchel, Mattias Duytschaever, and Haran Burri

The ESC Textbook of Vascular Biology
Edited by Robert Krams and Magnus Bäck

The ESC Textbook of Cardiovascular Development
Edited by José Maria Pérez-Pomares and Robert Kelly

The EACVI Textbook of Cardiovascular Magnetic Resonance
Edited by Massimo Lombardi, Sven Plein, Steffen Petersen, Chiara Bucciarelli-Ducci, Emanuela Valsangiacomo Buechel, Cristina Basso, and Victor Ferrari

The ESC Textbook of Sports Cardiology
Edited by Antonio Pelliccia, Hein Heidbuchel, Domenico Corrado, Mats Borjesson, and Sanjay Sharma

The ESC Handbook of Cardiac Rehabilitation: *A practical clinical guide*
Edited by Ana Abreu, Jean-Paul Schmid, and Massimo Piepoli

The ESC Textbook of Intensive and Acute Cardiovascular Care (Third Edition)
Edited by Marco Tubaro, Pascal Vranckx, Susanna Price, Christiaan Vrints, and Eric Bonnefoy

The ESC Textbook of Cardiovascular Imaging (Third Edition)
Edited by José Luis Zamorano, Jeroen J. Bax, Juhani Knuuti, Patrizio Lancellotti, Fausto J. Pinto, Bogdan A. Popescu, and Udo Sechtem

The ESC Textbook of Cardiovascular Nursing
Edited by Catriona Jennings, Felicity Astin, Donna Fitzsimons, Ekaterini Lambrinou, Lis Neubeck, and David R. Thompson

The EHRA Book of Pacemaker, ICD, and CRT Troubleshooting Vol. 2: *Case-based learning with multiple choice questions*
Edited by Haran Burri, Jens Brock Johansen, Nicholas J. Linker, and Dominic Theuns

The EACVI Handbook of Cardiovascular CT
Edited by Oliver Gaemperli, Pál Maurovich-Horvat, Koen Nieman, Gianluca Pontone, and Francesca Pugliese

The ESC Textbook of Heart Failure
Edited by Petar M. Seferović, Andrew J.S. Coats, Gerasimos Filippatos, Stefan Anker, Johann Bauersachs, and Giuseppe Rosano

The ESC Textbook of
Thrombosis

Edited by

Raffaele De Caterina
Cardiovascular Division, Pisa University Hospital, and University of Pisa, Pisa, Italy

David J. Moliterno
Division of Cardiovascular Medicine, Gill Heart and Vascular Institute, University of Kentucky, Lexington, Kentucky, USA

Steen Dalby Kristensen
Consultant Cardiologist and Head of the Cardiovascular Research Centre in the Department of Cardiology, Aarhus University Hospital Skejby, Denmark

OXFORD
UNIVERSITY PRESS

ESC
Working Group
Thrombosis

OXFORD
UNIVERSITY PRESS

Great Clarendon Street, Oxford, OX2 6DP,
United Kingdom

Oxford University Press is a department of the University of Oxford.
It furthers the University's objective of excellence in research, scholarship,
and education by publishing worldwide. Oxford is a registered trade mark of
Oxford University Press in the UK and in certain other countries

First Edition published in 2023

Published in the United States of America by Oxford University Press
198 Madison Avenue, New York, NY 10016, United States of America

British Library Cataloguing in Publication Data
Data available

Library of Congress Control Number: 2023936949

ISBN 978–0–19–286922–7

DOI: 10.1093/med/9780192869227.001.0001

Printed in the UK by
Bell & Bain Ltd., Glasgow

Foreword

While the evolution of knowledge in the field of thrombosis and antithrombotic therapies began quite slowly centuries ago, it has dramatically accelerated in recent decades. Many early key scientific findings in atherosclerosis, vascular biology, thrombosis, and focused therapeutics were made by European physicians and scientists. As but a few historic examples, in the mid-19th century the investigations of Rudolf Virchow (Germany) and Jean Cruveilhier (France) led to a now classic description of the prothrombotic triad—vascular injury, abnormal blood flow, and heightened coagulability. Later in the 19th century, the earliest recognized anticoagulant was suspected to be in the (leech) saliva of *Hirudo medicinalis* and was termed 'hirudine' by John Haycraft (UK), and acetylsalicylic acid was formulated by Felix Hoffman (Germany). This evolution in the understanding of thrombotic pathways, the discovery of novel therapeutic targets, and the clinical testing and application of new treatments continue aggressively in the present day. This has obligated clinical practice guidelines to be revised frequently by cardiac societies in order to keep pace with these exciting and progressive advancements.

At the same time, textbooks as the repositories of medical knowledge needed to more rapidly evolve with electronic platforms for near-instant access, information retrieval, sharing of knowledge, and continuous updating. A greater recognition of the global burden of atherothrombotic vascular disease and a global approach and partnership to studying and improving vascular health is now taking place. Considering together the discovery of medical advancements, electronic publishing, and the global burden of cardiovascular health, one can see the proof that science is truly social.

My personal journey in medicine has occurred during these recent evolutions. I have been fortunate to witness and participate first-hand in the growth and refinement in our understanding of vascular diseases and their treatments, the digitization and widespread dissemination of published information, and the pursuit in approaching the elements of vascular health from a global perspective. With these thoughts in mind, I feel privileged and honoured to write the foreword message for this third edition by these editors in a textbook now under the auspices of the European Society of Cardiology (ESC). *The ESC Textbook of Thrombosis* is an appropriate and needed addition to the ESC family of textbooks.

At present there are a number of available books covering the biology and pathology of thrombosis and its treatment. Likewise, there are books covering ischaemic vascular disorders involving the cerebral, coronary, and peripheral vessels or focused on venous, arterial, or structural heart interventions. This book has as a key attraction its comprehensive coverage of these topics—so-called one-stop shopping. The editors—Drs De Caterina, Kristensen, and Moliterno—have partnered with 78 expert authors from 12 countries to describe and explain the basis for thrombotic disorders and their treatments in carefully focused chapters. The layout of the book is logically organized and carefully divided into sections covering pathophysiology, pharmacology of antithrombotic therapies, clinical treatment strategies, and special care situations. From drug discovery to regulatory approval to clinical care delivery, this textbook covers the entire spectrum for practitioners.

In addition to foundational knowledge, the authors highlight timely information in the field as well as its appropriate clinical application. This information is made more practical by linking recommendations with the ESC Guidelines on the corresponding care pathways. From looking to the immediate past with 'What's new' to immediately forward with 'What's next' sections, the authors bring the reader up to date and engaged in looking ahead. Examples of new or refined topic areas include the development and testing of anti-factor XIa drugs, the genetics of drug metabolism, the antithrombotic therapies used for new interventional procedures and for patients undergoing transcatheter valve repair and replacement, and practical strategies to avoid and treat bleeding associated with antithrombotic therapies.

In summary, *The ESC Textbook of Thrombosis*, which is also available in an electronic, easy-to-consult platform, is a needed and welcome state-of-the-art compilation of the field of thrombocardiology, providing information for practitioners in multiple areas of medicine. The editors have done a terrific job of minimizing the obligatory overlap among chapters and keeping the text focused on the latest findings and clinical applications. I am confident to say this is a very helpful textbook at the present time. While it will undoubtedly need future editions to keep pace with our dynamic and progressive field, it will stand as a landmark compendium.

Valentin Fuster, MD, PhD
Physician-in-Chief, Mount Sinai Hospital, New York, USA
Director, Centro Nacional de Investigaciones Cardiovasculares, Madrid, Spain

Preface

Wherever the art of medicine is loved, there is also a love of humanity.

Hippocrates

Over the past several decades, knowledge regarding the pathobiology of thrombotic cardiovascular disease has substantially increased. The crux of ischaemic vascular disease is well established to be a complex interplay of atherosclerosis, inflammation, and thrombosis. The understanding of venous thromboembolism, hypercoagulable states, and atrial fibrillation has also witnessed impressive progress, and these disorders have become important areas of investigation with translation into several aspects of clinical medicine. At the same time, the number of therapeutic agents that have become available has dramatically increased, in parallel with the discovery of new biological targets and pathways.

We have undertaken this textbook edition keeping in mind the marked evolution in our understanding of the pathobiological background of thrombosis as well as the tremendous growth in therapeutic options. We edited a first edition of this textbook (*Therapeutic Strategies in Thrombosis*, by Clinical Publishing) in 2006 and a second edition (*Therapeutic Advances in Thrombosis*, by Wiley-Blackwell) in 2012. The expansion in the number of available intravenous and oral antithrombotic agents has been particularly remarkable in recent years: direct and specific coagulation factor inhibitors, as well as new antiplatelet agents have been developed and are quickly finding their place in daily practice. In creating a third textbook edition, now endorsed by the European Society of Cardiology (ESC) and the ESC Working Group on Thrombosis, we have partnered with expert authors globally for a complete rewriting of chapters. The book includes 30 chapters and is divided into four key sections: pathophysiology of thrombosis, clinical pharmacology of antithrombotic drugs, therapeutic strategies, and special situations. The chapters address virtually all thrombotic and antithrombotic aspects of atherosclerotic disease, venous disease, valvular and structural heart disease, and atrial fibrillation. Great efforts have been made to present contemporary data on each of these topics, emphasizing the newest developments ('What's new'), providing practical guidance by including ESC Guideline recommendations, and summarizing foreseeable developments ('What's next'). In an era of rapid access to online information and declining attention to hardcover books, we believe that a comprehensive effort to put together the best and most up-to-date knowledge in an important therapeutic area is needed, worthwhile, and welcome.

We are very grateful and most indebted to all the contributors who have made this textbook possible. Their commitment to scholarly activity and education has certainly been inspired by an unrelented passion for a discipline—clinical thrombocardiology—that brings together cardiology, internal medicine, haematology, neurology, vascular and cardiac surgery, vascular and molecular biology, and pharmacology.

We edited this textbook with passion, in the belief that passionate interest in this topic is important for preventing and treating a substantial number of current medical conditions.

Raffaele De Caterina, MD, PhD, FESC
David J. Moliterno, MD, FESC
Steen Dalby Kristensen, MD, DMSc, FESC

Contents

Contributors

Walter Ageno
Dipartimento di Medicina e Chirurgia, Università degli Studi dell'Insubria, Varese, Italy

Stefan Agewall
Department of Clinical Sciences, Danderyd Hospital, Karolinska Institutet, Stockholm, Sweden; Institute of Clinical Sciences, University of Oslo, Oslo, Norway

John H. Alexander
Division of Cardiology and Duke Clinical Research Institute, Duke University, Durham, North Carolina, USA

Mohamad Alkhouli
Department of Cardiovascular Medicine, Mayo Clinic, Rochester, Minnesota, USA

Asger Andersen
Department of Cardiology, Aarhus University Hospital, Aarhus; Institute of Clinical Medicine, Faculty of Health, Aarhus University, Aarhus, Denmark

Dominick J. Angiolillo
Division of Cardiology, University of Florida College of Medicine, Jacksonville, Florida, USA

Lina Badimon
Cardiovascular Program-ICCC, IR-Hospital de la Santa Creu i Sant Pau–IIB SantPau and CiberCV, Barcelona, Spain

Gorav Batra
Department of Medical Sciences, Cardiology, and Uppsala Clinical Research Center, Uppsala University, Uppsala, Sweden

Craig J. Beavers
Department of Pharmacy Practice and Science, University of Kentucky, College of Pharmacy, Lexington, Kentucky, USA

Alexander P. Benz
Department of Cardiology, University Medical Center Mainz, Johannes Gutenberg-University, Mainz, Germany; Population Health Research Institute, Hamilton Health Sciences and McMaster University, Hamilton, Ontario, Canada

Deepak L. Bhatt
Mount Sinai Heart, Icahn School of Medicine at Mount Sinai Health System, New York, NY, USA

Marc A. Brouwer
Department of Cardiology, Radboud University Medical Center, Nijmegen, The Netherlands

Harry R. Buller
Department of Vascular Medicine, Amsterdam University Medical Center, Amsterdam, The Netherlands

Peter Calvert
Liverpool Centre for Cardiovascular Science at University of Liverpool, Liverpool John Moores University and Liverpool Heart & Chest Hospital, Liverpool; Liverpool Heart & Chest NHS Foundation Trust, Liverpool, UK

Davide Cao
Center for Interventional Cardiovascular Research and Clinical Trials, Mount Sinai Heart, Icahn School of Medicine at Mount Sinai Health System, New York, NY, USA; Department of Biomedical Sciences, Humanitas University, Pieve Emanuele-Milan, Italy

Davide Capodanno
Division of Cardiology, Azienda Ospedaliero-Universitaria Policlinico 'G. Rodolico – San Marco', University of Catania, Catania, Italy

Alexander T. Cohen
Department of Haematological Medicine, Guy's and St Thomas' NHS Foundation Trust, King's College London, London, UK

Yazan Daaboul
Division of Cardiovascular Diseases, Department of Medicine, Beth Israel Deaconess Medical Center, Harvard Medical School, Boston; Baim Institute for Clinical Research, Boston, Massachusetts, USA

George Dangas
Center for Interventional Cardiovascular Research and Clinical Trials, Mount Sinai Heart, Icahn School of Medicine at Mount Sinai Health System, New York, NY, USA

Raffaele De Caterina
Cardiovascular Division, Pisa University Hospital, and University of Pisa, Pisa, Italy

Gentian Denas
Thrombosis Research Laboratory, Cardiology Clinic University of Padova, Padova, Italy

Marcello Di Nisio
Department of Medicine and Ageing Sciences, University 'G. d'Annunzio' of Chieti-Pescara, Chieti, Italy

Hans Christoph Diener
Department of Neuroepidemiology, Institute for Medical Informatics, Biometry and Epidemiology, Medical Faculty of the University Duisburg-Essen, Essen, Germany

Steven P. Dunn
Department of Pharmacy Services and Division of Cardiovascular Medicine, UVA Health, University of Virginia, Charlottesville, Virginia, USA

John W. Eikelboom
Department of Medicine, McMaster University, Hamilton, and Population Health Research Institute, Hamilton, Canada

Chaozer Er
Department of General Medicine, Woodlands Health, Singapore

Alexander C. Fanaroff
Penn Cardiovascular Outcomes, Quality and Evaluative Research Center, Leonard Davis Institute, and Cardiovascular Medicine Division, University of Pennsylvania, Philadelphia, USA

James C. Fredenburgh
Department of Medicine, McMaster University, Hamilton; Thrombosis and Atherosclerosis Research Institute, McMaster University, Hamilton, Ontario, Canada

Tobias Geisler
Department of Cardiology and Angiology, University Hospital Tübingen, Germany

C. Michael Gibson
Division of Cardiovascular Diseases, Department of Medicine, Beth Israel Deaconess Medical Center, Harvard Medical School, Boston; Baim Institute for Clinical Research, Boston, Massachusetts, USA

Antonio Greco
Division of Cardiology, Azienda Ospedaliero-Universitaria Policlinico 'G. Rodolico – San Marco', University of Catania, Catania, Italy

Erik Lerkevang Grove
Department of Cardiology, Aarhus University Hospital, Aarhus; Department of Clinical Medicine, Health, Aarhus University, Aarhus, Denmark

Graeme J. Hankey
Perron Institute for Neurological and Translational Science, Perth, Australia; Medical School, Centre for Neurological and Neuromuscular Diseases, The University of Western Australia, Perth, Australia

Ziad Hijazi
Department of Medical Sciences, Cardiology, and Uppsala Clinical Research Center, Uppsala University, Uppsala, Sweden

Stefan H. Hohnloser
Department of Cardiology, J.W. Goethe University, Frankfurt, Germany

Serge Korjian
Division of Cardiovascular Diseases, Department of Medicine, Beth Israel Deaconess Medical Center, Harvard Medical School, Boston; Baim Institute for Clinical Research, Boston, Massachusetts, USA

Kasper Korsholm
Department of Cardiology, Aarhus University Hospital, Aarhus; Institute of Clinical Medicine, Faculty of Health, Aarhus University, Aarhus, Denmark

Steen Dalby Kristensen
Department of Cardiology, Aarhus University Hospital, Aarhus; Department of Clinical Medicine, Health, Aarhus University, Aarhus, Denmark

Johan Lindbäck
Uppsala Clinical Research Center, Uppsala University, Uppsala, Sweden

Gregory Y.H. Lip
Liverpool Centre for Cardiovascular Science at University of Liverpool, Liverpool John Moores University and Liverpool Heart & Chest Hospital, Liverpool, UK; Danish Center for Clinical Health Services Research, Department of Clinical Medicine, Aalborg University, Aalborg, Denmark

Renato D. Lopes
Division of Cardiology and Duke Clinical Research Institute, Duke University, Durham, North Carolina, USA

Michael Maeng
Department of Cardiology, Aarhus University Hospital, Aarhus; Department of Clinical Medicine, Health, Aarhus University, Aarhus, Denmark

Rossella Marcucci
Department of Experimental and Clinical Medicine, University of Florence and Atherothrombosis Center, Careggi Hospital, Florence, Italy

Francisco Marín
Hospital Clínico Universitario Virgen de la Arrixaca, University of Murcia, IMIB-Arrixaca, CIBERCV, Murcia, Spain

Roxana Mehran
Center for Interventional Cardiovascular Research and Clinical Trials, Mount Sinai Heart, Icahn School of Medicine at Mount Sinai Health System, New York, NY, USA

Erica Michelotti
Cardiovascular Division, Pisa University Hospital, and University of Pisa, Pisa, Italy

Naoki Misumida
Division of Cardiovascular Medicine, Gill Heart and Vascular Institute, University of Kentucky, Lexington, Kentucky, USA

David J. Moliterno
Division of Cardiovascular Medicine, Gill Heart and Vascular Institute, University of Kentucky, Lexington, Kentucky, USA

Jens Erik Nielsen-Kudsk
Department of Cardiology, Aarhus University Hospital, Aarhus; Institute of Clinical Medicine, Faculty of Health, Aarhus University, Aarhus, Denmark

Renske H. Olie
Department of Internal Medicine and Thrombosis Expertise Center, Maastricht University Medical Center, Maastricht; Cardiovascular Research Institute Maastricht (CARIM), Maastricht University, The Netherlands

Luis Ortega-Paz
Division of Cardiology, University of Florida College of Medicine, Jacksonville, Florida, USA

Manan Pareek
Center for Translational Cardiology and Pragmatic Randomized Trials, Department of Biomedical Sciences, Faculty of Health and Medical Sciences, University of Copenhagen and Copenhagen University Hospital – Herlev and Gentofte, Copenhagen; Department of Cardiology, The Heart Center, Copenhagen University Hospital – Rigshospitalet, Copenhagen, Denmark

William A.E. Parker
Cardiovascular Research Unit, University of Sheffield, Sheffield, UK

Carlo Patrono
Division of Pharmacology, Department of Safety and Bioethics, Catholic University School of Medicine, Rome, Italy

Vittorio Pengo
Thrombosis Research Laboratory, Department of Cardiac, Thoracic, Vascular Sciences and Public Health, University of Padova, Padova, and Arianna Foundation on Anticoagulation, Bologna, Italy

Nicola Potere
Department of Medicine and Ageing Sciences, Center for Advanced Studies and Technology, 'G. d'Annunzio' University, Chieti, Italy

Paul M. Ridker
Center for Cardiovascular Disease Prevention, Divisions of Preventive Medicine and Cardiovascular Diseases, Brigham and Women's Hospital, and Harvard Medical School, Boston, Massachusetts, USA

Konstantinos D. Rizas
Medizinische Klinik und Poliklinik I, LMU University Hospital Munich, Munich; German Centre for Cardiovascular Research (DZHK), partner site Munich Heart Alliance, Munich, Germany

Bianca Rocca
Division of Pharmacology, Department of Safety and Bioethics, Catholic University School of Medicine, Rome, Italy

Vanessa Roldán
Hospital Universitario Morales Meseguer, University of Murcia, Murcia, Spain

Dirk Sibbing
Privatklinik Lauterbacher Mühle am Ostersee, Seeshaupt & Medizinische Klinik und Poliklinik I, LMU University Hospital Munich, Munich; German Centre for Cardiovascular Research (DZHK), partner site Munich Heart Alliance, Munich, Germany

Agneta Siegbahn
Department of Medical Sciences, Clinical Chemistry, and Uppsala Clinical Research Center, Uppsala University, Uppsala, Sweden

Jolanta M. Siller-Matula
Department of Internal Medicine II, Division of Cardiology, Medical University of Vienna, Vienna, Austria

Peter R. Sinnaeve
Department of Cardiovascular Medicine, University Hospitals Leuven, and Department of Cardiovascular Sciences, University of Leuven, Belgium

Alessandro Spirito
Center for Interventional Cardiovascular Research and Clinical Trials, Mount Sinai Heart, Icahn School of Medicine at Mount Sinai Health System, New York, NY, USA

Robert F. Storey
Department of Infection, Immunity and Cardiovascular Disease, University of Sheffield, Sheffield, UK

Peter J. Svensson
Department of Translational Medicine Clinical Coagulation Research Unit, Skåne University Hospital, Lund University, Malmö, Sweden

Jur M. ten Berg
St. Antonius Hospital, Department of Cardiology, Nieuwegein, and Cardiovascular Research Institute Maastricht (CARIM), Maastricht, The Netherlands

Hugo ten Cate
Department of Internal Medicine and Thrombosis Expertise Center, Maastricht University Medical Center, Maastricht; Cardiovascular Research Institute Maastricht (CARIM), Maastricht University, The Netherlands

Nicola Tidbury
Liverpool Centre for Cardiovascular Science at University of Liverpool, Liverpool John Moores University and Liverpool Heart & Chest Hospital, Liverpool; Liverpool Heart & Chest NHS Foundation Trust, Liverpool, UK

Frans Van de Werf
Department of Cardiovascular Medicine, University Hospital Leuven, and Department of Cardiovascular Sciences, University of Leuven, Belgium

Wout W.A. van den Broek
St. Antonius Hospital, Department of Cardiology, Nieuwegein, The Netherlands

Nick van Es
Department of Vascular Medicine, Amsterdam University Medical Center, Amsterdam, The Netherlands

Freek W.A. Verheugt
Department of Cardiology, Heartcenter, Onze Lieve Vrouwe Gasthuis, Amsterdam, The Netherlands

Gemma Vilahur
Cardiovascular Program-ICCC, IR-Hospital de la Santa Creu i Sant Pau–IIB SantPau and CiberCV, Barcelona, Spain

Håkan Wallén
Division of Cardiovascular Medicine, Department of Clinical Sciences, Danderyd Hospital, Karolinska Institutet, Stockholm, Sweden

Lars Wallentin
Department of Medical Sciences, Cardiology, and Uppsala Clinical Research Center, Uppsala University, Uppsala, Sweden

Jeffrey I. Weitz
Department of Medicine, McMaster University, Hamilton; Thrombosis and Atherosclerosis Research Institute, McMaster University, Hamilton; Department of Biochemistry and Biomedical Sciences, McMaster University, Hamilton, Ontario, Canada

Symbols and abbreviations

➔	cross-reference
~	approximately
≥	equal to or greater than
≤	equal to or less than
>	greater than
<	less than
ABC	Age, Biomarkers, Clinical history
ABI	ankle–brachial index
ACC	American College of Cardiology
ACCP	American College of Chest Physicians
ACR	Academic Research Consortium
ACS	acute coronary syndrome
ACT	activated clotting time
ADMA	asymmetric dimethylarginine
ADP	adenosine diphosphate
AHA	American Heart Association
AIS	acute ischaemic stroke
aPL	antiphospholipid antibodies
APS	antiphospholipid syndrome
aPTT	activated partial thromboplastin time
ASA	American Stroke Association
ASCO	American Society of Clinical Oncology
ASCVD	atherosclerotic cardiovascular disease
ASH	American Society of Haematology
AT	antithrombin
ATP	adenosine triphosphate
AUC	area under the curve
BARC	Bleeding Academic Research Consortium
BMI	body mass index
BNP	B-type natriuretic peptide
CABG	coronary artery bypass graft
CAC	coronary artery calcium
CAD	coronary artery disease
cAMP	cyclic adenosine monophosphate
CAPS	catastrophic antiphospholipid syndrome
CAT	cancer-associated thrombosis
CCS	chronic coronary syndrome
CDER	Center for Drug Evaluation and Research
CF-LVAD	continuous flow left ventricular assist device
CHD	coronary heart disease
CHMP	Committee for Medicinal Products for Human Use
CI	confidence interval
CMR	cardiac magnetic resonance imaging
COC	combined oral contraceptive
COR	class of recommendation
COX	cyclooxygenase
CPB	cardiopulmonary bypass
CPIC	Clinical Pharmacogenetics Implementation Consortium
CRC	colorectal cancer
CrCl	creatinine clearance
CRP	C-reactive protein
CTA	clinical trial application
c-TCD	contrast-enhanced transcranial Doppler
CTEPH	chronic thromboembolic pulmonary hypertension
cTn	cardiac troponin
c-TOE	contrast-enhanced transoesophageal echocardiography
c-TTE	contrast-enhanced transthoracic echocardiography
CYP	cytochrome P450
DAPT	dual antiplatelet therapy
DAT	dual antithrombotic therapy
DDI	drug–drug interaction
DM	diabetes mellitus
DOAC	direct oral anticoagulant
DRT	device-related thrombosis
DSMB	Drug Safety and Monitoring Board
DVT	deep vein thrombosis
EACTS	European Association for Cardio-Thoracic Surgery
ECG	electrocardiogram
ECLS	extracorporeal life support
ECMO	extracorporeal membrane oxygenation
EM	extensive metabolizer
EMA	European Medicines Agency
eNOS	endothelial nitric oxide synthase
ESC	European Society of Cardiology

ESO	European Stroke Organisation
ESUS	embolic stroke of unknown source
ET	essential thrombocythaemia
EU	European Union
EV	extracellular vesicle
FLAIR	fluid-attenuated inversion recovery
FVL	factor V Leiden
GCS	graded compression stocking
GDF	growth differentiation factor
GFR	glomerular filtration rate
GP	glycoprotein
GPI	glycoprotein IIb/IIIa inhibitor
GUSTO	Global Use of Strategies for Opening Occluded Coronary Arteries
HALT	hypoattenuated leaflet thickening
HAM	hypoattenuation affecting motion
HBR	high bleeding risk
HIT	heparin-induced thrombocytopenia
HPR	high platelet reactivity
HR	hazard ratio
hs-cTn	high-sensitivity cardiac troponin
HTS	high-throughput screening
ICH	intracranial haemorrhage
ICU	intensive care unit
IM	intermediate metabolizer
IMPROVE	International Medical Prevention Registry on Venous Thromboembolism
IND	Investigational New Drug
INR	international normalized ratio
IPC	intermittent pneumatic compressor
ISTH	International Society on Thrombosis and Haemostasis
IV	intravenous
LA	left atrium/atrial
LAA	left atrial appendage
LAAC	left atrial appendage closure
LAAO	left atrial appendage occluder/occlusion
LMWH	low-molecular-weight heparin
LOE	level of evidence
LoF	loss of function
LPR	low platelet reactivity
LTA	light transmission aggregometry
LV	left ventricle/ventricular
LVAD	left ventricular assist device
MAA	Marketing Authorization Application
MACE	major adverse cardiovascular event
MAD	multiple ascending dose
MHV	mechanical heart valve
MI	myocardial infarction
MINS	myocardial injury after non-cardiac surgery
miRNA	microribonucleic acid
MMP	matrix metalloproteinase
MR	mitral regurgitation
MRI	magnetic resonance imaging
mRNA	messenger RNA
MVR	mitral valve replacement
NACE	net adverse clinical events
NCS	non-cardiac surgery
NDA	New Drug Application
NET	neutrophil extracellular trap
NICE	National Institute for Health and Care Excellence
NIHSS	National Institutes of Health Stroke Scale
NO	nitric oxide
NOAC	non-vitamin K antagonist oral anticoagulant
NSAID	non-steroidal anti-inflammatory drug
NSTE	non-ST-segment elevation
NSTEMI	non-ST-elevation myocardial infarction
NT-proBNP	N-terminal pro B-type natriuretic peptide
OAC	oral anticoagulation/anticoagulant
OPR	optimal platelet reactivity
OR	odds ratio
PAD	peripheral artery disease
PAI-1	plasminogen activator inhibitor-1
PAR-1	protease-activated receptor-1
PASCAL	PFO-Associated Stroke Causal Likelihood
PCI	percutaneous coronary intervention
PDE	phosphodiesterase
PE	pulmonary embolism
PESI	Pulmonary Embolism Severity Index
PFO	patent foramen ovale
PG	prostaglandin
PGHS	prostaglandin H-synthase
P-gp	permeability-glycoprotein
PI	pharmacoinvasive
PM	poor metabolizer
PPC	prothrombin complex concentrate
PPI	proton pump inhibitor
PT	prothrombin time
PTA	percutaneous transluminal angioplasty
PVT	prosthetic valve thrombosis or polycythaemia vera
RAM	risk assessment model
RCT	randomized controlled trial
RoPE	Risk of Paradoxical Embolism
SAD	single ascending dose
SAPT	single antiplatelet therapy
SAVR	surgical aortic valve replacement
SEC	spontaneous echo contrast
SEVE	serious vascular event
sPESI	simplified Pulmonary Embolism Severity Index
STE	ST-elevation
STEMI	ST-elevation myocardial infarction
SVD	structural valve degeneration
SVT	superficial venous thrombosis
TAT	triple antiplatelet therapy
TAVI	transcatheter aortic valve implantation
TAVR	transcatheter aortic valve replacement

TEER	transcatheter edge-to edge repair
TEG	thromboelastography
TF	tissue factor
TIA	transient ischaemic attack
TIMI	Thrombolysis in Myocardial Infarction
TIMP	tissue inhibitor of matrix metalloproteinase
TMVR	transcatheter mitral valve replacement
tPA	tissue plasminogen activator
TX	thromboxane
UFH	unfractionated heparin
VASP	vasodilator-stimulated phosphoprotein
ViV	valve-in-valve
VKA	vitamin K antagonist
VTE	venous thromboembolism
VWF	von Willebrand factor

SECTION 1

Pathophysiology of thrombosis

CHAPTER 1

Arterial thrombosis: pathophysiological background

Lina Badimon and Gemma Vilahur

Contents

Summary

The formation of a complex blood clot within a coronary artery triggers the thrombotic events. Arterial thrombosis comprises four basic pathways: platelet activation and aggregation, blood coagulation with fibrin formation, inflammation, and fibrinolysis. These pathways interact with each other and with the vessel wall, in the special regulatory conditions set by the local blood flow to trigger the formation of a thrombus with a determined growth rate, mass, and stability on top of an atherosclerotic plaque. In this chapter, cellular and molecular mechanisms of thrombus formation, from platelet aggregation to coagulation, fibrinolysis, and inflammation, are described. Determinants of thrombus growth, comprising both local factors, as well as severity and type of exposed atherosclerotic tissue, and systemic thrombogenic risk factors and comorbidities, are also conveyed as important drivers in the final thrombotic episode. The thrombus mass and stability at the time of coronary plaque disruption/destabilization influences the severity of clinical symptoms.

Pathophysiology of thrombosis: cellular and molecular mechanisms of thrombus formation

Regulation of platelet adhesion, activation, and aggregation

Platelets originate from the cytoplasm of bone marrow megakaryocytes. Although platelets do not have genomic DNA, they contain messenger RNA (mRNA), derived from the megakaryocytes and from the translation machinery necessary for protein synthesis (ribosomes), that enables them to synthesize a subset of proteins, a function that is found to be enhanced upon platelet activation.[1,2] Circulating platelets are discoid in shape, with dimensions of approximately 2.0–4.0 by 0.5 μm, and an average volume of 7–11 fL. Their shape and small size allow them to be pushed to the edges of blood vessels, placing them in an optimal position for constant monitoring of vascular integrity. Platelets circulate in concentrations of 150,000–450,000 cells/μL. Of the total number of platelets in the body, 70% are maintained in the circulation, while the other 30% remain transiently but constantly in the spleen, staying in circulation for an average of 10 days. Under physiological conditions, platelets circulate without adhering to a healthy vascular endothelium. ➲ Figure 1.1 details the multiple antithrombotic mechanisms that prevent platelets from

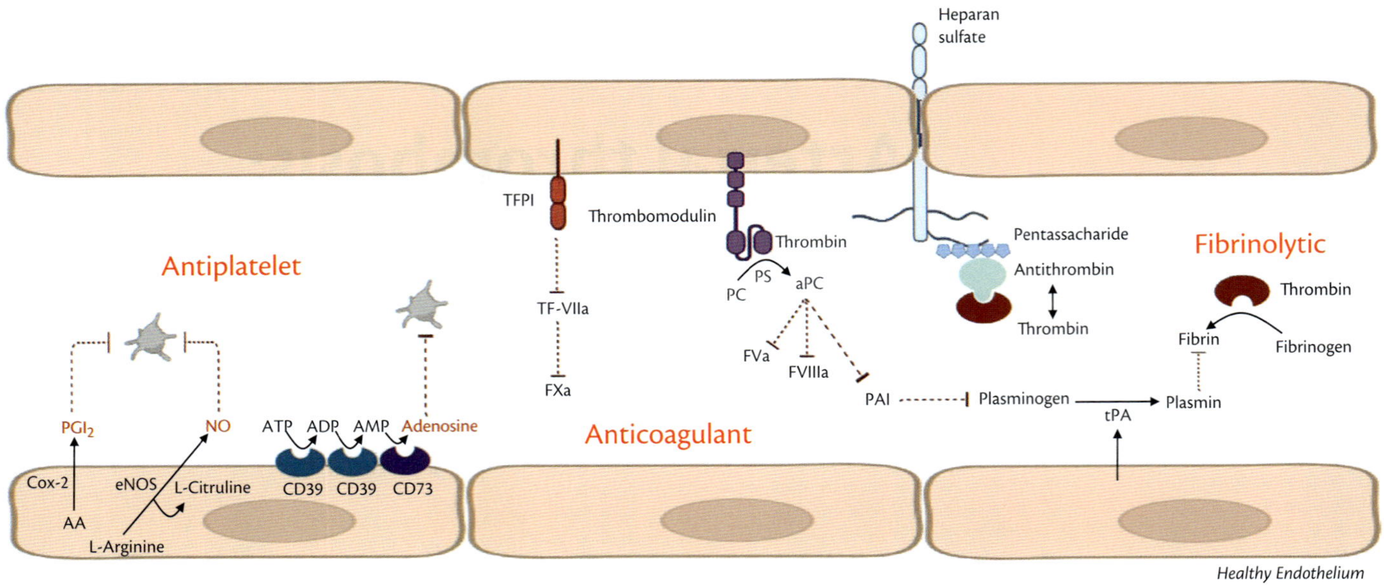

Figure 1.1 Mechanisms by which a healthy endothelium prevents thrombus formation. aPC, activated protein C; CD, cluster of differentiation; Cox2, cyclooxygenase-2; eNOS, endothelial nitric oxide synthase; NO, nitric oxide; PAI-1, plasminogen activator inhibitor-1; PC, protein C; PGI2, prostacyclin; PS, protein S; TF, tissue factor; TFPI, tissue factor pathway inhibitor; tPA, tissue plasminogen activator.

sticking to the vessel wall. However, exposure of deeper vascular layers or atherosclerotic plaque components triggers a series of events that involve the interplay between platelets and the coagulation cascade, leading to thrombus formation.

The initial recognition of damaged vessel wall by platelets involves the adhesion, activation, and adherence to recognition sites on the thrombogenic substrate; the spreading of the platelet on the surface; and eventual aggregation of platelets to form a platelet plug or white thrombus.[3]

At sites of vascular or plaque disruption, platelets sense small amounts of agonists, which induce changes in their surface receptors towards a high-affinity state favouring platelet adherence. Several key checkpoints within the platelet molecular machinery need to be passed to switch platelets to such a pro-adhesive state. These are located at the level of receptor stimulation, intracellular calcium (Ca^{2+}) elevation, activation of small GTPases [e.g. Ras-proximate-1 (RAP1)], and outside-in signalling.[4,5]

Platelet adhesion is brought about by multiple membrane surface receptors, which interact with the damaged endothelium, other platelets, and leucocytes. According to protein structure, function, and ligand properties, platelet receptors involved in adhesion have been classified as integrins (β1, β2, and β3), leucine-rich repeat receptors, immunoglobulin superfamily receptors, selectins, and miscellaneous (➔ Table 1.1).

Table 1.1 Different platelet membrane receptors involved in platelet adhesion to the vessel and leucocytes through the interaction with different ligands

		Receptor	Ligand
Integrins	β_1	$\alpha_2\beta_1$ (GPIa/IIa)	Collagen
		$\alpha_5\beta_1$ (GPIc/IIa)	Fibronectin
		α6β1	Laminin
	β2	αLβ2	Neutrophils
	β3	αVβ3	Vitronectin
			Fibronectin
			Fibronectin
			Von Willebrand factor
		αIIβ3 (GPIIb/IIIa)	Von Willebrand factor
			Vitronectin
			Fibronectin
Leucine-rich repeat receptors		GP Ib–IX–V	Von Willebrand factor
Immunoglobulin superfamily receptors		GP VI–FcRY	Collagen
Selectins		P-selectin	Neutrophils and monocytes
Miscellaneous		GP IV	Thrombospondin

Glycoprotein (GP)-Ib–IX–V, GPVI, and integrin αIIbβ3 have been shown to play a dominant role in platelet–vessel interaction, with the support of von Willebrand factor (VWF). VWF is a multimeric GP built from identical subunits that contain binding sites for both platelet GP receptors and collagen.[6] As such, platelet adhesion to the site of vascular injury is mainly driven by the interaction of the VWF anchored to collagen via the A3 domain with the platelet GPIbα receptor (from the GPIb–IX–V platelet complex) via the VWF A1 domain (➔ Figure 1.2).[7,8] The adhesive activity of VWF depends on the size of its multimers, with high-molecular-weight multimers the most effective in supporting interactions with collagen and platelet receptors.[6] Although endothelial cells and megakaryocytes synthesize VWF, only endothelial cell-derived VWF, not the platelet pool of VWF, seems to contribute to platelet adhesion.[9] Recent studies have shown that

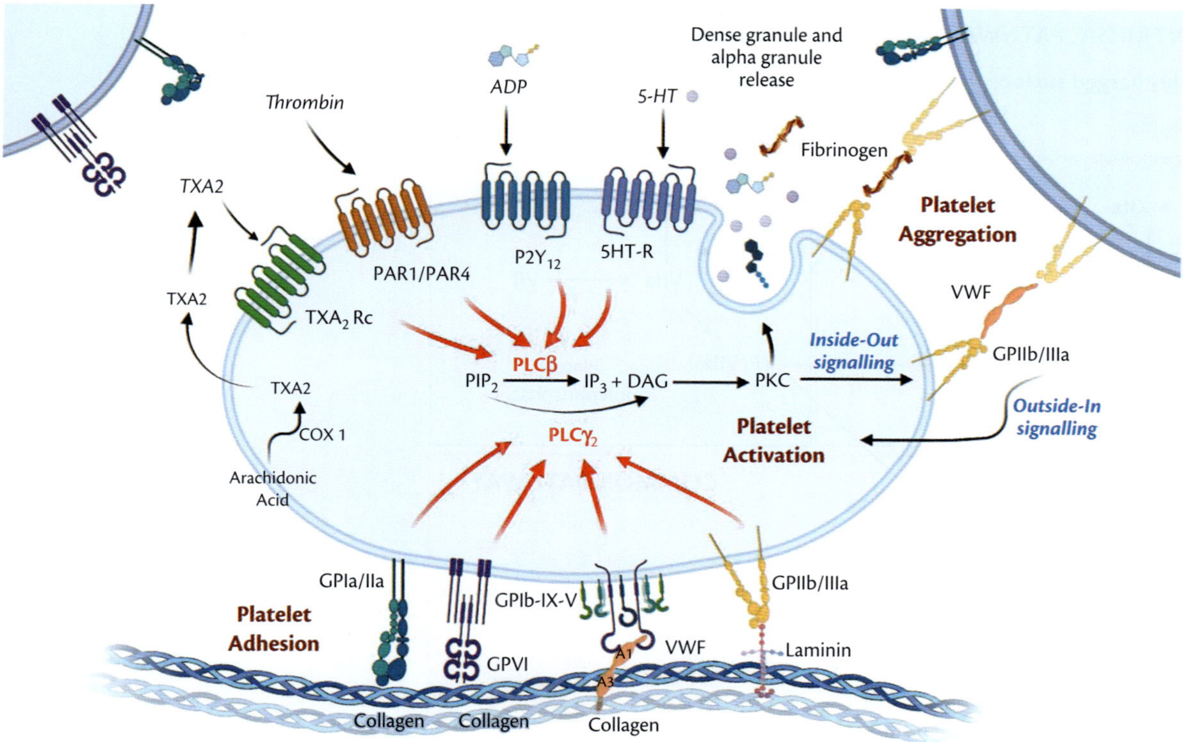

Figure 1.2 Mechanisms involved in platelet adhesion, activation, and aggregation. ADP, adenosine diphosphate; COX, cyclooxygenase; GP, glycoprotein; PAR, proteolytic activated receptor; PK, protein kinase; PLC, phospholipase C; TX, thromboxane; VWF, von Willebrand factor.

the intracellular adaptor signalling molecule 14-3-3ζ, found associated with the cytoplasmic domain of GPIb subunit, regulates VWF binding to GPIb–IX–V and mediates VWF/GPIb–IX–V-dependent signalling.[10,11] GPIb–IX–V interaction is enough to promote binding of platelets to the subendothelium. However, the transient nature of this interaction results in the rapid dislocation of platelets from the site of injury.[8] A stronger platelet–vessel interaction is mainly driven by GPVI. GPVI, although initially expressed as a monomer, when it forms a dimer displays a high affinity for collagen, favouring a persistent adhesion of platelets to the vessel surface. Furthermore, GPVI also triggers the activation of integrins $\alpha_2\beta_1$ (or GPIa/IIa) and $\alpha IIb\beta_3$ (GPIIb/IIIa) (➔ Figure 1.2),[12,13] which further support adhesion, activation, and platelet aggregation by binding to collagen or to laminin, fibrinogen, or VWF, respectively. Although to a lesser extent, fibronectin, vitronectin, and thrombospondin also contribute to platelet adhesion by binding to GPIc/IIa, vitronectin receptors, and to GPIV, respectively.

Platelet adhesion and further activation modify platelet morphology and stimulate the release of platelet granule content, which is rich in platelet-activating factors (ADP, ATP, histamine, ionized Ca^{2+}, serotonin, glutamate, magnesium, platelet polyphosphate), adhesion molecules (P-selectin, CD63, VEGF, PDGF, IGF-1, TGFβ, EGF, interleukin 1β, MIP-1α, CD40L), chemokines [CXCL1 (GRO-8), CXCL4 (PF4), CXCL5 (ENA-78), CXCL7, CCL5 (RANTES), CCL3 (MIP1-α)], and haemostatic and coagulation factors (fibrinogen, VWF, fibronectin, kininogens, multimerin, protein S, plasminogen, prothrombin, vitronectin, factors V, VII, XI, XIII) among others, all of which amplify the thrombotic response.

Besides tethering platelets to the damaged vascular wall, GPIa/IIa has also been suggested to induce arachidonic acid release from the phospholipid platelet membrane through phospholipase A_2 enzymes.[14] Arachidonic acid is a main precursor of thromboxane A_2 (TXA_2) through cyclooxygenase-1 (COX-1).[15] TXA_2 exerts platelet-activating and vasoconstrictive effects by interacting with thromboxane receptors on platelets and endothelial cells, respectively.[15] In contrast, platelet activation induces the translocation of phosphatidylserine from the internal to the external platelet membrane leaflet, which facilitates the assembly of Xase (tenase) and prothrombinase complexes, playing a key role in the activation of the coagulations cascade, as detailed below (➔ Figure 1.3).[16]

Overall, platelet activation induced by the binding of adhesive ligands (e.g. collagen, VWF, and fibrinogen) or soluble agonists (e.g. ADP, thrombin, serotonin, and TXA_2) to their respective platelet receptors (mainly G protein-coupled receptors; ➔ Figure 1.2)[8] triggers platelet signalling transduction pathways that involve key proteins such as phospholipase C (PLC) and protein kinase C (PKC), so-called *inside-out* signalling, which culminates in GPIIb/IIIa conformational change and its consequent transformation into an active state with high affinity for its ligands VWF and fibrinogen. In turn, ligand binding to active GPIIb/IIIa triggers an *outside-in* signalling, which leads to cytoskeletal reorganization and platelet spreading, platelet aggregation, and thrombus stabilization and growth.[17,18]

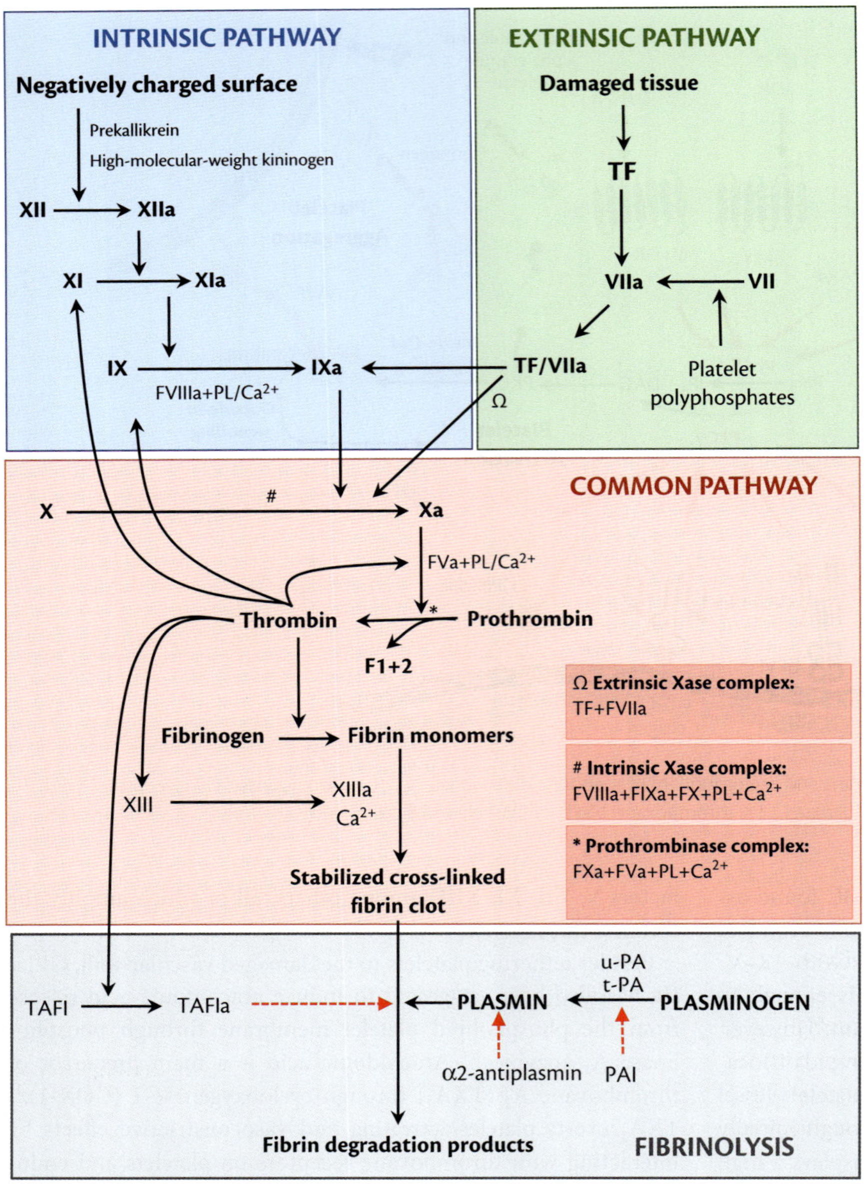

Figure 1.3 Coagulation and fibrinolytic pathways. PAI-1, plasminogen activator inhibitor-1; PL, platelet phospholipid membrane; TF, tissue factor; tPA, tissue plasminogen activator; TFPI, tissue factor pathway inhibitor; uPA, urokinase plasminogen activator.

Coagulation and fibrinolysis

The blood coagulation system involves a sequence of reactions integrating zymogens (proteins susceptible to activation into enzymes via limited proteolysis) and cofactors (non-proteolytic enzyme activators), and involves two distinct, yet cross-talking pathways: the extrinsic, or tissue factor (TF)-dependent, pathway; and the intrinsic, or contact activation, pathway[19] (➔ Figure 1.3).

During atherosclerotic plaque rupture, blood elements interact with inner components of the atherosclerotic lesions or vascular bed, mostly TF. In fact, TF exposure is considered the initial trigger of arterial thrombosis, since it induces the formation of a fibrin monolayer that covers the culprit lesion onto which circulating platelets interact and attach.[3,20,21] TF is highly expressed in deep vascular layers, atherosclerotic plaque components (macrophages, foam cells, and vascular smooth muscle cells), neutrophil extracellular traps (NETs), platelets, monocytes, and microparticles.[22–25] Concurrently, platelet-released polyphosphates activate factor (F)-VII into FVIIa, which binds to TF and forms the FVIIa/TF complex (the extrinsic tenase complex; ➔ Figure 1.3). In the presence of calcium, the intrinsic tenase complex activates FX into FXa, which consequently activates prothrombin into thrombin in the presence of its cofactor FVa.

In the intrinsic pathway, FXII may become activated by interacting with negatively charged surfaces such as the phospholipid surface of the platelet membrane or with polyphosphates released from platelet dense granules.[26,27] Activated FXII, in combination with plasma prekallikrein and high-molecular-weight kininogen, cleaves FXI, producing FXIa, which activates FIX to FIXa, in the presence of Ca^{2+} and FVIIIa. FVIII is produced by endothelial and liver cells and forms a complex with circulating VWF. Upon plaque disruption, FVIIIa dissociates from VWF and binds to FIX. FVIIIa and FIXa form the intrinsic tenase complex. Yet, the TF–FVIIa complex through the intrinsic pathway (➔ Figure 1.3) can also activate FIX. Both the extrinsic and the intrinsic tenase complexes converge in the common coagulation pathway and catalyse the activation of FX to FXa. Then, FXa and FVa assemble on negatively charged phospholipid membranes in the presence of Ca^{2+} forming the prothrombinase complex, which converts prothrombin into thrombin. Hence, as stated above, activated platelets play a key role in the coagulation cascade since they provide the required procoagulant surface for the assembly and expression of tenases and prothrombinase enzymatic complexes.[3] Once formed, thrombin converts fibrinogen to fibrin. Furthermore, thrombin also activates FV, FVIII, and FXI, amplifying the activation of the coagulation cascade; activates thrombin-activatable fibrinolysis inhibitor (TAFI) preventing fibrinolysis; and activates FXIII, which catalyses the intertwining between fibrin monomers, contributing to the formation of the stabilized cross-linked fibrin clot (➔ Figure 1.3).[28,29]

Importantly, however, thrombin may also exert anticoagulant effects and promote endogenous fibrinolysis. As such, once the platelet plug is formed and fibrin expands to the intact endothelium, thrombin binds to endothelial-derived thrombomodulin, thereby shifting from a procoagulant to an anticoagulant state. As such, thrombin/thrombomodulin binding induces protein C (PC) activation in the presence of protein S. Activated PC exerts anticoagulant effects by proteolytic inactivation of FVa and FVIIIa (➔ Figure 1.1).[30] In contrast, thrombin may also bind to heparan sulfate-bound antithrombin through a pentasaccharide (➔ Figure 1.1). Once bound, antithrombin undergoes a conformational change that enhances its reactivity with thrombin, promoting the formation of antithrombin/thrombin complexes. Thrombin has also been shown to stimulate the subsequent release of tissue plasminogen activator (tPA) via TAFI-mediated mechanisms,[31] thus initiating endogenous lysis through plasmin generation from plasminogen. Thrombin therefore plays a critical role in maintaining the complex balance of initial prothrombotic reparative events and subsequent endogenous anticoagulant and thrombolytic pathways.

Proteolysis of fibrin by plasmin induces the generation of fibrin degradation products. The most specific of stabilized fibrin degradation products are D-dimers. Elevated plasma levels of D-dimers are a marker for increased thrombin formation and fibrin degradation turnover.[32] However, fibrinolysis is found to be limited to the culprit site, the atheromatous core—a rich source of plasminogen activator inhibitor (PAI-1), a powerful endogenous antifibrinolytic molecule.

Determinants of thrombus growth by local and systemic factors

Local determinants of thrombosis in atherosclerotic arteries

The dynamics of platelet deposition and thrombus growth following vascular damage are locally modulated by the type of vascular injury and the geometry at the site damage (degree of stenosis).

Type of vascular injury

The degree of atheroma plaque rupture (ulceration, fissure, or erosion) is key to determining local arterial thrombogenicity. It is likely that, when injury to the vessel wall is mild (erosion), the thrombogenic stimulus is relatively limited, and the resulting thrombotic occlusion is transient, as occurs in unstable angina. In contrast, deep vessel injury secondary to plaque rupture or ulceration results in the exposure of collagen, TF, and other elements of the vessel matrix, leading to relatively persistent thrombotic occlusion and myocardial infarction. Consequently, exposure of a de-endothelialized vessel wall, native collagen fibres with a rough surface, or atherosclerotic plaque components at similar blood shear rate conditions lead to increasing degrees of platelet deposition.[33,34]

The nature of the substrate exposed after spontaneous or mechanically induced plaque rupture is one factor determining whether an unstable plaque proceeds rapidly to an occlusive thrombus or persists as non-occlusive mural thrombus. The analysis of the relative contribution of different components of human atherosclerotic plaques (fatty streaks, sclerotic plaques, fibro-lipid plaques, lipid-rich atheromatous plaques, hyperplasic cellular plaques, and normal intima) to the formation of an acute thrombus revealed that the atheromatous plaques exposing the lipid core were up to sixfold more active than the other substrates in triggering thrombosis.[34,35] As proof of concept, we showed that local tissue blockade of TF by treatment with TF pathway inhibitor significantly reduces thrombosis. The use of active site-inhibited recombinant FVIIa (TF–rFVIIa) has been shown to significantly reduce thrombus growth on damaged vessels devoid of TF, indicating that blockage of blood-borne TF at the site of a growing thrombus has therapeutic implications. The importance of TF is also underscored by the fact that high levels are found in the circulation of those coronary artery disease patients who are most prone to thrombotic complications, such as diabetic and dyslipidaemic patients, and smokers. The contribution of TF from the atherosclerotic plaque with regard to systemic TF to overall thrombus growth remains, however, yet to be determined. Overall, plaques with a large atheromatous lipid-rich core content are at high risk of leading to acute coronary events after spontaneous or mechanically induced rupture due to their increased thrombogenicity.[36] Importantly, powerful pharmacological interventions addressing lipid lowering and the use of imaging techniques to characterize plaque subtypes have confirmed these data. The GLAGOV trial demonstrated that the PCSK9 inhibitor evolocumab, added to optimal treatment with statins, reduced the lipid-rich atheroma volume, with a greater percentage of patients demonstrating plaque regression. One year later, evolocumab was shown to reduce clinical outcomes in the FOURIER trial. Further, the recently published PACMAN trial has reported that the addition of another PCSK9 inhibitor, alirocumab, to statins to intensively reduce low-density lipoprotein cholesterol levels, that equally showed reduction of cardiovascular events in the ODISSEY trial, has also shown—by multimodality serial imaging—a coronary plaque regression in non–infarct-related lesions and a reduction of lesion lipid content greater than with statins. Therefore, a reduction of lipid-rich plaques is a key objective to reduce the risk of atherothrombotic events.

Local geometry and flow: the haemodynamic regulation

Platelet deposition is directly related to the degree of stenosis in the presence of the same degree of injury, indicating a shear-induced platelet activation.[37] In addition, analysis of the axial distribution of platelet deposition indicates that the apex, and not the flow recirculation zone distal to the apex, is the segment of greatest platelet accumulation.[33] These data suggest that the severity of the acute platelet response to plaque disruption depends in part on the sudden changes in geometry following rupture.

Geometry changes are also occurring due to the dynamic nature of coronary thrombosis. Spontaneous lysis of thrombus occurs not only in unstable angina, but also in acute myocardial infarction. In these patients, as well as in those undergoing thrombolysis for an acute infarction, the presence of a residual mural thrombus predisposes to recurrent thrombotic vessel occlusion. Two main contributing factors for the development of rethrombosis have been identified. First, a residual mural thrombus may encroach into the vessel lumen, resulting in increased shear rates, which facilitate the activation and deposition of platelets on the lesion (➔ Figure 1.4). Hence, although a gradual increase in platelet deposition in the area of maximal stenosis may be followed by an abrupt decrease in platelet deposition, probably because of spontaneous embolization of the thrombus or platelet de-aggregation, this episode is likely to be immediately followed by a rapid new increase in platelet deposition. In fact, platelet deposition is increased two to four times on a residual thrombus compared with that on the deeply injured arterial wall. Second, a fragmented thrombus appears to be one of the most powerful thrombogenic surfaces. Thus, following lysis, thrombin becomes exposed to the circulating blood, leading to activation of platelets and coagulation, further enhancing thrombosis.

Local fluid dynamics (shear stress and tensile stress) also modulate thrombus progression (➔ Figure 1.4). High shear stress (a force that acts parallel to the surface) favours a conformational change in ultra-large VWF from its globular to an elongated form exposing the VWF A1 binding site domain to platelet GPIb, favouring the occurrence of platelet adhesion.[38] On the other hand, tensile stress (a force that acts perpendicular to the surface) has been shown to influence the localization of ADAMTS13, a metalloproteinase known to cleave unusually large prothrombotic multimers of VWF.[39]

Systemic determinants of thrombosis on atherosclerotic arteries

In one-third of acute coronary events, particularly in cases of sudden death, there is no rupture of a mildly stenotic plaque rich

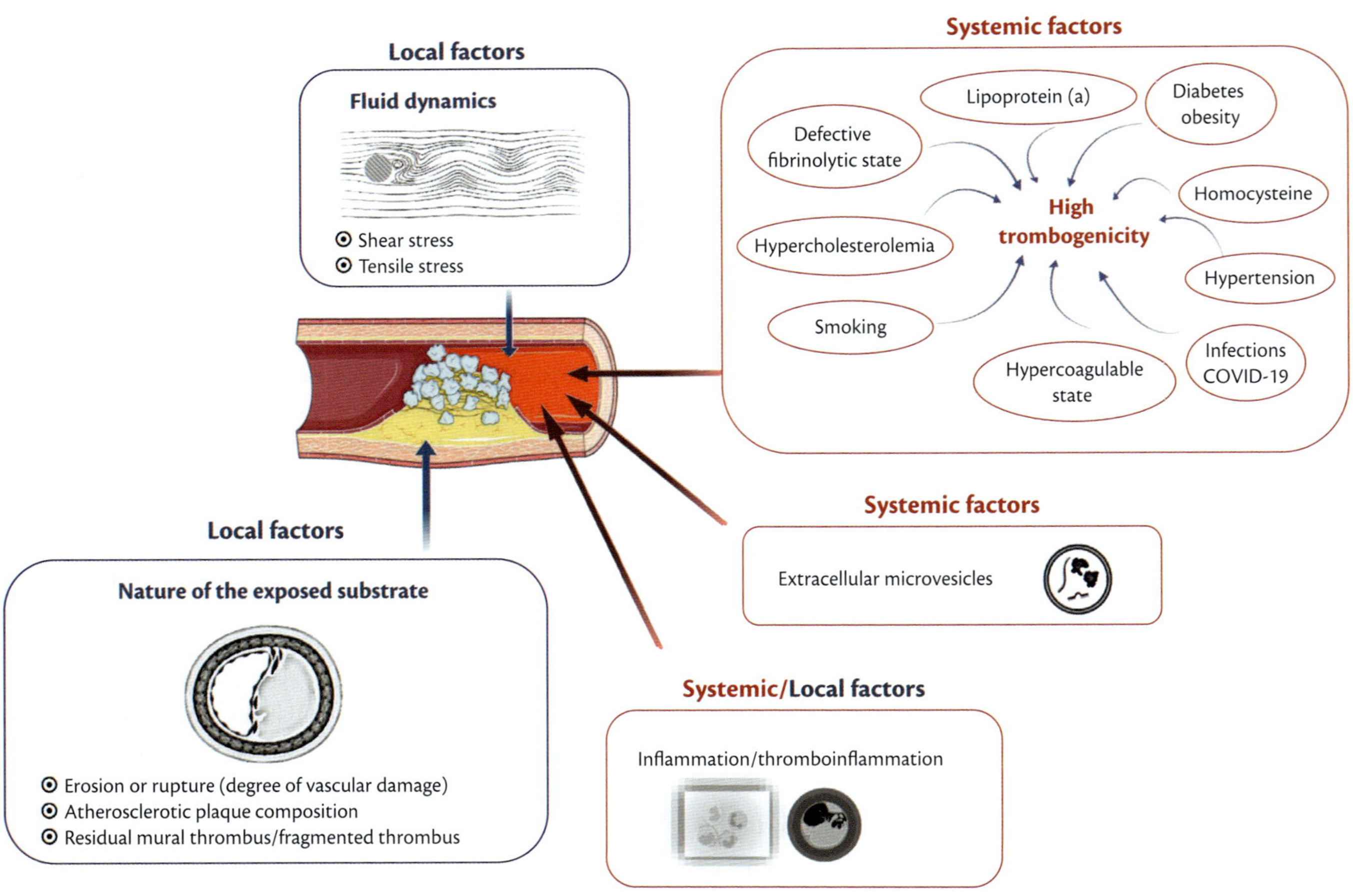

Figure 1.4 Local and systemic factors that modulate thrombus formation.

in lipids, but rather the superficial erosion of a markedly stenotic and fibrotic plaque. Furthermore, postmortem studies have evidenced the presence of repeated and healed thrombotic episodes within the same lesion.[40] These observations support that, in addition to local factors implicated in coronary thrombosis, thrombus formation may depend on the overall 'systemic thrombogenic state' (the so-called *vulnerable* or *high-risk blood*).[41] In this regard, several systemic factors have been identified to modulate blood thrombogenesis, as detailed in ➔ Figure 1.4.[42,43] Importantly, however, the effective management of these risk factors through lifestyle changes and improved medical therapies has been shown to lower the prothrombotic tendency besides reducing plaque vulnerability.[44–46] Among those systemic factors known to enhance thrombotic risk, special attention has been recently paid to viral infections, particularly, SARS-CoV-2. Thrombotic events that frequently occur in COVID-19 are predominantly venous thromboembolic. Yet, arterial thrombotic events, including myocardial infarction, stroke, and mesenteric artery occlusion, have all been reported to occur in COVID-19 patients.[47,48] The hyperinflammatory response induced by SARS-CoV-2 has been shown to induce microvascular dysfunction and endothelial injury, the increased production of NETs (NETosis), hypercoagulability, and hypofibrinolysis, overall favouring thrombus formation.[49–51]

Extracellular vesicles (EVs), small lipid-bilayer membrane vesicles released by most cellular types, exert pivotal and multifaceted roles in atherothrombosis.[52] Emerging evidence emphasizes the importance of EVs in intercellular communication processes, with key effects on inflammation, and thrombosis.[53,54] As such, EVs behave as signalling molecules able to both derail vascular homeostasis and induce vascular dysfunction, inflammation, plaque progression, and platelet activation; and support coagulation as well as drive anti-inflammation, vascular repair, and atheroprotection.[52,54] As per the role of EVs in thrombosis, circulating and platelet-derived EVs have been shown to enhance thrombosis on atherosclerotic plaques.[55] Moreover, circulating, platelet-, and monocyte/leucocyte-related EVs are found to be enhanced in patients with complete coronary thrombotic occlusion [i.e. ST-elevation myocardial infarction (STEMI) patients] as compared to those with partial coronary thrombotic occlusion (i.e. non-STEMI), thereby serving as a marker of thrombus burden. Additionally, erythrocyte-derived microparticles, which are continuously released from evolving growing thrombi, have been suggested to serve as a potential biomarker of ongoing thrombosis.[56]

Inflammation, thrombosis, and thromboinflammation

Molecular and histological analyses of the aspirated thrombi have improved our current understanding of thrombus composition and growth dynamics. Characterization of intracoronary thrombus from STEMI patients within the first hours after the onset of pain to a percutaneous coronary intervention revealed a rapid (3 hours) recruitment of neutrophils and monocytes and a late appearance (6 hours) of T and B lymphocytes along with progenitor cells.[57] Moreover, the content of fibrin increased over time, contrary to the pattern observed for platelet content.[57] Additionally, application of proteomic approaches allowed the identification of potential biomarkers of ischaemic damage, such as profilin-1, a cytoskeleton-associated protein likely released by thrombin-activated platelets at the atherosclerotic culprit site.[57,58] Furthermore, the high content of inflammatory cells in old thrombi indicated the important role of innate immunity cells in the dynamics of thrombus growth.

The concept of 'thromboinflammation' has been proposed as a link to include the various systems that have a role in triggering thrombosis, including humoral inflammatory mediators, innate immune response, coagulation, fibrinolysis, and the complement system. Activation of these systems subsequently induces, or results from, the activation of endothelial cells, leucocytes, and platelets, finally triggering thrombotic and inflammatory reactions.[59]

Vessel wall and inflammation

Vascular damage, endothelial dysfunction, and inflammation are the major facilitators of atherothrombotic disease. Inflammatory processes decisively contribute to the progression of atherosclerotic lesions, but also to their acute thrombotic complications, as shown by the fact that many inflammatory mediators can augment TF gene expression in endothelial cells, thus triggering the coagulation cascade.[60]

Platelets and inflammation

Platelets can both produce and respond to chemoattractant cytokines,[61] or express CD40 ligand, a molecule that regulates TF gene expression in atherosclerotic cells, particularly in vascular smooth muscle cells, and foam cells.[62] Similarly, P-selectin, a transmembrane protein present in the alpha granules of platelets, can quickly move to the platelet surface after activation, where it interacts with the P-selectin glycoprotein ligand-1 (PSGL-1) on leucocytes, forming aggregates and upregulating TF formation. Endothelial cells and platelets can also bind to one another via this interaction, which exposes P-selectin on endothelial cells which then binds to platelet PSGL-1 receptors. Activated platelets can also deposit chemokines [e.g. RANTES, platelet factor 4 (PF4)] onto endothelial cells during transient interactions, thereby promoting further monocyte recruitment and arrest. In addition, several studies have shown that platelets, via chemokine release, are capable of interacting with and to mediate the recruitment of circulating stem or progenitor cells[63] thereby contributing to vessel repair at the site of injury and the formation of a neointima.[64,65] Additionally, it has been demonstrated that the functional relevance of interactions between platelets or platelet-derived factors is not only restricted to the recruitment of circulating stem/progenitor cells; they may also influence important progenitor cell functions, such as migration or differentiation.[66]

Humoral inflammation

C-reactive protein (CRP) is a member of the highly conserved pentraxin superfamily of proteins, and is often used in clinical practice as a marker of inflammation. There is now increasing evidence that CRP is not only a marker of inflammation, but also that destabilized isoforms of CRP possess proinflammatory and prothrombotic properties.[67,68] CRP circulates as a functionally inert pentameric form (pCRP), which relaxes its conformation after binding to phosphocholine-enriched membranes and then dissociates to monomeric CRP (mCRP). Exposure of GPIIb/IIIa on the platelet surface has been shown to support the dissociation of the pentameric form into monomeric subunits,[69] which in turn exert a significant effect on platelet adhesion and thrombus growth.[70] Besides the contribution to thrombus formation, CRP has been shown to exert other significant biological effects in regulating many of the aspects central to the pathogenesis of atherothrombosis.[71]

Immune cells: neutrophil extracellular traps

Neutrophils play a key role in the development of different forms of acute organ injuries, and the release of NETs is emerging as a common pathogenic mechanism. NETs are essential in controlling pathogens, and their defective release or increased degradation leads to a higher risk of infection. However, NETs also contain several proinflammatory and cytotoxic molecules that can exacerbate thromboinflammation. Interestingly the molecular signature of in-stent thrombosis indicates the participation of oxidative stress and innate immune cells. In fact, an imbalance in redox-related proteins is suggestive of an exacerbated oxidative stress that leads to an accumulation of oxidative products in in-stent thrombosis. Moreover, the coordinated increase in chaperones and regulatory proteins reflects the activation of intracellular protection mechanisms to maintain protein integrity in in-stent thrombosis. Failure to counterbalance the stress situation could trigger cellular apoptosis leading to destabilization of the thrombus and to a worse prognosis of in-stent thrombosis in STEMI patients.[72]

Summary

The cellular and molecular mechanisms at play in the formation, growth, and stabilization of arterial thrombosis are being investigated, and many of the platelet receptor–ligand interactions and platelet signal transduction pathways have been identified. Inflammation has been revealed as a key player in the local, systemic, and diffuse pattern of atherothrombotic disease. Strategies combining dietary, pharmacological/medical, and interventional/surgical strategies have shown considerable success in the prevention and treatment of major cardiovascular events. These regimens focus on inhibiting the various pathways involved in thrombus generation. Novel therapeutic approaches based on a deeper understanding of the biochemistry of platelet aggregation and the coagulation processes, as well as the geometric conditions encountered in the circulation, are currently in different stages of development and of testing in clinical trials. Advances in non-invasive imaging methodologies will allow the identification of vulnerable atherosclerotic plaques and a reduction in the clinical impact of atherothrombosis.

References

1. Mills EW, Green R, Ingolia NT. Slowed decay of mRNAs enhances platelet specific translation. Blood. 2017;129:e38–48.
2. Fountain JH, Lappin SL. Physiology, Platelet. Treasure Island, FL: StatPearls; 2020.
3. Badimon L, Vilahur G. Thrombosis formation on atherosclerotic lesions and plaque rupture. J Intern Med. 2014;276:618–32.
4. Stefanini L, Bergmeier W. RAP GTPases and platelet integrin signaling. Platelets. 2019;30:41–7.
5. Stefanini L, Bergmeier W. Negative regulators of platelet activation and adhesion. J Thromb Haemost. 2018;16:220–30.
6. Stockschlaeder M, Schneppenheim R, Budde U. Update on von Willebrand factor multimers: focus on high-molecular-weight multimers and their role in hemostasis. Blood Coagul Fibrinolysis. 2014;25:206–16.
7. Badimon L, Badimon JJ, Turitto VT, Fuster V. Role of von Willebrand factor in mediating platelet-vessel wall interaction at low shear rate; the importance of perfusion conditions. Blood. 1989;73:961–7.
8. Vilahur G, Gutierrez M, Arzanauskaite M, Mendieta G, Ben-Aicha S, Badimon L. Intracellular platelet signalling as a target for drug development. Vasc Pharmacol. 2018;111:22–5.
9. Doddapattar P, Dhanesha N, Chorawala MR, et al. Endothelial cell-derived von Willebrand factor, but not platelet-derived, promotes atherosclerosis in apolipoprotein E-deficient mice. Arterioscler Thromb Vasc Biol. 2018;38:520–8.
10. Chen Y, Ruggeri ZM, Du X. 14-3-3 proteins in platelet biology and glycoprotein Ib-IX signaling. Blood. 2018;131:2436–48.
11. Zhang Y, Ehrlich SM, Zhu C, Du X. Signaling mechanisms of the platelet glycoprotein Ib-IX complex. Platelets. 2022;33:823–32.
12. Manne BK, Badolia R, Dangelmaier C, et al. Distinct pathways regulate Syk protein activation downstream of immune tyrosine activation motif (ITAM) and hemITAM receptors in platelets. J Biol Chem. 2015;290:11557–68.
13. Fuentes E. Modulation of glycoprotein VI and its downstream signaling pathways as an antiplatelet target. Int J Mol Sci. 2022;23:9882.
14. Wong DA, Kita Y, Uozumi N, Shimizu T. Discrete role for cytosolic phospholipase A(2)alpha in platelets: studies using single and double mutant mice of cytosolic and group IIA secretory phospholipase A(2). J Exp Med. 2002;196:349–57.
15. Badimon L, Vilahur G, Rocca B, Patrono C. The key contribution of platelet and vascular arachidonic acid metabolism to the pathophysiology of atherothrombosis. Cardiovasc Res. 2021;117:2001–15.
16. Reddy EC, Rand ML. Procoagulant phosphatidylserine-exposing platelets in vitro and in vivo. Front Cardiovasc Med. 2020;7:15.

17. Stefanini L, Bergmeier W. RAP1-GTPase signaling and platelet function. J Mol Med. 2016;94:13–19.
18. Laurent PA, Severin S, Gratacap MP, Payrastre B. Class I PI 3-kinases signaling in platelet activation and thrombosis: PDK1/Akt/GSK3 axis and impact of PTEN and SHIP1. Adv Biol Regul. 2014;54:162–74.
19. Chaudhry R, Usama SM, Babiker HM. Physiology, Coagulation Pathways. Treasure Island, FL: StatPearls; 2020.
20. Grover SP, Mackman N. Tissue factor in atherosclerosis and atherothrombosis. Atherosclerosis. 2020;307:80–6.
21. Camera M, Toschi V, Brambilla M, et al. The role of tissue factor in atherothrombosis and coronary artery disease: insights into platelet tissue factor. Semin Thromb Hemost. 2015;41:737–46.
22. Badimon L, Vilahur G. Neutrophil extracellular traps: a new source of tissue factor in atherothrombosis. Eur Heart J. 2015;36:1364–6.
23. Stakos DA, Kambas K, Konstantinidis T, et al. Expression of functional tissue factor by neutrophil extracellular traps in culprit artery of acute myocardial infarction. Eur Heart J. 2015;36:1405–14.
24. Muller I, Klocke A, Alex M, et al. Intravascular tissue factor initiates coagulation via circulating microvesicles and platelets. FASEB J. 2003;17:476–8.
25. Rauch U, Bonderman D, Bohrmann B, et al. Transfer of tissue factor from leukocytes to platelets is mediated by CD15 and tissue factor. Blood. 2000;96:170–5.
26. Rai V, Balters MW, Agrawal DK. Factors IX, XI, and XII: potential therapeutic targets for anticoagulant therapy in atherothrombosis. Rev Cardiovasc Med. 2019;20:245–53.
27. Szekely O, Borgi M, Lip GYH. Factor XI inhibition fulfilling the optimal expectations for ideal anticoagulation. Expert Opin Emerg Drugs. 2019;24:55–61.
28. Al-Amer OM. The role of thrombin in haemostasis. Blood Coagul Fibrinolysis. 2022;33:145–8.
29. Malkhassian D, Sabir S, Sharma S. Physiology, Factor XIII. Treasure Island, FL: StatPearls; 2022.
30. Dahlback B, Villoutreix BO. Regulation of blood coagulation by the protein C anticoagulant pathway: novel insights into structure-function relationships and molecular recognition. Arterioscler Thromb Vasc Biol. 2005;25:1311–20.
31. Ni R, Neves MAD, Wu C, et al. Activated thrombin-activatable fibrinolysis inhibitor (TAFIa) attenuates fibrin-dependent plasmin generation on thrombin-activated platelets. J Thromb Haemost. 2020;18:2364–76.
32. Olson JD. D-dimer: an overview of hemostasis and fibrinolysis, assays, and clinical applications. Adv Clin Chem. 2015;69:1–46.
33. Badimon L, Badimon JJ. Mechanisms of arterial thrombosis in nonparallel streamlines: platelet thrombi grow on the apex of stenotic severely injured vessel wall. Experimental study in the pig model. J Clin Invest. 1989;84:1134–44.
34. Fernandez-Ortiz A, Badimon JJ, Falk E, et al. Characterization of the relative thrombogenicity of atherosclerotic plaque components: implications for consequences of plaque rupture. J Am Coll Cardiol. 1994;23:1562–9.
35. Badimon L, Badimon JJ, Turitto VT, Vallabhajosula S, Fuster V. Platelet thrombus formation on collagen type I. A model of deep vessel injury. Influence of blood rheology, von Willebrand factor, and blood coagulation. Circulation. 1988;78:1431–42.
36. Toschi V, Gallo R, Lettino M, et al. Tissue factor modulates the thrombogenicity of human atherosclerotic plaques. Circulation. 1997;95:594–9.
37. Lassila R, Badimon JJ, Vallabhajosula S, Badimon L. Dynamic monitoring of platelet deposition on severely damaged vessel wall in flowing blood. Effects of different stenoses on thrombus growth. Arteriosclerosis. 1990;10:306–15.
38. Bryckaert M, Rosa JP, Denis CV, Lenting PJ. Of von Willebrand factor and platelets. Cell Mol Life Sci. 2015;72:307–26.
39. Shida Y, Swystun LL, Brown C, et al. Shear stress and platelet-induced tensile forces regulate ADAMTS13-localization within the platelet thrombus. Res Pract Thromb Haemost. 2019;3:254–60.
40. Ziada KM, Misumida N. In vivo identification of healed plaques in culprit lesions: is what we're seeing really there? J Am Coll Cardiol. 2019;73:2264–6.
41. Arbab-Zadeh A, Fuster V. From detecting the vulnerable plaque to managing the vulnerable patient: JACC state-of-the-art review. J Am Coll Cardiol. 2019;74:1582–93.
42. Boffa MB, Koschinsky ML. Lipoprotein (a): truly a direct prothrombotic factor in cardiovascular disease? J Lipid Res. 2016;57:745–57.
43. Lacey B, Herrington WG, Preiss D, Lewington S, Armitage J. The role of emerging risk factors in cardiovascular outcomes. Curr Atheroscler Rep. 2017;19:28.
44. Sambola A, Osende J, Hathcock J, et al. Role of risk factors in the modulation of tissue factor activity and blood thrombogenicity. Circulation. 2003;107:973–7.
45. Nilsson J. Atherosclerotic plaque vulnerability in the statin era. Eur Heart J. 2017;38:1638–44.
46. Osende JI, Badimon JJ, Fuster V, et al. Blood thrombogenicity in type 2 diabetes mellitus patients is associated with glycemic control. J Am Coll Cardiol. 2001;38:1307–12.
47. Shi S, Qin M, Shen B, et al. Association of cardiac injury with mortality in hospitalized patients with COVID-19 in Wuhan, China. JAMA Cardiol. 2020;5:802–10.
48. Romero M, Cardenas AM, Fuentes AB, Barragan AAS, Gomez DBS, Jimenez MT. Acute mesenteric arterial thrombosis in severe SARS-Co-2 patient: a case report and literature review. Int J Surg Case Rep. 2021;86:106307.
49. Cenko E, Badimon L, Bugiardini R, et al. Cardiovascular disease and COVID-19: a consensus paper from the ESC Working Group on Coronary Pathophysiology & Microcirculation, ESC Working Group on Thrombosis and the Association for Acute CardioVascular Care (ACVC), in collaboration with the European Heart Rhythm Association (EHRA). Cardiovasc Res. 2021;117:2705–29.
50. Sutelman P, Vilahur G. An obscure myocardial blood flow may illuminate post-acute sequelae of COVID-19 cardiovascular syndrome. Eur J Clin Invest. 2022;52:e13884.
51. Gorog DA, Storey RF, Gurbel PA, et al. Current and novel biomarkers of thrombotic risk in COVID-19: a consensus statement from the International COVID-19 Thrombosis Biomarkers Colloquium. Nat Rev Cardiol. 2022;19:475–95.
52. Suades R, Greco MF, Padro T, Badimon L. Extracellular vesicles as drivers of immunoinflammation in atherothrombosis. Cells. 2022;11:11.
53. Suades R, Padro T, Vilahur G, Badimon L. Platelet-released extracellular vesicles: the effects of thrombin activation. Cell Mol Life Sci. 2022;79:190.
54. Badimon L, Suades R, Vilella-Figuerola A, et al. Liquid biopsies: microvesicles in cardiovascular disease. Antioxid Redox Signal. 2020;33:645–62.
55. Suades R, Padro T, Vilahur G, Badimon L. Circulating and platelet-derived microparticles in human blood enhance thrombosis on atherosclerotic plaques. Thromb Haemost. 2012;108:1208–19.
56. Suades R, Padro T, Vilahur G, et al. Growing thrombi release increased levels of CD235a(+) microparticles and decreased levels of activated platelet-derived microparticles. Validation in ST-elevation myocardial infarction patients. J Thromb Haemost. 2015;13:1776–86.

57. Ramaiola I, Padro T, Pena E, et al. Changes in thrombus composition and profilin-1 release in acute myocardial infarction. Eur Heart J. 2015;36:965–75.
58. Helseth R, Seljeflot I, Opstad T, et al. Genes expressed in coronary thrombi are associated with ischemic time in patients with acute myocardial infarction. Thromb Res. 2015;135:329–33.
59. Ekdahl KN, Teramura Y, Asif S, Jonsson N, Magnusson PU, Nilsson B. Thromboinflammation in therapeutic medicine. Adv Exp Med Biol. 2015;865:3–17.
60. Libby P, Simon DI. Inflammation and thrombosis: the clot thickens. Circulation. 2001;103:1718–20.
61. Abi-Younes S, Sauty A, Mach F, Sukhova GK, Libby P, Luster AD. The stromal cell-derived factor-1 chemokine is a potent platelet agonist highly expressed in atherosclerotic plaques. Circ Res. 2000;86:131–8.
62. Henn V, Slupsky JR, Grafe M, et al. CD40 ligand on activated platelets triggers an inflammatory reaction of endothelial cells. Nature. 1998;391:591–4.
63. Jin DK, Shido K, Kopp HG, et al. Cytokine-mediated deployment of SDF-1 induces revascularization through recruitment of CXCR4+ hemangiocytes. Nat Med. 2006;12:557–67.
64. Stellos K, Bigalke B, Langer H, et al. Expression of stromal-cell-derived factor-1 on circulating platelets is increased in patients with acute coronary syndrome and correlates with the number of CD34+ progenitor cells. Eur Heart J. 2009;30:584–93.
65. Hristov M, Zernecke A, Bidzhekov K, et al. Importance of CXC chemokine receptor 2 in the homing of human peripheral blood endothelial progenitor cells to sites of arterial injury. Circ Res. 2007;100:590–7.
66. Langer H, May AE, Daub K, et al. Adherent platelets recruit and induce differentiation of murine embryonic endothelial progenitor cells to mature endothelial cells in vitro. Circ Res. 2006;98:e2–10.
67. Vilahur G, Hernandez-Vera R, Molins B, et al. Short-term myocardial ischemia induces cardiac modified C-reactive protein expression and proinflammatory gene (cyclo-oxygenase-2, monocyte chemoattractant protein-1, and tissue factor) upregulation in peripheral blood mononuclear cells. J Thromb Haemost. 2009;7:485–93.
68. Yaron G, Brill A, Dashevsky O, et al. C-reactive protein promotes platelet adhesion to endothelial cells: a potential pathway in atherothrombosis. Br J Haematol. 2006;134:426–31.
69. de la Torre R, Pena E, Vilahur G, Slevin M, Badimon L. Monomerization of C-reactive protein requires glycoprotein IIb-IIIa activation: pentraxins and platelet deposition. J Thromb Haemost. 2013;11:2048–58.
70. Molins B, Pena E, Vilahur G, Mendieta C, Slevin M, Badimon L. C-reactive protein isoforms differ in their effects on thrombus growth. Arterioscler Thromb Vasc Biol. 2008;28:2239–46.
71. Badimon L, Padro T, Arderiu G, Vilahur G, Borrell-Pages M, Suades R. Extracellular vesicles in atherothrombosis: from biomarkers and precision medicine to therapeutic targets. Immunol Rev. 2022;312:6–19.
72. Cubedo J, Blasco A, Padro T, et al. Molecular signature of coronary stent thrombosis: oxidative stress and innate immunity cells. Thromb Haemost. 2017;117:1816–27.

CHAPTER 2

Venous thrombosis and thromboembolism: pathophysiological background

Marcello Di Nisio, Nicola Potere, Harry R. Buller, and Nick van Es

Contents

Summary

Venous thromboembolism (VTE) is a leading cause of morbidity and mortality worldwide, especially among the elderly and cancer patients, with an overall incidence of 1–2 per 1000 patient-years. About half of VTEs occur with no identifiable risk factors (unprovoked), while the remainder are associated with major or minor risk factors (transient or persistent). These risk factors can affect one or more components of Virchow's triad, comprising blood stasis, vessel wall damage, and hypercoagulability. Uncontrolled activation of the immune system was also recently implicated in VTE pathogenesis. Endothelial cell activation by inflammatory stimuli leads to expression of adhesion molecules that facilitate the binding of circulating leucocytes, platelets, erythrocytes, and extracellular vesicles. Subsequent leucocyte activation induces tissue factor expression and generation of neutrophil extracellular traps that trigger and propagate thrombosis. Further understanding of VTE pathophysiology may improve risk stratification and foster the development of novel therapeutic approaches to VTE complementary to anticoagulation.

Introduction

The most common site of deep venous thrombosis (DVT) is the lower extremities, where thrombi usually develop around venous valves due to blood stasis, endothelial damage, or hypercoagulability.[1] When thrombi in these locations grow and extend in the deep venous system, they can eventually break loose and embolize to the pulmonary circulation causing pulmonary embolism (PE). Therefore, DVT and PE are considered part of the same disease, named venous thromboembolism (VTE), and consequently require a similar diagnostic and treatment approach.[1]

DVT occurs in the deep veins, that is, within the fascia of the muscles, as opposed to superficial vein thrombosis that occurs in subcutaneous veins.[1] Patients with DVT usually present with a combination of pain, redness, and swelling of an extremity, causing significant discomfort and reduced mobility.[1] DVT of the lower extremities can

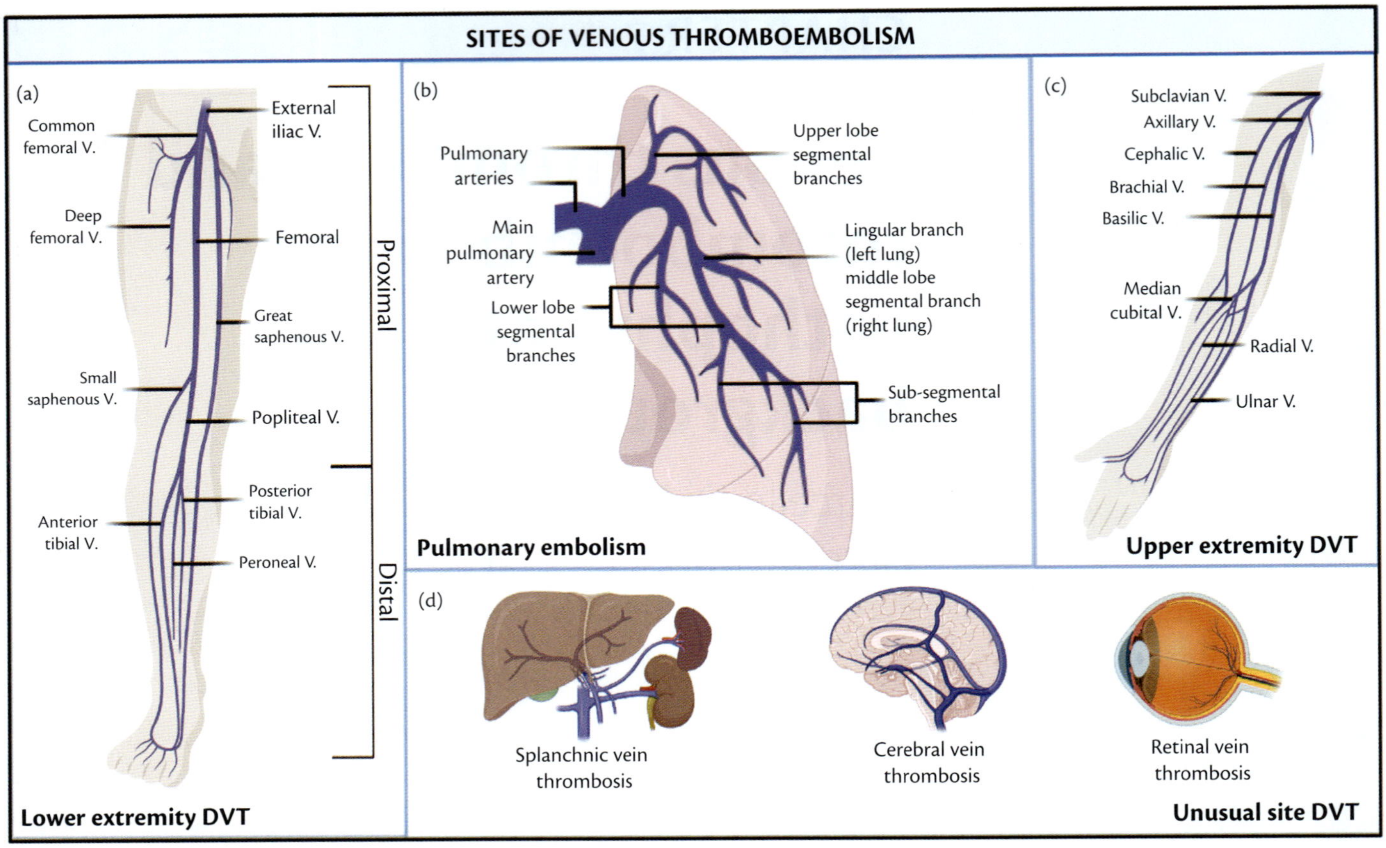

Figure 2.1 Sites of venous thromboembolism. Panel (a) shows the deep venous system of the lower extremities. Deep vein thrombosis (DVT) of the lower extremities is classified into proximal or distal if occurring above or below the knee joint, respectively. Panel (b) illustrates the anatomy and distribution of the pulmonary arteries with segmental and subsegmental branches. Panel (c) displays the deep venous system of the upper extremity (vein, V.). Panel (d) shows unusual sites of DVT, which include the splanchnic venous circulation (e.g. hepatic, portal, superior mesenteric, inferior mesenteric, and splenic veins), the cerebral venous system (e.g. the dural sinus and cerebral veins), and the retinal vein.
Created with BioRender.com.

be classified into distal and proximal. Isolated distal DVT is restricted to the infrapopliteal veins, that is, below the knee joint, including the peroneal, posterior tibial, and anterior tibial veins, as well as the calf muscle veins (i.e. the gastrocnemius and soleus muscles), whereas proximal DVT involves the popliteal, femoral, iliac veins and the inferior vena cava (➔ Figure 2.1a).[1] The distinction between distal and proximal DVT is clinically relevant, since the risk of embolization, extension, and recurrence is lower in patients with isolated distal DVT than in those with proximal DVT.[2,3] Albeit less frequent, DVT can also occur at unusual sites, including the deep veins of the upper extremity or of the neck (e.g. the internal jugular, subclavian, axillary, brachial, radial, and ulnar veins), the abdomen (e.g. the hepatic, portal, superior mesenteric, inferior mesenteric, and splenic veins), the renal veins, the retinal veins, or the cerebral sinus veins (➔ Figure 2.1c,d).[1]

Superficial vein thrombosis of the lower extremities usually involves the great or small saphenous veins, but also any other subcutaneous veins or venous varices. Patients typically exhibit pain, induration, and redness along the course of the thrombosed vein, which can be identified as a palpable cord.[1] The risk of embolization of superficial vein thrombosis is generally low, unless it extends by proximity into the deep venous system.[4]

PE mainly results from embolization of lower extremity deep vein thrombi.[1] PE can be located in central, lobar, segmental, or subsegmental pulmonary arteries, and can be unilateral or bilateral (➔ Figure 2.1b).[1] PE can manifest with dyspnoea, pleuritic chest pain, fatigue, and, less frequently, coughing, with or without haemoptysis.[5] Extensive or central pulmonary artery thrombi can result in haemodynamic alterations due to right ventricle overload, causing tachycardia, hypotension, and syncope. PE is classified as 'high risk' if associated with haemodynamic instability, defined as cardiac arrest, obstructive shock, or persistent systolic blood pressure below 90 mmHg without another cause.

Epidemiology of venous thromboembolism

VTE is a common disease with an overall incidence of about 1–2 per 1000 person-years.[6] The risk appears to be higher in Black than in White people, but is significantly lower among Asian individuals.[7,8] VTE risk increases exponentially with age, and is therefore rare in children and young adults.[9] Among younger individuals, VTE occurs more often in women than in men due to hormone-related risk factors, such as pregnancy and exposure to oral contraceptives, while the risk is higher in older men than in women of the same age. When adjusted for female reproductive risk factors, the overall risk of developing a first VTE event is about twofold higher in males than in females.[10] About half of cases of VTE are unprovoked, while the other half is provoked by major or minor risk factors that can be transient or persistent (➔ Risk factors for venous thromboembolism).

Historically, DVT was more frequently diagnosed than PE; however, the incidence of PE has been steadily rising over the last decades.[11] For example, PE incidence in Denmark increased threefold between 1999 and 2018.[12] This trend may be the result of increased awareness among physicians; a lower threshold for imaging in suspected patients[13]; and improved spatial resolution of modern, high-sensitivity computed tomography scanners that allow detection of smaller thrombi in pulmonary subsegmental arteries.[14]

Short- and long-term sequelae of pulmonary embolism

PE is a potentially fatal condition when haemodynamic decompensation occurs due to acute right ventricular failure. In the first month after PE diagnosis, the case fatality rate ranges from 12% in high-risk patients to 5% in those with non-high-risk PE.[15] At the population level, PE is responsible for about 7 deaths per 100,000 individuals in Europe, with substantial differences across countries.[16] Several registry-based studies have independently demonstrated a consistent decrease in PE-related mortality in the last decades, which is likely the result of earlier diagnosis, improved management, and increased detection of small thrombi (e.g. subsegmental PE) with fewer clinically relevant consequences.[12,16,17]

A substantial proportion of patients with acute PE develops the so-called post-PE syndrome, characterized by persistent exertional dyspnoea after 3 months of adequate treatment. This syndrome can be the result of chronic thromboembolic pulmonary hypertension, chronic thromboembolic pulmonary disease, cardiac dysfunction, or functional impairment.[18] Among such conditions, chronic thromboembolic pulmonary hypertension has the worse long-term prognosis; however, it is relatively uncommon, with a 2-year cumulative incidence of about 2%.[18] It is caused by persistent obstruction of pulmonary arteries leading to right ventricular dysfunction. Awareness among physicians and early diagnosis are crucial, since timely pulmonary endarterectomy may be curative.

Short- and long-term sequelae of deep vein thrombosis

Among patients with DVT, the most feared early complication is a compromised arterial or microcirculation leading to critical limb ischaemia. This rare condition, which is termed 'phlegmasia cerulea dolens', is usually the result of extensive venous thrombi, venous hypertension, and subsequent oedema and fluid sequestration in the affected limb. The increased interstitial and compartmental pressure compromises the arterial circulation, ultimately leading to acute ischaemia and gangrene. Rapid treatment with thrombolytic agents is required.

In the long term, a common complication of DVT is the post-thrombotic syndrome, which is defined as chronic venous insufficiency caused by venous obstruction, valvular reflux, and inflammation.[1] About 20–50% of patients develop the post-thrombotic syndrome after a proximal DVT, with the highest rates observed in those with extensive iliofemoral DVT, obesity, or severe symptoms at diagnosis.[19] The diagnosis and grading of severity of post-thrombotic syndrome is based on the Villalta score, which combines five subjective symptoms (pain, cramps, heaviness, paraesthesia, and pruritus) with seven objective signs (pretibial oedema, skin induration, hyperpigmentation, redness, venous ectasia, pain on calf compression, and venous ulcer). Post-thrombotic syndrome frequently leads to impaired quality of life and treatment options are limited at present.

Pathophysiological mechanisms of venous thrombosis

Venous thrombosis is believed to occur at the valve pocket sinus of large, deep veins, where the local turbulent blood flow and relative hypoxia favour the formation of small thrombi that progressively extend along the lumen, eventually leading to vessel occlusion and thrombus embolization.[20] In contrast to arterial thrombosis, which typically forms on a damaged blood vessel surface (e.g. a ruptured atherosclerotic plaque) at high shear stress, venous thrombosis tends to arise from a largely intact endothelium under low shear stress, and contains many red blood cells (the so-called red thrombi) in a fibrin mesh.[20] Venous thrombi also contain other trapped blood cellular elements, such as platelets and white blood cells, mainly neutrophils and monocytes, according to the proportion found in peripheral blood that actively participate to thrombogenesis.[21]

Mechanisms of blood coagulation activation and control

Activation of the blood coagulation cascade, comprising the extrinsic and intrinsic pathways, culminates in the activation of factor X and prothrombin (i.e. the common pathway), with subsequent fibrin formation from fibrinogen (➔ Figure 2.2).[20] The extrinsic coagulation pathway, which is usually initiated by a complex formation between tissue factor (TF) and activated factor VII, appears to play a central role in venous thrombosis, although the contribution of the intrinsic (contact activation) pathway is increasingly recognized. Under pathological conditions, activated monocytes and tumour cells can be sources of intravascular TF by expressing this protein on their cell membrane, or by releasing TF-exposing extracellular vescicles.[20] Increased levels of these extracellular vesicles have been observed in patients with cancer and in those undergoing major surgery, and may thus be implicated in the development of VTE in these settings.[22–24] In addition, extracellular material including nucleic

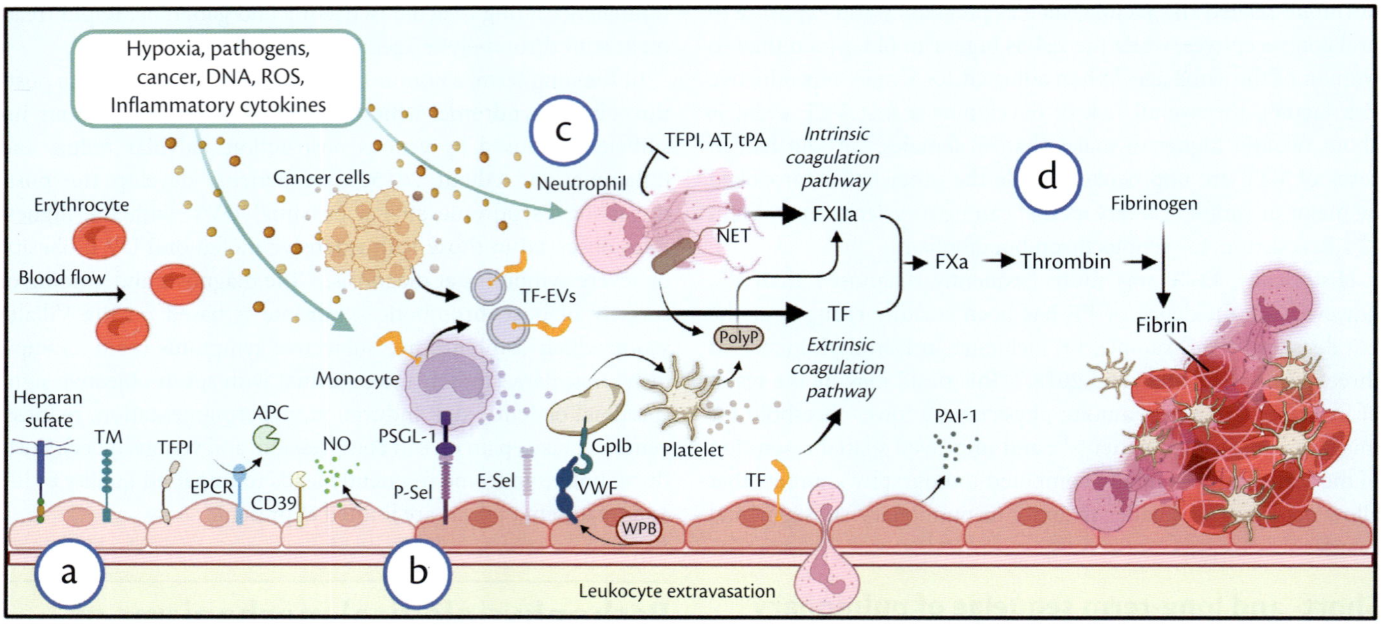

Figure 2.2 Overview of the pathophysiological mechanisms of vein thrombosis. (a) Under physiological conditions, the endothelium lining the vein wall is an antithrombotic surface. Quiescent endothelial cells prevent coagulation through the expression of glycosaminoglycans (e.g. heparan sulfate), tissue factor pathway inhibitor (TFPI), the ectonucleotidase CD39, as well as through the release of tissue-type plasminogen activator (tPA), nitric oxide (NO), and prostacyclin. In addition, thrombomodulin (TM) and the endothelial protein C receptor (EPCR) producing activated protein C (APC) have anti-inflammatory activity, and negatively modulate activation of coagulation. (b) In response to local hypoxia and blood flow perturbations, particularly at the valve pocket sinus, vascular damage, and a wide range of inflammatory signals including proinflammatory cytokines (e.g. IL-1, IL-6, TNF-α, and reactive oxygen species (ROS)), the endothelium undergoes a phenotypic shift to a prothrombotic surface that expresses leucocyte (P-selectin (P-Sel), E-selectin (E-Sel)) and platelet (von Willebrand factor (VWF)) adhesion molecules, promoting the rolling and endothelial binding of leucocytes and platelets. (c) Bound leucocytes, primarily monocytes, become activated and express tissue factor (TF) or release TF-positive extracellular vesicles (TF-EVs) that, together with perivascular TF and cancer cell-derived TF, trigger the extrinsic coagulation pathway. Extracellular nucleic acids and polyphosphate (PolyP) released from pathogens and activated platelets activate factor (F) XIIa of the intrinsic coagulation pathway. Immune activation also results in the generation of neutrophil extracellular traps (NETs), which further support coagulation and downregulate endogenous anticoagulants (TFPI, antithrombin (AT)), and fibrinolytics (tPA). (d) Altogether, these changes ultimately result in thrombin generation, fibrin accumulation, and venous thrombus formation. GpIb, glycoprotein Ib; PSGL-1, P-selectin glycoprotein ligand-1; WPB, Weibel–Palade body.
Created with BioRender.com.

acids [i.e. DNA, RNA, and neutrophil extracellular traps (NETs)] as well as polyphosphates generated during tissue injury and infection can activate factor XII and trigger the intrinsic coagulation pathway to support venous thrombogenesis.[20] A complex regulatory system comprising endogenous anticoagulant proteins together with anticoagulant effects of endothelial cells prevents undesired clotting under physiological conditions. For example, antithrombin inactivates several coagulation proteases, while TF pathway inhibitor blocks the TF/factor VIIa complex and factor Xa.[20] Binding of thrombin to thrombomodulin on the endothelial surface dramatically changes thrombin specificity from fibrinogen to protein C, thus boosting protein C activation. In turn, activated protein C together with its cofactor protein S inactivate factors VIIIa and Va.[20] Once formed, clots are physiologically removed by the fibrinolytic system, the activation of which results in the proteolytic digestion of fibrin by plasmin. Production of plasmin is also tightly regulated: tissue plasminogen activator (tPA) and urokinase promote the conversion of plasminogen into plasmin, which is antagonized by plasminogen activator inhibitor 1 (PAI-1).[20] Other regulatory mechanisms include α_2-antiplasmin and α_2-macroglobulin, which bind and inactivate plasmin, and thrombin-activatable fibrinolysis inhibitor (TAFI), which prevents binding of plasminogen to fibrin.

Numerous local and systemic factors can, either alone or synergistically, alter the physiological balance between coagulation and anticoagulation. These factors have been traditionally illustrated by Virchow's triad, comprising reduced blood flow or stasis, procoagulant changes occurring in the blood (hypercoagulability), and vessel wall damage (➔ Table 2.1).[20] However, in the last decades, studies have unravelled additional cellular and molecular thrombogenic mechanisms that have expanded our current understanding of the pathophysiology of venous thrombosis. A proposed model for the formation and propagation of venous thrombosis is shown in ➔ Figure 2.2.[20,25,26]

The endothelium, erythrocytes, and platelets in venous thrombosis

The intact endothelium maintains vascular homeostasis and blood fluidity by expressing natural anticoagulants, including TF pathway inhibitor, endothelial protein C receptor, thrombomodulin, and glycosaminoglycans (e.g. heparan sulfate), and the endogenous fibrinolytics tPA and urokinase-type

Table 2.1 Risk factors for venous thromboembolism

Non-heritable risk factors		
Hypercoagulability	**Vascular damage**	**Venous stasis/immobilization**
Increasing age	Surgery	Hospitalization for acute medical illness or exacerbation of chronic illness (e.g. congestive heart failure, infections, or rheumatological disorders)
Active cancer	Trauma or fracture	Nursing-home residence
Antiphospholipid syndrome	Central venous catheter or pacemaker	Long-haul travel for >4 hours
Hormone therapy		Paresis or paralysis
Pregnancy or puerperium		Venous insufficiency
Personal or family history of venous thromboembolism		Reduced mobility
Obesity		
Autoimmune and chronic inflammatory diseases		
Heparin-induced thrombocytopenia		
Heritable risk factors		
Factor V Leiden		
Prothrombin 20210A mutation		
Antithrombin deficiency		
Protein C deficiency		
Protein S deficiency		
Non-0 blood group		

plasminogen activator.[26] Quiescent endothelial cells also produce platelet inhibitors such as nitric oxide, prostacyclin, and CD39, a vascular ectonucleotidase that dissipates extracellular ATP and ADP. Proinflammatory cytokines [e.g. tumour necrosis factor α (TNFα), interleukin (IL)-1β, and IL-6], complement system components (e.g. C3a and C5a), reactive oxygen species, autoantibodies, microbial products, turbulent blood flow, and hypoxia are all able to induce a phenotypic switch from the quiescent venous endothelium into a highly thrombogenic surface.[26,26a] Simultaneous with the loss of anticoagulant properties, several adhesion molecules [P-selectin, E-selectin, intracellular cell adhesion molecule-1 (ICAM-1), vascular cell adhesion molecule-1 (VCAM-1)] are rapidly mobilized to the luminal surface on the activated endothelium, where they mediate the docking of circulating leucocytes, platelets, and blood cell-derived procoagulant extracellular vesicles through ligand-specific receptors such as P-selectin glycoprotein ligand-1 (PSGL-1) and the integrin very late antigen 4 (VLA4).[26] In addition, endothelial activation promotes the exocytosis of Weibel–Palade bodies containing von Willebrand factor (VWF) that sequesters platelets by binding to the glycoprotein Ibα receptor. Binding of circulating platelets to VWF results in platelet activation and shape change, with release of platelet-derived granules containing procoagulant, proangiogenic, and proinflammatory molecules.[27] Among others, thrombin, ADP, and thromboxane A_2 further promote platelet activation during thrombogenesis. Once activated, platelets aggregate by linkage to fibrinogen via the $\alpha_{IIb}\beta_3$ receptor and form leucocyte–platelet aggregates. Aggregated platelets within the forming thrombus also provide a phospholipid surface that sustains the activation of the coagulation cascade.[27] VWF also interacts with PSGL-1 and β_2 integrins on leucocytes, and enhances endothelial permeability favouring leucocyte extravasation and recruitment.[20]

Once considered passive bystanders, erythrocytes are increasingly recognized contributors to venous thrombosis.[28] Recent studies suggest that erythrocytes can form stacked rouleaux structures that enhance blood viscosity and directly enhance local thrombin generation. Once incorporated within venous thrombi, erythrocytes contribute to increase thrombus size, decrease thrombus permeability, and hinder thrombus lysis.[28]

Leucocyte contribution to venous thrombosis

Immunothrombosis refers to the complex interplay between immunity and coagulation, whereby coagulation triggers the activation of immune cells and these, in turn, sustain coagulation.[26,29,29a] While serving as an evolutionarily conserved mechanism to limit the dissemination of pathogens, accumulating evidence identified uncontrolled activation of immune cells as key contributors to venous thrombosis.[26,29a] The local increase in proinflammatory mediators produced by recruited leucocytes works in an autocrine and paracrine fashion to trigger TF exposure on monocytes and the release of TF-positive extracellular vesicles that initiate coagulation.[20] This inflammatory milieu is also capable of inducing 'NETosis', the generation of NETs from dying neutrophils.[30,30a] NETs are extruded web-like structures composed of a DNA backbone decorated with histones and proteins with antimicrobial activity. NETs are emerging central players in venous thrombosis. NETs favour the activation of coagulation factors (e.g. factor XII), present coagulation factors (e.g. TF, factor XI, and thrombin) to blood, degrade anticoagulant (e.g. TF pathway inhibitor and antithrombin) and fibrinolytic (e.g. tPA) molecules, and entrap platelets and erythrocytes, thus providing an essential scaffold for thrombus extension and organization.[30] NETs are abundant in venous thrombi, and circulating markers of NETosis such as extracellular DNA and histones are significantly increased in patients with VTE, although the routine clinical use of NETs as biomarkers of VTE is not yet established.[29] During thrombogenesis, leucocyte activation, NETosis, as well as complement system engagement can be boosted by platelets through the release of platelet-derived mediators such as platelet factor 4 (PF4) and high mobility group protein B1 (HMGB1).[27] In summary, studies over the last decades have unravelled novel molecular mechanisms that contribute to the pathogenesis of venous thrombosis, which may provide the basis for the identification of novel preventive and therapeutic strategies in VTE.

Risk factors for venous thromboembolism

VTE is a multifactorial disease in which multiple risk factors additively or multiplicatively contribute to overcome the so-called thrombosis threshold. However, the relative contribution of each of these risk factors remains only partially understood and clinically difficult to disentangle, as several risk factors likely contribute simultaneously to the development of thrombosis within an individual.

➔ Table 2.2 provides a list of inherited and acquired risk factors for VTE. Importantly, in one-third to one-half of patients with a first VTE episode, no apparent risk factors can be identified, and such events are classified as 'unprovoked'.[1,25]

The risk of VTE increases exponentially with age, which may be the result of additive effects of age-specific and conventional risk factors of VTE accumulating during the lifetime. Elderly patients often have multiple comorbidities, such as cancer, heart failure, or rheumatological disorders, which all increase VTE risk.[31] In addition, age-specific risk factors such as frailty, nursing-home residence, reduced mobility, and reduced muscle strength and calf muscle pump function may increase blood stasis and viscosity, resulting in increased VTE risk.[31] The actual relevance of these risk factors remains difficult to establish, because other concomitant risk factors, such as hospitalization for a medical illness or surgery, may confound these associations. Ageing is also accompanied by increased concentrations of several circulating procoagulant factors, such as factors VII and VIII, and is often characterized by remodelling of the venous wall, which may lead to or be associated with venous insufficiency and endothelial dysfunction that could contribute to thrombosis.[31,32]

VTE has a strong hereditary susceptibility, which has been estimated to be as high as 50% in recent genetic epidemiological studies.[33] The most common forms of inherited thrombophilia are factor V Leiden and the prothrombin 20210A mutation,

Table 2.2 Categorization of risk factors for venous thromboembolism based on the associated risk of recurrence

Estimated risk for long-term recurrence after completion of at least 3 months of anticoagulant treatment	Risk factor category	Examples
Low risk (<3% per year)	Major transient or reversible factors associated with >10-fold increased risk for the index VTE event compared to patients without the risk factor	Surgery with general anaesthesia for >30 min Hospitalization due to an acute illness, or acute exacerbation of a chronic illness with confinement to bed for ≥3 days Major trauma
Intermediate risk (3–8% per year)	Transient or reversible factors associated with ≤10-fold increased risk for first (index) VTE compared to patients without the risk factor	Minor surgery with general anaesthesia for <30 min Admission to hospital for <3 days with an acute illness Confined to bed out of hospital for ≥3 days with an acute illness Hormone therapy Pregnancy or puerperium Leg injury (without fracture) associated with reduced mobility for ≥3 days Long-haul flight
	Non-malignant persistent risk factors	Inflammatory bowel disease Active autoimmune disease
	No identifiable risk factor	
High risk (>8% per year)		Active cancer One or more previous episodes of VTE in the absence of a major transient or reversible factor Antiphospholipid antibody syndrome

Source data from Konstantinides SV, Meyer G, Becattini C, et al.; ESC Scientific Document Group. 2019 ESC Guidelines for the diagnosis and management of acute pulmonary embolism developed in collaboration with the European Respiratory Society (ERS). Eur Heart J. 2020;41(4):543–603. doi:10.1093/eurheartj/ehz405 which increase the risk of thrombosis by two- to fivefold.[1,25,33] Other well-known inherited thrombophilias include deficiency of antithrombin, protein C, and protein S. Novel genotyping and sequencing technologies have revealed several other genetic variations associated with VTE risk. Nevertheless, these polymorphisms seem to account for only a modest percentage of disease heritability, suggesting that additional genetic loci are yet to be identified.[33] This hypothesis is further supported by the observation that family history remains a strong VTE risk factor even among first-degree relatives without evident hereditary thrombophilic defects. Polygenic risk scores have been developed that can identify high-risk patients beyond the traditional inherited thrombophilia, but they are currently not used in practice.[34]

The antiphospholipid syndrome is an acquired form of thrombophilia that is characterized by persistently detectable lupus anticoagulant, anti-beta-2-glycoprotein or anti-cardiolipin IgM/IgG antibodies on two or more occasions (at least 12 weeks apart) in association with venous, arterial, or microvascular thrombosis (thrombotic antiphospholipid syndrome), or pregnancy complications such as recurrent pregnancy loss, intrauterine growth restriction, or severe preeclampsia (obstetrical antiphospholipid syndrome). Patients with thrombotic antiphospholipid syndrome have a considerable 2-year risk of recurrent VTE, which is estimated to be 5.4% if anticoagulant therapy is withdrawn.[35]

Current international guidelines do not recommend routine screening for inherited thrombophilia or antiphospholipid syndrome in most patients with unprovoked VTE.[36,37,37a] Although controversy exists about the indications and added value of thrombophilia testing, this may be considered in patients with VTE occurring at a young age (e.g. <50 years), unprovoked VTE against a background of a strong family history of VTE in first-degree relatives, and in patients with recurrent VTE.[36] In such cases, testing may help in tailoring the type, regimen, and duration of anticoagulant treatment. Testing for thrombophilia may also help to inform female family members about the potential risks of VTE associated with hormonal therapy or pregnancy.

In addition to age and thrombophilia, several other risk factors contribute to the development of VTE including surgery, trauma, cancer, hospitalization for acute medical illness, congestive heart failure, infection, as well as autoimmune and rheumatological diseases (➔ Table 2.1). Epidemiological studies conducted over the past two decades suggested that VTE and arterial thrombosis may be considered as part of a cardiovascular disease continuum.[38] VTE and atherosclerosis share common risk factors such as obesity, smoking, and diabetes mellitus, although these associations have been inconsistently reported.[39] Patients with VTE exhibit an increased risk of subsequent myocardial infarction, stroke, or peripheral arterial embolization and, conversely, patients with myocardial infarction or heart failure have an increased tendency to develop VTE.[38]

Patients with cancer

About 20% of all VTEs occur in patients with cancer. Recent epidemiological studies found that overall VTE risk is about 12-fold higher in cancer patients compared with individuals without cancer, but the risk increase varies considerably between 7- and 20-fold across tumour types.[40] While cancers of the pancreas, ovary, lung, stomach, and brain and non-Hodgkin lymphoma have the highest relative risk of VTE, other more prevalent tumour types, such as breast or colorectal cancer, contribute most to the overall burden of VTE. Compared with the general population, the risk of VTE is further increased up to 23-fold by anticancer therapies such as cancer surgery and chemotherapy.[40] Novel anticancer treatments, including immune checkpoint inhibitors, chimeric antigen receptor T cells, and angiogenesis inhibitors, have revolutionized the approach to many cancer types and led to improved survival, but may increase VTE risk by three- to fourfold.[37] Prior VTE, the presence of metastases, advanced or progressive disease, reduced mobility, frequent hospitalizations or invasive procedures, and infections may further augment VTE risk in patients with cancer.

Women

The risk of VTE is increased during pregnancy, the postpartum period, and in women using hormone replacement therapy or oestrogen-containing oral contraceptives. While the underlying pathophysiology remains incompletely understood, hormone-related increases in plasma concentrations of procoagulant factors together with reduced levels of anticoagulant proteins (e.g. antithrombin or protein S) may contribute to explain the association between these female-specific risk factors and VTE.[41] Venous stasis during pregnancy and caesarean sections also increase the risk, which is highest during the postpartum period.

The reported risk of VTE in women using hormonal therapy varied substantially across studies, probably due to the heterogeneity of the populations included and the type, intensity, and duration of hormonal therapies. The type and dose of hormonal therapy seem to be relevant with respect to VTE risk, as the latter appears to be higher in women using formulations containing higher oestrogen doses or combinations of an oestrogen and a progestogen, especially desogestrel or gestodene.[41] Hormone-releasing intrauterine devices and contraceptives containing only progesterone have not been associated with a significant increase in VTE risk, and may be preferable options in women with a personal or strong family history of VTE. Another source of variability of VTE risk in women using hormonal therapy is likely represented by the presence of other concomitant risk factors, such as personal or strong family history of VTE or inherited thrombophilia.[41]

Major or minor transient or persistent risk factors

The risk of VTE recurrence is highly variable and strongly influenced by risk factors that were present around the time of the initial VTE event. Therefore, understanding and categorizing risk factors according to the associated probability of recurrence is key for personalized VTE recurrence risk assessment. Patients in whom no precipitating factor for VTE can be identified are often categorized as having unprovoked VTE. In all other patients in whom a precipitating cause of the event can be identified, VTE is categorized as provoked. However, due to the high variability in the risk of recurrent VTE, this binary categorization using the descriptors 'provoked' and 'unprovoked' VTE is no longer supported by the European Society of Cardiology (ESC) guideline for the diagnosis and management of acute PE.[3] The most recent categorization proposed by the ESC classifies patients as having VTE with no identifiable risk factors or VTE associated with major transient, minor transient, or persistent risk factors. This classification provides a framework to group VTE risk factors based on similar estimated risks of recurrence (i.e. high, intermediate, or low), which is relevant for making decisions about the duration of anticoagulant treatment (➔ Table 2.2).

Patients who develop VTE in association with transient major risk factor such as trauma, surgery, joint replacements, or spinal cord injury are expected to have a risk of recurrence following discontinuation of anticoagulation as low as 1% at 1 year.[37] Therefore, a short course of anticoagulant treatment of 3 months is generally recommended in these patients. At the other end of the spectrum, patients with recurrent VTE and no identifiable risk factor, as well as patients with VTE associated with persistent risk factors such as malignancy or severe thrombophilia, have a higher VTE recurrence risk. Therefore, in these patients, a long-term or indefinite treatment duration is usually recommended. Severe hereditary thrombophilia generally encompasses antithrombin deficiency, deficiency of protein C or protein S, or homozygosity for factor V Leiden or prothrombin G20210A mutation. For patients with mild hereditary thrombophilia such as heterozygous factor V Leiden or prothrombin 20210A mutation, there is currently no evidence of a clinical benefit for extended anticoagulant treatment.[1,25] International guidelines consistently recommend indefinite anticoagulation for VTE patients with antiphospholipid syndrome, based on their high risk of recurrence.[35,37,42–44]

Estimating the risk of recurrence and making decisions on duration of anticoagulation is less clear-cut and more challenging in patients in whom the initial VTE event occurred in the context of an intermediate risk factor. This represents a rather common scenario and therapeutic quandary, since over half of patients with VTE have no identifiable risk factor or minor transient risk factors such as minor surgery, hospitalization, leg injury with reduced mobility, hormonal therapy, or pregnancy. The risk of recurrent VTE in these patients has been estimated to be in the range of 3–8%.[36] This relatively large interval may be the consequence of differences in patient populations or concomitant VTE risk factors.

In a recent systematic review and individual patient meta-analysis of randomized controlled trials and prospective cohort studies, the risk of recurrence in patients with first VTE and no identifiable risk factor was 10% at 1 year, 25% at 5 years, and 36% at 10 years after completion of at least 3 months of anticoagulant treatment.[45] According to the ESC guidelines, extension of anticoagulation beyond 3 months should be considered in these patients, consistent with the indication of most guidelines, which consider these estimates to be high enough for recommending indefinite anticoagulation.[37] Another important factor to take into consideration when deciding about the duration of anticoagulation is the risk of bleeding, but this is beyond the scope of this chapter.

It remains controversial whether VTE events occurring in association with oestrogen-containing oral contraceptives can be considered within the group of VTE with no identifiable risk factor or be categorized as VTE associated with minor or intermediate risk factors. The guideline of the International Society of Thrombosis and Haemostasis and the guideline of the American Society of Hematology define the use of oestrogen-containing oral contraceptives as a minor transient risk factor, whereas the ESC guidelines consider oestrogen use as an intermediate risk factor for VTE.[37,42,43] A recent meta-analysis concluded that the risk of recurrence after stopping anticoagulation is low in women with VTE associated with oestrogen-containing contraceptives, although there was evidence of high heterogeneity and results could not exclude a substantial residual risk in women using specific types or formulations of contraceptives, different lengths of contraceptive use, or in women with additional risk factors for VTE.[46]

Conclusion

VTE comprises DVT and PE, and is a common disease with an incidence of 1–2 per 1000 patient-years. Traditionally, the main drivers of development of VTE were thought to be venous stasis, vessel well damage, or hereditary or acquired hypercoagulability, but recent evidence indicates that the immune system also plays an important role. Various transient or persistent risk factors contribute to the development of VTE (e.g. cancer, surgery, and hereditary thrombophilia) and, if present, result in the classification of VTE as 'provoked'. Anticoagulant treatment is indicated to prevent disease progression or recurrence, wherein the duration of treatment (limited-duration vs indefinite) is based on the estimated risk of VTE recurrence after stopping anticoagulation.

References

1. Di Nisio M, van Es N, Büller HR. Deep vein thrombosis and pulmonary embolism. Lancet. 2016;388(10063):3060–73. doi:10.1016/S0140-6736(16)30514-1
2. Stein PD, Matta F, Musani MH, Diaczok B. Silent pulmonary embolism in patients with deep venous thrombosis: a systematic review. Am J Med. 2010;123(5):426–31. doi:10.1016/J.AMJMED.2009.09.037
3. Eichinger S, Heinze G, Jandeck LM, Kyrle PA. Risk assessment of recurrence in patients with unprovoked deep vein thrombosis or pulmonary embolism: the Vienna prediction model. Circulation. 2010;121(14):1630–6. doi:10.1161/CIRCULATIONAHA.109.925214
4. Galanaud JP, Sevestre MA, Pernod G, et al. Long-term risk of venous thromboembolism recurrence after isolated superficial vein

thrombosis. J Thromb Haemost. 2017;15(6):1123–31. doi:10.1111/JTH.13679

5. Pollack CV, Schreiber D, Goldhaber SZ, et al. Clinical characteristics, management, and outcomes of patients diagnosed with acute pulmonary embolism in the emergency department: initial report of EMPEROR (Multicenter Emergency Medicine Pulmonary Embolism in the Real World Registry). J Am Coll Cardiol. 2011;57(6):700–6. doi:10.1016/J.JACC.2010.05.071
6. Raskob GE, Angchaisuksiri P, Blanco AN, et al. Thrombosis. Arterioscler Thromb Vasc Biol. 2014;34(11):2363–71. doi:10.1161/ATVBAHA.114.304488
7. White RH, Zhou H, Romano PS. Incidence of idiopathic deep venous thrombosis and secondary thromboembolism among ethnic groups in California. Ann Intern Med. 1998;128(9):737–40. doi:10.7326/0003-4819-128-9-199805010-00006
8. Stein PD, Kayali F, Olson RE, Milford CE. Pulmonary thromboembolism in Asians/Pacific Islanders in the United States: analysis of data from the National Hospital Discharge Survey and the United States Bureau of the Census. Am J Med. 2004;116(7):435–42. doi:10.1016/J.AMJMED.2003.11.020
9. Næss IA, Christiansen SC, Romundstad P, Cannegieter SC, Rosendaal FR, Hammerstrøm J. Incidence and mortality of venous thrombosis: a population-based study. J Thromb Haemost. 2007;5(4):692–9. doi:10.1111/J.1538-7836.2007.02450.X
10. Roach REJ, Lijfering WM, Rosendaal FR, Cannegieter SC, Le Cessie S. Sex difference in risk of second but not of first venous thrombosis: paradox explained. Circulation. 2014;129(1):51–6. doi:10.1161/CIRCULATIONAHA.113.004768
11. Huang W, Goldberg RJ, Anderson FA, Kiefe CI, Spencer FA. Secular trends in occurrence of acute venous thromboembolism: the Worcester VTE study (1985–2009). Am J Med. 2014;127(9):829–39.e5. doi:10.1016/J.AMJMED.2014.03.041
12. Sonne-Holm E, Kjærgaard J, Bang LE, Fosbøl E, Carlsen J, Winther-Jensen M. Pulmonary embolism: age specific temporal trends in incidence and mortality in Denmark 1999–2018. Thromb Res. 2022;210:12–19. doi:10.1016/J.THROMRES.2021.12.011
13. Wang RC, Miglioretti DL, Marlow EC, et al. Trends in imaging for suspected pulmonary embolism across US health care systems, 2004 to 2016. JAMA Netw Open. 2020;3(11):e2026930. doi:10.1001/JAMANETWORKOPEN.2020.26930
14. Wiener RS, Schwartz LM, Woloshin S. When a test is too good: how CT pulmonary angiograms find pulmonary emboli that do not need to be found. BMJ. 2013;347(7915):f3368. doi:10.1136/BMJ.F3368
15. Blondon M, Jimenez D, Robert-Ebadi H, et al. Comparative clinical prognosis of massive and non-massive pulmonary embolism: a registry-based cohort study. J Thromb Haemost. 2021;19(2):408–16. doi:10.1111/JTH.15146
16. Barco S, Mahmoudpour SH, Valerio L, et al. Trends in mortality related to pulmonary embolism in the European Region, 2000–15: analysis of vital registration data from the WHO Mortality Database. Lancet Respir Med. 2020;8(3):277–87. doi:10.1016/S2213-2600(19)30354-6
17. Hoskin S, Brieger D, Chow V, Kritharides L, Ng ACC. Trends in acute pulmonary embolism admission rates and mortality outcomes in Australia, 2002–2003 to 2017–2018: a retrospective cohort study. Thromb Haemost. 2021;121(9):1237–45. doi:10.1055/S-0041-1725932/ID/JR200845-6
18. Valerio L, Mavromanoli AC, Barco S, et al. Chronic thromboembolic pulmonary hypertension and impairment after pulmonary embolism: the FOCUS study. Eur Heart J. 2022;43(36):3387–98. doi:10.1093/EURHEARTJ/EHAC206
19. Rabinovich A, Ducruet T, Kahn SR, et al. Development of a clinical prediction model for the postthrombotic syndrome in a prospective cohort of patients with proximal deep vein thrombosis. J Thromb Haemost. 2018;16(2):262–70. doi:10.1111/jth.13909
20. Mackman N. New insights into the mechanisms of venous thrombosis. J Clin Invest. 2012;122(7):2331. doi:10.1172/JCI60229
21. von Brühl ML, Stark K, Steinhart A, et al. Monocytes, neutrophils, and platelets cooperate to initiate and propagate venous thrombosis in mice in vivo. J Exp Med. 2012;209(4):819–35. doi:10.1084/jem.20112322
22. Johnson GJ, Leis LA, Bach RR. Tissue factor activity of blood mononuclear cells is increased after total knee arthroplasty. Thromb Haemost. 2009;102(4):728–34. doi:10.1160/TH09-04-0261
23. Tesselaar MET, Romijn FPHTM, Van Der Linden IK, Bertina RM, Osanto S. Microparticle-associated tissue factor activity in cancer patients with and without thrombosis. J Thromb Haemost. 2009;7(8):1421–3. doi:10.1111/J.1538-7836.2009.03504.X
24. Zwicker JI, Liebman HA, Neuberg D, et al. Tumor-derived tissue factor-bearing microparticles are associated with venous thromboembolic events in malignancy. Clin Cancer Res. 2009;15(22):6830–40. doi:10.1158/1078-0432.CCR-09-0371
25. Khan F, Tritschler T, Kahn SR, Rodger MA. Venous thromboembolism. Lancet. 2021;398(10294):64–77. doi:10.1016/S0140-6736(20)32658-1
26. Colling ME, Tourdot BE, Kanthi Y. Inflammation, infection and venous thromboembolism. Circ Res. 2021;128(12):2017–36. doi:10.1161/CIRCRESAHA.121.318225

26a. Potere N, Abbate A, Kanthi Y, Carrier M, Porreca E, Di Nisio M. Inflammasome signaling, thromboinflammation, and venous thromboembolism. J Am Coll Cardiol Basic Trans Science. Jun 07, 2023. doi: 10.1016/j.jacbts.2023.03.017

27. Koupenova M, Clancy L, Corkrey HA, Freedman JE. Circulating platelets as mediators of immunity, inflammation, and thrombosis. Circ Res. 2018;122(2):337–51. doi:10.1161/CIRCRESAHA.117.310795
28. Byrnes JR, Wolberg AS. Red blood cells in thrombosis. Blood. 2017;130(16):1795–9. doi:10.1182/BLOOD-2017-03-745349
29. Foley JH, Conway EM. Cross talk pathways between coagulation and inflammation. Circ Res. 2016;118(9):1392–408. doi:10.1161/CIRCRESAHA.116.306853

29a. Potere N, Garrad E, Kanthi Y, et al. NLRP3 inflammasome and interleukin-1 contributions to COVID-19-associated coagulopathy and immunothrombosis. Cardiovasc Res. 2023; May 30;cvad084. doi: 10.1093/cvr/cvad084

30. Thålin C, Hisada Y, Lundström S, Mackman N, Wallén H. Neutrophil extracellular traps: villains and targets in arterial, venous, and cancer-associated thrombosis. Arterioscler Thromb Vasc Biol. 2019;39(9):1724–38. doi:10.1161/ATVBAHA.119.312463

30a. Potere N, Abbate A, Kanthi Y, Carrier M, Porreca E, Di Nisio M. Inflammasome signaling, thromboinflammation, and venous thromboembolism. J Am Coll Cardiol Basic Trans Science. Jun 07, 2023. Epublished doi: 10.1016/j.jacbts.2023.03.017

31. Engbers MJ, van Hylckama Vlieg A, Rosendaal FR. Venous thrombosis in the elderly: incidence, risk factors and risk groups. J Thromb Haemost. 2010;8(10):2105–12
32. Wang H, Rosendaal FR, Cushman M, van Hylckama Vlieg A. Procoagulant factor levels and risk of venous thrombosis in the elderly. J Thromb Haemost. 2021;19(1):186–93. doi:10.1111/jth.15127
33. Morange PE, Suchon P, Trégouët DA. Genetics of venous thrombosis: update in 2015. Thromb Haemost. 2015;114(5):910–19. doi:10.1160/th15-05-0410
34. Klarin D, Busenkell E, Judy R, et al. Genome-wide association analysis of venous thromboembolism identifies new risk loci and genetic overlap with arterial vascular disease. Nat Genet. 2019;51(11):1574–9. doi:10.1038/s41588-019-0519-3

35. Ortel TL, Meleth S, Catellier D, et al. Recurrent thrombosis in patients with antiphospholipid antibodies and an initial venous or arterial thromboembolic event: a systematic review and meta-analysis. J Thromb Haemost. 18(9):2274–86. doi:10.1111/jth.14936
36. Klok FA, Ageno W, Ay C, et al. Optimal follow-up after acute pulmonary embolism: a position paper of the European Society of Cardiology Working Group on Pulmonary Circulation and Right Ventricular Function, in collaboration with the European Society of Cardiology Working Group on Atherosclerosis and Vascular Biology, endorsed by the European Respiratory Society. Eur Heart J. 2022;43(3):183–9. doi:10.1093/eurheartj/ehab816
37. Konstantinides SV, Meyer G, Becattini C, et al. 2019 ESC Guidelines for the diagnosis and management of acute pulmonary embolism developed in collaboration with the European Respiratory Society (ERS): The Task Force for the diagnosis and management of acute pulmonary embolism of the European Society of Cardiology (ESC). Eur Respir J. 2019;54(3):1901647. doi:10.1183/13993003.01647-2019
37a. Middeldorp S, Nieuwlaat R, Baumann Kreuziger L, et al. American Society of Hematology 2023 Guidelines for Management of Venous Thromboembolism: Thrombophilia Testing. Blood Adv. 2023; May 17. doi: 10.1182/bloodadvances.2023010177
38. Becattini C, Vedovati MC, Ageno W, Dentali F, Agnelli G. Incidence of arterial cardiovascular events after venous thromboembolism: a systematic review and a meta-analysis. J Thromb Haemost. 2010;8(5):891–7. doi:10.1111/j.1538-7836.2010.03777.x
39. Ageno W, Becattini C, Brighton T, Selby R, Kamphuisen PW. Cardiovascular risk factors and venous thromboembolism: a meta-analysis. Circulation. 2008;117(1):93–102. doi:10.1161/CIRCULATIONAHA.107.709204
40. Mulder FI, Horváth-Puhó E, van Es N, et al. Venous thromboembolism in cancer patients: a population-based cohort study. Blood. 2021;137(14):1959–69. doi:10.1182/blood.2020007338
41. van Hylckama Vlieg A, Middeldorp S. Hormone therapies and venous thromboembolism: where are we now? J Thromb Haemost. 2011;9(2):257–66.
42. Ortel TL, Neumann I, Ageno W, et al. American Society of Hematology 2020 guidelines for management of venous thromboembolism: treatment of deep vein thrombosis and pulmonary embolism. Blood Adv. 2020;4(19):4693–738. doi:10.1182/bloodadvances.2020001830
43. Kearon C, Ageno W, Cannegieter SC, et al. Categorization of patients as having provoked or unprovoked venous thromboembolism: guidance from the SSC of ISTH. J Thromb Haemost. 2016;14(7):1480–1483.
44. Stevens SM, Woller SC, Baumann Kreuziger L, et al. Executive summary: antithrombotic therapy for VTE disease: second update of the CHEST guideline and expert panel report. Chest. 2021;160(6):2247–59. doi:10.1016/j.chest.2021.07.056
45. Khan F, Rahman A, Carrier M, et al. Long term risk of symptomatic recurrent venous thromboembolism after discontinuation of anticoagulant treatment for first unprovoked venous thromboembolism event: systematic review and meta-analysis. BMJ. 2019;366:l4363. doi:10.1136/bmj.l4363
46. Wiegers HMG, Knijp J, van Es N, et al. Risk of recurrence in women with venous thromboembolism related to estrogen-containing contraceptives: systematic review and meta-analysis. J Thromb Haemost. 2022;20(5):1158–65. doi:10.1111/jth.15661

CHAPTER 3

Thrombosis and thromboembolism in atrial fibrillation: pathophysiological background

Peter Calvert, Nicola Tidbury, and Gregory Y.H. Lip

Contents

Summary

Atrial fibrillation presents a situation whereby all three elements of Virchow's triad of thrombosis are met within the left atrium. Chronic endothelial injury and dysfunction results in fibrotic remodelling of the left atrium, and fibrillation impairs contractile function, resulting in blood stasis. Meanwhile, the coagulation system activates abnormally, and fibrinolysis is impaired. This creates a prothrombotic state for thrombus formation, particularly within the left atrial appendage, which may lead to systemic thromboembolism and stroke.

Introduction

Atrial fibrillation (AF) is the most common cardiac rhythm disorder. It affects 1–2% of adults, with an increasing global prevalence, in part—but not entirely—due to the ageing population.[1,2] Indeed, adults over 40 years old have an approximate 25% lifetime risk of developing AF. Patients with AF have increased morbidity and mortality, in part due to an up to fivefold higher risk of thromboembolic events compared to the general population.[3]

Multiple studies suggest that AF confers a hypercoagulable state. Abnormal activation of the coagulation cascade has been reported for patients with both paroxysmal[4–6] and sustained AF.[7,8] In fact, hypercoagulability may occur in as little as 6 hours from the onset of AF.[4]

AF develops due to endothelial inflammation and structural remodelling, which are caused by underlying cardiovascular comorbidities such as hypertension, diabetes mellitus, obesity, and smoking. The higher risk of thromboembolic events directly relates to these processes.

In this chapter, we will explore the mechanisms underlying thrombosis and thromboembolism in AF and how they tie into Virchow's triad of blood stasis, vessel wall abnormalities, and hypercoagulability.

Endothelial inflammation

The endothelium consists of a monolayer of cells that line the peripheral vasculature as well as the endocardial surface of the heart. It has a multitude of roles, not only in allowing selective movement of macromolecules, but in mediating inflammation, vascular tone, and haemostasis. A healthy endothelium promotes an antiplatelet and anticoagulant state. When dysfunctional, activated endothelial cells express adhesion molecules and promote a prothrombotic state.

Chronic endothelial inflammation is well recognized as the major pathophysiological abnormality underlying atherosclerotic cardiovascular disease; however, it also plays a key role in initiation and progression of AF.

Endothelial abnormalities in AF are well described in histopathological studies. These include thickening and wrinkling of the endocardium, fibrosis and fibroelastosis,[9] neutrophilic infiltration and inflammation,[10] myocyte hypertrophy, and thrombotic aggregations,[11] all of which are seen far more frequently in those with AF compared with controls.[12,13] These changes appear specific to the atria, with the majority of concurrent ventricular biopsies being normal[13]—hence the term 'atrial cardiopathy'.

In one postmortem series, 16 of 17 AF cases showing 'rough endothelium' in the left atrium (LA) demonstrated mural thrombi.[12] The endothelium was found to be irregular with evidence of injury and regenerative processes, compared with non-AF controls where the endothelium was flat and polygonal. These abnormalities were strongly associated with thrombosis.

A number of inflammatory biomarkers have been linked with AF and thromboembolic risk, with varying levels of evidence. These include C-reactive protein, interleukins (IL-2, -6, and -8), and tumour necrosis factor-α (TNF-α).[14]

Evidence for these biomarkers tends to be variable, with some studies finding positive associations with thromboembolic risk and others reporting that such associations disappear after multivariable regression.[15,16] This suggests that pre-existing cardiovascular comorbidities may explain the risk associated with inflammation. It follows that AF results from inflammatory changes, and the combination significantly increases thromboembolic risk.

Inflammation results in upregulation of prothrombotic factors—including tissue factor (TF),[16] von Willebrand factor (VWF),[17] fibrinogen, and factor VIII.[14] Furthermore, elevated IL-6 may also reduce levels of protein S—an endogenous antithrombotic molecule.[17] Inflammation also results in abnormal function of the endothelium, as described below.

Endothelial dysfunction

Chronic inflammation of the endothelium results in endothelial dysfunction. This is well described in AF and further ties into the increased thromboembolic risk.

Under normal circumstances, healthy endothelium synthesizes nitric oxide (NO) via endothelial nitric oxide synthase (eNOS). NO exerts an antithrombotic effect by inhibiting platelet activation and supressing production of the prothrombotic molecules plasminogen activator inhibitor-1 (PAI-1) and prostacyclin. Studies in porcine models of AF demonstrate significantly reduced levels of eNOS and NO in the LA,[18] correlating with a 1.8-fold increase in PAI-1. PAI-1 inhibits conversion of plasminogen to plasmin—an endogenous fibrinolytic—hence increased levels of PAI-1 may contribute to thrombosis in AF.

Human studies have confirmed reduced NO production, though there is conflicting evidence regarding circulating PAI-1 levels—with some finding similar levels to controls[19] and others finding raised levels in AF patients.[20,21] This disparity may relate to the degree of LA endothelial dysfunction; one might expect that, in earlier disease, PAI-1 levels may be altered only locally in the LA. This is indeed what the aforementioned porcine study found—right atrial and aortic levels of NO, NOS, and PAI-1 were not altered.[18] Similar findings have been observed in a canine model.[22]

Beyond the above, AF has been shown to cause increased levels of angiotensin-II, which upregulates production of PAI-1.[23] This process is normally counter-regulated by apelin. Apelin levels in AF, however, may be lower than controls, further contributing to increased PAI-1 levels.[24]

An increase in asymmetric dimethylarginine (ADMA) concentration has been observed in patients with AF in several studies,[25–27] and increases further in the presence of cardiovascular comorbidities.[28] ADMA is a competitive inhibitor of NOS,[29] and therefore may cause a reduction in NO and an increase in PAI-1 as described above. Elevated ADMA may also result in excessive platelet aggregation and monocyte adhesion to the endothelium.[30] Studies have identified that an increased ADMA concentration is associated with thromboembolic risk and mortality in AF patients.[31,32]

Hence inflammation and coagulation—and, thereby, thromboembolic risk—are intricately linked. These chronic changes result in structural remodelling of the atria, which are described in the next section.

Structural remodelling and blood flow abnormalities

Fibrosis and remodelling

There is a well-established link between AF and LA fibrosis.[33,34] Matrix metalloproteinases (MMPs) are involved in the modulation of extracellular matrix through the degradation of its components. There are several subgroups of MMPs which all have different substrate specificity due to slight structural differences.[35] For example, MMP-1 breaks down collagens type I, II, and III, while MMP-9 degrades type IV and V collagens. The actions of MMPs are inhibited by tissue inhibitors of matrix metalloproteinase (TIMPs). Any change to the balance of these proteins may promote fibrosis via abnormal extracellular matrix degradation.

Several studies have analysed MMPs and TIMPs in the setting of AF. One study found levels of MMP-1 were lower—and TIMP-1 levels were higher—than controls, with a significant correlation between MMP/TIMP and prothrombotic biomarkers.[36,37] MMP-9 concentrations also appear higher in AF patients compared with controls[38] and have been implicated in the structural remodelling process.[39,40] This correlates with the finding of atrial and left atrial appendage (LAA) fibrosis on magnetic resonance imaging (MRI), which has been associated with spontaneous echo contrast (SEC)—a smoke-like appearance seen on ultrasound associated with thrombogenesis[41,42]—and LAA thrombosis.[43] Analysis of resected LAA following cardiac surgery further confirms this.[44]

LA connective tissue abnormalities have also been noted in some studies, with increased volumes of thickened collagen and interstitial fibrosis in those with AF.[45–47] This is supported by evidence of raised collagen turnover markers in AF.[20] There is conflicting evidence, with some proposing that structural disease itself, rather than AF per se, is the cause of such abnormalities.[48]

Left atrial structural abnormalities

It has long been recognized that atrial enlargement occurs with prolonged AF.[49] Evidence shows that, as the LA enlarges, contractile function impairs, and both of these factors progress with increased arrhythmia burden.[50] This results in blood stasis within the LA, which promotes thrombogenesis.[51,52]

Enlargement of the LA has been linked to the appearance of SEC. Furthermore, LA enlargement itself is independently associated with stroke risk[51,53,54] and failure of anticoagulation therapy.[55]

In patients with AF, even a normal size LA may have impaired contractile function, which may persist even when the patient is in sinus rhythm.[50] This emphasizes the fact that thromboembolic risk is still elevated even with effective rhythm control—that is, fixing the rhythm does not resolve the endothelial abnormalities described above.

Left atrial appendage abnormalities

The LAA is a blind-ended structure arising from the LA and is well recognized as the most common site of thrombus formation in patients with AF.[56,57] The LAA may be structurally abnormal in AF, with postmortem studies showing enlargement, increased luminal surface area, and reduced pectinate musculature.[9]

Larger LAA orifice area has been shown to correlate with reduced flow velocities,[58] SEC,[59] and stroke.[60] Patients with larger LAA orifices tend to be older and more often have hypertension and AF, with longer duration of AF further correlating with increased area.[59] At least one study, however, found the inverse—that smaller LAA orifice was associated with stroke[61]—so the exact relationship may not be completely clear.

During AF, the LAA loses contractile function, resulting in blood stasis and risk of thrombus formation. This has been demonstrated in transoesophageal echocardiographic studies, where reduced LAA function assessed by pulsed-wave Doppler (or other methods) was significantly linked to the presence of SEC or thrombus[62] and stroke risk.[41]

Three LAA blood flow patterns have been described. Type 1 (biphasic) is found only in sinus rhythm while types 2 (multiphasic) and 3 (low flow) are found only in AF.[63,64] Type 3 represents the poorest LAA contractile function and is the only type significantly associated with thrombosis.[63–65] Cardioversion to sinus rhythm significantly improves LAA and LA mechanical function[66,67] though there is minimal evidence that maintenance of sinus rhythm reduces the long-term risk of thromboembolism. Indeed, thromboembolic risk is increased in the peri-cardioversion period.[68]

LAA peak flow velocity ≤ 20 cm/s has been associated with thromboembolism,[41] and this correlates with other factors such as LA volume index, left ventricular (LV) mass index, and clinical risk scores.[69] Raised LA pressure may also contribute to impairment of LAA flow velocity,[70] which may explain correlations between heart failure and thromboembolic risk in AF.[71]

Left atrial appendage—anatomical morphology

Irrespective of AF, LAA anatomy varies between individuals. Recognized anatomical variants are described based on their structural appearance: cactus, chicken wing, windsock, and cauliflower[72] (➔ Figure 3.1). Different LAA morphologies have been directly associated with flow velocity, orifice area, and stroke risk.

The highest flow velocity and smallest orifice area are seen in the chicken-wing type, and lowest flow and largest orifice area are seen in the cauliflower type.[73,74] This neatly fits with the finding that chicken-wing morphology is associated with the lowest risk of stroke, with cauliflower type having up to an eightfold increased likelihood in comparison.[60,72,75] Although conflicting evidence exists,[61,76] two meta-analyses with a combined total of over 6000 patients demonstrated that patients with non-chicken-wing morphology are at higher thromboembolic risk.[77,78] An additional study found that an anatomically superior LAA 'take-off' was associated with higher stroke risk.[76]

The effects of structural remodelling

In summary, the effect of chronic inflammation, and resultant structural and electrical remodelling, increases the risk of thromboembolic events and leads to the development of AF itself. AF is an independent risk factor for thromboembolism due to blood stasis and abnormal blood flow within the LAA—further worsened in those with non-chicken-wing morphology.

This sets the stage for thrombogenesis and thromboembolism, however the story is not yet complete. Beyond the above, abnormalities in clotting mechanisms have been observed in AF. These are described in the next section.

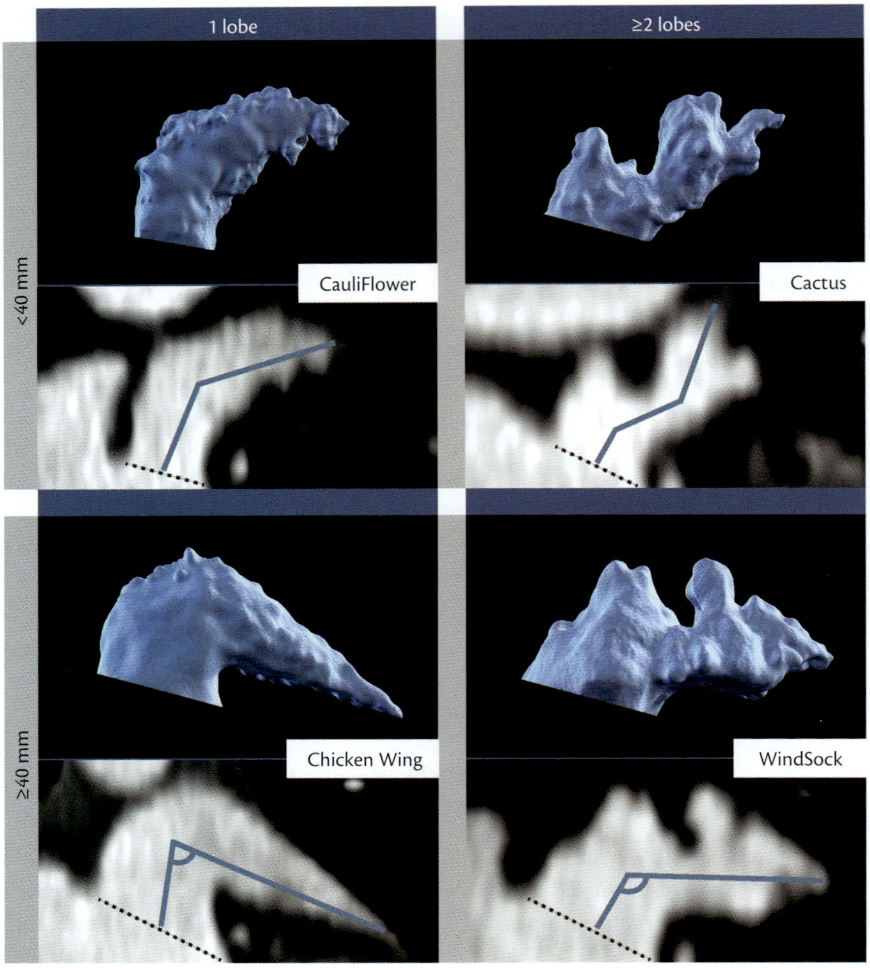

Figure 3.1 Common anatomical morphologies of the LAA.

Reproduced from Korhonen M, Parkkonen J, Hedman M, Muuronen A, Onatsu J, Mustonen P, Vanninen R, Taina M. Morphological features of the left atrial appendage in consecutive coronary computed tomography angiography patients with and without atrial fibrillation. PLoS One. 2017 Mar 13;12(3):e0173703. doi: 10.1371/journal.pone.0173703. https://creativecommons.org/licenses/by/4.0/

Abnormalities of the coagulation system

Enhanced initiation of the coagulation cascade

As described above, inflammation leads to increased levels of factors involved in initiation of the coagulation cascade, such as VWF and TF.

VWF is a crucial component in haemostasis, mediating adhesion at sites of vascular injury and promoting platelet aggregation during high shear stress. Several studies have demonstrated elevated VWF concentrations in AF patients, correlating with an increased risk of LAA thrombus,[79] stroke, and mortality.[80,81] This is strongly supported by meta-analyses.[82,83]

TF is equally important in haemostasis, being a primary initiator of the extrinsic pathway of the coagulation cascade. It is upregulated by inflammation which, as described above, occurs in the atrial endocardium in AF. A histopathological study found significantly elevated endothelial TF—and VWF—in those with cardiogenic thromboembolism.[10] Conversely, another study found that, despite 60% of ischaemic stroke patients having detectable active TF levels at baseline, this was not significant after multivariable adjustment.[84] Another study found that TF levels were elevated only in non-anticoagulated AF patients, which may partly explain this disparity.[85]

Additionally, levels of certain clotting factors (VIIa, XIa, and XIIa) are increased compared with non-AF controls.[4]

Endothelial adhesion molecules are upregulated during inflammation. These molecules are expressed on the surface of endothelial cells and mediate the adhesion of a variety of leucocytes as part of the inflammatory response. This is well recognized in the setting of atherosclerosis, which shares risk factors with AF and equally involves endothelial inflammation. Vascular cell adhesion molecule-1 (VCAM-1) levels have been independently linked to atrial thrombosis.[86,87] Similarly, elevated E-selectin levels have been associated with increased risk of adverse cardiovascular events in patients with AF.[88]

Enhanced platelet activation may be another mechanism of thrombosis in AF. Markers of platelet activation, including P-selectin, β-thromboglobulin, and CD40 ligand, have been studied. While some small studies have found elevated levels of these biomarkers,[85,89,90] larger studies have demonstrated that they are not clinically useful. The overall theme is that enhanced platelet activation probably relates to underlying cardiovascular comorbidities rather than AF, per se[91]; however, they are still likely to contribute to thromboembolic risk.

Abnormal fibrinolysis

Increased thrombosis, mediated by the above mechanisms, results in increased activity of endogenous fibrinolytic systems. Several biomarkers of increased fibrinolysis have been demonstrated in AF, including D-dimer, fibrinogen, soluble fibrin monomer complex, and prothrombin fragments 1 and 2.[36,92,93]

Concentrations of antithrombotic molecules—such as antithrombin III and tissue plasminogen activator (tPA)—also increase, in an attempt to mitigate the increase in thrombosis.[21] Thrombomodulin, which is also increased in AF, binds thrombin. This has two effects, both inhibiting fibrinolysis by activating thrombin-activatable fibrinolysis inhibitor (TAFI), and enhancing anticoagulation by activating protein C (an endogenous anticoagulant).

The balance, unfortunately, remains biased towards thrombosis. This is, in part, due to inhibition of tPA by elevated levels of PAI-1 as described above. Furthermore, while TAFI levels increase,[94] studies have shown that protein C activity—as well as protein S activity—is reduced in AF.[95] The end result is a prolonged clot lysis time.[94]

It should be noted that this is a fairly simplistic overview of a highly complex topic. There are studies with conflicting evidence, and research is ongoing to attempt to fully understand the underlying mechanisms. What appears clear is that fibrinolysis increases due to the prothrombotic state in AF, however such protective systems are not sufficient to mitigate the risk of thromboembolism, as evidenced by clinical outcomes.

Summary

Chronic endothelial inflammation—mostly due to cardiovascular comorbidities—is well observed in the setting of AF. This results in endothelial dysfunction and structural remodelling, which promotes blood stasis. Altered levels of protective factors such as NO and increasing levels of procoagulants such as PAI-1 are compounded by enhanced initiation of the coagulation cascade and platelet activation, coupled with abnormalities in protective fibrinolytic mechanisms. The result is a prothrombotic state, fulfilling all three aspects of Virchow's triad, and resulting in a propensity to thrombosis and thromboembolism in AF (➔ Figure 3.2).

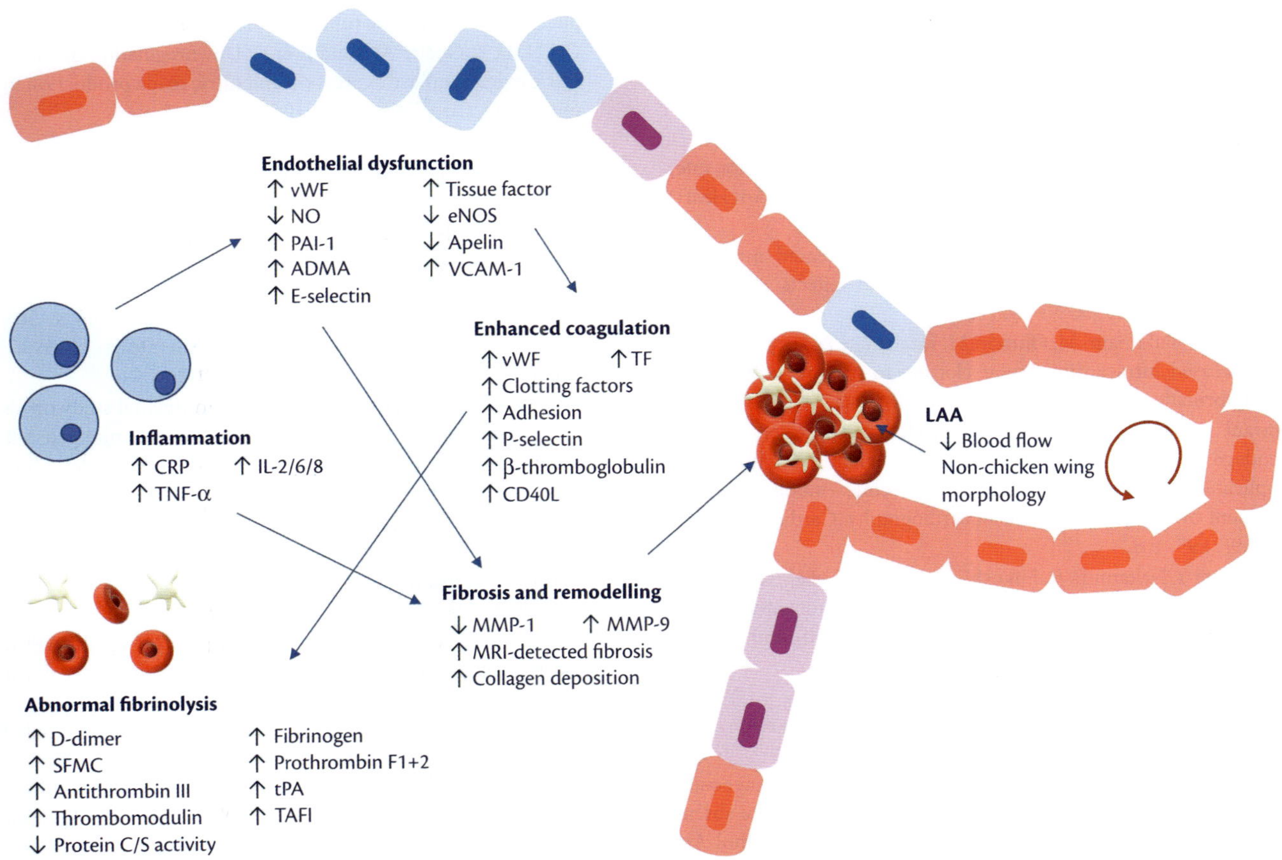

Figure 3.2 Schematic diagram showing the interrelation of factors promoting thrombosis and thromboembolism in atrial fibrillation. ADMA, asymmetric dimethylarginine; CD40L, CD40 ligand; CRP, C-reactive protein; eNOS, endothelial nitric oxide synthase; IL, interleukin; MMP, matrix metalloproteinase; MRI, magnetic resonance imaging; NO, nitric oxide; PAI-1, plasminogen activator inhibitor 1; SFMC, soluble fibrin monomer complex; TAFI, thrombin-activatable fibrinolysis inhibitor; TF, tissue factor; tPA, tissue plasminogen activator; VCAM-1, vascular cell adhesion molecule 1; VWF, von Willebrand factor.

What's new

- Many individual mechanisms underlying thrombosis in AF have been known about for decades—more recently appreciated are the links between these mechanisms.
- Understanding of fibrosis, LA remodelling, and the flow dynamics of the LAA has evolved in recent years.
- Increasing numbers of biomarkers associated with inflammation, endothelial dysfunction, and hypercoagulability in AF are being recognized.

What's next

- Research into new drug targets for thromboembolic protection.
- Research into potential drug targets for reducing endothelial injury and LA cardiopathy.

References

1. Lloyd-Jones DM, Wang TJ, Leip EP, et al. Lifetime risk for development of atrial fibrillation. Circulation. 2004;110(9):1042–6.
2. Heeringa J, van der Kuip DAM, Hofman A, et al. Prevalence, incidence and lifetime risk of atrial fibrillation: the Rotterdam study. Eur Heart J. 2006;27(8):949–53.
3. Wolf PA, Abbott RD, Kannel WB. Atrial fibrillation as an independent risk factor for stroke: the Framingham Study. Stroke. 1991;22(8):983–8.
4. Negreva M, Zarkova A, Prodanova K, Petrov P. Paroxysmal atrial fibrillation: insight into the intimate mechanisms of coagulation. Cardiol Res. 2020;11(1):22–32.
5. Sohara H, Amitani S, Kurose M, Miyahara K. Atrial fibrillation activates platelets and coagulation in a time-dependent manner: a study in patients with paroxysmal atrial fibrillation. J Am Coll Cardiol. 1997;29(1):106–12.
6. Lip GYH, Lowe GDO, Rumley A, Dunn FG. Fibrinogen and fibrin D-dimer levels in paroxysmal atrial fibrillation: evidence for intermediate elevated levels of intravascular thrombogenesis. Am Heart J. 1996;131(4):724–30.
7. Lip GY, Lowe GD, Rumley A, Dunn FG. Increased markers of thrombogenesis in chronic atrial fibrillation: effects of warfarin treatment. Heart. 1995;73(6):527–33.
8. Kumagai K, Fukunami M, Ohmori M, Kitabatake A, Kamada T, Hoki N. Increased intracardiovascular clotting in patients with chronic atrial fibrillation. J Am Coll Cardiol. 1990;16(2):377–80.
9. Shirani J, Alaeddini J. Structural remodeling of the left atrial appendage in patients with chronic non-valvular atrial fibrillation: implications for thrombus formation, systemic embolism, and assessment by transesophageal echocardiography. Cardiovasc Pathol. 2000;9(2):95–101.
10. Nakamura Y, Nakamura K, Fukushima-Kusano K, et al. Tissue factor expression in atrial endothelia associated with nonvalvular atrial fibrillation: possible involvement in intracardiac thrombogenesis. Thromb Res. 2003;111(3):137–42.
11. Goldsmith I, Kumar P, Carter P, Blann AD, Patel RL, Lip GY. Atrial endocardial changes in mitral valve disease: a scanning electron microscopy study. Am Heart J. 2000;140(5):777–84.
12. Masawa N, Yoshida Y, Yamada T, Joshita T, Ooneda G. Diagnosis of cardiac thrombosis in patients with atrial fibrillation in the absence of macroscopically visible thrombi. Virchows Arch A Pathol Anat Histopathol. 1993;422(1):67–71.
13. Frustaci A, Chimenti C, Bellocci F, Morgante E, Russo MA, Maseri A. Histological substrate of atrial biopsies in patients with lone atrial fibrillation. Circulation. 1997;96(4):1180–4.
14. Guo Y, Lip GYH, Apostolakis S. Inflammation in atrial fibrillation. J Am Coll Cardiol. 2012;60(22):2263–70.
15. Conway DSG, Buggins P, Hughes E, Lip GYH. Relation of interleukin-6, C-reactive protein, and the prothrombotic state to transesophageal echocardiographic findings in atrial fibrillation. Am J Cardiol. 2004;93(11):1368–73.
16. Conway DSG, Buggins P, Hughes E, Lip GYH. Relationship of interleukin-6 and C-Reactive protein to the prothrombotic state in chronic atrial fibrillation. J Am Coll Cardiol. 2004;43(11):2075–82.
17. Burstein SA, Peng J, Friese P, et al. Cytokine-induced alteration of platelet and hemostatic function. Stem Cells. 1996;14(S1):154–62.
18. Cai H, Li Z, Goette A, Mera F, et al. Downregulation of endocardial nitric oxide synthase expression and nitric oxide production in atrial fibrillation. Circulation. 2002;106(22):2854–8.
19. Minamino T, Kitakaze M, Sato H, et al. Plasma levels of nitrite/nitrate and platelet cGMP levels are decreased in patients with atrial fibrillation. Arterioscler Thromb Vasc Biol. 1997;17(11):3191–5.
20. Jabati S, Fareed J, Liles J, et al. Biomarkers of inflammation, thrombogenesis, and collagen turnover in patients with atrial fibrillation. Clin Appl Thromb Hemost. 2018;24(5):718–23.
21. Roldán V, Marín F, Marco P, Martínez JG, Calatayud R, Sogorb F. Hypofibrinolysis in atrial fibrillation. Am Heart J. 1998;136(6):956–60.
22. Han W, Li WM, Song LY, et al. [The experimental study on changes of endothelial nitric oxide synthase and plasminogen activator inhibitor-1 protein in the canine atrial fibrillation model]. Zhonghua Xin Xue Guan Bing Za Zhi. 2005;33(1):69–72.
23. Siddiquee K, Hampton J, Khan S, et al. Apelin protects against angiotensin II-induced cardiovascular fibrosis and decreases plasminogen activator inhibitor type-1 production. J Hypertens. 2011;29(4):724–31.
24. Cheng H, Chen Y, Li X, et al. Involvement of apelin/APJ axis in thrombogenesis in valve heart disease patients with atrial fibrillation. Int Heart J. 2019;60(1):145–50.
25. Ramuschkat M, Appelbaum S, Atzler D, et al. ADMA, subclinical changes and atrial fibrillation in the general population. Int J Cardiol. 2016;203:640–6.
26. Cengel A, Sahinarslan A, Biberoğlu G, et al. Asymmetrical dimethylarginine level in atrial fibrillation. Acta Cardiol. 2008;63(1):33–7.
27. Goette A, Hammwöhner M, Bukowska A, et al. The impact of rapid atrial pacing on ADMA and endothelial NOS. Int J Cardiol. 2012;154(2):141–6.

28. Lim HS, Willoughby SR, Schultz C, et al. Thrombogenic risk in patients with atrial fibrillation. JACC Clin Electrophysiol. 2015;1(3):210–7.
29. Leone A, Moncada S, Vallance P, Calver A, Collier J. Accumulation of an endogenous inhibitor of nitric oxide synthesis in chronic renal failure. Lancet. 1992;339(8793):572–5.
30. Böger RH. Association of asymmetric dimethylarginine and endothelial dysfunction. Clin Chem Lab Med. 2003;41(11):1467–72.
31. Xia W, Wang Y, Duan T, Rong Y, Chi Y, Shao Y. Asymmetric dimethylarginine predicts left atrial appendage thrombus in patients with non-valvular atrial fibrillation. Thromb Res. 2015;136(6):1156–9.
32. Horowitz JD, de Caterina R, Heresztyn T, et al. Asymmetric and symmetric dimethylarginine predict outcomes in patients with atrial fibrillation. J Am Coll Cardiol. 2018;72(7):721–33.
33. Benito EM, Cabanelas N, Nuñez-Garcia M, et al. Preferential regional distribution of atrial fibrosis in posterior wall around left inferior pulmonary vein as identified by late gadolinium enhancement cardiac magnetic resonance in patients with atrial fibrillation. Europace. 2018;20(12):1959–65.
34. Lee DK, Shim J, Choi JI, Kim YH, Oh YW, Hwang SH. Left atrial fibrosis assessed with cardiac MRI in patients with paroxysmal and those with persistent atrial fibrillation. Radiology. 2019;292(3):575–82.
35. Klein T, Bischoff R. Physiology and pathophysiology of matrix metalloproteases. Amino Acids. 2011;41(2):271–90.
36. Marîn F, Roldán V, Climent V, Garcîa A, Marco P, Lip GYH. Is thrombogenesis in atrial fibrillation related to matrix metalloproteinase-1 and its inhibitor, TIMP-1? Stroke. 2003;34(5):1181–6.
37. Liu Y, Xu B, Wu N, et al. Association of MMPs and TIMPs with the occurrence of atrial fibrillation: a systematic review and meta-analysis. Can J Cardiol. 2016;32(6):803–13.
38. Nakano Y, Niida S, Dote K, et al. Matrix metalloproteinase-9 contributes to human atrial remodeling during atrial fibrillation. J Am Coll Cardiol. 2004;43(5):818–25.
39. Li M, Yang G, Xie B, Babu K, Huang C. Changes in matrix metalloproteinase-9 levels during progression of atrial fibrillation. J Int Med Res. 2013;42(1):224–30.
40. Lewkowicz J, Knapp M, Tankiewicz-Kwedlo A, et al. MMP-9 in atrial remodeling in patients with atrial fibrillation. Ann Cardiol Angeiol (Paris). 2015;64(4):285–91.
41. Zabalgoitia M, Halperin JL, Pearce LA, Blackshear JL, Asinger RW, Hart RG. Transesophageal echocardiographic correlates of clinical risk of thromboembolism in nonvalvular atrial fibrillation. Stroke Prevention in Atrial Fibrillation III Investigators. J Am Coll Cardiol. 1998;31(7):1622–6.
42. Leung DY, Black IW, Cranney GB, Hopkins AP, Walsh WF. Prognostic implications of left atrial spontaneous echo contrast in nonvalvular atrial fibrillation. J Am Coll Cardiol. 1994;24(3):755–62.
43. Akoum N, Fernandez G, Wilson B, Mcgann C, Kholmovski E, Marrouche N. Association of atrial fibrosis quantified using LGE-MRI with atrial appendage thrombus and spontaneous contrast on transesophageal echocardiography in patients with atrial fibrillation. J Cardiovasc Electrophysiol. 2013;24(10):1104–9.
44. Miyauchi S, Tokuyama T, Uotani Y, et al. Association between left atrial appendage fibrosis and thrombus formation: a histological approach. J Cardiovasc Electrophysiol. 2022;33(4):677–87.
45. Boldt A, Wetzel U, Lauschke J, et al. Fibrosis in left atrial tissue of patients with atrial fibrillation with and without underlying mitral valve disease. Heart. 2004;90(4):400–5.
46. Corradi D, Callegari S, Maestri R, et al. Differential structural remodeling of the left-atrial posterior wall in patients affected by mitral regurgitation with or without persistent atrial fibrillation: a morphological and molecular study. J Cardiovasc Electrophysiol. 2012;23(3):271–9.
47. Mitrofanova LB, Orshanskaya V, Ho SY, Platonov PG. Histological evidence of inflammatory reaction associated with fibrosis in the atrial and ventricular walls in a case-control study of patients with history of atrial fibrillation. Europace. 2016;18(Suppl 4):iv156–62.
48. Smorodinova N, Lantová L, Bláha M, et al. Bioptic study of left and right atrial interstitium in cardiac patients with and without atrial fibrillation: interatrial but not rhythm-based differences. PLoS One. 2015;10(6):e0129124.
49. Sanfilippo AJ, Abascal VM, Sheehan M, et al. Atrial enlargement as a consequence of atrial fibrillation. A prospective echocardiographic study. Circulation. 1990;82(3):792–7.
50. Gupta DK, Shah AM, Giugliano RP, et al. Left atrial structure and function in atrial fibrillation: ENGAGE AF-TIMI 48. Eur Heart J. 2014;35(22):1457–65.
51. Hamatani Y, Ogawa H, Takabayashi K, et al. Left atrial enlargement is an independent predictor of stroke and systemic embolism in patients with non-valvular atrial fibrillation. Sci Rep. 2016;6:31042.
52. Vincelj J, Sokol I, Jaksić O. Prevalence and clinical significance of left atrial spontaneous echo contrast detected by transesophageal echocardiography. Echocardiography. 2002;19(4):319–24.
53. Predictors of thromboembolism in atrial fibrillation: II. Echocardiographic features of patients at risk. The Stroke Prevention in Atrial Fibrillation Investigators. Ann Intern Med. 1992;116(1):6–12.
54. di Tullio MR, Sacco RL, Sciacca RR, Homma S. Left atrial size and the risk of ischemic stroke in an ethnically mixed population. Stroke. 1999;30(10):2019–24.
55. Dakay K, Chang AD, Hemendinger M, et al. Left atrial enlargement and anticoagulation status in patients with acute ischemic stroke and atrial fibrillation. J Stroke Cerebrovasc Dis. 2018;27(1):192–7.
56. Blackshear JL, Odell JA. Appendage obliteration to reduce stroke in cardiac surgical patients with atrial fibrillation. Ann Thorac Surg. 1996;61(2):755–9.
57. Stoddard MF, Dawkins PR, Prince CR, Ammash NM. Left atrial appendage thrombus is not uncommon in patients with acute atrial fibrillation and a recent embolic event: a transesophageal echocardiographic study. J Am Coll Cardiol. 1995;25(2):452–9.
58. Chen L, Xu C, Chen W, Zhang C. Left atrial appendage orifice area and morphology is closely associated with flow velocity in patients with nonvalvular atrial fibrillation. BMC Cardiovasc Disord. 2021;21(1):442.
59. Miki Y, Uchida Y, Tanaka A, et al. Clinical significance of the left atrial appendage orifice area. Intern Med. 2022;61(12):1801–7.
60. Kong B, Liu Y, Hu H, et al. Left atrial appendage morphology in patients with atrial fibrillation in China: implications for stroke risk assessment from a single center study. Chin Med J (Engl). 2014;127(24):4210–4.
61. Khurram IM, Dewire J, Mager M, et al. Relationship between left atrial appendage morphology and stroke in patients with atrial fibrillation. Heart Rhythm. 2013;10(12):1843–9.
62. Sahin T, Ural D, Kilic T, et al. Evaluation of left atrial appendage functions according to different etiologies of atrial fibrillation with a tissue Doppler imaging technique by using transesophageal echocardiography. Echocardiography. 2009;26(2):171–81.
63. Li YH, Lai LP, Shyu KG, et al. Clinical implications of left atrial appendage function: its influence on thrombus formation. Int J Cardiol. 1994;43(1):61–6.
64. García-Fernández MA, Torrecilla EG, San Román D, et al. Left atrial appendage Doppler flow patterns: implications on thrombus formation. Am Heart J. 1992;124(4):955–61.

65. Mügge A, Kühn H, Nikutta P, Grote J, Lopez JA, Daniel WG. Assessment of left atrial appendage function by biplane transesophageal echocardiography in patients with nonrheumatic atrial fibrillation: identification of a subgroup of patients at increased embolic risk. J Am Coll Cardiol. 1994;23(3):599–607.
66. Ito T, Suwa M, Otake Y, et al. Assessment of left atrial appendage function after cardioversion of atrial fibrillation: relation to left atrial mechanical function. Am Heart J. 1998;135(6 Pt 1):1020–6.
67. Mazzone C, Pandullo C, Scardi S, et al. Left atrial and appendage mechanical function after pharmacological or electrical cardioversion in patients with chronic atrial fibrillation: a multicenter, randomized study. Ital Heart J. 2000;1(2):128–36.
68. McIntyre WF, Connolly SJ, Wang J, et al. Thromboembolic events around the time of cardioversion for atrial fibrillation in patients receiving antiplatelet treatment in the ACTIVE trials. Eur Heart J. 2019;40(36):3026–32.
69. Harada M, Tabako S, Fujii Y, et al. Correlation between plasma brain natriuretic peptide levels and left atrial appendage flow velocity in patients with non-valvular atrial fibrillation and normal left ventricular systolic function. J Echocardiogr. 2018;16(2):72–80.
70. Tabata T, Oki T, Fukuda N, et al. Influence of left atrial pressure on left atrial appendage flow velocity patterns in patients in sinus rhythm. J Am Soc Echocardiogr. 1996;9(6):857–64.
71. Kang SH, Kim J, Park JJ, et al. Risk of stroke in congestive heart failure with and without atrial fibrillation. Int J Cardiol. 2017;248:182–7.
72. di Biase L, Santangeli P, Anselmino M, et al. Does the left atrial appendage morphology correlate with the risk of stroke in patients with atrial fibrillation? Results from a multicenter study. J Am Coll Cardiol. 2012;60(6):531–8.
73. Fukushima K, Fukushima N, Kato K, et al. Correlation between left atrial appendage morphology and flow velocity in patients with paroxysmal atrial fibrillation. Eur Heart J Cardiovasc Imaging. 2016;17(1):59–66.
74. Lee Y, Park HC, Lee Y, Kim SG. Comparison of morphologic features and flow velocity of the left atrial appendage among patients with atrial fibrillation alone, transient ischemic attack, and cardioembolic stroke. Am J Cardiol. 2017;119(10):1596–604.
75. Kimura T, Takatsuki S, Inagawa K, et al. Anatomical characteristics of the left atrial appendage in cardiogenic stroke with low CHADS2 scores. Heart Rhythm. 2013;10(6):921–5.
76. Nedios S, Koutalas E, Kornej J, et al. Cardiogenic stroke despite low CHA2 DS2 -VASc score: assessing stroke risk by left atrial appendage anatomy (ASK LAA). J Cardiovasc Electrophysiol. 2015;26(9):915–21.
77. Lupercio F, Carlos Ruiz J, Briceno DF, et al. Left atrial appendage morphology assessment for risk stratification of embolic stroke in patients with atrial fibrillation: a meta-analysis. Heart Rhythm. 2016;13(7):1402–9.
78. Anan AR, Fareed J, Suhaib J, et al. Left atrial appendage morphology as a determinant for stroke risk assessment in atrial fibrillation patients: systematic review and meta-analysis. J Atr Fibrillation. 2019;12(2):2183.
79. Heppell RM, Berkin KE, McLenachan JM, Davies JA. Haemostatic and haemodynamic abnormalities associated with left atrial thrombosis in non-rheumatic atrial fibrillation. Heart. 1997;77(5):407–11.
80. Ancedy Y, Berthelot E, Lang S, et al. Is von Willebrand factor associated with stroke and death at mid-term in patients with non-valvular atrial fibrillation? Arch Cardiovasc Dis. 2018;111(5):357–69.
81. García-Fernández A, Roldán V, Rivera-Caravaca JM, et al. Does von Willebrand factor improve the predictive ability of current risk stratification scores in patients with atrial fibrillation? Sci Rep. 2017;7(1):41565.
82. Zhong C, Xin M, He L, Sun G, Shen F. Prognostic value of von Willebrand factor in patients with atrial fibrillation. Medicine. 2018;97(27):e11269.
83. Ye YZ, Chang YF, Wang BZ, Ma YT, Ma X. Prognostic value of von Willebrand factor for patients with atrial fibrillation: a meta-analysis of prospective cohort studies. Postgrad Med J. 2020;96(1135):267–76.
84. Ząbczyk MT, Hanarz M, Malinowski KP, et al. Active FXI can independently predict ischemic stroke in anticoagulated atrial fibrillation patients: a cohort study. Thromb Haemost. 2022;122(8):1397–406.
85. Choudhury A, Freestone B, Patel J, Lip GYH. Relationship of soluble CD40 ligand to vascular endothelial growth factor, angiopoietins, and tissue factor in atrial fibrillation. Chest. 2007;132(6): 1913–9.
86. Hammwöhner M, Ittenson A, Dierkes J, et al. Platelet expression of CD40/CD40 ligand and its relation to inflammatory markers and adhesion molecules in patients with atrial fibrillation. Exp Biol Med (Maywood). 2007;232(4):581–9.
87. Katoh S, Honda S, Watanabe T, et al. Atrial endothelial impairment through Toll-like receptor 4 signaling causes atrial thrombogenesis. Heart Vessels. 2014;29(2):263–72.
88. Krishnamoorthy S, Khoo CW, Lim HS, et al. Prognostic role of plasma von Willebrand factor and soluble E-selectin levels for future cardiovascular events in a 'real-world' community cohort of patients with atrial fibrillation. Eur J Clin Invest. 2013;43(10):1032–8.
89. Choudhury A, Chung I, Blann AD, Lip GYH. Elevated platelet microparticle levels in nonvalvular atrial fibrillation. Chest. 2007;131(3):809–15.
90. Minamino T, Kitakaze M, Asanuma H, et al. Plasma adenosine levels and platelet activation in patients with atrial fibrillation. Am J Cardiol. 1999;83(2):194–8.
91. Feinberg WM, Pearce LA, Hart RG, et al. Markers of thrombin and platelet activity in patients with atrial fibrillation: correlation with stroke among 1531 participants in the stroke prevention in atrial fibrillation III study. Stroke. 1999;30(12):2547–53.
92. Rivera-Caravaca JM, Roldán V, Romera M, et al. Soluble fibrin monomer complex and prediction of cardiovascular events in atrial fibrillation: the Observational Murcia Atrial Fibrillation Project. J Gen Intern Med. 2018;33(6):847–54.
93. Weymann A, Sabashnikov A, Ali-Hasan-Al-Saegh S, et al. Predictive role of coagulation, fibrinolytic, and endothelial markers in patients with atrial fibrillation, stroke, and thromboembolism: a meta-analysis, meta-regression, and systematic review. Med Sci Monit Basic Res. 2017;23:97–140.
94. Ząbczyk M, Majewski J, Lelakowski J. Thromboembolic events are associated with prolonged clot lysis time in patients with permanent atrial fibrillation. Pol Arch Med Wewn. 2011;121(11):400–7.
95. Negreva M, Georgiev S, Vitlianova K. Decreased activity of the protein C anticoagulant pathway in the early hours of paroxysmal atrial fibrillation. Clin Appl Thromb Hemost. 2017;23(7):793–9.
96. Korhonen M, Parkkonen J, Hedman M, et al. Morphological features of the left atrial appendage in consecutive coronary computed tomography angiography patients with and without atrial fibrillation. PLoS One. 2017;12(3):e0173703.

CHAPTER 4

Thrombosis on foreign surfaces and devices

Tobias Geisler

Contents

Summary

Thrombosis on artificial surfaces is a crucial condition and dependent on the material properties of the device and patient adherent factors. This chapter discusses the pathophysiology of device-related thrombosis and gives an overview of the clinical relevance and diagnostic and treatment algorithms.

Pathophysiology of device-related thrombosis and strategies against it

Surfaces on devices can activate the coagulation system by enhanced adsorption of proteins, adhesion of platelets, leucocytes, and red blood cells, activation of the extrinsic coagulation cascade leading to thrombin generation, and activation of the complement system. Similar to physiological conditions, thrombotic alterations on foreign material rely on Virchow's triad. Low-flow conditions (*stasis*) can induce a prothrombotic situation with activation of coagulation factors, *endothelial dysfunction* by reactive injury and cellular interactions with the device, and device-related thrombogenicity. These factors and patient comorbidities lead to *hypercoagulability*. The surface of cardiac implants provides a prothrombotic environment. Depending on the device material and on the location of the implant, development of device-related thrombosis (DRT) and its timely occurrence is variable. The cardiac conditions can promote the development of DRT, for example, due to impaired circulation and stasis in association with heart failure. The negatively charged hydrophilic surface of devices can cause protein adsorption independently from flow velocity.[1,2] As a consequence of fibrinogen, fibronectin, and von Willebrand factor (VWF) adhesion to the surface of foreign material, platelets can adhere and are activated. Factor (F)-XII activation to FXIIa is promoted by negatively charged surfaces and polyphosphates, thus initiating the intrinsic pathway (➔ Figure 4.1).[1,2] FXIIa leads to subsequent activation of FXI, FIX, FX, and prothrombin. In addition, factor XIIa triggers complement activation to promote thrombin amplification. Previous studies have shown in contact phase-initiated thrombosis animal models (e.g. catheter-induced thrombosis and cardiopulmonary bypass) that inhibiting FXIa/FXIIa (e.g. by Ixodes ricinus contact phase inhibitor) effectively attenuates thrombosis on foreign surfaces without promoting bleeding.[3,4] Adhesion of leucocytes including neutrophils mainly to fibrinogen immobilized on the device surface via CD11b/CD18 [macrophage-1 antigen 1 (MAC-1)] is a further critical step to foster a thromboinflammatory milieu. Platelets can interact with leucocytes mainly via cross-linking of P-selectin with P-selectin glycoprotein

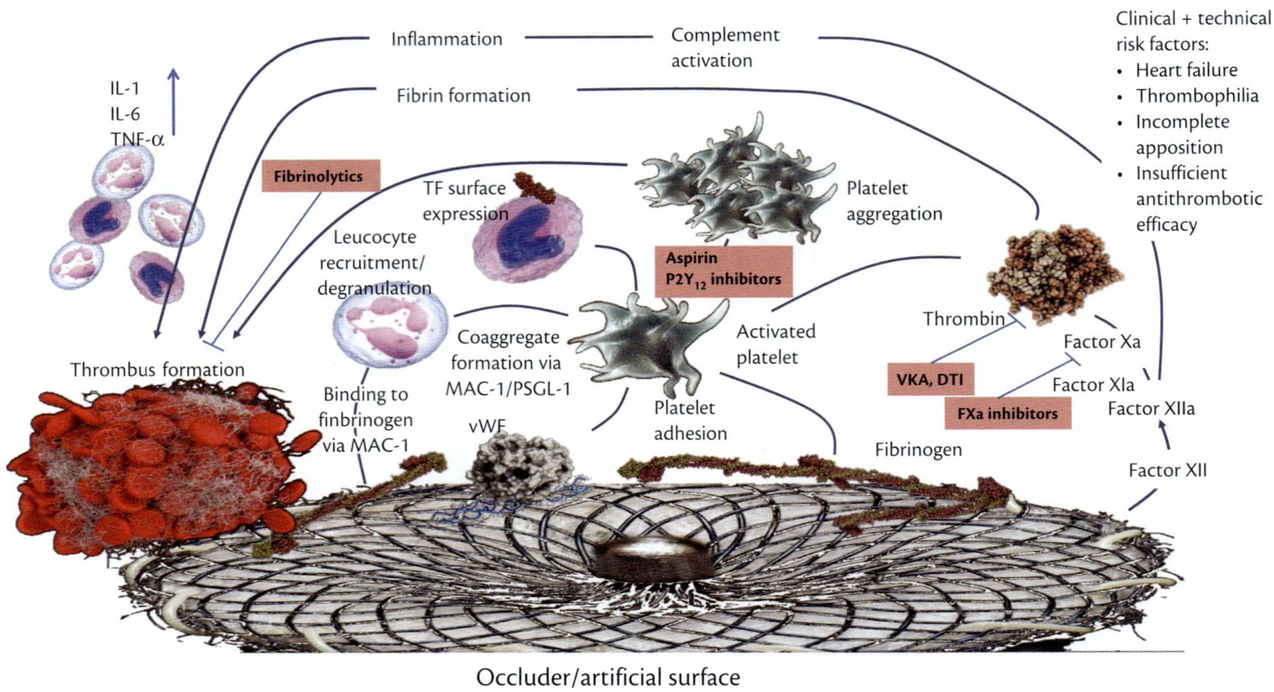

Figure 4.1 Pathophysiology of thrombus formation on an artificial surface leading to device thrombosis.
Source data from Geisler T, Jorbenadze R, Popov AF, et al. Thrombogenicity and antithrombotic strategies in structural heart interventions and nonaortic cardiac device therapy—current evidence and practice. Thromb Haemost. 2019;119(10):1590–605. doi: 10.1055/s-0039-1694751.

ligand-1 (PSGL-1) and MAC-1 with glycoprotein 1b-α (GP1bα) thus forming platelet–leucocyte aggregates. Leucocyte degranulation further maintains a prothrombotic and proinflammatory milieu by generating free radicals, releasing cytokines [e.g. interleukin (IL)-1 and IL6 and tumour necrosis factor-α (TNF-α)], and activating monocytes, causing tissue factor expression and consequent initiation of the coagulation cascade. Modification of the surface of foreign materials aims at reducing blood–biomaterial surface interaction. This can be achieved by modifications of hydrophilic characteristics of the polymer surface or by mimicking the endothelium and increasing the haemocompatibility. Electrostatic and hydrophobic interactions leading to protein surface interactions have been hampered by synthetic and natural materials including polyethylene oxide, phosphorylcholine, pyrolytic carbon, albumin, and elastin-inspired protein polymers.[1] In addition, attempts have been made to immobilize anticoagulants like heparin[5] or thrombomodulin[6] and to alter the surface chemistry and/or morphology[7,8] as well as to achieve active release of antithrombotic compounds from the device surface (e.g. heparin, nitric oxide, and direct thrombin inhibitors).[9–11]

Clinical aspects of device-related thrombosis in specific conditions

Left atrial appendage occluder

The location of the left atrial appendage (LAA) is particularly thrombogenic due to impaired flow condition in association with atrial fibrillation (AF), atriopathy, and heart failure. There is a large variety of available closure device systems (➔ Figure 4.2); however, the most frequently used devices with the largest body of evidence from clinical trials and post-marketing registries include the Watchman/Watchman FLX™, the Amplatzer Cardiac Plug™, and the second-generation Amplatzer Amulet™ left atrial appendage occluder (LAAO). The Watchman/Watchman FLX device consists of a self-expanding nitinol frame with fixation barbs and a permeable polyester fabric cover. The Amplatzer Amulet occluder is composed of nitinol wire mesh and a polyester patch and consists of a lobe and a disc connected by a central waist. Thrombosis on LAA closure devices has been reported in up to 17%.[12] In a pooled analysis of available trials and registries the incidence of DRT was reported at 3.7% for the Watchman and was associated with a higher rate of stroke and systemic embolism.[13] In a randomized controlled trial (Amulet IDE) comparing both devices, the incidence of DRT was 3.3% with the Amplatzer Amulet LAAO compared to 4.5% with the Watchman device at 18 months.[14] Possible risk factors for DRT include device type or positioning, LAA anatomy, postprocedural antithrombotic regimen, and clinical risk factors. Older age and a history of stroke were identified as predictors of DRT in a recent registry, whereas effective antithrombotic therapy [either dual antiplatelet or oral anticoagulation (OAC)] at discharge were protective against it. Importantly, DRT was independently associated with ischaemic strokes and transient ischaemic attacks at follow-up.[15] Suboptimal LAAO was proposed as the main factor for thrombus formation.[16] Specifically for the Amplatzer Amulet LAAO, incomplete coverage of the limbus by the Amulet disc, a lower left ventricular ejection fraction, larger left atrial diameter, greater spontaneous echocardiogram contrast, and lower peak

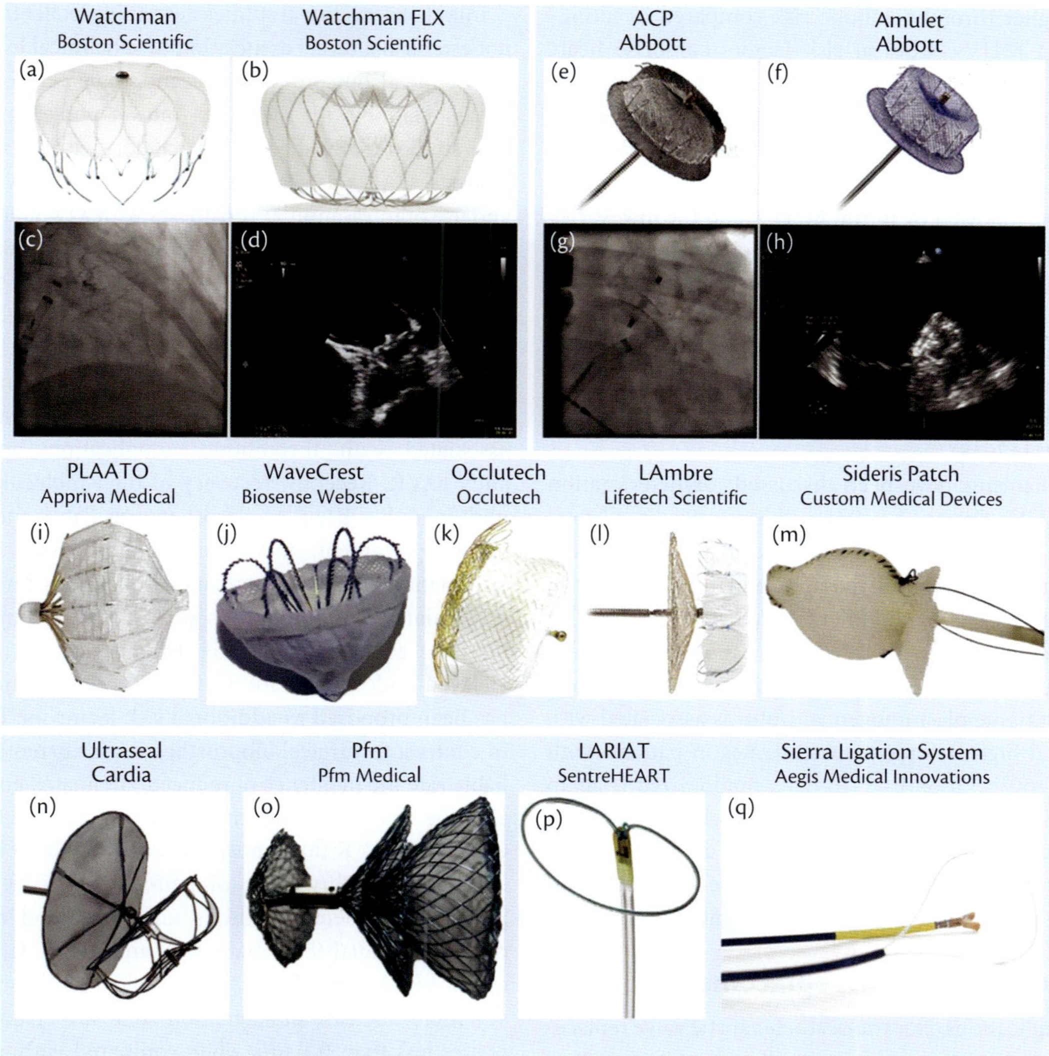

Figure 4.2 Percutaneous LAAO devices. The Watchman™ and Watchman FLX™ devices (a, b). Fluoroscopic and echocardiographic images of the Watchman™ device (c, d). Amplatzer Cardiac Plug™ (ACP) and Amplatzer Amulet™ (e, f). Fluoroscopic and echocardiographic views of the ACP device (g, h). PLAATO™ device (i). WaveCrest™ LAAO device (j). Occlutech™ LAA occluder (k). LAmbre™ LAA closure system (l). Sideris™ transcatheter patch (m). Ultraseal™ LAAO device (n). Pfm™ device (o). Lariat™ device (p). Sierra™ ligation system (q).

Reproduced from Asmarats L, Rodés-Cabau J. Percutaneous Left Atrial Appendage Closure: Current Devices and Clinical Outcomes. Circ Cardiovasc Interv. 2017 Nov;10(11):e005359. doi: 10.1161/CIRCINTERVENTIONS.117.005359 with permission from Wolters Kluwer.

LAA emptying velocity have been identified as predictors of DRT in a case–control study.[16] In addition, higher AF burden is a potential risk factor for LAAO DRT.[13] The role of on-treatment platelet reactivity is uncertain. Clopidogrel non-responsiveness measured by platelet function testing was higher in patients experiencing DRT in one study[17] whereas there was no association of high on-treatment platelet reactivity with DRT but low on-treatment platelet reactivity with bleeding events in another observational study.[18] A recent echocardiographic study found that thrombi were predominantly observed within the untrabeculated region of the LAA ostium between the left upper pulmonary vein ridge and the occluder disc. Other locations of the thrombus included the occluder disc of the Amplatzer occluder or the polyethylene terephthalate fabric of the Watchman device.[19] The observed incidence of LAAO DRT is dependent on the imaging modality and duration of follow-up. In a computed tomography (CT) study including 117 patients with both Watchman and Amplatzer (Cardiac Plug and Amulet) devices, the DRT prevalence was reported at 16% at 3 months after implantation.[20] In a recent systematic registry differentiating between time occurrence of DRT, early (within 1.5 months), late (between 1.5 and 6 months), and very late (between 6 and 12 months) LAAO thrombosis occurred in 28.6%, 28.6% and 42.9% of the cases, respectively.[21] Of note, not the duration of dual antiplatelet therapy but rather patient-related risk factors were associated with the incidence of DRT.

Mechanical valves

Prosthetic valve thrombosis (PVT) is associated with a high mortality. Ineffective anticoagulation is one of the major drivers for PVT of mechanical heart valves (MHVs). The risk of long-term thromboembolic events is almost twice as high with MHVs in mitral compared to aortic position prostheses.[22,23] Cage-ball MHVs carry a much higher thromboembolic risk compared to tilting-disc and bileaflet MHVs. Clinical risk factors comprise heart failure with left ventricular ejection fraction of less than 35%, AF, older age, coagulation disorders, and a history of thromboembolic events.[24] Thromboembolic risk is also dependent on prosthesis type and location. The thromboembolic risk is highest for double MHVs, followed by mitral MHVs, and the lowest risk occurs with aortic MHVs.[25,26] Newer-generation pyrolytic carbon aortic heart valves (On-X®; Artivion, formerly CryoLife) have been approved by the US Food and Drug Administration for a reduced target international normalized ratio of 1.5–2. Currently, the efficacy of safety of apixaban versus warfarin is being investigated in a randomized trial (PROACT Xa; ClinicalTrials.gov Identifier: NCT04142658).[27]

Different mechanisms have been discussed for deterioration of function of MHVs. Pannus formation characterized as fibrotic tissue growing around artificial valves, usually in an annular location, as a consequence of local inflammation and impaired haemostasis after surgery needs to be differentiated from sole PVT.[28] Thrombolytic therapy and surgery are both possible management strategies of PVT. A recent observational study suggests that low-dose infusions of tissue plasminogen activator is associated with low mortality and high treatment success rates in patients with obstructive PVT over 3 months.[29] To date, randomized trials to compare fibrinolysis and surgical therapy are lacking. Surgery is still the first-line option in patients with PVT and cardiogenic shock, extensive pannus formation as the cause of thrombosis, and in patients with contraindication(s) to thrombolysis.

Transcatheter aortic valve replacement

Thrombotic complications after transcatheter aortic valve replacement (TAVR) including stroke are potentially devastating and associated with high morbidity and mortality. There is increasing recognition of TAVR thrombosis that might be associated with thrombotic complications and early valve degeneration. Clinically manifest TAVR thrombosis is rare (0.6–2.8%)[30,31] and can usually be detected by echocardiography. Patients may suffer from progressive symptoms of heart failure (progressive dyspnoea, peripheral oedema) or arterial embolization (i.e. stroke, acute limb ischaemia, acute mesenteric ischaemia, and acute ischaemic kidney injury). Subclinical TAVR thrombosis is typically detected by four-dimensional multidetector CT and is characterized by reduced leaflet mobility (➔ Figure 4.3a). Substantial increases in gradient are indicators and should lead to a further workup using transoesophageal echocardiography imaging and CT imaging (➔ Figure 4.3b). Based on the CT findings, two phenomena have been described: (1) hypoattenuated leaflet thickening (HALT) referring to enhanced opacity with hypoattenuation at the base of valve leaflets and (2) hypoattenuation affecting motion (HAM) referring to a reduction of leaflet motion related to HALT (➔ Figure 4.3a). Of note, it is challenging to differentiate subclinical valve thrombosis from other causes of prosthesis leaflet dysfunction including structural (e.g. calcification) and non-structural valve deterioration (e.g. prothesis malposition or prosthesis–patient mismatch) and endocarditis.[32,33]

Initial observational studies describing leaflet thrombosis could not establish a direct association of subclinical leaflet thrombosis with clinical outcomes.[34] A recent single-centre study reported an association with mortality[35] and a pooled analysis of available studies established an association with stroke. In the latter analysis, OAC was associated with a 58% relative risk reduction and use of intra-annular prostheses with a twofold greater risk for subclinical leaflet thrombosis.[36] Of note, the occurrence of HALT is very dynamic with 50% of patients showing spontaneous regression in up to 1 year, and new incidence in about 20% of patients at 1 year among patients with no prior HALT.[37,38]

Clinical factors including older age, left ventricular failure, severe aortic calcification, chronic kidney disease, and AF are associated with thrombotic complications including stroke after TAVR. Recently, recovery of high-molecular-weight VWF multimers has been reported between day 8 and 22 post aortic valve replacement, and patients characterized in a VWF predominant state showed enhanced thrombus formation.[39] High-molecular-weight multimers of VWF contributed not only to bleeding events but also to thrombotic events after TAVR.[40] Delayed endothelialization of the TAVR prosthesis stent frame has been proposed as additional risk factor for TAVR. However, in contrast to surgical bioprostheses it is currently difficult to reliably rate the incidence of reduced/attenuated endothelialization and the diagnostic algorithms are uncertain. Procedural predictors of TAVR thrombosis included height of annular deployment and width/volume of neo-sinuses, valve-in-valve (ViV) procedures/patient–prosthesis mismatch, and reduced cardiac output.[33] By analysing anatomical and TAVR deployment geometries, supra-annular prosthesis deployment resulted in a nearly sevenfold decrease in stagnation zone size characterized by velocities less than 0.1 m/s when compared with an intra-annular deployment.[41] For ViV procedures, the risk appears to be higher in prostheses implanted in stented porcine valves compared to bovine pericardial valves.[23,31]

Current guidelines recommend long-term single antiplatelet therapy in patients without indication for OAC and long-term OAC for patients with indication for anticoagulation (e.g. AF) undergoing TAVR (class I recommendation).[26] The underlying trial evidence is discussed in ➔ Chapter 17.

Although the general use of anticoagulants after TAVR in patients with no other indication for OAC has been questioned by recent randomized trials,[42,43] the use of OAC including non-vitamin K antagonist oral anticoagulants (NOACs) effectively reduced the incidence of HALT/HAM after TAVR.[36,43,44] There have been several reports that showed resolution of clinical and subclinical leaflet thrombosis after 1–6 months of treatment with OAC (both vitamin K antagonists (VKAs) and NOACs) (➔ Figure 4.4).[45]

Transcatheter edge-to edge repair, transcatheter mitral valve replacement, and transcatheter tricuspid valve replacement

Transcatheter techniques to treat atrioventricular valve regurgitation are rapidly evolving. Transcatheter edge-to edge repair

(a)

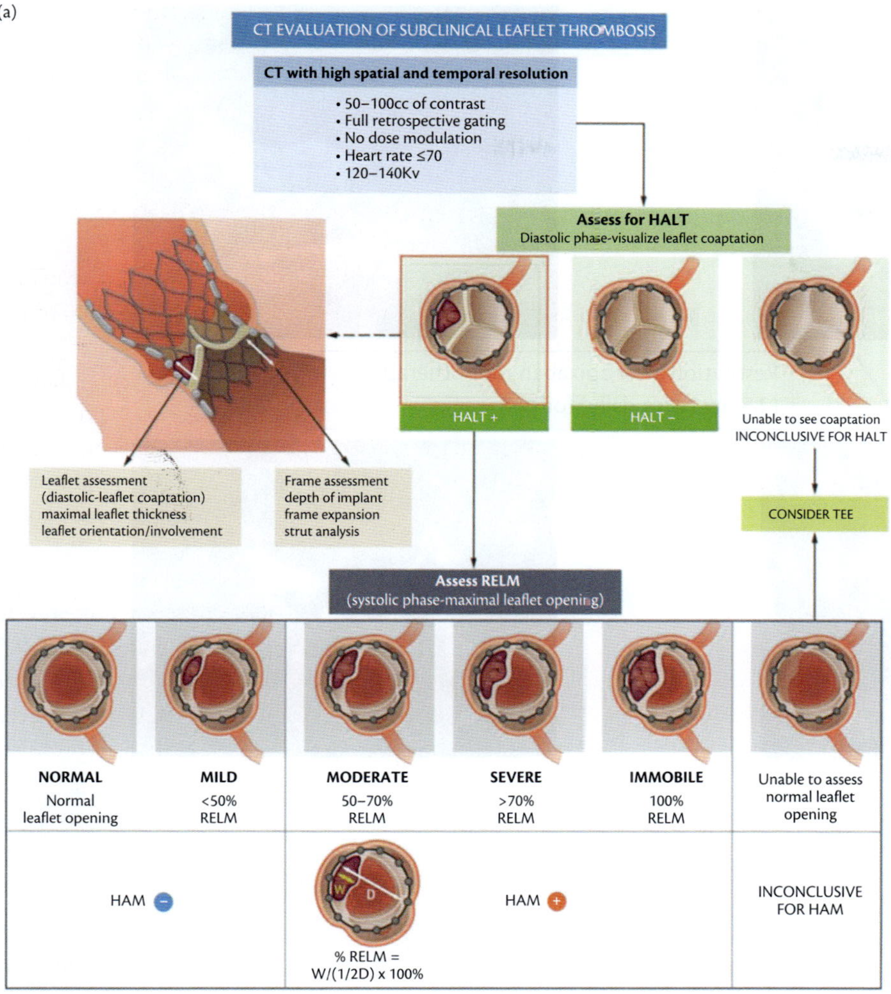

(b)

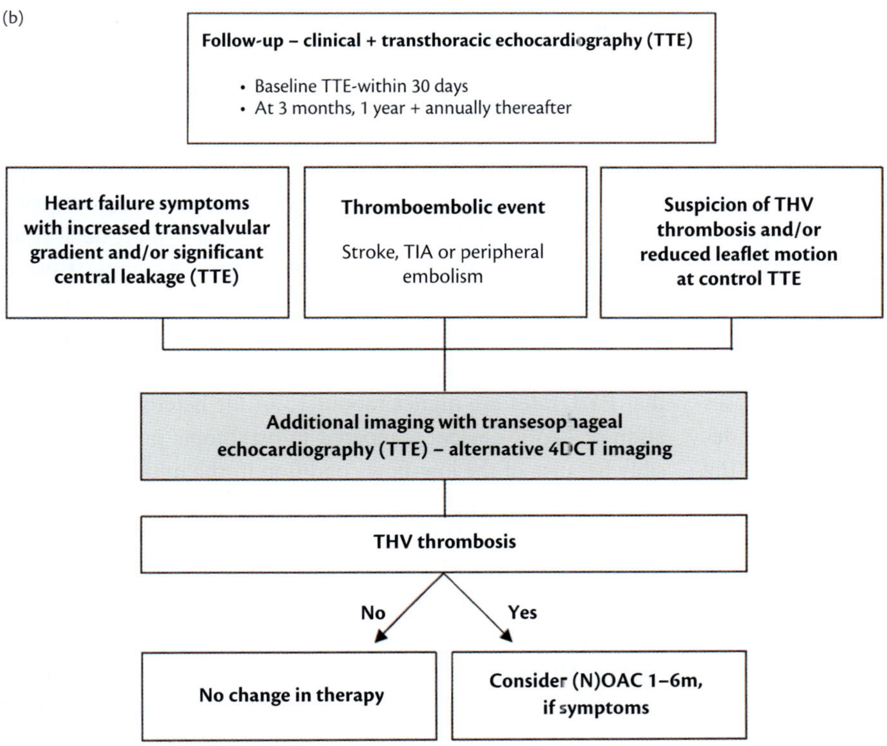

Figure 4.3 (a) Systematic CT methodology for the evaluation of subclinical leaflet thrombosis. HALT, hypoattenuated leaflet thickening; HAM, hypoattenuation affecting motion; RELM, reduced leaflet motion. (b) Algorithm for the follow-up of TAVR patients considering the risk for clinical valve thrombosis and subclinical leaflet thrombosis.

(a) Reproduced from Jilaihawi H, Asch FM, Manasse E, et al. Systematic CT Methodology for the Evaluation of Subclinical Leaflet Thrombosis. JACC Cardiovasc Imaging. 2017 Apr;10(4):461–470. doi: 10.1016/j.jcmg.2017.02.005 with permission from Elsevier.

(b) Reproduced from Rosseel L, De Backer O, Søndergaard L. Clinical Valve Thrombosis and Subclinical Leaflet Thrombosis Following Transcatheter Aortic Valve Replacement: Is There a Need for a Patient-Tailored Antithrombotic Therapy? Front Cardiovasc Med. 2019 Apr 18;6:44. doi: 10.3389/fcvm.2019.00044 https://creativecommons.org/licenses/by/4.0/.

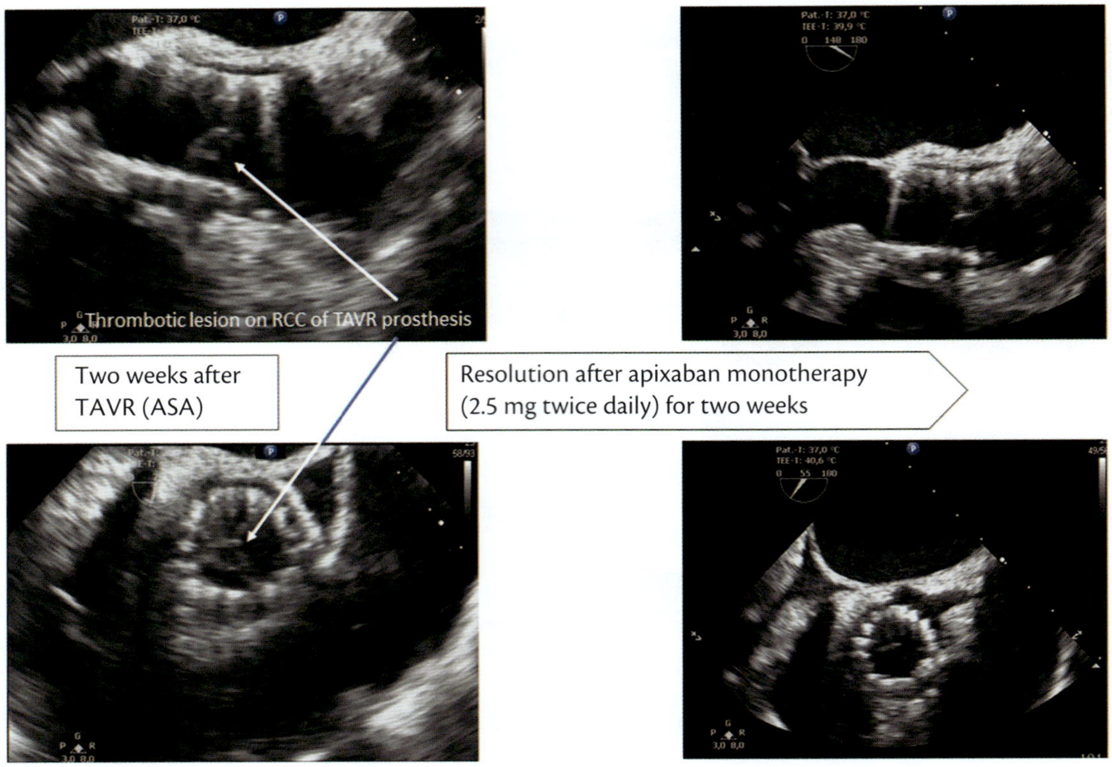

Figure 4.4 Example of a patient developing thrombosis of the TAVR prosthesis (CoreValve Evolute) after temporary modfication of antithrombotic treatment (full dose OAC to aspirin monotherapy) due to major bleeding, complete thrombus resolution after 2 weeks of apixaban 2.5 mg twice daily without bleeding recurrence.

(TEER) of the mitral valve has gained a class IIa, level of evidence B recommendation for secondary mitral regurgitation (MR) and a class IIb, level of evidence B recommendation for primary MR in patients who are deemed at high surgical risk in current guidelines.[26] Heart failure, in particular atriopathy as underlying condition for secondary MR and AF showing a prevalence of up to 50% of the patients are associated with increased risk for thromboembolism and stroke.[46] Altered haemodynamics, impaired endothelial function, and different blood composition are predisposing factors for increased thrombogenicity in heart failure. To date, systematic evaluations of DRT formation after TEER procedures using either the MitraClip® (Abbot), or the PASCAL® (Edwards Lifesciences) are missing. The annual stroke risk after TEER has been reported as between 1% and 2.1% in trials and registries[47,48] considering that not all strokes are cardioembolic strokes and there is no information about device relatedness. A series of cases has documented thrombotic alterations associated with the device or the procedure. Thrombus formation was observed in the region of the Clip system or the delivery system respectively,[49,50] in the left atrium[51], in the LAA,[52] or left ventricle.[53] Thrombi in or on the trans-septal guide sheath have also been reported in single case reports for the MitraClip procedure.[54] There are no reported cases for the PASCAL system, so far. Altered haemodynamics by the TEER may lead to stasis in the LA and LAA, thus increasing thrombogenicity which can be directly measured by thromboelastography in blood taken from the left atrium during the procedure (➔ Figure 4.5a). In a series of patients undergoing TEER, we found a large intraindividual variability of platelet aggregation and thromboelastography parameters before and after device implantation (➔ Figure 4.5b). The clinical impact of these alterations remains to be investigated in future. Possible explanations include acute dramatic haemodynamic alterations in the left atrium related to the reductions in MR and effects caused by mild to moderate mitral stenosis. Recently, transcatheter mitral valve replacement (TMVR) has gained importance in treating high-risk surgical patients by using TAVR devices (e.g. Sapien XT™/3™, Edwards Lifesciences) in heterotopic position in patients with previous mitral valve prosthesis, annuloplasty ring, or calcified mitral disease. In addition, novel TMVR devices are approved or are currently being investigated for clinical use in feasibility trials including the CardiAQ™ (Edwards Lifesciences), Tiara™ (Neovasc), Tendyne™ (Abbott), Intrepid™ (Medtronic), and HighLife™ (Highlife Medical). A few observational studies suggest that PVT rates are higher (about 15%) for heterotopic implantation of TAVR devices compared to orthotopic positioning possibly because of the low-flow condition in the mitral position.[23,55] The overall rate of PVT was reported up to 7%.[56,57] The risk of thrombosis after TMVR is defined by procedure- and patient-related risk factors (➔ Figure 4.6). ViV procedures seem to be associated with a higher thrombogenic risk compared to valve-in-ring procedures.[23] Currently, there are limited data available on mid- and long-term follow-up to evaluate the risk of valve thrombosis after TMVR. The global rate of PVT with orthotopic TMVR devices has been reported at 1.7% at short-term follow-up and 4.0% at mid-term (up to 12 months) follow-up in early feasibility studies.[58] The TMVR programme with the Fortis valve (Edwards

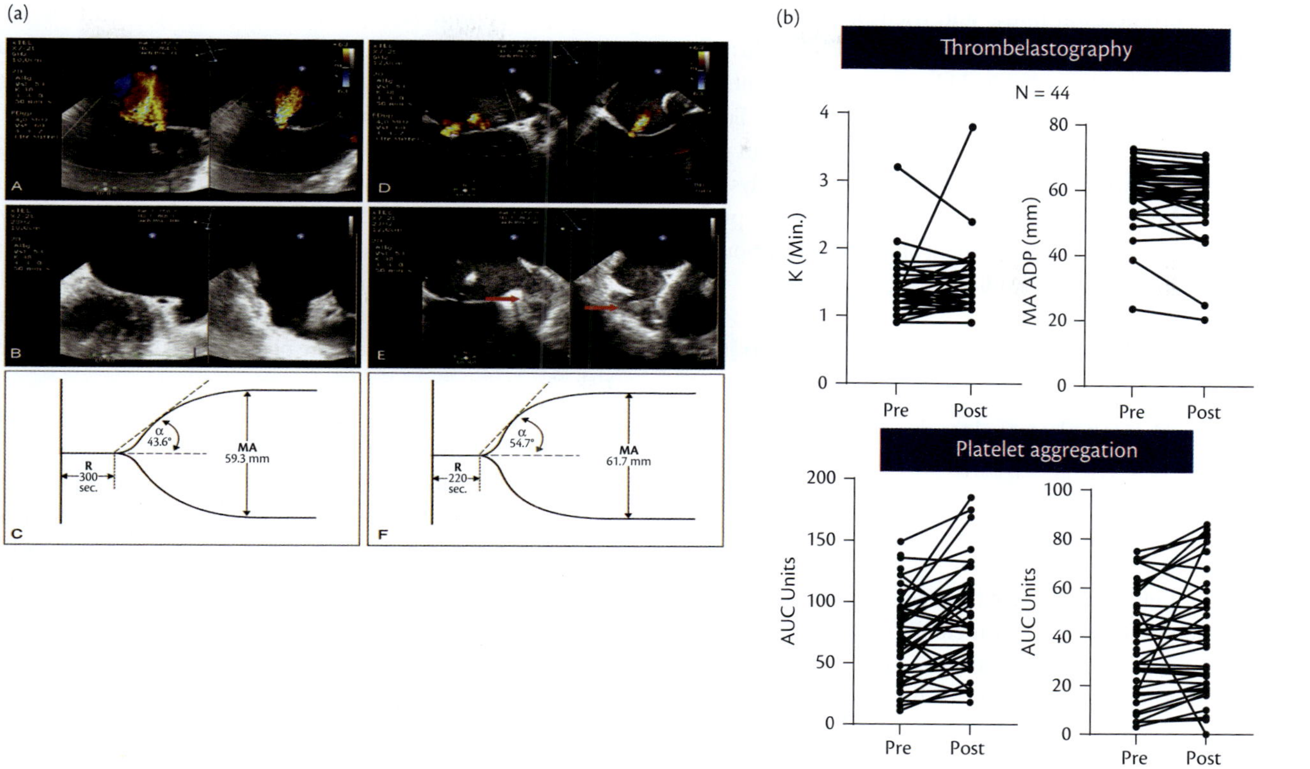

Figure 4.5 (a) Example of periprocedural thrombosis in the left atrium due to altered haemodynamics after MitraClip TEER procedure; haemodynamic changes lead to altered thromboelastography. (b) Intraindividual changes of thromboelastography and platelet aggregation after TEER (PASCAL) in a consecutive series of 44 patients (unpublished data).

(a) Reproduced from Glatthaar A, Seizer P, Patzelt J, Langer H, Schreieck J, Gawaz M. Formation of a left atrial thrombus during percutaneous mitral valve edge-to-edge repair induced by acute reduction of mitral regurgitation. J Cardiol Cases. 2017 Sep 22;17(1):33–35. doi: 10.1016/j.jccase.2017.09.001 with permission from Elsevier.

Lifesciences) was prematurely terminated due to cumulative cases of valve thrombosis.[58a] For the Tendyne transapical device, prosthetic leaflet thrombosis was detected in 1% at 30-day and 6% at mid-term follow-up. All PVTs occurred within the first year after implantation suggesting the risk of late thromboses as low and most of them resolved after temporary (3–6 months) OAC with VKAs.[59,60] Based on expert opinion rather than systematic trials, 3–6 months of OAC (preferably VKA) is currently recommended for

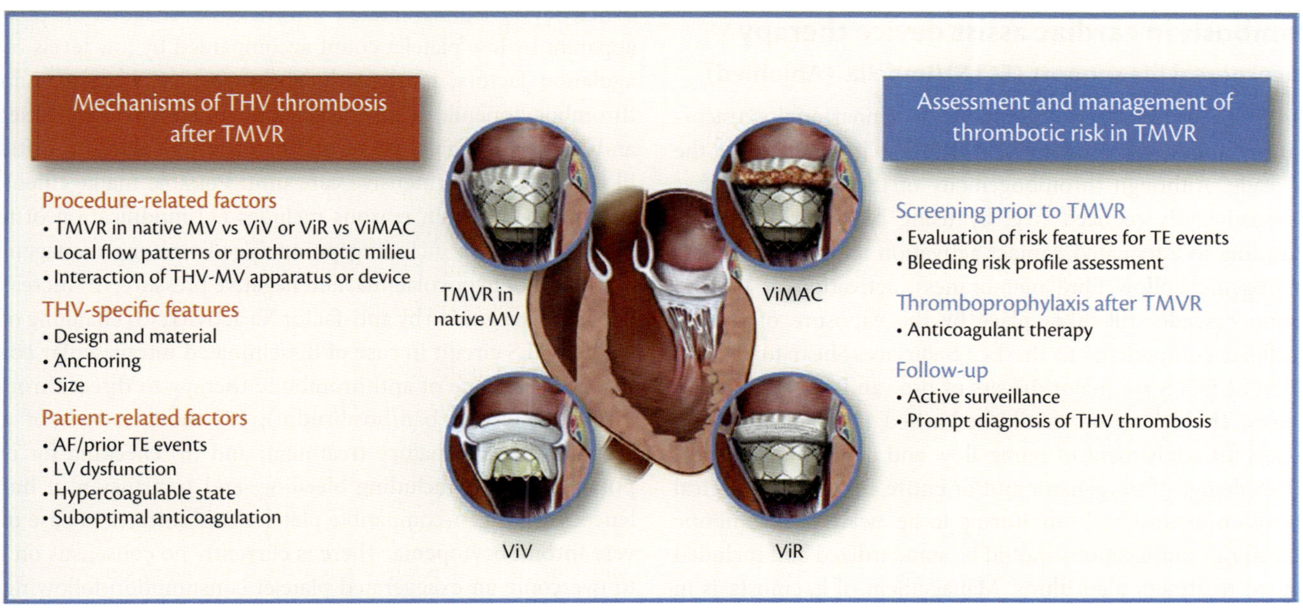

Figure 4.6 Risk factors after transcatheter mitral valve replacement (TMVR). AF, atrial fibrillation; LV, left ventricular; MV, mitral valve; ViMAC, valve-in-mitral annular calcification; ViR, valve-in-ring; ViV, valve-in-valve.

Reproduced from Pagnesi M, Moroni F, Beneduce A, Giannini F, Colombo A, Weisz G, Latib A. Thrombotic Risk and Antithrombotic Strategies After Transcatheter Mitral Valve Replacement. JACC Cardiovasc Interv. 2019 Dec 9;12(23):2388–2401. doi: 10.1016/j.jcin.2019.07.055 with permission from Elsevier.

transcatheter protheses in mitral and tricuspid positions regardless of previous indication for OAC followed by an antithrombotic therapy according to the individual bleeding risk (e.g. antiplatelet therapy in patients with high bleeding risk under OAC). For long-term treatment, there are no adverse signals of NOACs in patients previously treated with bioprostheses from pooled analyses from randomized trials in AF patients.[61] Thus, NOACs might present a suitable option for long-term treatment after TMVR, although this needs to be proven in future studies.

Thrombosis of prostheses in tricuspid position

The incidence of thrombosis of prosthetic (mechanical) tricuspid valves is highest among heart valves due to low-flow velocity in the right heart and the usually larger size and surface of tricuspid valve prostheses. Transcatheter tricuspid edge–edge repair has recently emerged as treatment option in patients with severe tricuspid regurgitation. Transcatheter tricuspid valve replacement (TTVR) although in its infancy has been applied using different valve prostheses. These can be principally classified in heterotopic and orthotopic transcatheter valves. Heterotopic transcatheter valves include the Sapien XT (Edwards Lifesciences), the TricValve™ (P+F Products + Features), and the Tricento™ device (New Valve Technology). Orthotopic valves comprise the following prostheses: the Cardiovalve™ (Boston Medical), the Evoque™ (Edwards Lifesciences), the LUX-Valve™ (Jenscare Biotechnology), the NaviGate™ (NaviGate Cardiac Structures Inc.), the Trisol™ (Trisol Medical), the Intrepid (Medtronic) and the Tricares™ device (TRiCares SAS). Due to the limited use and experience from large registries it is too early to define the true risk of thrombosis of these devices. In a registry evaluating adverse events in 306 patients undergoing ViV or valve-in-ring TTVR, clinically relevant valve thrombosis occurred in 2.6%.[62] The current guidelines follow the recommendations for TMVR.[26]

Thrombosis in cardiac assist device therapy

Extracorporeal life support (ECLS)/Impella® (Abiomed)

Use of ECLS using either venovenous or venoarterial extracorporeal membrane oxygenation (ECMO) has increased over the last decade. Although thrombogenicity of the components has been significantly reduced (e.g. by using biocompatible coatings leading to attenuated contact activation and the use of less thrombogenic hollow fibre membranes), activation of the coagulation cascade still takes place by the exposure of plasma and cellular components to the ECLS surface. Shear forces and duration of ECLS are major drivers of pro- and anticoagulatory processes. Thus, duration should be limited to a minimum and protocols for adjustment of pump flow and cardiac decompression,[63] exchange of oxygenator and/or entire circuit, and surgical intervention to treat and monitoring to be aware of thrombotic and bleeding complications should be standardized and included in patient treatment algorithms. Management of haemostasis in long-term ECLS recipients is still challenging as often there is a small window between bleeding and thrombosis. Bleeding risk is mainly driven by consumption of coagulation factors, in particular factor VIII, consumption of platelets after activation leading to thrombocytopenia, and shear-dependent loss of high-molecular-weight VWF bands. In contrast, the large artificial surface area of the ECMO can stimulate a number of prothrombotic and proinflammatory processes. Several components have been identified to influence platelet-activating and procoagulation pathways. In artificial models, the pump was identified at highest risk for platelet activation and thrombus formation, followed by the reinfusion cannula and the connector.[64] Beside the pump system itself, hypothermia, despite neutral/negative clinical trial results, is still frequently used in cardiogenic shock patients undergoing ECLS, can activate platelets and enhances thrombotic risk.[65–67]

There are few reported cases of thrombotic complications with the Impella ventricular assist device (2.5, CP, 5.0, RP). These events mostly occurred in patients with pre-existing left ventricular thrombosis due to poor ventricular function and/or left ventricular aneurysm. According to the instruction for use, Impella should not be implanted in patients with known ventricular thrombus.

Prevention and management of thrombosis under ECLS/Impella

During ECLS, heparinization with a target activated clotting time of 180–220 seconds is effective to reduce thrombotic complications; some clinical scenarios in patients at high bleeding risk may require modifications of these target values. There is still uncertainty how to manage overshooting platelet consumption occurring under ECSL. Diagnosis of a true prothrombotic cause of thrombocytopenia under ECLS affecting the therapeutic consequences is often challenging. Possible causes include (1) haemolysis to be monitored by elevated plasma-free haemoglobin and lactate dehydrogenase levels; (2) ineffective anticoagulation by unfractionated heparin leading to intervascular and pump thrombosis caused by too low heparin doses or acquired antithrombin deficiency; (3) disseminated intravascular coagulation possibly apparent by low platelet count accompanied by low levels of coagulation factors, particularly fibrinogen; (4) heparin-induced thrombocytopenia, ideally detected by functional tests; (5) sepsis; and (6) physiological stress and/or occult bleeding in critically ill patients in the intensive care unit. Possible management according to the main reasons includes (1) modification of technical parameters including pump speed, volume management, avoidance of hypovolaemia, and negative pressure; (2) increase of heparin dose guided by anti-factor Xa activity; (3) changing of the whole ECLS circuit in case of disseminated intravascular coagulation; (4) change of antithrombotic therapy to direct thrombin inhibitors (argatroban/bivalirudin); (5) modifications of antibiotic/anti-inflammatory treatment; and (6) checking for other possible reasons including bleeding, and transfusion of human leucocyte antigen-compatible platelet concentrates in case of severe thrombocytopenia. There is currently no consensus on how to overcome an exaggerated platelet consumption following activation under ECLS. Once other treatable causes have been excluded, pharmacological platelet inhibition using short-acting compounds (e.g. intravenous cangrelor, a $P2Y_{12}$ inhibitor) have been reported as beneficial in a few cases including patients with heparin-induced thrombocytopenia under careful evaluation of the bleeding risk.[68–70] Of note, infusion of cangrelor led to a significant decrease of platelet activation and subsequent increase of platelet count under hypothermia in an animal model and *in vitro* model of extracorporeal circulation (Chandler loop).[71] Currently, standardized anticoagulation protocols during haemodynamic support with the Impella system are lacking. According to the manufacturer's recommendations, an activated clotting time of 160–180 seconds should be targeted. Guiding of heparinization according to factor Xa levels (window between 0.3 and 0.5 U/mL) and aPTT is currently recommended and has been associated with a low rate of thrombotic and bleeding complications.[72,72a]

Left ventricular assist devices (LVADs)

Implantation of LVADs is becoming more frequent due to the limited availability of cardiac transplants, increasing numbers of recipients, and technical improvement of the devices. Different concepts for use of LVADs exist which are bridge to recovery, bridge to transplant, bridge to destination, and bridge to candidacy.[73,74] The most frequently used system is LVAD with continuous-flow (CF-LVAD) which is available as an axial or centrifugal flow pump. CF-LVADs have a more favourable safety profile with regard to durability, fewer surgical complications, and less thrombogenicity. Although the technology advances and indications improve, complications are common and related to a high morbidity and mortality. Bleeding and device thrombosis are among the most frequent and serious adverse events.[75]

Besides this, LVAD thrombosis is a serious and, in many cases, life-threatening complication that can lead to haemodynamic instability and thromboembolic events including stroke. Depending on the device, the incidence has been reported between 1.4% and 11.8%.[76–79] For the HeartMate II™ device (Abbott), thrombosis occurred in up to 8.4% in a recent registry with a median time from implantation to thrombosis of 18.6 months.[79] Improvement of implant techniques, postoperative management, and technical advances like the magnetically levitated miniaturized centrifugal-flow pump (HeartMate III™) contributed to the substantial reduction of pump thrombosis.[80] The latter device was investigated in the MOMENTUM 3 trial. Pump thrombosis was observed in 1.1% of the patients compared to 15.7% in patients receiving an axial flow pump (hazard ratio 0.06, 95% confidence interval 0.01–0.26; P <0.001).[81]

Risk factors for LVAD pump thrombosis include high shear stress, device and surface characteristics, chronic inflammation and infections, surgical factors (e.g. inadequate device positioning of the inflow cannula and inadequate sizing of the pump pocket), and ineffective anticoagulation. Patient-related factors include pre-existing intracardiac thrombi, non-compliance, coagulation disorders, and poorly controlled blood pressure. The diagnosis of LVAD thrombosis should be made by an interdisciplinary approach using standardized algorithms (➔ Figure 4.7)[82]

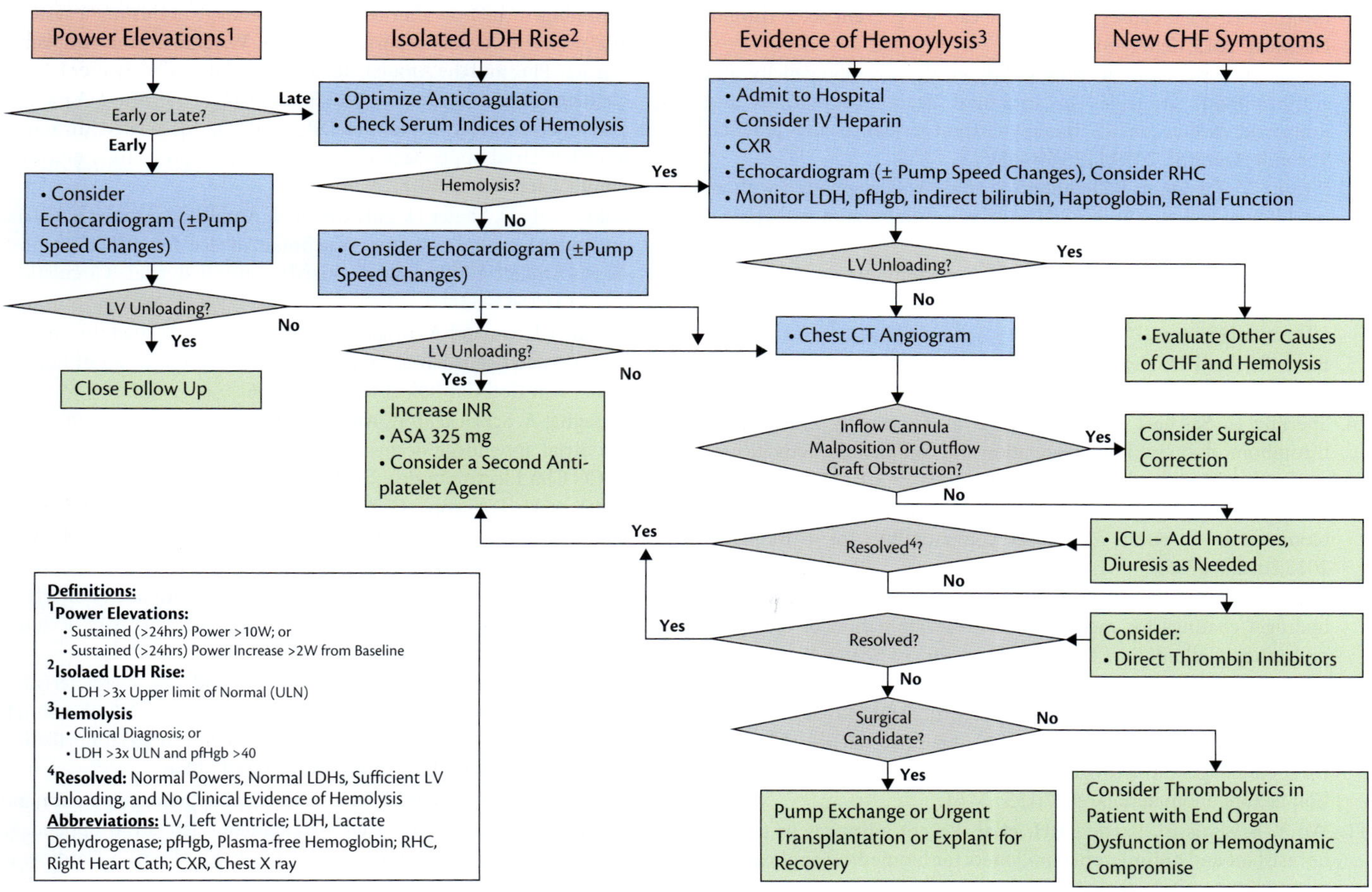

Figure 4.7 Algorithm for the diagnosis and management of suspected pump thrombus.

Reproduced from Goldstein DJ, John R, Salerno C, et al.; Algorithm for the diagnosis and management of suspected pump thrombus. J Heart Lung Transplant. 2013 Jul;32(7):667–70. doi: 10.1016/j.healun.2013.05.002 with permission from Elsevier.

usually on the basis of laboratory findings combined with changes in LVAD physical parameters (power consumption, speed, and estimated flow). In case of a clear diagnosis of CF-LVAD thrombosis, LVAD exchange is often necessary. Non-surgical options include thrombolytic and antithrombotic strategies (e.g. direct thrombin inhibitor, tissue plasminogen activator, or glycoprotein IIb/IIIa antagonist).[83–87] Direct thrombolytic therapy (tissue plasminogen activator) has been used to treat LVAD thrombosis in some cases.[88] However, thrombolytic therapy is associated with a higher risk of recurrence[89] and bleeding complications including haemorrhagic strokes.[90] In a recent meta-analysis, surgical pump exchange was superior to medical therapy with a higher success rate of pump thrombosis resolution, lower mortality, and lower recurrence rate.[91] OAC with a VKA is mandatory for long-term treatment after LAVD. The international normalized ratio target should be between 2.0 and 3.5 depending on the particular manufacturer's recommendations for modern LVADs. There is still controversy whether additional antiplatelet therapy is beneficial and at what dose. Recently, a systematic review has revealed that a majority of centres use a combination therapy with aspirin initiated 24–72 hours postoperatively without any complications.[92]

Summary and future perspectives

DRT is of high clinical impact with the increasing number of cardiac devices in daily clinical practice. Early and specific recognition is crucial to modify antithrombotic treatment and thus reduce the risk of serious complications and mortality. Further development and engineering of new surface and barrier coatings, cardiac tissue engineering assisted by computational modelling,[93] and the use of biodegradable nanopolymers mimicking the natural cardiovascular tissue are promising to reduce thrombotic risk in future. In addition, the advent of novel antithrombotics targeting the contact-activation pathway with a favourable safety profile (e.g. factor XIa/XIIa inhibitors) will offer individualized strategies in high-bleeding-risk patients and these compounds should be investigated in clinical trials addressing the issues of thrombotic complications after implantation of cardiac devices and in patients undergoing extracorporeal cardiac support.[3,4]

References

1. Jaffer IH, Fredenburgh JC, Hirsh J, et al. Medical device-induced thrombosis: what causes it and how can we prevent it? J Thromb Haemost. 2015;13:S72–81.
2. Geisler T, Jorbenadze R, Popov A-F, et al. Thrombogenicity and antithrombotic strategies in structural heart interventions and nonaortic cardiac device therapy-current evidence and practice. Thromb Haemost. 2019;119:1590–605.
3. Pireaux V, Tassignon J, Demoulin S, et al. Anticoagulation with an inhibitor of factors XIa and XIIa during cardiopulmonary bypass. J Am Coll Cardiol. 2019;74:2178–89.
4. Demoulin S, Godfroid E, Hermans C. Dual inhibition of factor XIIa and factor XIa as a therapeutic approach for safe thromboprotection. J Thromb Haemost. 2021;19:323–9.
5. Biran R, Pond D. Heparin coatings for improving blood compatibility of medical devices. Adv Drug Deliv Rev. 2017;112:12–23.
6. Sperling C, Salchert K, Streller U, et al. Covalently immobilized thrombomodulin inhibits coagulation and complement activation of artificial surfaces in vitro. Biomaterials. 2004;25:5101–13.
7. de Mel A, Cousins BG, Seifalian AM. Surface modification of biomaterials: a quest for blood compatibility. Int J Biomater. 2012;2012:e707863.
8. Butruk-Raszeja BA, Łojszczyk I, Ciach T, et al. Athrombogenic hydrogel coatings for medical devices—examination of biological properties. Colloids Surf B Biointerfaces. 2015;130:192–8.
9. Lu B, Han X, Zhao A, et al. Intelligent H2S release coating for regulating vascular remodeling. Bioact Mater. 2020;6:1040–50.
10. Maitz MF, Zitzmann J, Hanke J, et al. Adaptive release of heparin from anticoagulant hydrogels triggered by different blood coagulation factors. Biomaterials. 2017;135:53–61.
11. Wo Y, Brisbois EJ, Bartlett RH, et al. Recent advances in thromboresistant and antimicrobial polymers for biomedical applications: just say yes to nitric oxide (NO). Biomater Sci. 2016;4:1161–83.
12. Lempereur M, Aminian A, Freixa X, et al. Device-associated thrombus formation after left atrial appendage occlusion: a systematic review of events reported with the Watchman, the Amplatzer Cardiac Plug and the Amulet: device-related thrombosis after LAAO. Catheter Cardiovasc Interv. 2017;90:E111–21.
13. Dukkipati SR, Kar S, Holmes DR, et al. Device-related thrombus after left atrial appendage closure: incidence, predictors, and outcomes. Circulation. 2018;138:874–85.
14. Lakkireddy D, Thaler D, Ellis CR, et al. Amplatzer Amulet left atrial appendage occluder versus Watchman device for stroke prophylaxis (Amulet IDE): a randomized, controlled trial. Circulation. 2021;144:1543–52.
15. Fauchier L, Cinaud A, Brigadeau F, et al. Device-related thrombosis after percutaneous left atrial appendage occlusion for atrial fibrillation. J Am Coll Cardiol. 2018;71:1528–36.
16. Sedaghat A, Schrickel J-W, Andrié R, et al. Thrombus formation after left atrial appendage occlusion with the Amplatzer Amulet device. JACC Clin Electrophysiol. 2017;3:71–5.
17. Ketterer U, D'Ancona G, Siegel I, et al. Percutaneous left atrial appendage occlusion: device thrombosis in clopidogrel non-responders. Int J Cardiol. 2016;204:196–7.
18. Dannenberg L, Mourikis P, Naguib D, et al. Antiplatelet effects of aspirin and clopidogrel after left atrial appendage (LAA) occluder implantation. Int J Cardiol. 2019;275:95–100.
19. Kubo S, Mizutani Y, Meemook K, et al. Incidence, characteristics, and clinical course of device-related thrombus after Watchman left atrial appendage occlusion device implantation in atrial fibrillation patients. JACC Clin Electrophysiol. 2017;3:1380–6.
20. Cochet H, Iriart X, Sridi S, et al. Left atrial appendage patency and device-related thrombus after percutaneous left atrial appendage occlusion: a computed tomography study. Eur Heart J Cardiovasc Imaging. 2018;19:1351–61.

21. Pracon R, Bangalore S, Dzielinska Z, et al. Device thrombosis after percutaneous left atrial appendage occlusion is related to patient and procedural characteristics but not to duration of postimplantation dual antiplatelet therapy. Circ Cardiovasc Interv. 2018;11:e005997.
22. Roudaut R, Serri K, Lafitte S. Thrombosis of prosthetic heart valves: diagnosis and therapeutic considerations. Heart. 2007;93:137–42.
23. Dangas GD, Weitz JI, Giustino G, et al. Prosthetic heart valve thrombosis. J Am Coll Cardiol. 2016;68:2670–89.
24. Nishimura RA, Otto CM, Bonow RO, et al. 2017 AHA/ACC focused update of the 2014 AHA/ACC guideline for the management of patients with valvular heart disease: a report of the American College of Cardiology/American Heart Association Task Force on Clinical Practice Guidelines. Circulation. 2017;135:e1159–95.
25. Whitlock RP, Sun JC, Fremes SE, et al. Antithrombotic and Thrombolytic Therapy for Valvular Disease: Antithrombotic Therapy and Prevention of Thrombosis, 9th ed: American College of Chest Physicians evidence-based clinical practice guidelines. Chest 2012;141:e576S–e600S.
26. Vahanian A, Beyersdorf F, Praz F, et al. 2021 ESC/EACTS Guidelines for the management of valvular heart disease. Eur Heart J. 2022;43:561–632.
27. Jawitz OK, Wang TY, Lopes RD, et al. Rationale and design of PROACT Xa: a randomized, multicenter, open-label, clinical trial to evaluate the efficacy and safety of apixaban vs. warfarin in patients with a mechanical On-X® Aortic Heart Valve. Am Heart J. 2020;227:91–9.
28. Tabet JY, Bouvier E, Cormier B, et al. Unusual cause of stroke after mitral valve replacement. Circulation. 2010;122:e484–5.
29. Özkan M, Gündüz S, Güner A, et al. Thrombolysis or surgery in patients with obstructive mechanical valve thrombosis: the multicenter HATTUSHA Study. J Am Coll Cardiol. 2022;79:977–89.
30. Latib A, Naganuma T, Abdel-Wahab M, et al. Treatment and clinical outcomes of transcatheter heart valve thrombosis. Circ Cardiovasc Interv. 2015;8:e001779.
31. Jose J, Sulimov DS, El-Mawardy M, et al. Clinical bioprosthetic heart valve thrombosis after transcatheter aortic valve replacement: incidence, characteristics, and treatment outcomes. JACC Cardiovasc Interv. 2017;10:686–97.
32. Capodanno D, Petronio AS, Prendergast B, et al. Standardized definitions of structural deterioration and valve failure in assessing long-term durability of transcatheter and surgical aortic bioprosthetic valves: a consensus statement from the European Association of Percutaneous Cardiovascular Interventions (EAPCI) endorsed by the European Society of Cardiology (ESC) and the European Association for Cardio-Thoracic Surgery (EACTS). Eur J Cardiothorac Surg. 2017;52:408–17.
33. Ng ACT, Holmes DR, Mack MJ, et al. Leaflet immobility and thrombosis in transcatheter aortic valve replacement. Eur Heart J. 2020;41:3184–97.
34. Vollema EM, Kong WKF, Katsanos S, et al. Transcatheter aortic valve thrombosis: the relation between hypo-attenuated leaflet thickening, abnormal valve haemodynamics, and stroke. Eur Heart J. 2017;38:1207–17.
35. Garcia S, Fukui M, Dworak MW, et al. Clinical impact of hypoattenuating leaflet thickening after transcatheter aortic valve replacement. Circ Cardiovasc Interv. 2022;15:e011480.
36. Bogyi M, Schernthaner RE, Loewe C, et al. Subclinical leaflet thrombosis after transcatheter aortic valve replacement: a meta-analysis. JACC Cardiovasc Interv. 2021;14:2643–56.
37. Makkar RR, Blanke P, Leipsic J, et al. Subclinical leaflet thrombosis in transcatheter and surgical bioprosthetic valves: PARTNER 3 cardiac computed tomography substudy. J Am Coll Cardiol. 2020;75:3003–15.
38. Blanke P, Leipsic JA, Popma JJ, et al. Bioprosthetic aortic valve leaflet thickening in the Evolut Low Risk sub-study. J Am Coll Cardiol. 2020;75:2430–42.
39. Yamashita K, Yagi H, Hayakawa M, et al. Rapid restoration of thrombus formation and high-molecular-weight von Willebrand factor multimers in patients with severe aortic stenosis after valve replacement. J Atheroscler Thromb. 2016;23:1150–8.
40. Matsushita K, Marchandot B, Trimaille A, et al. Paradoxical increase of stroke in patients with defect of high molecular weight multimers of the von Willebrand factors following transcatheter aortic valve replacement. Thromb Haemost. 2020;120:1330–8.
41. Midha PA, Raghav V, Sharma R, et al. The fluid mechanics of transcatheter heart valve leaflet thrombosis in the neosinus. Circulation. 2017;136:1598–609.
42. Dangas GD, Tijssen JGP, Wöhrle J, et al. A controlled trial of rivaroxaban after transcatheter aortic-valve replacement. N Engl J Med. 2020;382:120–9.
43. Collet J-P, Van Belle E, Thiele H, et al. Apixaban vs. standard of care after transcatheter aortic valve implantation: the ATLANTIS trial. Eur Heart J. 2022;43:2783–97.
44. De Backer O, Dangas GD, Jilaihawi H, et al. Reduced leaflet motion after transcatheter aortic-valve replacement. N Engl J Med. 2020;382:130–9.
45. Makkar RR, Fontana G, Jilaihawi H, et al. Possible subclinical leaflet thrombosis in bioprosthetic aortic valves. N Engl J Med. 2015;373:2015–24.
46. Adelborg K, Szépligeti S, Sundbøll J, et al. Risk of stroke in patients with heart failure: a population-based 30-year cohort study. Stroke. 2017;48:1161–8.
47. Puls M, Lubos E, Boekstegers P, et al. One-year outcomes and predictors of mortality after MitraClip therapy in contemporary clinical practice: results from the German transcatheter mitral valve interventions registry. Eur Heart J. 2016;37:703–12.
48. Webb JG, Hensey M, Szerlip M, et al. 1-Year outcomes for transcatheter repair in patients with mitral regurgitation from the CLASP study. JACC Cardiovasc Interv. 2020;13:2344–57.
49. Huntgeburth M, Müller-Ehmsen J, Brase C, et al. Thrombus formation at the MitraClip system during percutaneous mitral valve repair. JACC Cardiovasc Interve. 2014;7:e111–12.
50. Hamm K, Barth S, Diegeler A, et al. Stroke and thrombus formation appending to the MitraClip: what is the appropriate anticoagulation regimen? J Heart Valve Dis. 2013;22:713–15.
51. Bekeredjian R, Mereles D, Pleger S, et al. Large atrial thrombus formation after MitraClip implantation: is anticoagulation mandatory? J Heart Valve Dis. 2011;20:146–8.
52. Glatthaar A, Seizer P, Patzelt J, et al. Formation of a left atrial thrombus during percutaneous mitral valve edge-to-edge repair induced by acute reduction of mitral regurgitation. J Cardiol Cases. 2018;17:33–5.
53. Orban M, Braun D, Sonne C, et al. Dangerous liaison: successful percutaneous edge-to-edge mitral valve repair in patients with end-stage systolic heart failure can cause left ventricular thrombus formation. EuroIntervention. 2014;10:253–9.
54. Andrikopoulou E, Mitchell RNM, Kim AYK, et al. 496 A fatal case of MitraClip thrombosis. Eur Heart J Cardiovasc Imaging. 2020;21:jez319.260.
55. Eng MH, Greenbaum A, Wang DD, et al. Thrombotic valvular dysfunction with transcatheter mitral interventions for postsurgical failures: thrombotic valvular dysfunction mitral intervention. Cathet Cardiovasc Interv. 2017;90:321–8.
56. Yoon S-H, Whisenant BK, Bleiziffer S, et al. Outcomes of transcatheter mitral valve replacement for degenerated bioprostheses, failed annuloplasty rings, and mitral annular calcification. Eur Heart J. 2019;40:441–51.

57. Urena M, Brochet E, Lecomte M, et al. Clinical and haemodynamic outcomes of balloon-expandable transcatheter mitral valve implantation: a 7-year experience. Eur Heart J. 2018;39:2679–89.
58. Del Val D, Ferreira-Neto AN, Wintzer-Wehekind J, et al. Early experience with transcatheter mitral valve replacement: a systematic review. J Am Heart Assoc. 2019;8:e013332.
58a. Regueiro A, Granada JF, Dagenais F, Rodés-Cabau J. Transcatheter mitral valve replacement. J Am Coll Cardiol. 2017;69:2175–92.
59. Muller DWM, Farivar RS, Jansz P, et al. Transcatheter mitral valve replacement for patients with symptomatic mitral regurgitation. J Am Coll Cardiol. 2017;69:381–91.
60. Muller DWM, Sorajja P, Duncan A, et al. 2-Year outcomes of transcatheter mitral valve replacement in patients with severe symptomatic mitral regurgitation. J Am Coll Cardiol. 2021;78:1847–59.
61. Yokoyama Y, Briasoulis A, Ueyama H, et al. Direct oral anticoagulants versus vitamin K antagonists in patients with atrial fibrillation and bioprosthetic valves: a meta-analysis. J Thorac Cardiovasc Surg. 2023;165(6):2052–9.e4.
62. McElhinney DB, Aboulhosn JA, Dvir D, et al. Mid-term valve-related outcomes after transcatheter tricuspid valve-in-valve or valve-in-ring replacement. J Am Coll Cardiol. 2019;73:148–57.
63. Alhussein M, Moayedi Y, Posada JD, et al. Ventricular thrombosis post-venoarterial extracorporeal membrane oxygenation. Circ Heart Fail. 2017;10:e003757.
64. Fuchs G, Berg N, Broman LM, et al. Flow-induced platelet activation in components of the extracorporeal membrane oxygenation circuit. Sci Rep. 2018;8:13985.
65. Spiel AO, Kliegel A, Janata A, et al. Hemostasis in cardiac arrest patients treated with mild hypothermia initiated by cold fluids. Resuscitation. 2009;80:762–5.
66. Scharbert G, Kalb ML, Essmeister R, et al. Mild and moderate hypothermia increases platelet aggregation induced by various agonists: a whole blood in vitro study. Platelets. 2010;21:44–8.
67. Jeppesen AN, Kirkegaard H, Ilkjær S, et al. Influence of temperature on thromboelastometry and platelet aggregation in cardiac arrest patients undergoing targeted temperature management. Crit Care. 2016;20:118.
68. Ciolek AM, Ma K, Jennings DL, et al. Use of cangrelor during venoarterial extracorporeal membrane oxygenation following percutaneous coronary intervention. J Heart Lung Transplant. 2019;38:S307.
69. Droppa M, Vaduganathan M, Venkateswaran RV, et al. Cangrelor in cardiogenic shock and after cardiopulmonary resuscitation: a global, multicenter, matched pair analysis with oral P2Y12 inhibition from the IABP-SHOCK II trial. Resuscitation. 2019;137:205–12.
70. Gernhofer YK, Banks DA, Golts E, et al. Novel use of cangrelor with heparin during cardiopulmonary bypass in patients with heparin-induced thrombocytopenia who require cardiovascular surgery: a case series. Semin Thorac Cardiovasc Surg. 2020;32:763–9.
71. Krajewski S, Kurz J, Neumann B, et al. Short-acting P2Y12 blockade to reduce platelet dysfunction and coagulopathy during experimental extracorporeal circulation and hypothermia. Br J Anaesth. 2012;108:912–21.
72. Batra S, Kamran H, Lech T, et al. High thromboembolic event rate in patients supported with an Impella CP device with an anti-Xa level of less than 0.1 u/mL. J Heart Lung Transplant. 2018;37:S59.
72a. Vandenbriele C, Arachchillage DJ, Frederiks P, et al. Anticoagulation for percutaneous ventricular assist device-supported cardiogenic shock. J Am Coll Cardiol. 2022;79(19):1949–62. doi: 10.1016/j.jacc.2022.02.052. PMID: 35550692
73. Kirklin JK, Naftel DC, Pagani FD, et al. Long-term mechanical circulatory support (destination therapy): on track to compete with heart transplantation? J Thorac Cardiovasc Surg. 2012;144:584–603.
74. Rogers JG, Pagani FD, Tatooles AJ, et al. Intrapericardial left ventricular assist device for advanced heart failure. N Engl J Med. 2017;376:451–60.
75. Eckman PM, John R. Bleeding and thrombosis in patients with continuous-flow ventricular assist devices. Circulation. 2012;125:3038–47.
76. Kirklin JK, Naftel DC, Kormos RL, et al. Interagency Registry for Mechanically Assisted Circulatory Support (INTERMACS) analysis of pump thrombosis in the HeartMate II left ventricular assist device. J Heart Lung Transplant. 2014;33:12–22.
77. Miller LW, Pagani FD, Russell SD, et al. Use of a continuous-flow device in patients awaiting heart transplantation. N Engl J Med. 2007;357:885–96.
78. Pagani FD, Miller LW, Russell SD, et al. Extended mechanical circulatory support with a continuous-flow rotary left ventricular assist device. J Am Coll Cardiol. 2009;54:312–21.
79. Starling RC, Moazami N, Silvestry SC, et al. Unexpected abrupt increase in left ventricular assist device thrombosis. N Engl J Med. 2014;370:33–40.
80. Klodell CT, Massey HT, Adamson RM, et al. Factors related to pump thrombosis with the Heartmate II left ventricular assist device. J Card Surg. 2015;30:775–80.
81. Mehra MR, Goldstein DJ, Uriel N, et al. Two-year outcomes with a magnetically levitated cardiac pump in heart failure. N Engl J Med. 2018;378:1386–95.
82. Goldstein DJ, John R, Salerno C, et al. Algorithm for the diagnosis and management of suspected pump thrombus. J Heart Lung Transplant. 2013;32:667–70.
83. Sylvia LM, Ordway L, Pham DT, et al. Bivalirudin for treatment of LVAD thrombosis: a case series. ASAIO J. 2014;60:744–7.
84. Badiye A, Hernandez GA, Chaparro S. Argatroban as novel therapy for suspected thrombosis in patients with continuous-flow left ventricle assist device and hemolysis. ASAIO J. 2014;60:361–5.
85. Muthiah K, Robson D, Macdonald PS, et al. Thrombolysis for suspected Intrapump thrombosis in patients with continuous flow centrifugal left ventricular assist device: thoughts and progress. Artif Organs. 2013;37:313–18.
86. Tellor BR, Smith JR, Prasad SM, et al. The use of eptifibatide for suspected pump thrombus or thrombosis in patients with left ventricular assist devices. J Heart Lung Transplant. 2014;33:94–101.
87. Schlendorf K, Patel CB, Gehrig T, et al. Thrombolytic therapy for thrombosis of continuous flow ventricular assist devices. J Cardiac Fail. 2014;20:91–7.
88. Garbade J, Bittner HB, Mohr F-W, et al. Fluoroscopy-guided resolution of ingested thrombus leading to functional disturbance of a continuous-flow left ventricular assist device. Case Rep Surg. 2012;2012:1–3.
89. Köksel U, Erbasan O, Bayezid Ö, et al. Thrombosis in continuous flow left ventricular assist devices: our clinical experience with medical and surgical management. Transplant Proc. 2016;48:2162–7.
90. Bartoli CR, Ailawadi G, Kern JA. Diagnosis, nonsurgical management, and prevention of LVAD thrombosis. J Cardiac Surg. 2014;29:83–94.
91. Luc JGY, Tchantchaleishvili V, Phan K, Dunlay SM, Maltais S, Stulak JM. Medical therapy as compared to surgical device exchange for left ventricular assist device thrombosis: A systematic review and meta-analysis. ASAIO J. 2019;65(4):307–17.
92. Baumann Kreuziger LM, Kim B, Wieselthaler GM. Antithrombotic therapy for left ventricular assist devices in adults: a systematic review. J Thromb Haemost 2015;13(06):946–55.
93. Fioretta ES, Motta SE, Lintas V, et al. Next-generation tissue-engineered heart valves with repair, remodelling and regeneration capacity. Nat Rev Cardiol. 2021;18:92–116.

SECTION 2

Clinical pharmacology of antithrombotic drugs

CHAPTER 5

Aspirin

Carlo Patrono and Bianca Rocca

Contents

Summary

Aspirin represents a first choice for the acute treatment and long-term prevention of atherothrombotic events, with consistent recommendations in cardiovascular guidelines. This is based on a series of features reviewed in this chapter: (1) its relatively simple pharmacokinetics and platelet-specific pharmacodynamics make cumulative suppression of thromboxane production a highly predictable phenomenon in the vast majority of compliant patients; (2) the two- to threefold excess of the currently used dose as compared to the lowest daily dose necessary and sufficient to fully inactivate platelet cyclooxygenase-1 activity may accommodate most but extreme interindividual variations in body weight and platelet number; (3) acetylation of cyclooxygenase isozymes in the bone marrow precursors ensures long-lasting suppression of platelet cyclooxygenase activity throughout the dosing interval, and limits the consequences of occasionally missed drug intake, except in cases of accelerated platelet turnover; and (4) low-dose aspirin has undergone an unusual paradigm of independent drug development, characterized by a large number of phase II dose-finding studies and phase III randomized clinical trials, resulting in a very extensive efficacy and safety database for its use as an antiplatelet drug.

Historical background

Acetylsalicylic acid was synthesized for the first time within an industrial environment in 1897, rapidly tested as an analgesic/anti-inflammatory agent, and marketed as aspirin in 1899. Although its mechanism of action remained unknown until 1971, its classical pharmacological activities provided a template for the development of a large and successful class of similar agents, the non-steroidal anti-inflammatory drugs (NSAIDs). Emphasis on the gastrointestinal (GI) toxicity of aspirin and unjustified marketing claims of superior efficacy and/or safety of newer NSAIDs gradually displaced aspirin from its role in the symptomatic treatment of osteoarthritic conditions and confined it to the over-the-counter analgesic market. This coincided with fundamental discoveries about the mechanism of action of aspirin and aspirin-like drugs in the early 1970s. In particular, the discovery of a novel pro-aggregatory prostanoid, thromboxane (TX)-A_2, as the major product of platelet arachidonic acid metabolism via the cyclooxygenase (COX)-1 pathway, that could be inhibited by low concentrations of aspirin *in vitro*, provided the rationale for developing novel biomarkers of this particular mechanism of platelet activation and inhibition, beyond turbidimetric measurements of platelet aggregation (reviewed in reference 1). The use of mechanism-based biomarkers of platelet activation allowed the characterization of the clinical pharmacology of platelet inhibition by aspirin in health and disease, and provided the basis for the design of a number of placebo-controlled, randomized clinical trials (RCTs) to evaluate the clinical efficacy and safety of low-dose aspirin for cardiovascular disease treatment and prevention (reviewed in reference 2).

Mechanism of action

The best characterized mechanism of action of aspirin is represented by irreversible inactivation of the COX activity of prostaglandin H-synthase (PGHS)-1 and -2 (also referred to as COX-1 and COX-2), through the acetylation of serine529 in human COX-1 and serine516 in human COX-2 (➔ Figure 5.1).[3] This irreversible point modification permanently obstructs access of the substrate arachidonic acid to the COX catalytic site, thereby preventing its conversion to prostaglandin (PG)-G_2 and its further metabolism to various bioactive prostanoids.

PGHS-1 and -2 are bifunctional isozymes that sequentially convert arachidonic acid into PGG_2 and PGH_2 via the COX and hydroperoxidase (HOX) activities, respectively (➔ Figure 5.1).[4] The short-lived PGH_2 is the substrate of cell- and tissue-specific synthases generating various bioactive compounds, classified according to their cyclopentane ring structure as PGD_2, PGE_2, $PGF_{2\alpha}$, PGI_2, and TXA_2, the latter having an oxane ring structure.

Specifically, human platelets and vascular endothelial cells process PGH_2 to produce primarily TXA_2 and PGI_2, respectively.[5] TXA_2 induces platelet aggregation and vasoconstriction, while PGI_2 has the counterbalancing effect of inhibiting platelet aggregation and promoting vasodilation.[5] Under physiological conditions, PGI_2 is mainly derived from COX-2 constitutively expressed by vascular endothelial cells in response to laminar shear stress,[5] and largely unaffected by platelet-inhibiting aspirin regimens.[6] This may explain the substantial residual PGI_2 biosynthesis *in vivo* at daily doses of aspirin in the range of 30–100 mg.[7] Vascular PGI_2 is an important antithrombotic autacoid, as indicated by the prothrombotic phenotype of mice lacking the PGI_2 receptor, and by a meta-analysis of NSAID RCTs demonstrating enhanced risk of myocardial infarction (MI) associated with COX-2 inhibitors,[8] that support the concept of PGI_2 acting as an important mechanism of thromboresistance.[5,9]

Inhibition of COX-1-dependent platelet function can be achieved with low doses (i.e. ≤100 mg) of aspirin given once daily. In contrast, inhibition of COX-2-dependent pathophysiological processes (e.g. hyperalgesia and inflammation) requires larger doses, probably because acetylation is influenced by the oxidative state of the enzyme and is inhibited in cells with a high peroxide tone, and a much shorter dosing interval, because nucleated cells can rapidly resynthesize the enzyme.[3]

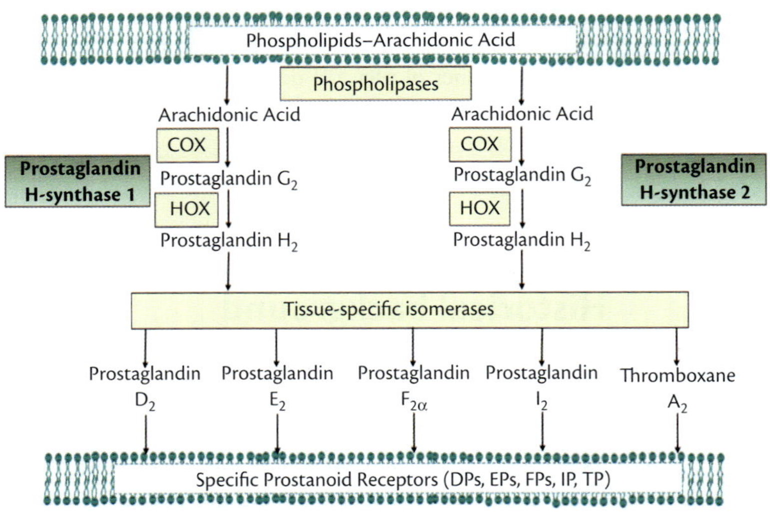

Figure 5.1 Mechanism of action of aspirin. Arachidonic acid, a 20-carbon fatty acid containing four double bonds, is liberated from the sn2 position of membrane phospholipids by several phospholipases, which are activated by chemical, physical, and other stimuli perturbing the cell membrane. Arachidonic acid is converted by the ubiquitous bifunctional enzymes, prostaglandin H-synthase (PGHS)-1 and -2, endowed with both cyclooxygenase (COX) and hydroperoxidase (HOX) activity, to the unstable intermediates PGG_2 and PGH_2. The PGHS-isozymes are colloquially referred to as COX-1 and COX-2. Low-dose aspirin selectively inhibits platelet COX-1, whereas high-dose aspirin inhibits both COX-1 and COX-2. PGH_2, a common intermediate in prostanoid biosynthesis, is converted by tissue-specific isomerases to multiple bioactive PGs and thromboxane (TX)-A_2. These lipid mediators activate specific cell membrane receptors of the superfamily of G protein-coupled receptors, such as the PGD_2 receptors (DPs), the PGE_2 receptors (EPs), the $PGF_{2\alpha}$ receptors (FPs), the prostacyclin (PGI_2) receptor (IP), and the TXA_2 receptor (TP).

Clinical pharmacology of platelet inhibition

Aspirin has a relatively simple pharmacokinetics that does not require metabolic activation by the liver cytochrome P450 (CYP450) isozymes, and thus is not influenced by their genetic polymorphisms nor is susceptible to CYP450-mediated drug–drug interactions. It is rapidly absorbed in the stomach and upper intestine without active transporters, by virtue of its weak acidic properties. Pharmacokinetic parameters, such as Cmax and Tmax, depend on the drug formulation and influence the rate at which inhibition of TXA_2-dependent platelet function becomes measurable, with enteric-coated aspirin requiring up to 4–5 hours to reach a maximum antiplatelet effect.[10] The oral systemic bioavailability of aspirin is approximately 50% over a wide range of doses.[11] A lower bioavailability has been reported for some enteric-coated tablets and sustained-release, microencapsulated preparations.

While aspirin half-life in the human circulation is 15–20 minutes,[10] its antiplatelet effect lasts for the lifespan (7–10 days) of the platelet because of permanent inactivation of COX-1,[12] allowing a once-daily dosing regimen. The pharmacodynamic target of low-dose aspirin is located in two distinct compartments, contributing to its sustained antiplatelet effect: (1) the pre-systemic compartment, in which acetylation of platelet COX-1 occurs during the first encounter of aspirin and platelets in the portal blood, is independent of systemic bioavailability, and is cumulative upon repeated daily dosing[6,11]; and (2) the systemic compartment, in which COX-1 and COX-2 are acetylated in the bone marrow platelet precursors, megakaryocytes, and pre- and proplatelets, whose inhibition is dependent on systemic bioavailability and contributes to long-lasting TXA_2 suppression.[12,13] In fact, new platelets entering the bloodstream from the bone marrow express acetylated COX isozymes during a substantial fraction of the 24-hour dosing interval, explaining the lack of a 10–12% recovery in the capacity to synthesize TXA_2, that would be expected from the platelet renewal rate. The relative selectivity of a low-dose aspirin regimen in targeting TXA_2 synthesis in platelets and their progenitors, while substantially sparing COX-1 activity in nucleated cells capable of replacing the acetylated COX-1 through new protein synthesis (e.g. epithelial cells of the GI mucosa and vascular endothelial cells), is reflected by the similar antithrombotic efficacy and GI safety of low-dose aspirin and a selective antagonist of the TXA_2 receptor (TP), terutroban, in a large randomized phase III trial (PERFORM).[14] These findings also support the current notion that the primary mechanism of action of low-dose aspirin in preventing atherothrombosis and enhancing GI bleeding is related to complete and selective blockade of platelet TXA_2 biosynthesis throughout the 24-hour dosing interval.[3]

With the development and marketing of newer antiplatelet agents, guided by platelet aggregation measurements, a commonly used narrative is that aspirin is a 'weak' antiplatelet agent and that newer $P2Y_{12}$-blockers—such as prasugrel or ticagrelor—are more 'potent' than aspirin.[15] Parenthetically, it should be emphasized that, in contrast to blood pressure, cholesterol, and glucose, platelet aggregation is not a physiological parameter with a range of 'normal' values, but rather a capacity index of what blood platelets can do if challenged *ex vivo* in response to various concentrations of a specific agonist [e.g. adenosine diphosphate (ADP), arachidonic acid, collagen] added to a platelet suspension (➔ Figure 5.2).[1] Therefore, antiplatelet agents cannot be compared for efficacy or potency, except among members of the same drug class working on the same platelet target. A comparative measure of potency of two drugs is the *in vitro* concentration or *in vivo* dose that causes 50% inhibition of a biochemical or functional response, namely their IC_{50} or ID_{50}. Such comparison of potency implies that both drugs share the same molecular target. This is clearly not the case for aspirin and $P2Y_{12}$ blockers, given their distinct molecular targets. As a matter of fact, aspirin is a potent antiplatelet agent, since it acts at low micromolar concentrations *in vitro* and low doses (as low as 30 mg daily) *in vivo* in acetylating platelet COX-1 and suppressing TXA_2 production.[6,10]

Pharmacological effectiveness indicates the maximum degree of activation or inhibition of a specific pharmacological response in a population of treated subjects. From this perspective, aspirin is the most effective inhibitor of platelet COX-1 activity among COX inhibitors, since it virtually completely suppresses platelet COX-1 activity in all compliant subjects. The same is not necessarily true for $P2Y_{12}$ blockers, depending on their individual pharmacokinetic and pharmacodynamic features.[16]

From an historical perspective, it should be mentioned that platelet aggregation measurements guided the choice of the high

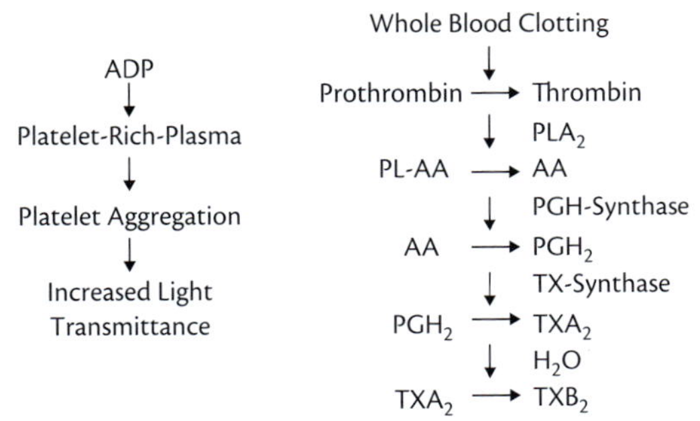

Figure 5.2 Electrical versus immunological signals of platelet activation. The principle of optical platelet aggregometry is shown in the left panel: as platelets aggregate in platelet-rich plasma (PRP), in response to a specific agonist (e.g. ADP), a non-specific electrical signal is generated as a consequence of plasma clearing and the resulting increase in light transmission through PRP.[1] This electrical signal is variably reduced by aspirin, depending on the specific agonist and its concentration, with marked inter- and intraindividual variability.[20] The right panel depicts the chain of enzymatic reactions triggered by endogenously formed thrombin during whole blood clotting. Thromboxane (TX)-A_2 is synthesized by blood platelets in a time- and temperature-dependent fashion, and is hydrolysed non-enzymatically to chemically stable TXB_2, reaching a steady-state concentration in serum after 60 minutes at 37°C.[17] TXB_2 can be easily measured in stored serum by immunoassay.[17] This specific immunological signal is consistently abolished by low concentrations of aspirin *in vitro* or by low-dose aspirin administered *in vivo*.[6,10]

daily doses (1000–1500 mg) used in the early clinical trials of aspirin for the secondary prevention of MI and stroke.[1] Moreover, the same functional measurements were the primary source of a popular (at the time) phenomenon labelled 'aspirin resistance' with over 3000 publications, peaking in 2008 with about 200 PubMed entries, now in the declining phase of the distribution curve.[1,3] In contrast, serum TXB_2 measurements, a highly specific and sensitive index of platelet COX-1 activity (➔ Figure 5.2),[17] were instrumental in (1) defining the dose, duration, and recovery slope of platelet TXA_2 inhibition by aspirin in health and disease[6,18,19]; (2) predicting the optimal dose necessary and sufficient to treat and prevent atherothrombotic complications[2,3]; and (3) demonstrating that the effect of aspirin is variably detected by functional assays, potentially leading to misclassification of 'responder' as 'resistant' phenotypes owing to poor reproducibility of functional measurements.[20]

At variance with the uniform effectiveness of low-dose aspirin in suppressing platelet COX-1 activity in healthy individuals, some clinical conditions are associated with suboptimal platelet inhibition, and variable residual serum TXB_2 levels during the 24-hour dosing interval of low-dose aspirin administration.[21–24] Patients with acute or chronic increase in platelet generation display suboptimal platelet inhibition by the standard aspirin regimen. Thus, aspirin 100 mg once daily does not fully inhibit platelet TXA_2 production in approximately 80% of patients with essential thrombocythaemia.[21] Accelerated platelet turnover is associated with a higher-than-normal fraction of newly released platelets with unacetylated COX-1 and/or COX-2, which accounts for incomplete inhibition as well as partial recovery of TXA_2-dependent platelet function during the 24-hour dosing interval.[21] The recent Aspirin Regimens in Essential Thrombocythemia Study (ARES) phase II trial showed that a twice-daily 100 mg aspirin regimen is superior to the standard once-daily regimen in suppressing platelet TXA_2 production, without inhibiting vascular PGI_2 biosynthesis.[25] Additional studies have consistently shown the superior biochemical efficacy of a shorter dosing interval versus a strategy of maintaining or increasing the once-daily dose of aspirin in a subgroup of patients with type 2 diabetes mellitus,[22] in the early weeks after coronary artery bypass grafting,[23] or in patients presenting with an acute coronary syndrome.[24]

Changes in the systemic bioavailability of the drug, as may occur with some enteric-coated aspirin formulations[26] and in association with obesity, may also impair the extent and duration of platelet TXA_2 suppression by low-dose aspirin.[27] According to the 2018 consensus document of the Working Group on Thrombosis of the European Society of Cardiology, it is reasonable to double the daily dose of aspirin or shorten its dosing interval (twice-daily dosing) in subjects with a body mass index of at least 40 kg/m^2.[28]

Finally, an additional assumption underlying the 'less-is-more' concept, and justifying the design of 'aspirin-free regimens' of antiplatelet therapy,[15] is that $P2Y_{12}$ blockers may inhibit platelet TXA_2 production to the same extent as low-dose aspirin, making the latter unnecessary and potentially harmful, as suggested by a small study in healthy subjects.[29] However, a more comprehensive study showed that neither genetic deficiency nor pharmacological blockade of platelet $P2Y_{12}$ impair the capacity of platelets to synthesize and release TXA_2.[30]

Available clinical evidence indicates that the COX-1/TXA_2 and ADP/$P2Y_{12}$ pathways of platelet activation are non-redundant and equally relevant.[9] The additive effects of inhibiting both pathways in terms of increased ischaemic protection and bleeding risk are consistent with this concept.[16]

Efficacy

The clinical efficacy of aspirin has been evaluated across the spectrum of atherosclerotic cardiovascular disease (ASCVD), from apparently healthy middle-aged subjects to patients presenting with acute MI or acute ischaemic stroke.[3,31,32] For each clinical indication, efficacy was established by one or more placebo-controlled RCTs[3,32] and their individual participant data meta-analyses performed by the Antithrombotic Trialists' Collaboration.[31] These include eight trials in patients with previous MI, ten trials in patients with previous stroke or transient ischaemic attack (TIA), three trials in unstable angina, one trial in chronic stable angina, one trial in suspected acute MI, and two trials in acute ischaemic stroke, totalling over 85,000 patients.[3,31,32] Treatment and follow-up ranged from a few weeks to 50 months. Overall, these RCTs established the following facts: (1) aspirin reduces the risk of a serious vascular event (SVE: non-fatal MI, non-fatal stroke, or vascular death) by about 25%; (2) this figure represents a composite of a one-third reduction in risk of non-fatal MI, one-quarter reduction in non-fatal stroke, and one-sixth reduction in vascular death; and (3) in the setting of an acute MI or ischaemic stroke, aspirin is a life-saving drug.[3,31,32] As shown in ➔ Figure 5.3, among a wide range of patients with ASCVD, in whom the annual risk of a SVE event ranged from 4% to 8%, aspirin prevented approximately 10–20 SVEs for every 1000 patients treated for 1 year.[3] It should be emphasized that these aspirin trials were completed some 30–40 years ago, at a time when other preventive strategies (e.g. statin therapy) and revascularization procedures were in their infancy, and SVE annual rates were at least twice as high as they are today. While this is unlikely to affect the relative risk reduction associated with current aspirin use, it would proportionally reduce the size of the absolute benefit of antiplatelet prophylaxis to about half of the above estimate, that is, five to ten SVEs prevented per 1000 patients treated with aspirin for 1 year, a benefit that clearly outweighs any potential harm in terms of bleeding complications in most patients (➔ Gastrointestinal safety).

Consistent with the clinical efficacy of aspirin being related to saturable molecular processes (i.e. acetylation of platelet COX-1 and consequent suppression of TXA_2 biosynthesis[10,12]) the proportional reduction in SVEs in high-risk trials appeared saturable at low doses.[31] Thus, in trials using daily doses in the range of 75–150 mg, 160–325 mg, and 500–1500 mg, the odds reductions in SVE were 32%, 26%, and 19%, respectively.[31] While any comparison among these trials suffers from the limitations of

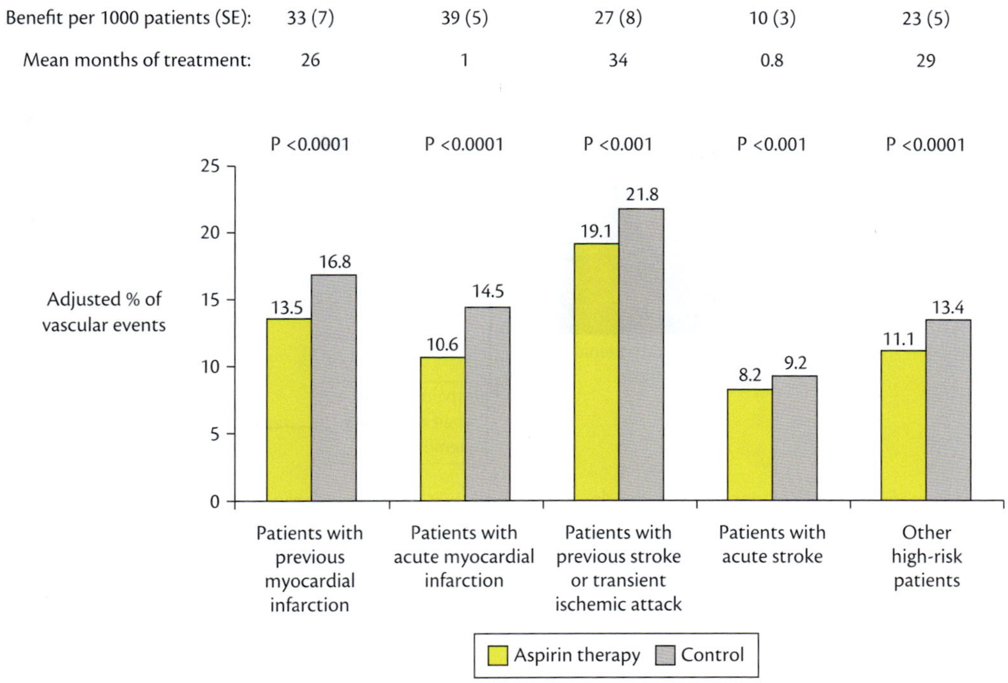

Figure 5.3 Absolute effects of antiplatelet therapy with aspirin on the risk of vascular events (non-fatal myocardial infarction, non-fatal stroke, or death from vascular causes) in five groups of high-risk patients.

Reproduced from Patrono C, García Rodríguez LA, Landolfi R, Baigent C. Low-dose aspirin for the prevention of atherothrombosis. N Engl J Med. 2005 Dec 1;353(22):2373–83. doi: 10.1056/NEJMra052717 with permission from Massachusetts Medical Society.

indirect comparisons, their results are consistent with a limited number of head-to-head randomized trials of low doses (75–100 mg) versus intermediate doses (300–325 mg) in over 40,000 patients with an acute coronary syndrome[33] and stable ASCVD,[34] showing no statistically significant differences in the primary SVE outcome, while reporting a better GI safety profile at lower doses (➔ Gastrointestinal safety).

Over the past 30 years, novel pharmacological strategies were developed targeting different platelet receptors, including oral blockers of glycoprotein IIb/IIIa, TP, and $P2Y_{12}$ receptors, with the aim of achieving superior antithrombotic efficacy versus aspirin in head-to-head phase III/IV RCTs.[16] In particular, three generations of $P2Y_{12}$ blockers were evaluated for superiority in nine RCTs in over 42,000 high-risk patients.[35] These trials were recently synthesized by a tabular data meta-analysis,[35] and the results showed that $P2Y_{12}$-blocker monotherapy is associated with similar risks of death, stroke, and major bleeding, and a marginally lower risk of MI—of borderline statistical significance despite the large number of patients analysed—as compared to aspirin monotherapy.[35]

Overall, there is no convincing evidence that any $P2Y_{12}$ blocker is clinically more effective than aspirin, and this is reflected by the fact that neither clopidogrel nor ticagrelor have a claim of superiority over aspirin approved by regulatory authorities. These clinical findings are mechanistically consistent with the hypothesis that the COX-1/TXA_2 and ADP/$P2Y_{12}$ pathways represent independent and non-redundant amplification mechanisms of platelet activation, that are equally relevant to primary haemostasis and atherothrombosis.[9]

Safety

Gastrointestinal safety

In the meta-analysis of RCTs in high-risk patients carried out by the Antithrombotic Trialists' Collaboration,[31] information was available on 787 major extracranial bleedings in 60 trials recording at least one such bleeding. These were generally defined as haemorrhages that were fatal (approximately 20%) or required transfusion. Overall, the proportional increase in risk of a major extracranial bleed with antiplatelet therapy was about one-half [odds ratio 1.6, 95% confidence interval (CI) 1.4–1.8]. After allowing for non-compliance in the trials, this estimate is compatible with the twofold excess observed in case–control studies.[36]

Aspirin-induced GI toxicity, as assessed in placebo-controlled RCTs, appears to be dose related in the range of 30–1300 mg daily. This is based largely on indirect comparisons of different trials and on a limited number of randomized, direct comparisons of different aspirin doses.[33,34,37] In the Dutch TIA Trial,[37] comparing aspirin 30 mg versus 283 mg daily in 3131 patients with TIA or minor stroke followed over 2.6 years, there were slightly fewer major bleeding complications in the lower-dose group than in the higher-dose group (40 vs 53), and a significantly lower number of minor bleedings [49 vs 84; hazard ratio (HR) 0.58; 95% CI 0.41–0.83]. Fewer patients receiving 30 mg of aspirin reported GI symptoms (164 vs 179) and other adverse effects (73 vs 90).[37] In the CURRENT-OASIS 7 trial,[33] comparing aspirin 75–100 mg versus 300–325 mg daily in 25,086 acute coronary syndrome patients followed for 30 days, the aspirin

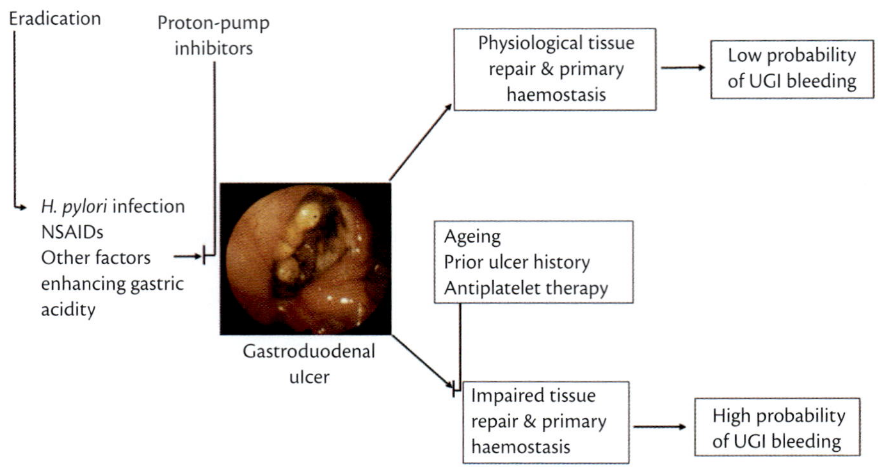

Figure 5.4 Mechanisms of formation and prevention of gastroduodenal ulcers and their bleeding complications. Platelet activation is involved in the physiological processes of tissue repair and primary haemostasis, thus limiting the probability of upper gastrointestinal (UGI) bleeding. Antiplatelet therapy, by impairing tissue repair and primary haemostasis, increases the risk of UGI bleeding, particularly in the elderly and those with prior ulcer history.[3]

dose groups did not differ significantly with respect to major bleeding. There was a nominally significant increase in the incidence of minor bleeding among patients who received higher-dose aspirin (HR 1.13, 95% CI 1.00–1.27; P = 0.04). There was also a small increase in the incidence of major GI bleeding among patients who received higher-dose aspirin, as compared with those who received lower-dose aspirin [47 patients (0.4%) vs 29 patients (0.2%); P = 0.04].[33] In the ADAPTABLE trial,[34] comparing a strategy of 81 mg or 325 mg of aspirin per day in 15,076 patients with ASCVD followed for 26 months, the primary safety outcome of hospitalization for major bleeding with an associated blood product transfusion had very stringent criteria and the overall incidence of events was low (0.6%), with no apparent difference between the two doses. Moreover, the ADAPTABLE investigators did not assess non-serious or minor bleeding adverse events. The fact that patients discontinued the 325 mg more often than the 81 mg dosing strategy, and dose switching was reported by 7% in the 81 mg group and 42% in the 325 mg group, makes interpretation of these findings quite problematic.[34]

A dose–response relationship in aspirin-induced GI toxicity is thought to reflect at least two COX-1-dependent components, that is, dose-dependent inhibition of COX-1 in the GI mucosa and dose-independent inhibition of COX-1 in platelets.[3] That incomplete and transient inhibition of COX-1-derived cytoprotective prostanoids by low-dose aspirin is not sufficient to induce new gastroduodenal ulcers was shown by a relatively large, placebo-controlled, double-blind endoscopic study of aspirin 81 mg in osteoarthritis patients, with repeat endoscopies performed at baseline and after 6 and 12 weeks of treatment.[38] Low-dose aspirin did not significantly increase ulcer incidence versus placebo, in contrast to a positive-control treatment with full-dose ibuprofen which tripled ulcer incidence.[38] Because of the high prevalence of GI mucosal lesions related to concurrent use of NSAIDs and/or *Helicobacter pylori* infection in the general population, it should be expected that any antiplatelet dose of aspirin (and any antiplatelet drug) would cause more bleeding from pre-existing lesions than placebo (➔ Figure 5.4). Consistent with this mechanistic interpretation, the relative risk of hospitalization due to upper GI bleeding and/or perforation associated with low-dose aspirin therapy was comparable to that of other antiplatelet agents in large population-based observational studies.[36] At variance with these observational findings, it has been claimed that clopidogrel is endowed with superior GI safety versus aspirin, largely based on the results of the CAPRIE trial that compared clopidogrel 75 mg daily and aspirin 325 mg daily in 19,185 patients with ASCVD followed for approximately 2 years.[39] The incidence of severe GI haemorrhage was significantly higher in the aspirin group than in the clopidogrel group (0.7 vs 0.5%; P = 0.05). This absolute excess of one severe GI bleeding per 1000 patients per year is likely to be due to the fourfold excess in the daily aspirin dose, as suggested by the aspirin dose comparison in the CURRENT OASIS-7 trial.[33] Consistent with this interpretation, Han et al. recently examined the effects of different antiplatelet regimens on GI mucosal injury by means of a novel magnetically controlled capsule endoscopy system in patients who had undergone percutaneous coronary intervention who were at low bleeding risk, and reported that low-dose aspirin and clopidogrel had similar effects.[40]

Cardiovascular safety

Although the risk of hospitalization due to heart failure was roughly doubled by all traditional NSAID and coxib regimens compared with placebo,[8] such a risk does not appear to be increased by low-dose aspirin therapy. In the two largest contemporary primary prevention trials of low-dose aspirin (100 mg daily) versus placebo, that is, ASCEND[41] (15,480 persons with diabetes mellitus followed for 7.4 years; mean age, 63 years) and ASPREE[42] (19,114 elderly persons followed for 4.7 years; median age, 74 years), the rate of fatal or non-fatal heart failure

Table 5.1 Effects of aspirin assignment on heart failure in recent primary prevention trials

Trial	Aspirin 100 mg	Placebo
ARRIVE*	NA	NA
ASCEND**	95 (1.2%)	113 (1.5%)
ASPREE***	88 (0.9%)	83 (0.9%)

* Any cardiac disorder: 216 (3.4%) versus 266 (4.2%) in aspirin versus placebo groups.
** Fatal or non-fatal heart failure.
*** Hospitalization for heart failure.

and hospitalization for heart failure did not differ to any statistically significant extent (➔ Table 5.1). No specific heart failure data were reported by the third largest primary prevention trial, ARRIVE[43] (12,546 patients at moderate cardiovascular risk followed for 5.0 years, mean age, 64 years), but compared with the placebo group, fewer patients in the aspirin group had at least one cardiac disorder (➔ Table 5.1). The finding that both NSAIDs and coxibs, but not low-dose aspirin, doubled the risk of heart failure causing hospital admission, is consistent with this being a COX-2-dependent hazard that is unrelated to variable platelet COX-1 inhibition, as would be expected from a serious cardiac complication most likely related to the haemodynamic consequences of COX-2 inhibition in the kidney and systemic vasculature.[44]

Cerebrovascular events are associated with cognitive impairment, and thus, low-dose aspirin may well prevent the development of dementia through the avoidance of ischaemic strokes, TIAs, and microinfarcts, but could accelerate cognitive impairment through an increased risk of intracranial haemorrhage and cerebral microbleeds.[45] However, the ASCEND trial reported that a broad dementia outcome occurred in a numerically lower percentage of participants in the aspirin group than in the placebo group: 548 participants (7.1%) versus 598 (7.8%) (rate ratio 0.91, 95% CI 0.81–1.02).[45] A meta-analysis of the effect of randomization to low-dose aspirin on dementia in the ASCEND, ASPREE, and JPAD trials, involving a total of 1,849 dementia cases, yielded a combined rate ratio of 0.92 (95% CI 0.84–1.01; $P = 0.09$),[45] thus excluding any major untoward vascular effect of long-term antiplatelet therapy.

Renal safety and blood pressure control

Low-dose aspirin has not been reported to affect renal function or blood pressure control, consistent with its lack of effect on the renal biosynthesis of prostanoids that derive primarily from constitutively expressed COX-2 in the human kidney (reviewed in reference 46). Moreover, at variance with traditional NSAIDs and coxibs,[46] aspirin 75 mg daily did not affect blood pressure control or the need for antihypertensive therapy in intensively treated hypertensive patients.[47] Similarly, the suggestion that the use of low-dose aspirin is associated with reduced benefit from enalapril and other angiotensin-converting enzyme inhibitors in patients with left ventricular systolic dysfunction is not supported by the results of a large meta-analysis of MI trials.[48]

Aspirin and cancer

Following the original observation of Kune et al.[49] of an association between use of aspirin and reduced risk of colorectal cancer (CRC), a very large body of observational evidence has accumulated confirming this association, with no clear evidence of a dose–effect relationship, and extending the finding to other NSAIDs.[50] A similar protective association has been reported for other digestive tract cancers (oesophagus and stomach),[51] as well as for a number of non-digestive tract cancers (including breast and prostate), though with a smaller effect size.[52] Although the involvement of COX-2-driven cellular events, including a local inflammatory response favouring CRC development and progression, has been established in experimental models of colorectal carcinogenesis, the lack of a dose–response relationship in the apparent chemopreventive effect of aspirin argues against COX-2 being a primary target of aspirin action, given the much higher doses and more frequent dosing required to exert an anti-inflammatory effect.[53] An alternative explanation is based on the hypothesis that platelet activation at sites of colorectal mucosal injury and the consequent release of inflammatory mediators and growth factors drives COX-2 expression and phenotypic changes in adjacent nucleated cells of the intestinal mucosa.[53] This would explain a similar chemopreventive effect exerted by low-dose aspirin acting upstream to downregulate platelet activation and COX-2 inhibitors acting downstream to restrain COX-2-driven events (➔ Figure 5.5). That low-dose aspirin may actually interfere with an early event in colorectal carcinogenesis, that is, the transition from an apparently healthy mucosa to an adenomatous lesion, was later shown by four placebo-controlled RCTs for the secondary prevention of sporadic adenoma recurrence and their meta-analysis, demonstrating a 17% reduction in any adenoma and approximately 30% reduction in advanced lesions.[54] However, the only prospective, randomized evidence for aspirin interfering with the transition to CRC comes from a placebo-controlled RCT in hereditary CRC (Lynch syndrome), with 10-year follow-up and registry-based 20-year data, the Colorectal Adenoma/Carcinoma Prevention Programme (CAPP)-2 study, suggesting a delayed benefit of 35% hazard reduction in adult carriers of a pathogenic mismatch repair gene defect.[55] The delayed protective effect of aspirin against CRC reported in patients with the Lynch syndrome is consistent with the hypothesis that aspirin interferes with an early event in colorectal carcinogenesis, and with similar observations made in post hoc analyses of aspirin trials for cardiovascular prevention[56] and in the prospective assessment of CRC incidence (a secondary endpoint) in the Women's Health Study.[57] The CAPP2 study tested the efficacy and safety of a single dose of aspirin (600 mg daily) and this study provides evidence that this dose was effective in long-term prevention of CRC.[55] However, whether such a high dose is indeed required, and whether this is the optimum aspirin dose to maximize the chemopreventive benefit with an acceptable GI bleeding risk, remains to be determined. To address this issue, the Cancer Prevention Programme (CaPP)-3 study was designed

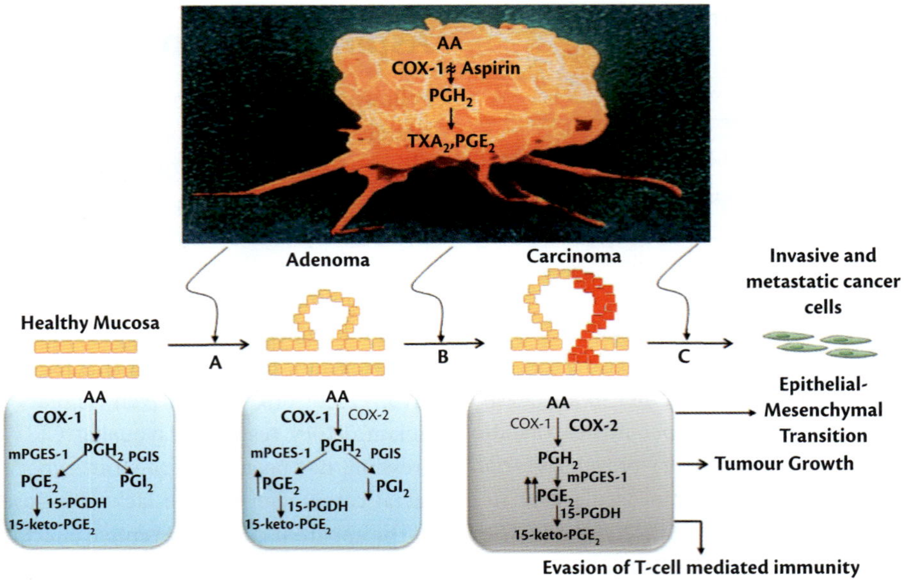

Figure 5.5 The potential role of local platelet activation and inhibition in the early and late stages of colorectal carcinogenesis. Platelet-derived lipid mediators that are inhibited by low-dose aspirin, such as thromboxane (TX)-A_2 and prostaglandin (PG)-E_2, PG-containing oxidized phospholipids, and sphingosine-1-phosphate, may contribute to the crosstalk among platelets, intestinal epithelial cells, cancer cells, and other cells of the colorectal cancer (CRC) microenvironment.[53,58] The proven efficacy of aspirin in reducing the transformation of an apparently healthy colorectal mucosa into an adenomatous lesion,[54] (stage A) and in reducing the risk of development of CRC (stage B) in patients with Lynch syndrome[55] is discussed in the text. The potential role of low-dose aspirin as adjuvant therapy in patients with CRC (stage C) is currently being evaluated by the Add-Aspirin trial.[59]

Reproduced from Patrignani P, Patrono C. Aspirin and Cancer. J Am Coll Cardiol. 2016 Aug 30;68(9):967–76. doi: 10.1016/j.jacc.2016.05.083 with permission from Elsevier.

as a randomized, non-inferiority trial of the 600 mg dose, compared with 300 mg and 100 mg, assigned in a blinded fashion for 2 years followed by open-label treatment for a further 3 years and assessment of Lynch syndrome cancers annually thereafter.[55]

Finally, low-dose aspirin might favourably influence later stages of CRC progression and metastatic spreading, as shown in Figure 5.5.[58] This hypothesis is currently being tested by the Add-Aspirin study, four parallel phase III trials in which approximately 8600 participants who had undergone primary treatment with curative intent for an early-stage common solid tumour (gastro-oesophageal, CRC, breast, prostate) were randomized to receive aspirin 100 mg, aspirin 300 mg, or placebo and are being followed for at least 5 years.[59] Primary outcome data are expected in 2025–2027.

Conclusions and perspective

Aspirin is unique among cardiovascular drugs in being 125 years old and still representing a first choice for the acute treatment and long-term prevention of atherothrombotic events, with consistent IA recommendations in European Society of Cardiology and other cardiovascular guidelines. This is probably due to a series of features: (1) its relatively simple pharmacokinetics and platelet-specific pharmacodynamics make cumulative suppression of TXA_2 biosynthesis a highly predictable phenomenon in the vast majority of compliant patients; (2) the two- to threefold excess of the currently used dose as compared to the lowest daily dose necessary and sufficient to fully inactivate platelet COX-1 activity may accommodate most but extreme interindividual variations in body weight and platelet number; (3) acetylation of COX isozymes in the bone marrow precursors ensures long-lasting suppression of platelet COX-1 activity throughout the dosing interval and limits the consequences of occasionally missed drug intake, except in cases of accelerated platelet turnover; and (4) low-dose aspirin has undergone an unusual paradigm of drug development independent of the pharmaceutical industry, carried out by the medical/scientific community with public funding, and characterized by a large number of phase II dose-finding studies and phase III RCTs, resulting in a very extensive efficacy and safety database for its use as an antiplatelet drug.[2,3]

In looking ahead, several open issues may require further basic and clinical investigation. These include (1) reconsidering the place of aspirin in the primary prevention of atherothrombosis, in light of the (low) current rate of SVEs in the at risk population, availability of alternative preventive measures, as well as the results of an ongoing individual patient data meta-analysis of the 14 RCTs that have evaluated its efficacy and safety in a variety of clinical settings ranging from middle-aged, perfectly healthy subjects to older patients with diabetes mellitus; (2) assessing the role of aspirin in CRC (and other cancer) treatment and prevention, beyond its current use in patients with the Lynch syndrome; and (3) exploiting the analytical tools for precision antiplatelet therapy in those patients characterized by abnormal TXA_2 biosynthesis[60,61] or accelerated renewal of the drug target, as exemplified by the extreme clinical paradigm of essential thrombocythaemia.[25]

What's new

- According to a recent report, based on long-term follow-up of participants in the Framingham Heart Study, systemic TX biosynthesis is an independent risk factor for all-cause and cardiovascular mortality irrespective of aspirin use.
- The totality of the evidence from RCTs is mechanistically consistent with the hypothesis that the COX-1/TXA_2 and ADP/$P2Y_{12}$ pathways represent independent and non-redundant amplification mechanisms of platelet activation and aggregation, that are equally relevant to primary haemostasis and atherothrombosis.
- Recent phase II trials and *in silico* modelling demonstrate the relevance of platelet turnover and body weight in modifying the antiplatelet pharmacodynamics of aspirin.
- Based on a large study with repeated magnetically controlled capsule endoscopy after percutaneous coronary intervention, in patients without GI ulcers or bleeding after 6 months of dual antiplatelet therapy, monotherapy with either aspirin or clopidogrel for additional 6 months resulted in a lower risk of GI mucosal injury compared with dual antiplatelet therapy through 12 months, with low-dose aspirin and clopidogrel causing similar lesions on the GI mucosa.
- Based on a recent meta-analysis of three primary prevention trials in older subjects, long-term treatment with low-dose aspirin is not associated with increased risk of dementia, and in fact a mild protective effect cannot be excluded.

Guideline recommendations

- Specific recommendations on the use of aspirin for the prevention of atherothrombosis in different clinical settings are covered by the individual disease-oriented chapters in this textbook.

What's next

- Analytical tools are available for precision antiplatelet therapy in those patients characterized by very high TXA_2 biosynthesis, accelerated renewal of the drug target, or severe obesity.
- The benefit/risk profile of low-dose aspirin for primary prevention in patients with biomarkers of or documented atherosclerotic vascular disease needs to be assessed. An ongoing trial is evaluating the impact of primary cardiovascular prevention with low-dose aspirin in patients with chronic kidney disease, a powerful risk factor for SVEs.
- Randomized, placebo-controlled clinical trials are ongoing to test the efficacy and safety of low-dose aspirin as adjuvant therapy in several types of solid cancer and for the prevention of CRC in patients with Lynch syndrome.

Drug dosing

- The standard maintenance dose of aspirin is 75–100 mg once daily, independent of the clinical setting.
- In aspirin-naïve patients experiencing an acute coronary syndrome, a single oral loading dose of 160–325 mg (to be reduced by half, if given intravenously) is indicated to ensure maximal suppression of platelet COX-1 activity on the first day of therapy.
- The use of a personalized, biomarker-guided, twice-daily regimen of low-dose aspirin should be considered experimental, in the absence of clinical evidence for its efficacy and safety.

References

1. Born G, Patrono C. Antiplatelet drugs. Br J Pharmacol. 2006;147 Suppl 1:S241–51.
2. Patrono C. Aspirin as an antiplatelet drug. N Engl J Med. 1994;330:1287–94.
3. Patrono C, Garcia Rodriguez LA, Landolfi R, Baigent C. Low-dose aspirin for the prevention of atherothrombosis. N Engl J Med. 2005;353:2373–83.
4. Smith WL, Malkowski MG. Interactions of fatty acids, nonsteroidal anti-inflammatory drugs, and coxibs with the catalytic and allosteric subunits of cyclooxygenases-1 and -2. J Biol Chem. 2019;294:1697–705.
5. Badimon L, Vilahur G, Rocca B, Patrono C. The key contribution of platelet and vascular arachidonic acid metabolism to the pathophysiology of atherothrombosis. Cardiovasc Res. 2021;117:2001–15.
6. Patrignani P, Filabozzi P, Patrono C. Selective cumulative inhibition of platelet thromboxane production by low-dose aspirin in healthy subjects. J Clin Invest. 1982;69:1366–72.
7. FitzGerald GA, Oates JA, Hawiger J, et al. Endogenous biosynthesis of prostacyclin and thromboxane and platelet function during chronic administration of aspirin in man. J Clin Invest. 1983;71:676–88.
8. Coxib and traditional NSAID Trialists' (CNT) Collaboration. Vascular and upper gastrointestinal effects of non-steroidal anti-inflammatory drugs: meta-analyses of individual participant data from randomised trials. Lancet. 2013;382:769–79.
9. Davì G, Patrono C. Platelet activation and atherothrombosis. N Engl J Med. 2007;357:2482–94.
10. Patrignani P, Tacconelli S, Piazuelo E, et al. Reappraisal of the clinical pharmacology of low-dose aspirin by comparing novel direct and traditional indirect biomarkers of drug action. J Thromb Haemost. 2014;12:1320–30.
11. Pedersen AK, FitzGerald GA. Dose-related kinetics of aspirin. Presystemic acetylation of platelet cyclooxygenase. N Engl J Med. 1984;311:1206–11.
12. Burch JW, Stanford N, Majerus PW. Inhibition of platelet prostaglandin synthetase by oral aspirin. J Clin Invest. 1978;61:314–19.
13. Patrono C, Ciabattoni G, Patrignani P, et al. Clinical pharmacology of platelet cyclooxygenase inhibition. Circulation. 1985;72:1177–84.
14. Bousser MG, Amarenco P, Chamorro A, et al. Terutroban versus aspirin in patients with cerebral ischaemic events (PERFORM): a randomised, double-blind, parallel-group trial. Lancet. 2011;377:2013–22.

15. Capodanno D, Mehran R, Valgimigli M, et al. Aspirin-free strategies in cardiovascular disease and cardioembolic stroke prevention. Nat Rev Cardiol. 2018;15:480–96.
16. Patrono C, Morais J, Baigent C, et al. Antiplatelet agents for the treatment and prevention of coronary atherothrombosis. J Am Coll Cardiol. 2017;70:1760–76.
17. Patrono C, Ciabattoni G, Pinca E, et al. Low dose aspirin and inhibition of thromboxane B2 production in healthy subjects. Thromb Res. 1980;17:317–27.
18. De Caterina R, Giannessi D, Bernini W, et al. Low-dose aspirin in patients recovering from myocardial infarction. Evidence for a selective inhibition of thromboxane-related platelet function. Eur Heart J. 1985;6:409–17.
19. Patrono C, Rocca B, De Stefano V. Platelet activation and inhibition in polycythemia vera and essential thrombocythemia. Blood. 2013;121:1701–11.
20. Santilli F, Rocca B, De Cristofaro R, et al. Platelet cyclooxygenase inhibition by low-dose aspirin is not reflected consistently by platelet function assays: implications for aspirin 'resistance'. J Am Coll Cardiol. 2009;53:667–77.
21. Pascale S, Petrucci G, Dragani A, et al. Aspirin-insensitive thromboxane biosynthesis in essential thrombocythemia is explained by accelerated renewal of the drug target. Blood. 2012;119: 3595–603.
22. Rocca B, Santilli F, Pitocco D, et al. The recovery of platelet cyclooxygenase activity explains interindividual variability in responsiveness to low-dose aspirin in patients with and without diabetes. J Thromb Haemost. 2012;10:1220–30.
23. Cavalca V, Rocca B, Veglia F, et al. On-pump cardiac surgery enhances platelet renewal and impairs aspirin pharmacodynamics: effects of improved dosing regimens. Clin Pharmacol Ther. 2017;102:849–58.
24. Parker WAE, Orme RC, Hanson J, et al. Very-low-dose twice-daily aspirin maintains platelet inhibition and improves haemostasis during dual-antiplatelet therapy for acute coronary syndrome. Platelets. 2019;30:148–57.
25. Rocca B, Tosetto A, Betti S, et al. A randomized double-blind trial of 3 aspirin regimens to optimize antiplatelet therapy in essential thrombocythemia. Blood. 2020;136:171–82.
26. Maree AO, Curtin RJ, Dooley M, et al. Platelet response to low-dose enteric-coated aspirin in patients with stable cardiovascular disease. J Am Coll Cardiol. 2005;46:1258–63.
27. Petrucci G, Zaccardi F, Giaretta A, et al. Obesity is associated with impaired responsiveness to once-daily low-dose aspirin and in vivo platelet activation. J Thromb Haemost. 2019;17:885–95.
28. Rocca B, Fox KAA, Ajjan RA, et al. Antithrombotic therapy and body mass: an expert position paper of the ESC Working Group on Thrombosis. Eur Heart J. 2018;39:1672–86.
29. Armstrong PC, Dhanji AR,Tucker AT, Mitchell JA, Warner TD. Reduction of platelet thromboxane A2 production ex vivo and in vivo by clopidogrel therapy. J Thromb Haemost. 2010;8:613–15.
30. Scavone M, Femia EA, Caroppo V, Cattaneo M. Inhibition of the platelet P2Y12 receptor for adenosine diphosphate does not impair the capacity of platelet to synthesize thromboxane A2. Eur Heart J. 2016;37:3347–56.
31. Antithrombotic Trialists Collaboration. Collaborative meta-analysis of randomised trials of antiplatelet therapy for prevention of death, myocardial infarction, and stroke in high risk patients. BMJ. 2002;324:71–86.
32. Patrono C, Baigent C, Hirsh J, Roth G. Antiplatelet drugs: American College of Chest Physicians Evidence-Based Clinical Practice Guidelines (8th Edition). Chest. 2008;133:199S–233S.
33. CURRENT-OASIS 7 Investigators, Mehta SR, Bassand JP, et al. Dose comparisons of clopidogrel and aspirin in acute coronary syndromes. N Engl J Med. 2010;363:930–42.
34. Jones WS, Mulder H, Wruck LM, et al. Comparative effectiveness of aspirin dosing in cardiovascular disease. N Engl J Med. 2021;384:1981–90.
35. Chiarito M, Sanz-Sanchez J, Cannata F, et al. Monotherapy with a P2Y12 inhibitor or aspirin for secondary prevention in patients with established atherosclerosis: a systematic review and meta-analysis. Lancet. 2020;395:1487–95.
36. Garcia Rodriguez LA, Lin KJ, Hernandez-Diaz S, Johansson S. Risk of upper gastrointestinal bleeding with low-dose acetylsalicylic acid alone and in combination with clopidogrel and other medications. Circulation. 2011;123:1108–15.
37. Dutch TIA Trial Study Group; van Gijn J, Algra A, Kappelle J, Koudstaal PJ, van Latum A. A comparison of two doses of aspirin (30 mg vs. 283 mg a day) in patients after a transient ischemic attack or minor ischemic stroke. N Engl J Med. 1991;325:1261–6.
38. Laine L, Maller ES, Yu C, Quan H, Simon T. Ulcer formation with low-dose enteric-coated aspirin and the effect of COX-2 selective inhibition: a double-blind trial. Gastroenterology. 2004;127:395–402.
39. CAPRIE Steering Committee. A randomised, blinded, trial of clopidogrel versus aspirin in patients at risk of ischaemic events (CAPRIE). Lancet. 1996;348:1329–39.
40. Han Y, Liao Z, Li Y, et al. Magnetically controlled capsule endoscopy for assessment of antiplatelet therapy-induced gastrointestinal injury. J Am Coll Cardiol. 2022;79:116–28.
41. The ASCEND Study Collaborative Group. Effects of aspirin for primary prevention in persons with diabetes mellitus. N Engl J Med. 2018;379:1529–39.
42. McNeil JJ, Wolfe R, Woods RL, et al. Effect of aspirin on cardiovascular events and bleeding in the healthy elderly. N Engl J Med. 2018;379:1509–18.
43. Gaziano JM, Brotons C, Coppolecchia R, et al. Use of aspirin to reduce risk of initial vascular events in patients at moderate risk of cardiovascular disease (ARRIVE): a randomised, double-blind, placebo-controlled trial. Lancet. 2018;392:1036–46.
44. Patrono C. Cardiovascular effects of cyclooxygenase-2 inhibitors: a mechanistic and clinical perspective. Br J Clin Pharmacol. 2016;82:957–64.
45. Parish S, Mafham M, Offer A, et al. Effects of aspirin on dementia and cognitive function in diabetic patients: the ASCEND trial. Eur Heart J. 2022;43:2010–19.
46. FitzGerald GA, Patrono C. The coxibs, selective inhibitors of cyclooxygenase-2. N Engl J Med. 2001;345:433–42.
47. Hansson L, Zanchetti A, Carruthers SG, et al. Effects of intensive blood-pressure lowering and low-dose aspirin in patients with hypertension: principal results of the Hypertension Optimal Treatment (HOT) randomised trial. HOT Study Group. Lancet. 1998;351:1755–62.
48. Latini R, Tognoni G, Maggioni AP, et al. Clinical effects of early angiotensin-converting enzyme inhibitor treatment for acute myocardial infarction are similar in the presence and absence of aspirin: systematic overview of individual data from 96,712 randomized patients. Angiotensin-converting Enzyme Inhibitor Myocardial Infarction Collaborative Group. J Am Coll Cardiol. 2000;35:1801–7.
49. Kune GA, Kune S, Watson LF. Colorectal cancer risk, chronic illnesses, operations, and medications: case control results from the Melbourne Colorectal Cancer Study. Cancer Res. 1988;48:4399–404.

50. Thun MJ, Henley SJ, Patrono C. Nonsteroidal anti-inflammatory drugs as anticancer agents: mechanistic, pharmacologic, and clinical issues. J Natl Cancer Inst. 2002;94:252–66.
51. Bosetti C, Santucci C, Gallus S, Martinetti M, La Vecchia C. Aspirin and the risk of colorectal and other digestive tract cancers: an updated meta-analysis through 2019. Ann Oncol. 2020;31:558–68.
52. Santucci C, Gallus S, Martinetti M, La Vecchia C, Bosetti C. Aspirin and the risk of nondigestive tract cancers: an updated meta-analysis to 2019. Int J Cancer. 2021;148:1372–82.
53. Patrono C, Patrignani P, Garcia Rodriguez LA. Cyclooxygenase-selective inhibition of prostanoid formation: transducing biochemical selectivity into clinical read-outs. J Clin Invest. 2001;108:7–13.
54. Cole BF, Logan RF, Halabi S, et al. Aspirin for the chemoprevention of colorectal adenomas: meta-analysis of the randomized trials. J Natl Cancer Inst. 2009;101:256–66.
55. Burn J, Sheth H, Elliott F, et al. Cancer prevention with aspirin in hereditary colorectal cancer (Lynch syndrome), 10-year follow-up and registry-based 20-year data in the CAPP2 study: a double-blind, randomised, placebo-controlled trial. Lancet. 2020;395:1855–63.
56. Rothwell PM, Wilson M, Elwin CE, et al. Long-term effect of aspirin on colorectal cancer incidence and mortality: 20-year follow-up of five randomised trials. Lancet. 2010;376:1741–50.
57. Cook NR, Lee IM, Zhang SM, Moorthy MV, Buring JE. Alternate-day, low-dose aspirin and cancer risk: long-term observational follow-up of a randomized trial. Ann Intern Med. 2013;159:77–85.
58. Patrignani P, Patrono C. Aspirin and cancer. J Am Coll Cardiol. 2016;68:967–76.
59. Joharatnam-Hogan N, Cafferty F, Hubner R, et al. Aspirin as an adjuvant treatment for cancer: feasibility results from the Add-Aspirin randomised trial. Lancet Gastroenterol Hepatol. 2019;4:854–62.
60. Patrono C, Rocca B. Measurement of thromboxane biosynthesis in health and disease. Front Pharmacol. 2019;10:1244.
61. Rade JJ, Barton BA, Vasan RS, et al. Association of thromboxane generation with survival in aspirin users and nonusers. J Am Coll Cardiol. 2022;80:233–50.

CHAPTER 6

Platelet $P2Y_{12}$ inhibitors

Manan Pareek and Deepak L. Bhatt

Contents

Summary

Adenosine diphosphate $P2Y_{12}$ receptor antagonists inhibit platelet activation and subsequent aggregation. These agents may be used either alone or as part of dual antiplatelet therapy regimens with aspirin. $P2Y_{12}$ inhibitors have proven useful in the treatment and prevention of several atherosclerotic cardiovascular conditions, including coronary, cerebrovascular, and peripheral artery disease. While clopidogrel served as the principal $P2Y_{12}$ inhibitor for a decade, the more potent agents, prasugrel and ticagrelor, are now preferred in many settings, particularly in patients with an acute coronary syndrome. This chapter summarizes the main pharmacological properties of contemporary oral and intravenous $P2Y_{12}$ inhibitors, and the major randomized controlled trials related to their clinical indications.

Introduction

Platelets play a central role in thrombus formation. Although aspirin remains a cornerstone in the treatment and prevention of thrombotic events through inhibition of the cyclooxygenase-1 enzyme, its variable efficacy and the existence of alternate pathways of platelet activation and aggregation have led to the development of complementary platelet inhibitors that may be used either alone or in combination with aspirin. Adenosine diphosphate (ADP) $P2Y_{12}$ receptor antagonists inhibit platelet activation and subsequent aggregation and have proven useful in the treatment of several atherosclerotic cardiovascular conditions.

The $P2Y_{12}$ receptor

ADP is secreted from storage granules upon platelet activation (➔ Figure 6.1). In turn, it stimulates purinergic, G protein-coupled, P2 receptors ($P2X_1$, $P2Y_1$, and $P2Y_{12}$) on the platelet surface (➔ Figure 6.2). Although the G_i-coupled $P2Y_{12}$ receptor plays the most significant role in platelet activation, a complete platelet response requires concomitant activation of the G_q-coupled $P2Y_1$ receptor. $P2Y_1$ receptor activation causes intracellular

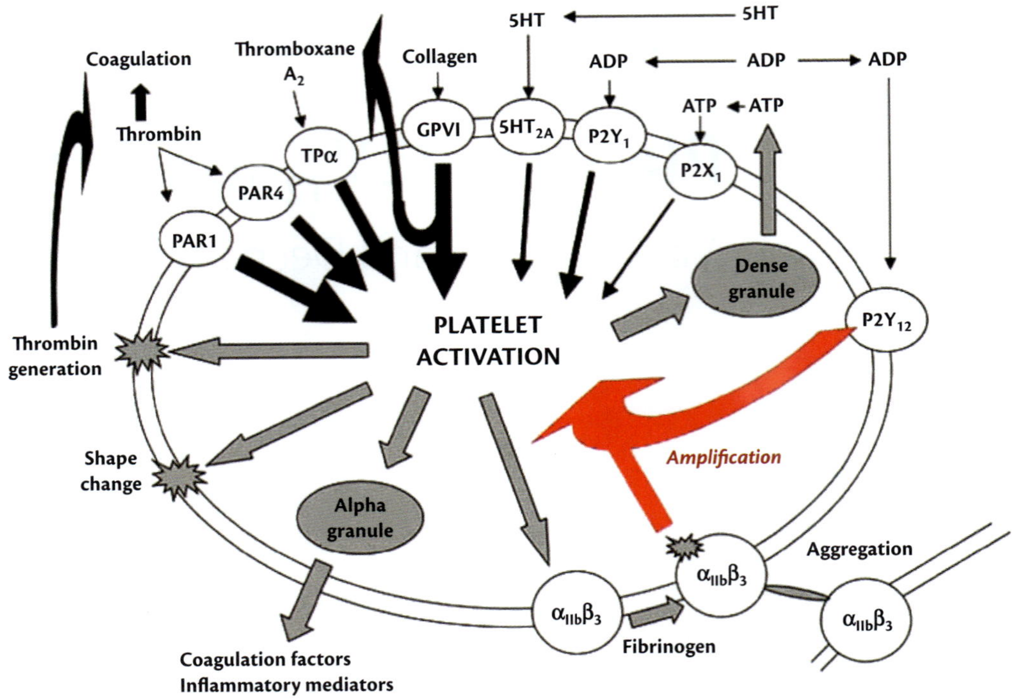

Figure 6.1 Platelet activation mechanisms.[3] 5HT, 5-hydroxytryptamine (serotonin); ADP, adenosine diphosphate; ATP, adenosine triphosphate.
Storey RF. Biology and pharmacology of the platelet P2Y12 receptor. Curr Pharm Des. 2006;12(10):1255–9. doi: 10.2174/138161206776361318

calcium mobilization, platelet shape change, and transient platelet aggregation whereas $P2Y_{12}$ receptor activation decreases intracellular cyclic adenosine monophosphate concentration through inhibition of adenylyl cyclase which helps sustain calcium mobilization. This potentiates downstream platelet aggregation by stimulation of the glycoprotein IIb/IIIa receptor and production of thromboxane.[1–4]

Thienopyridine and non-thienopyridine $P2Y_{12}$ inhibitors

$P2Y_{12}$ receptor antagonists are broadly divided into thienopyridine (ticlopidine, clopidogrel, and prasugrel) and non-thienopyridine agents (ticagrelor, elinogrel, cangrelor, and selatogrel).

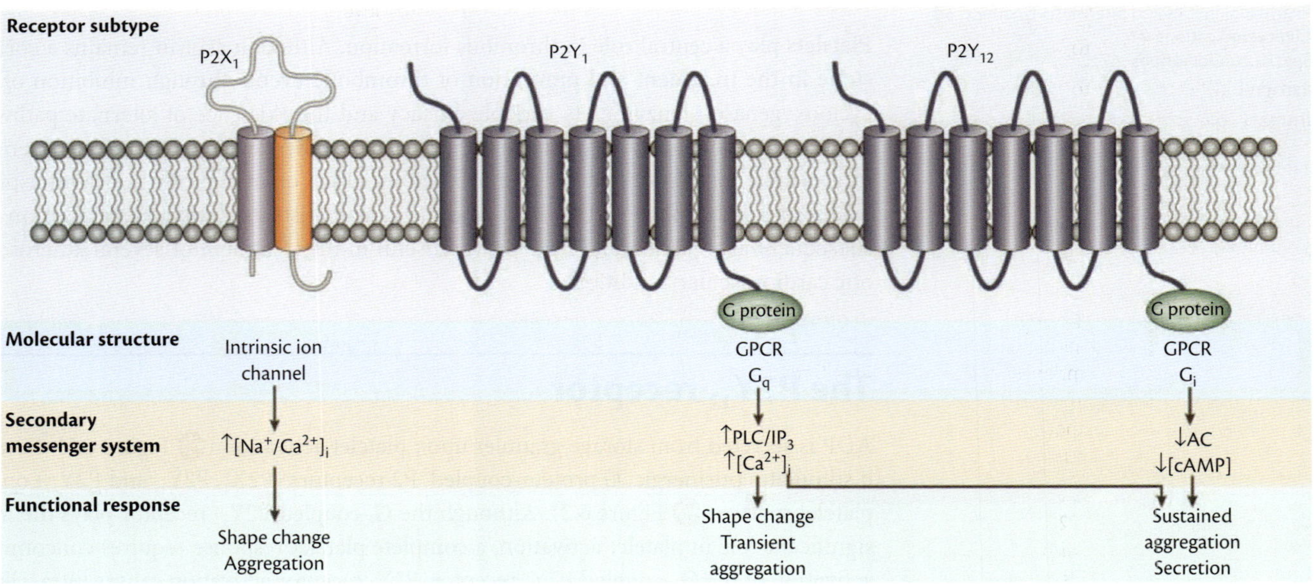

Figure 6.2 Subtypes of adenosine diphosphate receptors.[2] AC, adenylyl cyclase; cAMP, cyclic adenosine monophosphate; GPCR, G protein-coupled receptors; PLC, phospholipase C.
Bhatt DL, Topol EJ. Scientific and therapeutic advances in antiplatelet therapy. Nat Rev Drug Discov. 2003 Jan;2(1):15–28. doi: 10.1038/nrd985

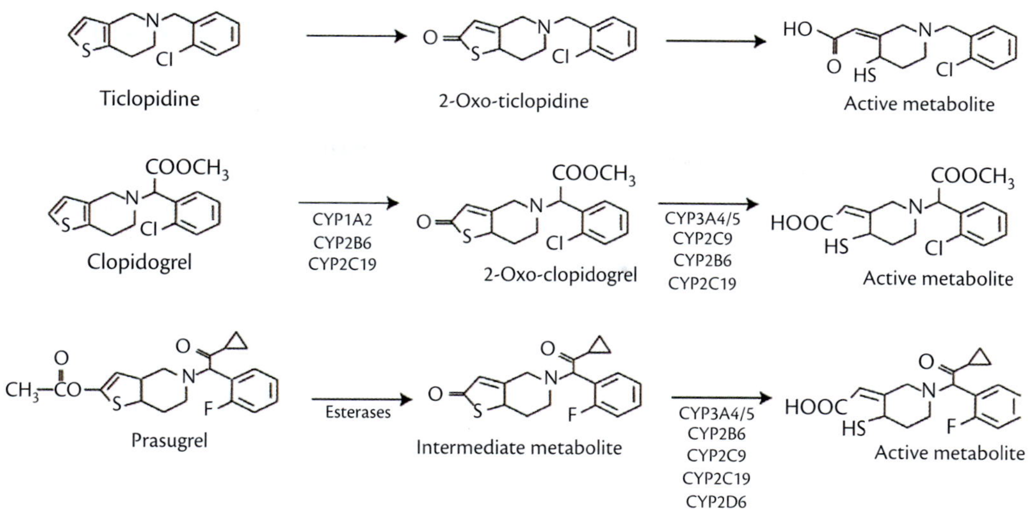

Figure 6.3 Activation of clopidogrel and prasugrel.[4]

Wallentin L. P2Y(12) inhibitors: differences in properties and mechanisms of action and potential consequences for clinical use. Eur Heart J. 2009 Aug;30(16):1964–77. doi: 10.1093/eurheartj/ehp296

Thienopyridines are prodrugs with no *in vitro* activity and require biotransformation by the hepatic cytochrome P450 (CYP) system (➔ Figure 6.3).[4,5] The resulting active metabolites irreversibly block the $P2Y_{12}$ receptor through covalent binding, leading to inhibition of ADP-induced platelet activation and aggregation. Conversely, non-thienopyridines are direct-acting agents that reversibly inhibit the $P2Y_{12}$ receptor.[4] The main pharmacological properties of contemporary $P2Y_{12}$ inhibitors are shown in ➔ Table 6.1.

Table 6.1 Main pharmacological properties of $P2Y_{12}$ inhibitors

	Clopidogrel	Prasugrel	Ticagrelor	Cangrelor
Drug class	Thienopyridine	Thienopyridine	Cyclopentyltriazolopyrimidine	ATP analogue
Administration	Oral	Oral	Oral	Intravenous
Bioactivation	Pro-drug, CYP-dependent, two steps	Pro-drug, CYP-dependent, one step	No	No
Reversibility	Irreversible	Irreversible	Reversible	Reversible
$P2Y_{12}$ receptor binding	Competitive	Competitive	Allosteric, non-competitive	Competitive
Onset of effect	2 to 6 hours	30 minutes to 4 hours	30 minutes to 2 hours	2 minutes
Time to peak effect	6 to 12 hours	2 hours	2 hours	2 to 30 minutes
Half-life	7 to 8 hours	7 to 8 hours	7 to 12 hours	3 to 6 minutes
Duration of effect	3 to 10 days	5 to 10 days	3 to 4 days	30 to 60 minutes
Clearance	Renal and biliary	Renal	Biliary	Plasma
Discontinue prior to surgery	5 days	7 days	5 days	1 to 6 hours
Major contraindications	Hypersensitivity to clopidogrel or any component of the formulation, active pathological bleeding, severe hepatic impairment (EMA)	Hypersensitivity to ticagrelor or any component of the formulation, active pathological bleeding, prior stroke or transient ischemic attack, severe hepatic impairment (EMA)	Hypersensitivity to prasugrel or any component of the formulation, active pathological bleeding, prior intracranial hemorrhage, severe hepatic impairment (EMA), coadministration with strong CYP3A4 inhibitors (EMA)	Hypersensitivity to cangrelor or any component of the formulation, prior stroke or transient ischemic attack (EMA), active pathological bleeding
Major interactions	CYP2C19 inducers, opioids, NSAIDs, warfarin, SSRIs, SNRIs, repaglinide	Opioids	Strong CYP3A inhibitors or inducers, opioids, simvastatin, lovastatin, digoxin	Thienopyridines

ATP, adenosine triphosphate; CYP, cytochrome P450; EMA, European Medicines Agency; NSAIDs, non-steroidal anti-inflammatory drugs; SNRIs, serotonin norepinephrine reuptake inhibitors; SSRIs, selective serotonin reuptake inhibitors.

Data from [4,43,44,57,58,97,98,105–109]

Ticlopidine

Ticlopidine was first approved for medical use in 1978. It was initially marketed for very specific settings in which platelet interaction with artificial surfaces may lead to thrombotic complications like cardiac surgery with extracorporeal circulation or haemodialysis.[6] Only later were its effects in patients with manifest vascular disease, including those undergoing percutaneous coronary intervention (PCI) with stent placement, evaluated.[7–10] However, because of delayed onset of action and haematological side effects like neutropenia and thrombotic thrombocytopenic purpura, its use is no longer recommended.[11,12]

Clopidogrel

Because of its superior safety and efficacy compared with ticlopidine, clopidogrel quickly became the preferred $P2Y_{12}$ inhibitor after its global launch in 1998.[6] Indeed, a meta-analysis of randomized and registry-based comparisons of clopidogrel and ticlopidine reported a significantly lower 30-day rate of both major adverse cardiac events [2.1% vs 4.0%, adjusted odds ratio (OR) 0.72, 95% confidence interval (CI) 0.59–0.89; P = 0.002] and death (0.5% vs 1.1%, adjusted OR 0.55, 95% CI 0.37–0.82; P = 0.003) with clopidogrel.[13]

Pharmacokinetics and pharmacodynamics

Clopidogrel is structurally related to ticlopidine, differing only by one additional methyl group.[5] Eighty-five per cent of clopidogrel is metabolized by circulating esterases to an inactive carboxylic acid derivate, and only one metabolite, H4, is metabolically active.[14] The metabolization of clopidogrel into the active metabolite is a two-step process for which particularly CYP2C19 is responsible for the first step and CYP2C19 and CYP3A4 for the second step. H4 likely blocks the $P2Y_{12}$ receptor through formation of a disulfide bridge between the reactive thiol group of the active metabolite and a cysteine residue of the $P2Y_{12}$ receptor.[15] Maximal platelet inhibition is achieved more rapidly by using a loading dose, with a 600 mg dose capable of resulting in faster and more pronounced effects than a 300 mg dose (➔ Figure 6.4).[16,17]

Clinical indications

Acute coronary syndrome

The Clopidogrel versus Aspirin in Patients at Risk of Ischemic Events (CAPRIE) trial tested the utility of clopidogrel monotherapy by randomizing 19,185 patients with recent ischaemic stroke, recent myocardial infarction (MI), or symptomatic peripheral artery disease to clopidogrel 75 mg once daily or aspirin 325 mg once daily for a mean of 1.9 years.[18] The composite of ischaemic stroke, MI, or vascular death was significantly reduced in

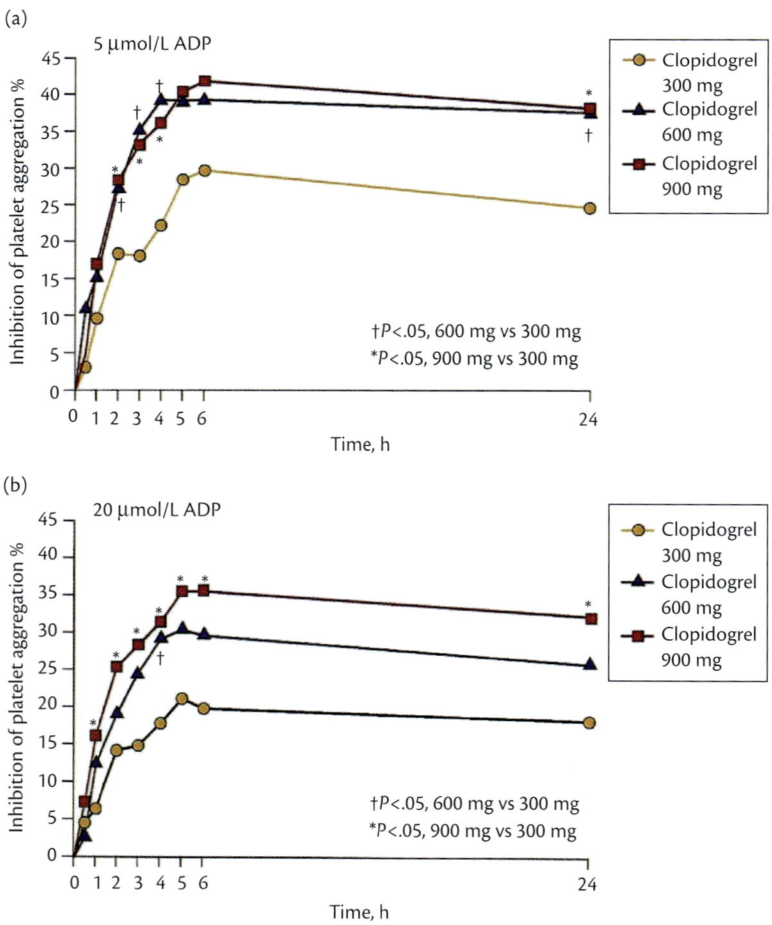

Figure 6.4 Percentage platelet inhibition with different loading doses of clopidogrel.[16] (a) Percentage inhibition of platelet aggregation after stimulation with 5 µmol/L adenosine diphosphate (ADP). (b) Percentage inhibition of platelet aggregation after stimulation with 20 µmol/L ADP.

Montalescot G, Sideris G, Meuleman C, et al.; ALBION Trial Investigators. A randomized comparison of high clopidogrel loading doses in patients with non-ST-segment elevation acute coronary syndromes: the ALBION (Assessment of the Best Loading Dose of Clopidogrel to Blunt Platelet Activation, Inflammation and Ongoing Necrosis) trial. J Am Coll Cardiol. 2006 Sep 5;48(5):931–8. doi: 10.1016/j.jacc.2006.04.090

Table 6.2 Major trials of P2Y$_{12}$ inhibitors in patients with acute and chronic coronary syndrome

Study	Intervention	Control	Key inclusion criteria	Sample size	Primary endpoint (intervention versus control)	Major bleeding (intervention versus control)
Acute coronary syndrome						
CURE[20]	Clopidogrel	Placebo	Age >18 years NSTE-ACS	12,562	Cardiovascular death, MI, or stroke: RR 0.80, 95% CI 0.72–0.90; P <0.001	RR 1.38, 95% CI 1.13–1.67; P = 0.001
TRITON–TIMI 38[50]	Prasugrel	Clopidogrel	Age ≥18 years STEMI or NSTE-ACS with planned PCI	13,608	Death from cardiovascular causes, MI, or stroke: HR 0.81, 95% CI 0.73–0.90; P <0.001	HR 1.32, 95% CI 1.03–1.68; P = 0.03
PLATO[64]	Ticagrelor	Clopidogrel	Age ≥18 years STEMI with planned PCI or NSTE-ACS	18,624	Death from vascular causes, MI, or stroke: HR 0.84, 95% CI 0.77–0.92; P <0.001	HR 1.04, 95% CI 0.95–1.13; P = 0.43
ISAR-REACT 5[71]	Ticagrelor	Prasugrel	Age ≥18 years STEMI or NSTE-ACS with planned invasive evaluation	4018	Death, MI, or stroke: HR 1.36, 95% CI 1.09–1.70; P = 0.006	HR 1.12, 95% CI 0.83–1.51; P = 0.46
Chronic coronary syndrome						
THEMIS[75]	Ticagrelor	Placebo	Age ≥50 years Stable coronary artery disease Type 2 diabetes	19,220	Cardiovascular death, MI, or stroke: HR 0.90, 95% CI 0.81–0.99; P = 0.04	HR 2.32, 95% CI 1.82–2.94; P <0.001
Acute or chronic coronary syndrome						
CHAMPION PHOENIX[95]	Cangrelor	Clopidogrel	Age ≥18 years Stable angina, STEMI, or NSTE-ACS undergoing PCI	11,145	Death, MI, ischaemia-driven revascularization, or stent thrombosis: adjusted OR 0.78, 95% CI 0.66–0.93; P = 0.005	Adjusted OR 1.50, 95% CI 0.53–4.22; P = 0.44

CI, confidence interval; HR, hazard ratio; MI, myocardial infarction; NSTE-ACS, non-ST-segment elevation acute coronary syndrome; OR, odds ratio; PCI, percutaneous coronary intervention; RR, relative risk; STEMI, ST-segment elevation myocardial infarction.

the clopidogrel group [annual risk 5.3% vs 5.8%, relative risk (RR) reduction 8.7%, 95% CI 0.3–16.5; P = 0.04], without any major differences in safety. Interestingly, when only considering individuals with a recent MI, clopidogrel was not associated with a reduction in composite ischaemic events (annual risk 5.0% vs 4.8%, RR increase 3.7%, 95% CI 22.1 to −12.0; P = 0.66; P-interaction = 0.04). In contrast, in the South Korean HOST-EXtended Antiplatelet Monotherapy (HOST-EXAM) trial, clopidogrel versus aspirin monotherapy during the chronic maintenance period after PCI [73% with an acute coronary syndrome (ACS)] was associated with net clinical benefit.[19]

The Clopidogrel in Unstable Angina to Prevent Recurrent Events (CURE) trial laid the foundation for long-term dual antiplatelet therapy (DAPT) in patients with a non-ST-segment-elevation ACS (n = 12,562) (➔ Table 6.2). Study participants were randomized to clopidogrel (300 mg immediately, followed by 75 mg once daily) or placebo, on top of aspirin (75–325 mg once daily), for a mean of 9 months.[20] The 1-year rate of cardiovascular death, MI, or stroke was significantly lower (9.3% vs 11.4%, RR 0.80, 95% CI 0.72–0.90; P <0.001), while the rate of major bleeding was significantly higher (3.7% vs 2.7%, RR 1.38, 95% CI 1.13–1.67; P = 0.001), with clopidogrel (➔ Figures 6.5 and 6.6). Importantly, fatal bleeding and haemorrhagic stroke were not increased in the DAPT group. In 2658 patients who underwent PCI, the composite of cardiovascular death, MI, or urgent target-vessel revascularization within 30 days of PCI was significantly reduced with clopidogrel (4.5% vs 6.4%, RR 0.70, 95% CI 0.50–0.97; P = 0.03).[21] Of note, subjects were treated with both aspirin and the study drug for a median of 6 days prior to PCI during initial hospitalization, and more than 80% in both study groups received open label thienopyridine for approximately 4 weeks after PCI.

Trials that extended the utility of clopidogrel to patients with ST-segment elevation MI included Clopidogrel for the Reduction of Events During Observation (CREDO), CLopidogrel as Adjunctive ReperfusIon TherapY–Thrombolysis In Myocardial Infarction 28 (CLARITY-TIMI 28), and the ClOpidogrel and Metoprolol in Myocardial Infarction Trial/Second Chinese Cardiac Study (COMMIT/CCS2).[22–24]

While prior studies had used a clopidogrel loading dose of 300 mg, the 600 mg dose was examined in the Clopidogrel and Aspirin Optimal Dose Usage to Reduce Recurrent Events–Seventh Organization to Assess Strategies in Ischemic Syndromes (CURRENT-OASIS 7) trial.[25,26] In this study of 25,086 patients with an ACS, a 600 mg clopidogrel loading dose followed by a

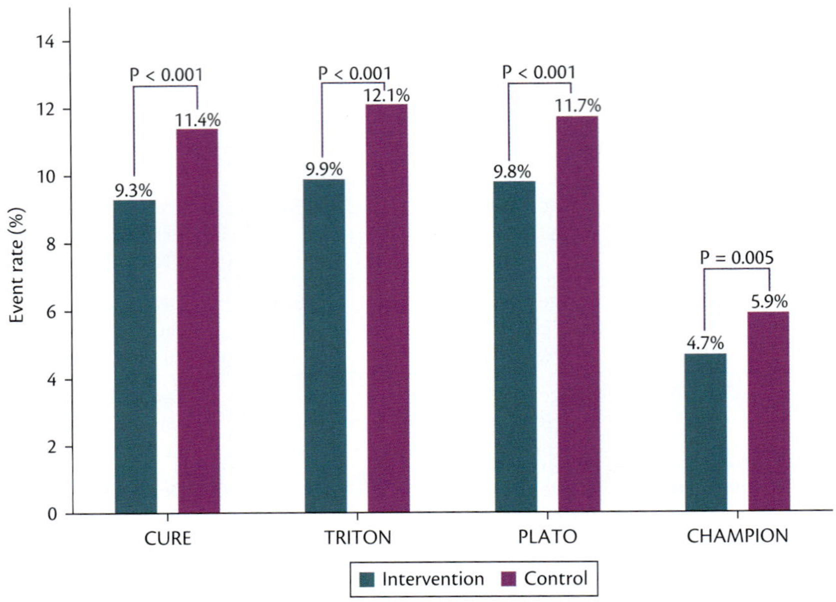

Figure 6.5 Ischaemic events with intervention versus control in selected trials of $P2Y_{12}$ inhibitors. For each trial, the rate of the primary endpoint was reported (12 months in CURE and PLATO, 15 months in TRITON, and 48 hours in CHAMPION). Please see the text and ➔ Table 6.2 for more details. CHAMPION, Cangrelor versus Standard Therapy to Achieve Optimal Management of Platelet Inhibition PHOENIX; CURE, The Clopidogrel in Unstable Angina to Prevent Recurrent Events trial; PLATO, Platelet Inhibition and Patient Outcomes; TRITON, The Trial to Assess Improvement in Therapeutic Outcomes by Optimizing Platelet Inhibition with Prasugrel-Thrombolysis in Myocardial Infarction 38.

150 mg maintenance dose versus conventional dosage during the first week did not reduce the primary composite outcome of cardiovascular death, MI, or stroke at 30 days in the overall study population [4.2% vs 4.4%, hazard ratio (HR) 0.94, 95% CI 0.83–1.06; P = 0.30], but did so in the 17,263 individuals undergoing PCI (3.9% vs 4.5%, adjusted HR 0.86, 95% CI 0.74–0.99; P = 0.04; P-interaction = 0.03). The risk of stent thrombosis was also reduced in the double dose group. As expected, the intervention

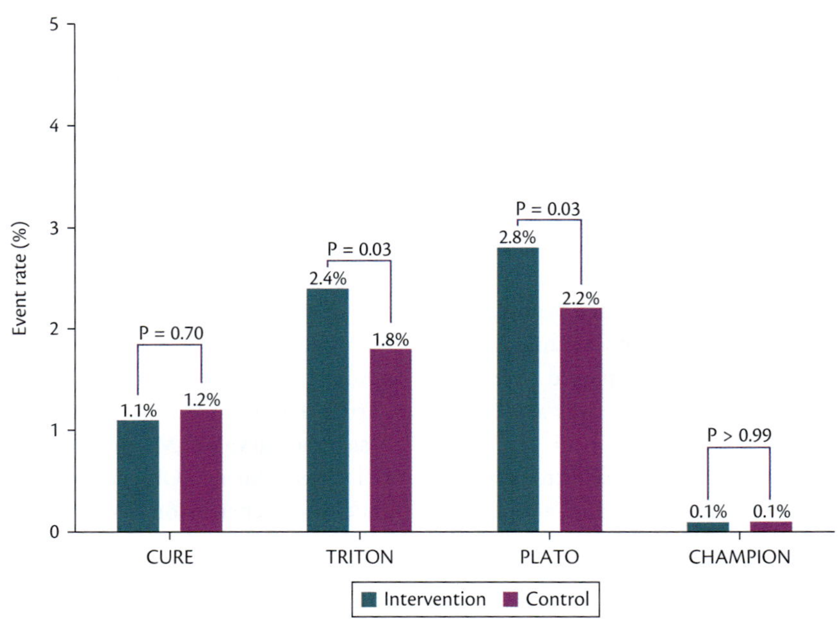

Figure 6.6 TIMI major bleeding events with intervention versus control in selected trials of $P2Y_{12}$ inhibitors. For each trial, the rate of TIMI major bleeding was chosen for standardization (12 months in CURE and PLATO, 15 months in TRITON, and 48 hours in CHAMPION). In TRITON, PLATO, and CHAMPION, this employed bleeding not related to coronary artery bypass grafting, while this was not specified in CURE. Please see the text and ➔ Table 6.2 for more details. CHAMPION, Cangrelor versus Standard Therapy to Achieve Optimal Management of Platelet Inhibition PHOENIX; CURE, The Clopidogrel in Unstable Angina to Prevent Recurrent Events trial; PLATO, Platelet Inhibition and Patient Outcomes; TIMI, Thrombolysis in Myocardial Infarction; TRITON, The Trial to Assess Improvement in Therapeutic Outcomes by Optimizing Platelet Inhibition with Prasugrel-Thrombolysis in Myocardial Infarction 38.

increased the risk of major bleeding (2.5% vs 2.0% in the overall study population, HR 1.24, 95% CI 1.05–1.46; P = 0.01).

Finally, the Dual Antiplatelet Therapy (DAPT) study randomly assigned 9961 patients who had undergone PCI with a drug-eluting stent (43% with an ACS) and completed 12 months of DAPT (65% clopidogrel, 35% prasugrel) to either continue thienopyridine treatment or to receive placebo for an additional 18 months.[27] The investigators found that prolonged DAPT lowered the risk of both coprimary endpoints, that is, stent thrombosis and major adverse cardiovascular and cerebrovascular events. While a reduction in thrombosis was seen in persons randomized to prolonged DAPT both with and without MI, the reduction in major adverse cardiovascular and cerebrovascular events was more pronounced in those with a prior MI or those on prasugrel.[27,28] Continued thienopyridine treatment increased the risk of moderate or severe bleeding, irrespective of clinical presentation.

Chronic coronary syndrome

Large, randomized studies of clopidogrel specifically targeting persons with chronic coronary syndrome (CCS) are lacking. Some conclusions may be drawn from the Clopidogrel for High Atherothrombotic Risk and Ischemic Stabilization, Management, and Avoidance (CHARISMA) trial, in which 15,603 patients with either established cardiovascular disease (documented coronary, cerebrovascular, or symptomatic peripheral artery disease) or multiple risk factors were randomized to receive clopidogrel 75 mg once daily plus aspirin 75–162 mg once daily or placebo plus aspirin.[29] At a median of 28 months, the rate of the primary composite endpoint of MI, stroke, or death from cardiovascular causes was 6.8% in the clopidogrel group and 7.3% in the placebo group (RR 0.93, 95% CI 0.83–1.05; P = 0.22). Rates of severe bleeding were 1.7% and 1.3%, respectively (RR 1.25, 95% CI 0.97–1.61; P = 0.09). Among individuals with established cardiovascular disease, approximately one in six of whom had CCS without prior MI, clopidogrel resulted in a significant reduction in the primary endpoint (6.9% vs 7.9%, RR 0.88, 95% CI 0.77–0.998; P = 0.046; P-interaction = 0.045). Furthermore, among patients with prior MI, stroke, or peripheral artery disease, clopidogrel significantly reduced the risk of the primary endpoint (7.3% vs 8.8%, HR 0.83, 95% CI 0.72–0.96; P = 0.01).[30]

In the HOST-EXAM trial, no difference in the effect of clopidogrel versus aspirin monotherapy was detected in subjects presenting without versus with CCS (27%).[19] Lastly, among the 57% of patients with CCS in the DAPT study, the risk of stent thrombosis was reduced to a similar extent as those with prior MI, but major adverse cardiovascular and cerebrovascular events were not lowered, with prolonged DAPT.[28]

Cerebrovascular disease

In patients with a recent stroke in CAPRIE, clopidogrel did not significantly reduce composite ischaemic events (annual risk 7.2% vs 7.7%, RR reduction 7.3%, 95% CI −5.7 to 18.7; P = 0.26; P-interaction = 0.04).[18] Conversely, in those with prior stroke in CHARISMA, DAPT was associated with a significant reduction in the primary endpoint (8.4% vs 10.7%, HR 0.78, 95% CI 0.62–0.98; P = 0.03).[30]

Several other randomized trials have examined the utility of clopidogrel in cerebrovascular disease with varying results. The Prevention Regimen for Effectively Avoiding Second Strokes (PRoFESS) trial randomized 20,332 patients with a recent ischaemic stroke to receive either aspirin 25 mg plus dipyridamole 200 mg twice daily or clopidogrel 75 mg once daily for a mean of 2.5 years. Stroke recurrence did not significantly differ between the two study groups (aspirin plus dipyridamole 9.0% vs clopidogrel 8.8%, HR 1.01, 95% CI 0.92–1.11), but there were more major haemorrhagic events in the combination therapy group (4.1% vs 3.6%, HR 1.15, 95% CI 1.00–1.32). The Secondary Prevention of Small Subcortical Strokes (SPS3) investigators did not find a reduction in recurrent stroke among subjects with recent symptomatic lacunar infarcts randomized to clopidogrel 75 mg once daily versus placebo, in addition to aspirin 325 mg once daily for a mean of 3.4 years.[31] However, the risk of major haemorrhage was significantly increased with DAPT, as was the risk of death. Triple antiplatelet therapy with aspirin 50–150 mg once daily, clopidogrel 75 mg once daily, and dipyridamole 200 mg twice daily was also not more effective than either clopidogrel alone or aspirin with dipyridamole, but did increase major bleeding, in the Triple Antiplatelets for Reducing Dependency after Ischaemic Stroke (TARDIS) trial.[32] Conversely, in both the Chinese Clopidogrel in High-Risk Patients with Acute Nondisabling Cerebrovascular Events (CHANCE) trial and the international Platelet-Oriented Inhibition in New TIA and Minor Ischemic Stroke (POINT) trial, DAPT with clopidogrel 75 mg once daily plus aspirin (75 mg once daily in CHANCE, 50–325 mg daily in POINT) compared with aspirin alone reduced the primary endpoint (stroke in CHANCE, a composite of ischaemic stroke, MI, or death from an ischaemic vascular event in POINT) at 90 days.[33,34] The risk of major haemorrhage was increased in POINT, but not in CHANCE.

Peripheral artery disease

The benefit of clopidogrel compared with aspirin monotherapy in CAPRIE was predominantly observed among patients with peripheral artery disease (annual risk 3.7% vs 4.9%, RR reduction 23.8%, 95% CI 8.9–36.2; P = 0.003; P-interaction = 0.04).[18] Furthermore, among those with prior MI, stroke, or peripheral artery disease in CHARISMA, DAPT significantly reduced the risk of the primary efficacy endpoint (7.3% vs 8.8%, HR 0.83, 95% CI 0.72–0.96; P = 0.01), though in the subgroup of individuals with peripheral artery disease alone, statistical significance was not achieved (7.6% vs 8.7%, HR 0.87, 95% CI 0.67–1.13; P = 0.29).[30]

Atrial fibrillation

Two landmark studies from the Atrial Fibrillation Clopidogrel Trial with Irbesartan for Prevention of Vascular Events (ACTIVE) investigators evaluated the utility of DAPT with clopidogrel and aspirin in patients with atrial fibrillation and at least one risk factor for stroke.[35,36] In ACTIVE W, warfarin was superior to clopidogrel plus aspirin, in reducing stroke, systemic embolus, MI, or vascular death, and was not associated with an increased risk of haemorrhage.[35] In the subsequently published ACTIVE A study, DAPT was superior to aspirin alone in reducing stroke, MI, systemic embolism, or death from vascular causes, but increased major bleeding.[36]

Special considerations

Genetic polymorphisms involving CYP2C19 may affect the response to clopidogrel.[37–39] These considerations are described in detail in ➔ Chapter 29. Early pharmacodynamic studies had suggested detrimental effects of administering omeprazole, a drug with potential CYP2C19-inhibitory properties, in patients on clopidogrel,[40,41] but the randomized Clopidogrel and the Optimization of Gastrointestinal Events Trial (COGENT) did not demonstrate an increased risk of ischaemic events with concomitant clopidogrel and omeprazole administration.[42] Nevertheless, COGENT was prematurely terminated for financial reasons, and the US and European drug labels still recommend avoiding omeprazole and esomeprazole in patients receiving clopidogrel.[43,44]

Prasugrel

Pharmacokinetics and pharmacodynamics

Prasugrel is hydrolysed by esterases in the intestines and blood to a thiolactone that in turn is metabolized by the CYP system (predominantly CYP3A and CYP2B6) in a rapid, single-step process to its active metabolite, R-138727.[45] This metabolite then inhibits ADP-induced platelet activation and aggregation through covalent linkage of a sulfhydryl group.[46] Compared with clopidogrel, prasugrel results in more rapid, pronounced, and consistent inhibition of platelet function.[47–49]

Clinical indications

Acute coronary syndrome

Findings of the Trial to Assess Improvement in Therapeutic Outcomes by Optimizing Platelet Inhibition with Prasugrel–Thrombolysis in Myocardial Infarction 38 (TRITON–TIMI 38) were reported in 2007 (➔ Table 6.2). The investigators randomly allocated 13,608 patients with an ACS scheduled for PCI to either prasugrel (60 mg loading dose, 10 mg once-daily maintenance dose) or clopidogrel (300 mg loading dose, 75 mg once-daily maintenance dose) for a median of 14.5 months.[50] All patients received aspirin at a dose of 75–162 mg once daily. Importantly, it was mandated that the coronary anatomy be known in study participants with a non-ST-segment elevation ACS or in those who had received medical treatment for an ST-segment elevation MI. The primary endpoint, a composite of death from cardiovascular causes, MI, or stroke, occurred in significantly fewer individuals in the prasugrel group (9.9% vs 12.1%, HR 0.81, 95% CI 0.73–0.90; P <0.001) in whom the risk of stent thrombosis was also decreased (➔ Figure 6.5). This came at the expense of an increased risk of major bleeding (2.4% vs 1.8%, HR 1.32, 95% CI 1.03–1.68; P = 0.03), including fatal bleeding (➔ Figure 6.6). Subjects with a previous stroke or transient ischaemic attack had net harm from prasugrel, while those aged 75 years or older, or those with a body weight less than 60 kg, had no net benefit.

Considering patients with medically managed ACS, the Targeted Platelet Inhibition to Clarify the Optimal Strategy to Medically Manage Acute Coronary Syndromes (TRILOGY ACS) did not show a benefit of prasugrel over clopidogrel.[51] However, in those who underwent angiography before enrolment and had confirmed coronary artery disease (CAD), there may have been an advantage of prasugrel.[52] Moreover, in the Comparison of Prasugrel at the Time of Percutaneous Coronary Intervention or as Pretreatment at the Time of Diagnosis in Patients with Non-ST Elevation Myocardial Infarction (ACCOAST) trial, pretreatment with prasugrel did not reduce ischaemic events, but increased major bleeding complications.[53]

Prasugrel-based de-escalation strategies after PCI for ACS were explored in two large, randomized trials conducted in Europe [Testing Responsiveness To Platelet Inhibition On Chronic Antiplatelet Treatment For Acute Coronary Syndromes (TROPICAL-ACS)] and South Korea [Harmonizing Optimal Strategy for Treatment of Coronary Artery Diseases Trial—Comparison of REDUCTION of PrasugrEl Dose & POLYmer TECHnology in ACS Patients (HOST-REDUCE-POLYTECH-ACS)], respectively.[54,55] The studies found that platelet function test guided de-escalation to clopidogrel from day 14, and reducing prasugrel maintenance dose from 10 mg to 5 mg after 1 month, reduced the risk of net clinical outcomes, without increasing ischaemic events.

Cerebrovascular disease

The PRAsugrel and clopidogrel in Japanese patients with ischemic STROke (PRASTRO-1) trial conducted in Japanese patients with a non-cardioembolic stroke was unable to confirm non-inferiority of prasugrel 3.75 mg daily versus clopidogrel 75 mg daily for the primary endpoint of ischaemic stroke, MI, or death from vascular causes.[56] Bleeding events occurred at similar rates in the two study groups.

Special considerations

On the basis of the results from TRITON–TIMI 38, prasugrel is contraindicated in patients with a prior stroke or transient ischaemic attack.[50,57,58]

Ticagrelor

Pharmacokinetics and pharmacodynamics

Ticagrelor belongs to the cyclopentyltriazolopyrimidine class of drugs.[59] It results in faster, greater, and more consistent $P2Y_{12}$ antagonism and thus stronger inhibition of platelet activation and aggregation than clopidogrel.[4,60,61] Although ticagrelor does not require bioactivation to exert its effects, it does have one active metabolite, AR-C124910XX, the potency of which is akin to the parent drug.[62] Ticagrelor also appears to provide stronger inhibition of platelet reactivity than prasugrel.[63]

Clinical indications

Acute coronary syndrome

The Platelet Inhibition and Patient Outcomes (PLATO) trial of hospitalized patients with an ACS was published in 2009 (➔ Table 6.2).[64] A total of 18,624 individuals were randomized to ticagrelor (180 mg loading dose, 90 mg twice-daily maintenance dose) versus clopidogrel (300-600 mg loading dose, 75 mg once-daily maintenance dose) in addition to aspirin (75 to 325 mg once daily). At 12 months, the occurrence of the primary composite efficacy endpoint of death from vascular causes, MI, or stroke was significantly reduced in those randomized to ticagrelor (9.8% vs 11.7%, HR 0.84, 95% CI 0.77–0.92; P <0.001) (➔ Figure 6.5). Ticagrelor also reduced the risk of death from vascular causes and from any cause. While no significant difference was found in the primary safety endpoint of major bleeding defined per study criteria (11.6% vs 11.2%, HR 1.04, 95% CI 0.95–1.13; P = 0.43), ticagrelor did increase the risk of non-coronary artery bypass graft-related bleeding and fatal intracranial bleeding (➔ Figure 6.6). Dyspnoea was also more common with ticagrelor. In a separate trial of individuals 70 years of age or older with non-ST-elevation ACS [Ticagrelor or prasugrel versus clopidogrel in elderly patients with an acute coronary syndrome: optimization of antiplatelet treatment in patients aged older than 70 years (POPular AGE)], clopidogrel reduced bleeding, without increasing thrombotic outcomes.[65] In that study, 95% of individuals randomized to intensive antiplatelet treatment had received ticagrelor.

Of note, although the safety of prehospital compared with in-hospital ticagrelor in patients with an ST-segment elevation MI was demonstrated in the Administration of Ticagrelor in the Cath Lab or in the Ambulance for New ST Elevation Myocardial Infarction to Open the Coronary Artery (ATLANTIC) trial, the prehospital strategy did not improve reperfusion outcomes.[66] Nevertheless, the median time difference between the two treatment strategies was only 31 minutes.

Various forms of unguided antiplatelet de-escalation involving ticagrelor were examined in the Clinical Study Comparing Two Forms of Anti-platelet Therapy After Stent Implantation (GLOBAL LEADERS), Ticagrelor with Aspirin or Alone in High-Risk Patients after Coronary Intervention (TWILIGHT), and the South Korean TicAgrelor Versus CLOpidogrel in Stabilized Patients With Acute Myocardial Infarction (TALOS-AMI) trials.[67–69] In general, de-escalation to either ticagrelor monotherapy or clopidogrel plus aspirin after a course of ticagrelor plus aspirin appeared safe(r), without loss of efficacy. A recent network meta-analysis also found that unguided compared with guided de-escalation of DAPT reduced bleeding, but did not increase ischaemic events, in patients with ACS.[70]

In 2019, the Intracoronary Stenting and Antithrombotic Regimen: Rapid Early Action for Coronary Treatment (ISAR-REACT) 5 investigators directly compared ticagrelor (180 mg loading dose, 90 mg twice-daily maintenance dose) and prasugrel (60 mg loading dose, 10 mg once-daily maintenance dose) in 4018 patients with an ACS scheduled to undergo coronary angiography, but without a history of stroke, transient ischaemic attack, or intracranial bleeding (➔ Table 6.2).[71] In the ticagrelor group, the loading dose was administered as soon as possible after randomization. Conversely, in the prasugrel group, the loading dose was given as soon as possible in patients with ST-segment elevation and after the coronary anatomy was known in those without ST-segment elevation. In addition, the maintenance dose was reduced to 5 mg in case of age of at least 75 years or body weight less than 60 kg. At 12 months, the occurrence of the primary endpoint of death, MI, or stroke was significantly higher among patients randomly allocated to ticagrelor (9.3% vs 6.9%, HR 1.36, 95% CI 1.09–1.70; P = 0.006), but there was no difference in the risk of major bleeding (5.4% vs 4.8%, HR 1.12, 95% CI 0.83–1.51; P = 0.46). Nevertheless, a subsequent network meta-analysis of randomized controlled trials did not report statistically significant differences between ticagrelor and prasugrel for any of the explored outcomes.[72]

Finally, the Prevention of Cardiovascular Events in Patients with Prior Heart Attack Using Ticagrelor Compared to Placebo on a Background of Aspirin–Thrombolysis in Myocardial Infarction 54 (PEGASUS–TIMI 54) trial investigated the utility of prolonged DAPT with ticagrelor (60 or 90 mg twice daily) plus aspirin (75 to 150 mg once daily) in patients with prior MI and found a reduced risk of ischaemic events and an increased risk of major bleeding at 3 years.[73] Prolonged DAPT also reduced the risk of death from cardiovascular causes and from any cause if ticagrelor (60 mg twice daily) was initiated 2 or less years from the MI (or ≤1 year after stopping the previous $P2Y_{12}$ inhibitor).[74]

Chronic coronary syndrome

The role of ticagrelor in patients with angiographically confirmed stable CAD and type 2 diabetes mellitus was tested in the Effect of Ticagrelor on Health Outcomes in Diabetes Mellitus Patients Intervention Study (THEMIS) (➔ Table 6.2).[75] A total of 19,220 participants without prior MI or stroke were randomized to ticagrelor or placebo on top of aspirin (75–150 mg daily). The ticagrelor dose was initially 90 mg twice daily but was later switched to 60 mg twice daily given the results from PEGASUS–TIMI 54.[73] At a median of 39.9 months, the incidence of composite ischaemic events (i.e. cardiovascular death, MI, or stroke) was significantly lower with ticagrelor (7.7% vs 8.5%, HR 0.90, 95% CI 0.81–0.99; P = 0.04). Conversely, the rates of TIMI major bleeding (2.2% vs 1.0%, HR 2.32, 95% CI 1.82–2.94; P <0.001) and of intracranial haemorrhage were higher. Results were generally comparable between patients who had a history of previous PCI and those who did not, though only those with prior PCI achieved net clinical benefit from DAPT (9.3% vs 11.0%, HR 0.85, 95% CI 0.75–0.95; P = 0.005; P-interaction = 0.01).[76]

A significant number of patients in both GLOBAL LEADERS (53%) and TWILIGHT (35% including asymptomatic patients) had CCS.[67,68] While the clinical presentation (i.e. ACS or CCS) did not modify the efficacy of de-escalation in either trial, there was evidence that early de-escalation to ticagrelor monotherapy in both trials reduced the risk of bleeding in individuals with ACS, but not in those with stable CAD.[77,78]

Cerebrovascular disease

The Acute Stroke or Transient Ischaemic Attack Treated with Aspirin or Ticagrelor and Patient Outcomes (SOCRATES), Acute Stroke or Transient Ischaemic Attack Treated with Ticagrelor and ASA for Prevention of Stroke and Death (THALES) trial, and Ticagrelor or Clopidogrel with Aspirin in High-Risk Patients with Acute Nondisabling Cerebrovascular Events II (CHANCE-2) trials tested various strategies involving ticagrelor in patients with non-severe acute stroke or transient ischaemic attack.[79–81] SOCRATES randomized study participants to ticagrelor or aspirin monotherapy for 90 days and detected no differences in ischaemic events (stroke, MI, or death) or major bleeding between the treatments.[79] In contrast, among 11,016 patients with mild-to-moderate acute non-cardioembolic ischaemic stroke or transient ischaemic attack in THALES, ticagrelor (180 mg loading dose, followed by 90 mg twice daily) plus aspirin (300–325 mg loading dose, followed by 75-100 mg once daily) significantly reduced the rate of stroke or death at 30 days (5.5% vs 6.6%, HR 0.83, 95% CI 0.71–0.96; P = 0.02), though this came at the expense of a higher rate of severe bleeding (0.5% vs 0.1%, HR 3.99, 95% CI 1.74–9.14; P = 0.001).[80] Moreover, the incidence of disability did not significantly differ between the two groups. Similarly, among 6412 patients in the Chinese CHANCE-2 trial with minor ischaemic stroke or transient ischaemic attack who were carriers of CYP2C19 loss-of-function alleles, ticagrelor (180 mg loading dose, 90 mg twice-daily maintenance dose) as compared with clopidogrel (300 mg loading dose, 75 mg once-daily maintenance dose) reduced the primary outcome of stroke at 90 days (6.0% vs 7.6%, HR 0.77, 95% CI 0.64–0.94; P = 0.008).[81] All patients received aspirin for 21 days (loading dose of 75–300 mg, followed by 75 mg once daily). While severe or moderate bleeding did not differ between the two groups, any bleeding was significantly increased with ticagrelor (5.3% vs 2.5%, HR 2.18, 95% CI 1.66–2.85).

Peripheral artery disease

Ticagrelor monotherapy (90 mg twice daily) was not superior to clopidogrel monotherapy (75 mg once daily) for the primary composite efficacy endpoint of cardiovascular death, MI, or ischaemic stroke in the Examining Use of Ticagrelor in Peripheral Artery Disease (EUCLID) trial of patients with symptomatic peripheral artery disease.[82] The risk of major bleeding did not differ between the two study groups.

Special considerations

In PEGASUS–TIMI 54, dyspnoea developed in more than 15% of individuals assigned to ticagrelor and led to drug discontinuation in a significant proportion.[73] In PLATO, bradyarrhythmic events occurred more commonly in the ticagrelor group within the first week after initiation, but they did not have clinical consequences.[83] Unlike the other $P2Y_{12}$ inhibitors, a specific antidote has been developed for ticagrelor. Among healthy volunteers who had been pretreated with ticagrelor for 48 hours, intravenous bentracimab administration provided rapid and sustained reversal of ticagrelor.[84] In a separate study, bentracimab was associated with haemostasis in 90% of ticagrelor-treated patients who required urgent surgery or had major bleeding, with approximately 5% experiencing potential post-reversal thrombotic events.[85]

Elinogrel

Elinogrel was a reversible $P2Y_{12}$ inhibitor available in both oral and intravenous formulations. The drug was shown to overcome high on-treatment platelet reactivity associated with the CYP2C19*2 genotype.[86] Furthermore, in a phase II randomized controlled trial, the combination of intravenous and oral elinogrel achieved more rapid and pronounced antiplatelet effects than clopidogrel in patients undergoing non-urgent PCI.[87] Bleeding requiring medical attention was significantly more common, while efficacy endpoints occurred with a similar rate, in the elinogrel group.[88] Although phase III studies had been planned, drug development was discontinued in 2012.

Cangrelor

Pharmacokinetics and pharmacodynamics

Cangrelor, an adenosine triphosphate (ATP) analogue, is the only intravenous $P2Y_{12}$ receptor antagonist currently available for clinical use.[89] The drug rapidly, predictably, and potently inhibits platelets.[59,90] Its half-life is very short due to rapid dephosphorylation to an inactive metabolite.[91] In a phase II randomized controlled trial of patients undergoing PCI, cangrelor resulted in similar platelet inhibition, and did not increase bleeding, compared with abciximab.[92] Moreover, platelet aggregation returned to baseline levels faster after termination of infusion with cangrelor versus abciximab.

Clinical indications

Acute coronary syndrome

In 2009, the Cangrelor versus Standard Therapy to Achieve Optimal Management of Platelet Inhibition (CHAMPION) investigators published two randomized controlled trials of cangrelor in patients undergoing PCI.[93,94] In CHAMPION PLATFORM, 5362 individuals (~95% with an ACS) who had not been treated with clopidogrel were randomly allocated to either cangrelor or placebo at the time of PCI, followed by a 600 mg dose of clopidogrel.[93] Clopidogrel was administered at the end of infusion in the cangrelor group (i.e. after 2–4 hours) and at the end of PCI in the placebo group. In CHAMPION PCI, 8877 subjects (~85% with an ACS) planned for PCI were randomized to cangrelor versus 600 mg of clopidogrel.[94] The rate of the primary endpoint, a composite of death, MI, or ischaemia-driven revascularization at 48 hours, did not differ between the two treatment groups in either trial. In CHAMPION PLATFORM, cangrelor reduced stent thrombosis and death, but increased major bleeding.[93] Conversely, in CHAMPION PCI, no significant differences for these endpoints were observed, though most bleeding outcomes occurred with a higher incidence in the cangrelor group.[94] Of note, the sample size in CHAMPION PLATFORM had originally been projected at 6400 participants, but enrolment was prematurely terminated based on an interim analysis concluding that the trial would be unlikely to show superiority of cangrelor.[93]

The subsequent CHAMPION PHOENIX trial assessed the utility of cangrelor versus 300 or 600 mg of clopidogrel in 11,145 patients undergoing PCI (~43% with an ACS) who had not received pretreatment with a $P2Y_{12}$ inhibitor (➔ Table 6.2).[95] A 600 mg dose of clopidogrel was also administered in the cangrelor group after infusion end. At 48 hours, the incidence of the primary composite efficacy endpoint of death, MI, ischaemia-driven revascularization, or stent thrombosis was significantly reduced in the cangrelor group (4.7% vs 5.9%, adjusted OR 0.78, 95% CI 0.66–0.93; P = 0.005) (➔ Figure 6.5). The individual endpoints of MI and stent thrombosis also occurred with a lower rate with cangrelor. The primary safety endpoint, severe bleeding at 48 hours, was not significantly increased (0.16% vs 0.11%, adjusted OR 1.50, 95% CI 0.53–4.22; P = 0.44) (➔ Figure 6.6), but more patients in the cangrelor group developed transient dyspnoea. Finally, in a pooled analysis of the three CHAMPION trials, cangrelor reduced the odds of death, MI, ischaemia-driven revascularization, or stent thrombosis at 48 hours (3.8% vs 4.7%; OR 0.81, 95% CI 0.71–0.91; P <0.001), but increased the risk of bleeding.[96]

Chronic coronary syndrome

In the combined CHAMPION cohort, 31% of patients had stable CAD. The efficacy of cangrelor was not modified by the type of coronary disease (stable CAD: 5.7% vs 7.3%, OR 0.77, 95% CI 0.64–0.93; non-ST-elevation ACS: 2.9% vs 3.5%, OR 0.82, 95% CI 0.68–0.99; ST-elevation MI: 2.9% vs 3.5%, OR 0.84, 95% CI 0.55–1.27; P-interaction = 0.87).[96]

Special considerations

Because the active metabolites of thienopyridines have short half-lives, it is recommended that these agents be administered immediately after and not during cangrelor infusion to allow for adequate $P2Y_{12}$ receptor binding.[89,97,98] However, prasugrel can be given up to 30 minutes before infusion end.[99] Ticagrelor may be administered before or during infusion.[100]

Selatogrel

Selatogrel is a new, potent, reversible $P2Y_{12}$ inhibitor available in oral and subcutaneous formulations.[101,102] Following subcutaneous administration, peak concentrations are achieved at approximately 30 minutes. Phase II studies of the subcutaneous formulation have demonstrated its safety in individuals with MI and CCS, respectively.[103,104] A phase III trial in patients with recent MI [Selatogrel Outcome Study in Suspected Acute Myocardial Infarction (SOS-AMI)] is currently ongoing (NCT04957719).

Summary

Platelet $P2Y_{12}$ receptor antagonists have been clinically available for more than 20 years. While clopidogrel served as the principal $P2Y_{12}$ inhibitor for a decade, the more potent agents, prasugrel and ticagrelor, are now preferred in many settings. Several randomized controlled trials have shed light on intensified DAPT strategies, single antiplatelet therapy with a $P2Y_{12}$ inhibitor, and optimal treatment duration. Ongoing studies will clarify the role of more individualized antiplatelet strategies in patients at high bleeding risk, drugs with alternative routes of administration, and specific reversal agents. As the indications for $P2Y_{12}$ inhibitors continue to be refined, this drug class will remain essential in the treatment of atherosclerotic cardiovascular disease for years to come.

What's new

- Prolonged DAPT after MI or PCI reduces ischaemic events, but increases major bleeding.
- Ticagrelor added to aspirin in patients with stable CAD and type 2 diabetes reduces ischaemic events, but increases major bleeding.

What's next

- Individualizing the choice and duration of $P2Y_{12}$ inhibitor in patients with CAD, particularly in those at high bleeding risk.
- Possible utility of a ticagrelor reversal agent, bentracimab, in daily clinical practice.
- Potential clinical role of a subcutaneously administered $P2Y_{12}$ inhibitor, selatogrel, after MI.

Drug dosing

	Clopidogrel	Prasugrel	Ticagrelor	Cangrelor
Loading dose	300–600 mg	60 mg	180 mg	30 mcg/kg bolus
Maintenance dose	75 mg once daily	10 mg once daily (5 mg once daily if body weight <60 kg or age ≥75 years)	90 mg twice daily (60–90 mg twice daily if continued after 12 months from diagnosis of an acute coronary syndrome)	4 mcg/kg/min infusion

Disclosures

Dr Pareek discloses the following relationships—Advisory Board: AstraZeneca, Janssen-Cilag; Grant Support: Danish Cardiovascular Academy funded by the Novo Nordisk Foundation and the Danish Heart Foundation (grant number: CPD5Y-2022004-HF); Speaker Honorarium: AstraZeneca, Bayer, Boehringer Ingelheim, Janssen-Cilag.

Dr Bhatt discloses the following relationships—Advisory Board: AngioWave, Bayer, Boehringer Ingelheim, Cardax, CellProthera, Cereno Scientific, Elsevier Practice Update Cardiology, High Enroll, Janssen, Level Ex, McKinsey, Medscape Cardiology, Merck, MyoKardia, NirvaMed, Novo Nordisk, PhaseBio, PLx Pharma, Regado Biosciences, Stasys; Board of Directors: AngioWave (stock options), Boston VA Research Institute, Bristol Myers Squibb (stock), DRS.LINQ (stock options), High Enroll (stock), Society of Cardiovascular Patient Care, TobeSoft; Chair: Inaugural Chair, American Heart Association Quality Oversight Committee; Consultant: Broadview Ventures; Data Monitoring Committees: Acesion Pharma, Assistance Publique-Hôpitaux de Paris, Baim Institute for Clinical Research (formerly Harvard Clinical Research Institute, for the PORTICO trial, funded by St. Jude Medical, now Abbott), Boston Scientific (Chair, PEITHO trial), Cleveland Clinic (including for the ExCEED trial, funded by Edwards), Contego Medical (Chair, PERFORMANCE 2), Duke Clinical Research Institute, Mayo Clinic, Mount Sinai School of Medicine (for the ENVISAGE trial, funded by Daiichi Sankyo; for the ABILITY-DM trial, funded by Concept Medical), Novartis, Population Health Research Institute; Rutgers University (for the NIH-funded MINT Trial); Honoraria: American College of Cardiology (Senior Associate Editor, Clinical Trials and News, ACC.org; Chair, ACC Accreditation Oversight Committee), Arnold and Porter law firm (work related to Sanofi/Bristol-Myers Squibb clopidogrel litigation), Baim Institute for Clinical Research (formerly Harvard Clinical Research Institute; RE-DUAL PCI clinical trial steering committee funded by Boehringer Ingelheim; AEGIS-II executive committee funded by CSL Behring), Belvoir Publications (Editor in Chief, Harvard Heart Letter), Canadian Medical and Surgical Knowledge Translation Research Group (clinical trial steering committees), Cowen and Company, Duke Clinical Research Institute (clinical trial steering committees, including for the PRONOUNCE trial, funded by Ferring Pharmaceuticals), HMP Global (Editor in Chief, Journal of Invasive Cardiology), Journal of the American College of Cardiology (Guest Editor; Associate Editor), K2P (Co-Chair, interdisciplinary curriculum), Level Ex, Medtelligence/ReachMD (CME steering committees), MJH Life Sciences, Oakstone CME (Course Director, Comprehensive Review of Interventional Cardiology), Piper Sandler, Population Health Research Institute (for the COMPASS operations committee, publications committee, steering committee, and USA national co-leader, funded by Bayer), Slack Publications (Chief Medical Editor, Cardiology Today's Intervention), Society of Cardiovascular Patient Care (Secretary/Treasurer), WebMD (CME steering committees), Wiley (steering committee); Other: Clinical Cardiology (Deputy Editor), NCDR-ACTION Registry Steering Committee (Chair), VA CART Research and Publications Committee (Chair); Patent: Sotagliflozin (named on a patent for sotagliflozin assigned to Brigham and Women's Hospital who assigned to Lexicon; neither I nor Brigham and Women's Hospital receive any income from this patent); Research Funding: Abbott, Acesion Pharma, Afimmune, Aker Biomarine, Amarin, Amgen, AstraZeneca, Bayer, Beren, Boehringer Ingelheim, Boston Scientific, Bristol-Myers Squibb, Cardax, CellProthera, Cereno Scientific, Chiesi, CinCor, CSL Behring, Eisai, Ethicon, Faraday Pharmaceuticals, Ferring Pharmaceuticals, Forest Laboratories, Fractyl, Garmin, HLS Therapeutics, Idorsia, Ironwood, Ischemix, Janssen, Javelin, Lexicon, Lilly, Medtronic, Merck, Moderna, MyoKardia, NirvaMed, Novartis, Novo Nordisk, Owkin, Pfizer, PhaseBio, PLx Pharma, Recardio, Regeneron, Reid Hoffman Foundation, Roche, Sanofi, Stasys, Synaptic, The Medicines Company, Youngene, 89Bio; Royalties: Elsevier (Editor, Braunwald's Heart Disease); Site Co-Investigator: Abbott, Biotronik, Boston Scientific, CSI, Endotronix, St. Jude Medical (now Abbott), Philips, SpectraWAVE, Svelte, Vascular Solutions; Trustee: American College of Cardiology; Unfunded Research: FlowCo, Takeda.

References

1. Storey RF, Sanderson HM, White AE, May JA, Cameron KE, Heptinstall S. The central role of the P(2T) receptor in amplification of human platelet activation, aggregation, secretion and procoagulant activity. Br J Haematol. 2000;110(4):925–34.
2. Bhatt DL, Topol EJ. Scientific and therapeutic advances in antiplatelet therapy. Nat Rev Drug Discov. 2003;2(1):15–28.
3. Storey RF. Biology and pharmacology of the platelet P2Y12 receptor. Curr Pharm Des. 2006;12(10):1255–9.
4. Wallentin L. P2Y(12) inhibitors: differences in properties and mechanisms of action and potential consequences for clinical use. Eur Heart J. 2009;30(16):1964–77.
5. Savi P, Herbert JM, Pflieger AM, et al. Importance of hepatic metabolism in the antiaggregating activity of the thienopyridine clopidogrel. Biochem Pharmacol. 1992;44(3):527–32.
6. Maffrand JP. The story of clopidogrel and its predecessor, ticlopidine: could these major antiplatelet and antithrombotic drugs be discovered and developed today? C R Chim. 2012;15(8):737–43.
7. Hass WK, Easton JD, Adams HP Jr, et al. A randomized trial comparing ticlopidine hydrochloride with aspirin for the prevention of stroke in high-risk patients. Ticlopidine Aspirin Stroke Study Group. N Engl J Med. 1989;321(8):501–7.
8. Schömig A, Neumann FJ, Kastrati A, et al. A randomized comparison of antiplatelet and anticoagulant therapy after the placement of coronary-artery stents. N Engl J Med. 1996;334(17):1084–9.
9. Becquemin JP. Effect of ticlopidine on the long-term patency of saphenous-vein bypass grafts in the legs. Etude de la Ticlopidine après Pontage Fémoro-Poplité and the Association Universitaire de Recherche en Chirurgie. N Engl J Med. 1997;337(24):1726–31.

10. Leon MB, Baim DS, Popma JJ, et al. A clinical trial comparing three antithrombotic-drug regimens after coronary-artery stenting. Stent Anticoagulation Restenosis Study Investigators. N Engl J Med. 1998;339(23):1665–71.
11. Haushofer A, Halbmayer WM, Prachar H. Neutropenia with ticlopidine plus aspirin. Lancet. 1997;349(9050):474–5.
12. Steinhubl SR, Tan WA, Foody JM, Topol EJ. Incidence and clinical course of thrombotic thrombocytopenic purpura due to ticlopidine following coronary stenting. EPISTENT Investigators. Evaluation of Platelet IIb/IIIa Inhibitor for Stenting. JAMA. 1999;281(9):806–10.
13. Bhatt DL, Bertrand ME, Berger PB, et al. Meta-analysis of randomized and registry comparisons of ticlopidine with clopidogrel after stenting. J Am Coll Cardiol. 2002;39(1):9–14.
14. Pereillo JM, Maftouh M, Andrieu A, et al. Structure and stereochemistry of the active metabolite of clopidogrel. Drug Metab Dispos. 2002;30(11):1288–95.
15. Savi P, Pereillo JM, Uzabiaga MF, et al. Identification and biological activity of the active metabolite of clopidogrel. Thromb Haemost. 2000;84(5):891–6.
16. Montalescot G, Sideris G, Meuleman C, et al. A randomized comparison of high clopidogrel loading doses in patients with non-ST-segment elevation acute coronary syndromes: the ALBION (Assessment of the Best Loading Dose of Clopidogrel to Blunt Platelet Activation, Inflammation and Ongoing Necrosis) trial. J Am Coll Cardiol. 2006;48(5):931–8.
17. Cuisset T, Frere C, Quilici J, et al. Benefit of a 600-mg loading dose of clopidogrel on platelet reactivity and clinical outcomes in patients with non-ST-segment elevation acute coronary syndrome undergoing coronary stenting. J Am Coll Cardiol. 2006;48(7):1339–45.
18. CAPRIE Steering Committee. A randomised, blinded, trial of clopidogrel versus aspirin in patients at risk of ischaemic events (CAPRIE). CAPRIE Steering Committee. Lancet. 1996;348(9038):1329–39.
19. Koo BK, Kang J, Park KW, et al. Aspirin versus clopidogrel for chronic maintenance monotherapy after percutaneous coronary intervention (HOST-EXAM): an investigator-initiated, prospective, randomised, open-label, multicentre trial. Lancet. 2021;397(10293):2487–96.
20. Yusuf S, Zhao F, Mehta SR, et al. Effects of clopidogrel in addition to aspirin in patients with acute coronary syndromes without ST-segment elevation. N Engl J Med. 2001;345(7):494–502.
21. Mehta SR, Yusuf S, Peters RJ, et al. Effects of pretreatment with clopidogrel and aspirin followed by long-term therapy in patients undergoing percutaneous coronary intervention: the PCI-CURE study. Lancet. 2001;358(9281):527–33.
22. Steinhubl SR, Berger PB, Mann JT 3rd, et al. Early and sustained dual oral antiplatelet therapy following percutaneous coronary intervention: a randomized controlled trial. JAMA. 2002;288(19):2411–20.
23. Sabatine MS, Cannon CP, Gibson CM, et al. Addition of clopidogrel to aspirin and fibrinolytic therapy for myocardial infarction with ST-segment elevation. N Engl J Med. 2005;352(12):1179–89.
24. Chen ZM, Jiang LX, Chen YP, et al. Addition of clopidogrel to aspirin in 45,852 patients with acute myocardial infarction: randomised placebo-controlled trial. Lancet. 2005;366(9497):1607–21.
25. CURRENT-OASIS 7 Investigators, Mehta SR, Bassand JP, et al. Dose comparisons of clopidogrel and aspirin in acute coronary syndromes. N Engl J Med. 2010;363(10):930–42.
26. Mehta SR, Tanguay JF, Eikelboom JW, et al. Double-dose versus standard-dose clopidogrel and high-dose versus low-dose aspirin in individuals undergoing percutaneous coronary intervention for acute coronary syndromes (CURRENT-OASIS 7): a randomised factorial trial. Lancet. 2010;376(9748):1233–43.
27. Mauri L, Kereiakes DJ, Yeh RW, et al. Twelve or 30 months of dual antiplatelet therapy after drug-eluting stents. N Engl J Med. 2014;371(23):2155–66.
28. Yeh RW, Kereiakes DJ, Steg PG, et al. Benefits and risks of extended duration dual antiplatelet therapy after PCI in patients with and without acute myocardial infarction. J Am Coll Cardiol. 2015;65(20):2211–21.
29. Bhatt DL, Fox KA, Hacke W, et al. Clopidogrel and aspirin versus aspirin alone for the prevention of atherothrombotic events. N Engl J Med. 2006;354(16):1706–17.
30. Bhatt DL, Flather MD, Hacke W, et al. Patients with prior myocardial infarction, stroke, or symptomatic peripheral arterial disease in the CHARISMA trial. J Am Coll Cardiol. 2007;49(19):1982–8.
31. SPS3 Investigators, Benavente OR, Hart RG, et al. Effects of clopidogrel added to aspirin in patients with recent lacunar stroke. N Engl J Med. 2012;367(9):817–25.
32. Bath PM, Woodhouse LJ, Appleton JP, et al. Antiplatelet therapy with aspirin, clopidogrel, and dipyridamole versus clopidogrel alone or aspirin and dipyridamole in patients with acute cerebral ischaemia (TARDIS): a randomised, open-label, phase 3 superiority trial. Lancet. 2018;391(10123):850–9.
33. Wang Y, Wang Y, Zhao X, et al. Clopidogrel with aspirin in acute minor stroke or transient ischemic attack. N Engl J Med. 2013;369(1):11–19.
34. Johnston SC, Easton JD, Farrant M, et al. Clopidogrel and aspirin in acute ischemic stroke and high-risk TIA. N Engl J Med. 2018;379(3):215–25.
35. ACTIVE Writing Group of the ACTIVE Investigators, Connolly S, Pogue J, et al. Clopidogrel plus aspirin versus oral anticoagulation for atrial fibrillation in the Atrial fibrillation Clopidogrel Trial with Irbesartan for prevention of Vascular Events (ACTIVE W): a randomised controlled trial. Lancet. 2006;367(9526):1903–12.
36. ACTIVE Investigators, Connolly SJ, Pogue J, et al. Effect of clopidogrel added to aspirin in patients with atrial fibrillation. N Engl J Med. 2009;360(20):2066–78.
37. Mega JL, Close SL, Wiviott SD, et al. Cytochrome p-450 polymorphisms and response to clopidogrel. N Engl J Med. 2009;360(4):354–62.
38. Simon T, Verstuyft C, Mary-Krause M, et al. Genetic determinants of response to clopidogrel and cardiovascular events. N Engl J Med. 2009;360(4):363–75.
39. Collet JP, Hulot JS, Pena A, et al. Cytochrome P450 2C19 polymorphism in young patients treated with clopidogrel after myocardial infarction: a cohort study. Lancet. 2009;373(9660):309–17.
40. Gilard M, Arnaud B, Cornily JC, et al. Influence of omeprazole on the antiplatelet action of clopidogrel associated with aspirin: the randomized, double-blind OCLA (Omeprazole CLopidogrel Aspirin) study. J Am Coll Cardiol. 2008;51(3):256–60.
41. Fontes-Carvalho R, Albuquerque A, Araújo C, Pimentel-Nunes P, Ribeiro VG. Omeprazole, but not pantoprazole, reduces the antiplatelet effect of clopidogrel: a randomized clinical crossover trial in patients after myocardial infarction evaluating the clopidogrel-PPIs drug interaction. Eur J Gastroenterol Hepatol. 2011;23(5):396–404.
42. Bhatt DL, Cryer BL, Contant CF, et al. Clopidogrel with or without omeprazole in coronary artery disease. N Engl J Med. 2010;363(20):1909–17.
43. US Food and Drug Administration. Clopidogrel product information. 2021. Available at: https://www.accessdata.fda.gov/drugsatfda_docs/label/2021/020839s074lbl.pdf
44. European Medicines Agency. Clopidogrel product information. 2008. Available at: https://www.ema.europa.eu/en/documents/product-information/plavix-epar-product-information_en.pdf

45. Niitsu Y, Jakubowski JA, Sugidachi A, Asai F. Pharmacology of CS-747 (prasugrel, LY640315), a novel, potent antiplatelet agent with in vivo P2Y12 receptor antagonist activity. Semin Thromb Hemost. 2005;31(2):184–94.
46. Wiviott SD, Antman EM, Braunwald E. Prasugrel. Circulation. 2010;122(4):394–403.
47. Jernberg T, Payne CD, Winters KJ, et al. Prasugrel achieves greater inhibition of platelet aggregation and a lower rate of non-responders compared with clopidogrel in aspirin-treated patients with stable coronary artery disease. Eur Heart J. 2006;27(10):1166–73.
48. Brandt JT, Payne CD, Wiviott SD, et al. A comparison of prasugrel and clopidogrel loading doses on platelet function: magnitude of platelet inhibition is related to active metabolite formation. Am Heart J. 2007;153(1):66.e9–16.
49. Wiviott SD, Trenk D, Frelinger AL, et al. Prasugrel compared with high loading- and maintenance-dose clopidogrel in patients with planned percutaneous coronary intervention: the Prasugrel in Comparison to Clopidogrel for Inhibition of Platelet Activation and Aggregation-Thrombolysis in Myocardial Infarction 44 trial. Circulation. 2007;116(25):2923–32.
50. Wiviott SD, Braunwald E, McCabe CH, et al. Prasugrel versus clopidogrel in patients with acute coronary syndromes. N Engl J Med. 2007;357(20):2001–15.
51. Roe MT, Armstrong PW, Fox KA, et al. Prasugrel versus clopidogrel for acute coronary syndromes without revascularization. N Engl J Med. 2012;367(14):1297–1309.
52. Wiviott SD, White HD, Ohman EM, et al. Prasugrel versus clopidogrel for patients with unstable angina or non-ST-segment elevation myocardial infarction with or without angiography: a secondary, prespecified analysis of the TRILOGY ACS trial. Lancet. 2013;382(9892):605–13.
53. Montalescot G, Bolognese L, Dudek D, et al. Pretreatment with prasugrel in non-ST-segment elevation acute coronary syndromes. N Engl J Med. 2013;369(11):999–1010.
54. Sibbing D, Aradi D, Jacobshagen C, et al. Guided de-escalation of antiplatelet treatment in patients with acute coronary syndrome undergoing percutaneous coronary intervention (TROPICAL-ACS): a randomised, open-label, multicentre trial. Lancet. 2017;390(10104):1747–57.
55. Kim HS, Kang J, Hwang D, et al. Prasugrel-based de-escalation of dual antiplatelet therapy after percutaneous coronary intervention in patients with acute coronary syndrome (HOST-REDUCE-POLYTECH-ACS): an open-label, multicentre, non-inferiority randomised trial. Lancet. 2020;396(10257):1079–89.
56. Ogawa A, Toyoda K, Kitagawa K, et al. Comparison of prasugrel and clopidogrel in patients with non-cardioembolic ischaemic stroke: a phase 3, randomised, non-inferiority trial (PRASTRO-I). Lancet Neurol. 2019;18(3):238–47.
57. European Medicines Agency. Ticagrelor product information. 2015. Available at: https://www.ema.europa.eu/en/documents/product-information/brilique-epar-product-information_en.pdf
58. US Food and Drug Administration. Prasugrel product information. 2020. Available at: https://www.accessdata.fda.gov/drugsatfda_docs/label/2020/022307s018lbl.pdf
59. van Giezen JJ, Humphries RG. Preclinical and clinical studies with selective reversible direct P2Y12 antagonists. Semin Thromb Hemost. 2005;31(2):195–204.
60. Husted S, Emanuelsson H, Heptinstall S, Sandset PM, Wickens M, Peters G. Pharmacodynamics, pharmacokinetics, and safety of the oral reversible P2Y12 antagonist AZD6140 with aspirin in patients with atherosclerosis: a double-blind comparison to clopidogrel with aspirin. Eur Heart J. 2006;27(9):1038–47.
61. Storey RF, Husted S, Harrington RA, et al. Inhibition of platelet aggregation by AZD6140, a reversible oral P2Y12 receptor antagonist, compared with clopidogrel in patients with acute coronary syndromes. J Am Coll Cardiol. 2007;50(19):1852–6.
62. Teng R, Butler K. Pharmacokinetics, pharmacodynamics, tolerability and safety of single ascending doses of ticagrelor, a reversibly binding oral P2Y(12) receptor antagonist, in healthy subjects. Eur J Clin Pharmacol. 2010;66(5):487–96.
63. Lemesle G, Schurtz G, Bauters C, Hamon M. High on-treatment platelet reactivity with ticagrelor versus prasugrel: a systematic review and meta-analysis. J Thromb Haemost. 2015;13(6):931–42.
64. Wallentin L, Becker RC, Budaj A, et al. Ticagrelor versus clopidogrel in patients with acute coronary syndromes. N Engl J Med. 2009;361(11):1045–57.
65. Gimbel M, Qaderdan K, Willemsen L, et al. Clopidogrel versus ticagrelor or prasugrel in patients aged 70 years or older with non-ST-elevation acute coronary syndrome (POPular AGE): the randomised, open-label, non-inferiority trial. Lancet. 2020;395(10233):1374–81.
66. Montalescot G, van 't Hof AW, Lapostolle F, et al. Prehospital ticagrelor in ST-segment elevation myocardial infarction. N Engl J Med. 2014;371(11):1016–27.
67. Vranckx P, Valgimigli M, Jüni P, et al. Ticagrelor plus aspirin for 1 month, followed by ticagrelor monotherapy for 23 months vs aspirin plus clopidogrel or ticagrelor for 12 months, followed by aspirin monotherapy for 12 months after implantation of a drug-eluting stent: a multicentre, open-label, randomised superiority trial. Lancet. 2018;392(10151):940–9.
68. Mehran R, Baber U, Sharma SK, et al. Ticagrelor with or without aspirin in high-risk patients after PCI. N Engl J Med. 2019;381(21):2032–42.
69. Kim CJ, Park MW, Kim MC, et al. Unguided de-escalation from ticagrelor to clopidogrel in stabilised patients with acute myocardial infarction undergoing percutaneous coronary intervention (TALOS-AMI): an investigator-initiated, open-label, multicentre, non-inferiority, randomised trial. Lancet. 2021;398(10308):1305–16.
70. Kuno T, Fujisaki T, Shoji S, et al. Comparison of unguided de-escalation versus guided selection of dual antiplatelet therapy after acute coronary syndrome: a systematic review and network meta-analysis. Circ Cardiovasc Interv. 2022;15(8):e011990.
71. Schüpke S, Neumann FJ, Menichelli M, et al. Ticagrelor or prasugrel in patients with acute coronary syndromes. N Engl J Med. 2019;381(16):1524–34.
72. Navarese EP, Khan SU, Kołodziejczak M, et al. Comparative efficacy and safety of oral P2Y(12) inhibitors in acute coronary syndrome: network meta-analysis of 52 816 patients from 12 randomized trials. Circulation. 2020;142(2):150–60.
73. Bonaca MP, Bhatt DL, Cohen M, et al. Long-term use of ticagrelor in patients with prior myocardial infarction. N Engl J Med. 2015;372(19):1791–800.
74. Dellborg M, Bonaca MP, Storey RF, et al. Efficacy and safety with ticagrelor in patients with prior myocardial infarction in the approved European label: insights from PEGASUS-TIMI 54. Eur Heart J Cardiovasc Pharmacother. 2019;5(4):200–6.
75. Steg PG, Bhatt DL, Simon T, et al. Ticagrelor in patients with stable coronary disease and diabetes. N Engl J Med. 2019;381(14):1309–20.
76. Bhatt DL, Steg PG, Mehta SR, et al. Ticagrelor in patients with diabetes and stable coronary artery disease with a history of previous percutaneous coronary intervention (THEMIS-PCI): a phase 3, placebo-controlled, randomised trial. Lancet. 2019;394(10204):1169–80.
77. Vranckx P, Valgimigli M, Odutayo A, et al. Efficacy and safety of ticagrelor monotherapy by clinical presentation: pre-specified analysis of the GLOBAL LEADERS Trial. J Am Heart Assoc. 2021;10(18):e015560.

78. Baber U, Dangas G, Angiolillo DJ, et al. Ticagrelor alone vs. ticagrelor plus aspirin following percutaneous coronary intervention in patients with non-ST-segment elevation acute coronary syndromes: TWILIGHT-ACS. Eur Heart J. 2020;41(37):3533–45.
79. Johnston SC, Amarenco P, Albers GW, et al. Ticagrelor versus aspirin in acute stroke or transient ischemic attack. N Engl J Med. 2016;375(1):35–43.
80. Johnston SC, Amarenco P, Denison H, et al. Ticagrelor and aspirin or aspirin alone in acute ischemic stroke or TIA. N Engl J Med. 2020;383(3):207–17.
81. Wang Y, Meng X, Wang A, et al. Ticagrelor versus clopidogrel in CYP2C19 loss-of-function carriers with stroke or TIA. N Engl J Med. 2021;385(27):2520–30.
82. Hiatt WR, Fowkes FG, Heizer G, et al. Ticagrelor versus clopidogrel in symptomatic peripheral artery disease. N Engl J Med. 2017;376(1):32–40.
83. Scirica BM, Cannon CP, Emanuelsson H, et al. The incidence of bradyarrhythmias and clinical bradyarrhythmic events in patients with acute coronary syndromes treated with ticagrelor or clopidogrel in the PLATO (Platelet Inhibition and Patient Outcomes) trial: results of the continuous electrocardiographic assessment substudy. J Am Coll Cardiol. 2011;57(19):1908–16.
84. Bhatt DL, Pollack CV, Weitz JI, et al. Antibody-based ticagrelor reversal agent in healthy volunteers. N Engl J Med. 2019;380(19):1825–33.
85. Bhatt DL, Pollack CV, Mazer CD, et al. Bentracimab for ticagrelor reversal in patients undergoing urgent surgery. NEJM Evid. 2022;1(3):EVIDoa2100047.
86. Gurbel PA, Bliden KP, Antonino MJ, et al. The effect of elinogrel on high platelet reactivity during dual antiplatelet therapy and the relation to CYP2C19*2 genotype: first experience in patients. J Thromb Haemost. 2010;8(1):43–53.
87. Angiolillo DJ, Welsh RC, Trenk D, et al. Pharmacokinetic and pharmacodynamic effects of elinogrel: results of the platelet function substudy from the intravenous and oral administration of elinogrel to evaluate tolerability and efficacy in nonurgent percutaneous coronary intervention patients (INNOVATE-PCI) trial. Circ Cardiovasc Interv. 2012;5(3):347–56.
88. Welsh RC, Rao SV, Zeymer U, et al. A randomized, double-blind, active-controlled phase 2 trial to evaluate a novel selective and reversible intravenous and oral P2Y12 inhibitor elinogrel versus clopidogrel in patients undergoing nonurgent percutaneous coronary intervention: the INNOVATE-PCI trial. Circ Cardiovasc Interv. 2012;5(3):336–46.
89. De Luca L, Steg PG, Bhatt DL, Capodanno D, Angiolillo DJ. Cangrelor: clinical data, contemporary use, and future perspectives. J Am Heart Assoc. 2021;10(13):e022125.
90. Storey RF, Wilcox RG, Heptinstall S. Comparison of the pharmacodynamic effects of the platelet ADP receptor antagonists clopidogrel and AR-C69931MX in patients with ischaemic heart disease. Platelets. 2002;13(7):407–13.
91. Akers WS, Oh JJ, Oestreich JH, Ferraris S, Wethington M, Steinhubl SR. Pharmacokinetics and pharmacodynamics of a bolus and infusion of cangrelor: a direct, parenteral P2Y12 receptor antagonist. J Clin Pharmacol. 2010;50(1):27–35.
92. Greenbaum AB, Grines CL, Bittl JA, et al. Initial experience with an intravenous P2Y12 platelet receptor antagonist in patients undergoing percutaneous coronary intervention: results from a 2-part, phase II, multicenter, randomized, placebo- and active-controlled trial. Am Heart J. 2006;151(3):689.e1–10.
93. Bhatt DL, Lincoff AM, Gibson CM, et al. Intravenous platelet blockade with cangrelor during PCI. N Engl J Med. 2009;361(24):2330–41.
94. Harrington RA, Stone GW, McNulty S, et al. Platelet inhibition with cangrelor in patients undergoing PCI. N Engl J Med. 2009;361(24):2318–29.
95. Bhatt DL, Stone GW, Mahaffey KW, et al. Effect of platelet inhibition with cangrelor during PCI on ischemic events. N Engl J Med. 2013;368(14):1303–13.
96. Steg PG, Bhatt DL, Hamm CW, et al. Effect of cangrelor on periprocedural outcomes in percutaneous coronary interventions: a pooled analysis of patient-level data. Lancet. 2013;382(9909):1981–92.
97. U.S. Food and Drug Administration. Cangrelor product information. 2019. Available at: https://www.accessdata.fda.gov/drugsatfda_docs/label/2019/204958s002lbl.pdf
98. European Medicines Agency. Cangrelor product information. 2019. Available at: https://www.ema.europa.eu/en/documents/product-information/kengrexal-epar-product-information_en.pdf
99. Schneider DJ, Seecheran N, Raza SS, Keating FK, Gogo P. Pharmacodynamic effects during the transition between cangrelor and prasugrel. Coron Artery Dis. 2015;26(1):42–8.
100. Schneider DJ, Agarwal Z, Seecheran N, Keating FK, Gogo P. Pharmacodynamic effects during the transition between cangrelor and ticagrelor. JACC Cardiovasc Interv. 2014;7(4):435–42.
101. Baldoni D, Bruderer S, Krause A, et al. A new reversible and potent P2Y12 receptor antagonist (ACT-246475): tolerability, pharmacokinetics, and pharmacodynamics in a first-in-man trial. Clin Drug Investig. 2014;34(11):807–18.
102. Juif PE, Boehler M, Dobrow M, Ufer M, Dingemanse J. Clinical pharmacology of the reversible and potent P2Y(12) receptor antagonist ACT-246475 after single subcutaneous administration in healthy male subjects. J Clin Pharmacol. 2019;59(1):123–30.
103. Sinnaeve P, Fahrni G, Schelfaut D, et al. subcutaneous selatogrel inhibits platelet aggregation in patients with acute myocardial infarction. J Am Coll Cardiol. 2020;75(20):2588–97.
104. Storey RF, Gurbel PA, Ten Berg J, et al. Pharmacodynamics, pharmacokinetics, and safety of single-dose subcutaneous administration of selatogrel, a novel P2Y12 receptor antagonist, in patients with chronic coronary syndromes. Eur Heart J. 2020;41(33):3132–40.
105. Sibbing D, Kastrati A, Berger PB. Pre-treatment with P2Y12 inhibitors in ACS patients: who, when, why, and which agent? Eur Heart J. 2016;37(16):1284–95.
106. Collet JP, Thiele H, Barbato E, et al. 2020 ESC Guidelines for the management of acute coronary syndromes in patients presenting without persistent ST-segment elevation. Eur Heart J. 2021;42(14):1289–367.
107. Ueno M, Rao SV, Angiolillo DJ. Elinogrel: pharmacological principles, preclinical and early phase clinical testing. Future Cardiol. 2010;6(4):445–53.
108. US Food and Drug Administration. Ticagrelor product information. 2021. Available at: https://www.accessdata.fda.gov/drugsatfda_docs/label/2021/022433s031lbl.pdf
109. European Medicines Agency. Prasugrel Product Information. 2013. Available at: https://www.ema.europa.eu/en/documents/product-information/efient-epar-product-information_en.pdf

CHAPTER 7

Dipyridamole, cilostazol, glycoprotein IIb/IIIa inhibitors, and protease-activated receptor-1 antagonists

Luis Ortega-Paz and Dominick J. Angiolillo

Contents

Summary

During the last decades of the 1900s, dipyridamole and cilostazol were introduced into clinical practice as antiplatelet agents. Although they were initially used for treating patients with coronary artery disease, they are used for preventing recurrent stroke in Asian countries. Cilostazol is also used worldwide for treating patients with peripheral artery disease. In 1998 and 2008, the glycoprotein IIb/IIIa inhibitors (GPIs) and protease-activated receptor-1 (PAR-1) antagonist were introduced into clinical practice, respectively. These drugs represent the beginning of the era of receptor-targeted antiplatelet drugs, which were the product of the discovery and better understanding of the role of platelet surface receptors. During the late 1990s and early 2000s, GPIs (abciximab, eptifibatide, tirofiban) were part of the standard of care in patients with coronary artery disease and undergoing percutaneous coronary intervention. However, with the introduction of newer-generation $P2Y_{12}$ inhibitors, their use has been mostly limited as a bail-out strategy in the presence of no-reflow or a thrombotic complication in patients undergoing percutaneous coronary intervention. Although PAR-1 antagonists reduce adverse cardiovascular events, they are associated with a higher risk of major bleeding, including intracranial bleeding. Currently, vorapaxar is the only available PAR-1 antagonist and is approved for preventing cardiovascular events in patients with a history of myocardial infarction or peripheral artery disease without a previous history of stroke, transient ischaemic attack, or intracranial haemorrhage. However, the clinical utilization of vorapaxar is limited. New drugs, including a PAR-1 inhibitor (PZ-128) and a GPI (zalunfiban) are undergoing phase II and III clinical investigations, respectively.

Introduction

Platelet activation and their accumulation at sites of vascular injury are the first steps in physiological haemostasis. However, excessive platelet activation after atherosclerotic plaque rupture or erosion may lead to thrombus formation. This phenomenon, known as atherothrombosis due to its atherosclerotic aetiology and its thrombotic consequences, clinically manifests as acute ischaemic events in the coronary, cerebrovascular, or peripheral artery territories.[1] Since the understanding of the critical role of platelets in atherothrombotic events, the development of drugs targeted to inhibit platelet activation and aggregation has been an area of extensive research. In the early 1900s, aspirin was the first antiplatelet agent introduced in clinical practice and represented a milestone in cardiovascular medicine.[1] Furthermore, during the last decades of the 1900s, the introduction of dipyridamole and cilostazol added more treatment options to achieve platelet inhibition.[1] A better understanding of platelet biology, surface receptors, and mechanism of activation and aggregation allowed a more precise development of antiplatelet drugs. Between the 1970s and 1980s, the discovery of the glycoprotein (GP)-IIb/IIIa receptor and understanding its role in platelet activation and aggregation was another pivotal milestone resulting in the development of a number of drugs targeting its inhibition.[1] Ultimately, in late 1990, the discovery of the protease-activated receptor-1 (PAR-1) receptor promoted the development of drugs targeting its inhibition.[1] This chapter will review the history, mechanism of action, and clinical evidence of dipyridamole, cilostazol, PAR-1 antagonist, and glycoprotein IIb/IIIa inhibitors (GPIs). Indications, future perspectives, and dosing regimens for each drug are reported at the end of the chapter.

Dipyridamole

Dipyridamole is a double ring structure compound formed from two pyrimidine rings and was discovered in 1951.[2] Early clinical studies show a marked increase in coronary blood flow without a significant increase in oxygen consumption.[2] It was introduced into clinical practice as a coronary vasodilator agent in 1959. The proposed mechanism leading to vasodilation was attributed to the inhibition of adenosine uptake.[2] Moreover, animal experiments showed that dipyridamole inhibits thrombus formation and has been considered an antiplatelet agent since the 1960s.[2] In 1968, studies reported that dipyridamole could provoke or aggravate anginal events when given intravenously to test coronary reserve or to treat unstable angina.[2] Subsequent studies revealed that in the presence of coronary obstruction, dipyridamole could induce a reduction in subendocardial blood flow and myocardial ischaemia.[3] Ultimately, dipyridamole was assessed as a coronary vasodilator used in nuclear stress testing in patients with suspected coronary artery disease (CAD).[4]

Mechanism of action

Dipyridamole was initially found to increase extracellular levels of adenosine by inhibiting adenosine uptake by red blood cells (➔ Figure 7.1).[4] At a clinically relevant dose, dipyridamole inhibits adenosine uptake by red blood cells by greater than 90%, increasing plasma adenosine levels by 60%.[4] Adenosine receptor activation by adenosine stimulates platelet adenylyl cyclase, increasing cyclic adenosine monophosphate (cAMP) intracellular levels, which ultimately acts as a potent inhibitor of platelet activation.[4] A second proposed mechanism of action is the increase in intracellular platelet levels of cAMP by preventing the breakdown of cAMP by the inhibition of phosphodiesterase (PDE) isoforms 3 and 5.[5]

Clinical evidence

Since 1968, dipyridamole has been studied in several randomized controlled trials (RCTs) among patients with cardiovascular disease, as summarized in ➔ Table 7.1.[4] In patients with CAD, dipyridamole did not reduce all-cause death or acute complications after percutaneous transluminal coronary angioplasty compared to aspirin. However, these early trials no longer reflect current clinical practice. More recently, dipyridamole has been used with oral anticoagulation (OAC) to prevent thromboembolic events in patients who underwent cardiac valve replacement with mechanical valves. In a meta-analysis of six RCTs, dipyridamole plus OAC was associated with a significant reduction in thromboembolic events (fatal and non-fatal) and mortality, without a difference in bleeding.[6] In 2002, the Antithrombotic Trialists' Collaboration meta-analysis analysed 25 trials that directly compared dipyridamole plus aspirin versus aspirin alone. There were no significant differences in serious vascular events between groups. However, in studies that indirectly compared both strategies, there was a benefit in vascular events in those treated with dipyridamole plus aspirin compared to aspirin alone.[7]

Dipyridamole has also been studied in the field of stroke in the European/Australasian Stroke Prevention in Reversible Ischaemia Trial (ESPRIT) and the Prevention Regimen for Effectively Avoiding Second Strokes (PRoFESS) trial.[8,9] In the ESPRIT trial, 2739 patients within 6 months of a TIA or minor stroke were randomized to dipyridamole plus aspirin or aspirin alone. Dipyridamole plus aspirin was associated with a significant reduction in the composite of death and major vascular complications compared to aspirin alone. Patients allocated to dipyridamole plus aspirin discontinued the study medication more frequently than those on aspirin alone.[8] In the PRoFESS trial, 20,332 patients were randomized to dipyridamole plus aspirin or clopidogrel. The predefined margin for non-inferiority was not met. The investigators concluded that there was no evidence that either of the two treatments was superior to the other in preventing recurrent stroke.[9]

Contraindications

Hypersensitivity to dipyridamole or any components. The American Society of Nuclear Cardiology has provided specific guidance for absolute and relative contraindications when it is used for stress testing.[10]

Cilostazol

During the 1980s, researchers from Japan synthesized a quinolone derivative, cilostamide, which inhibited platelet aggregation and

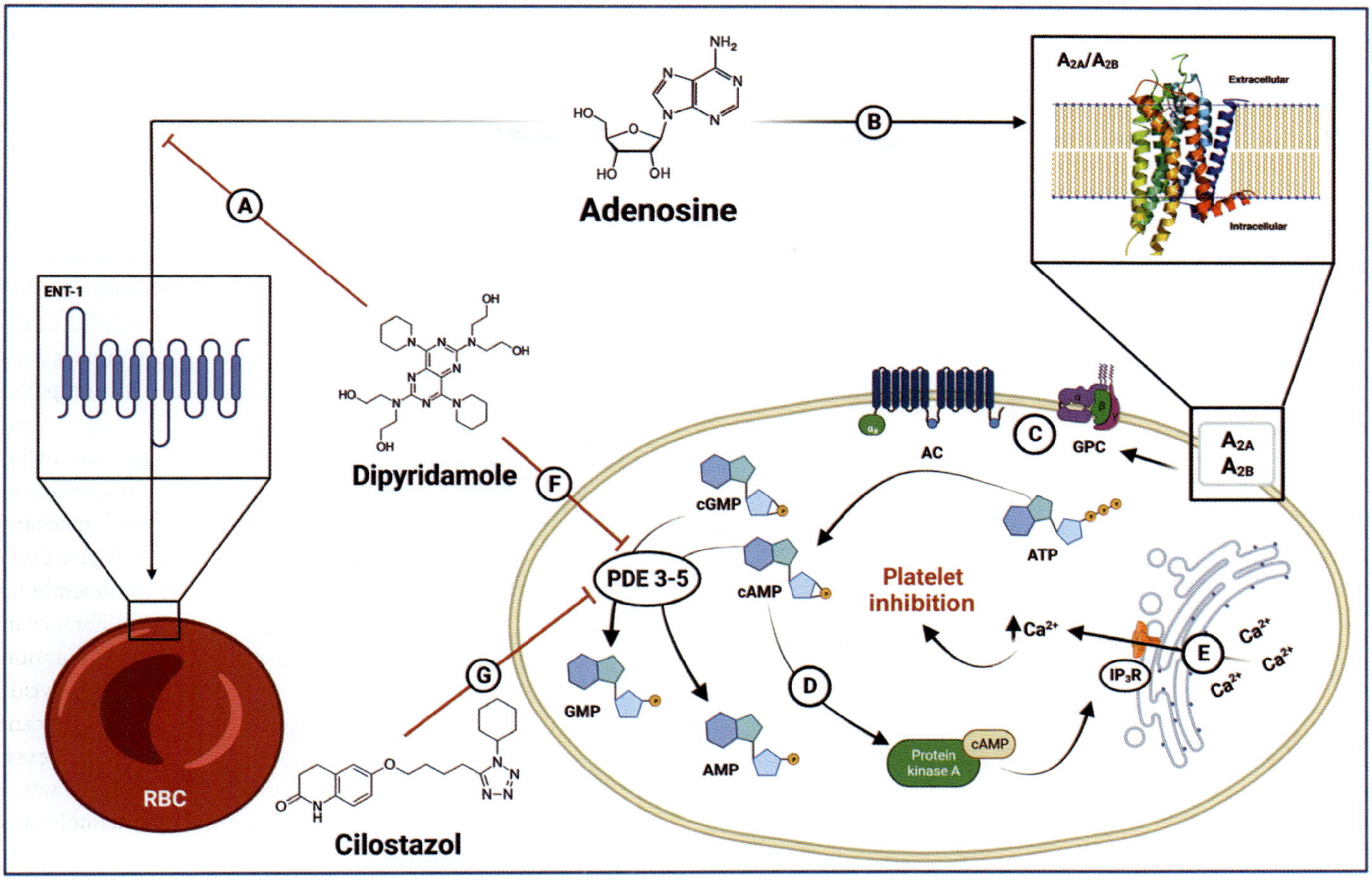

Figure 7.1 Mechanism of platelet inhibition of dipyridamole and cilostazol. A: at clinically relevant doses, dipyridamole can significantly inhibit the circulating adenosine recapture by the equilibrative nucleoside transporters (ENT)-1 in the red blood cells (RBC). B: circulating adenosine can activate the platelet adenosine A_{2A} and A_{2B} receptors, stimulating the G protein-coupled (GPC). C: GPC promotes the activation of the adenylyl cyclase (AC), which metabolizes cytosolic adenosine triphosphate (ATP) into cyclic adenosine monophosphate (cAMP). D: cAMP activates the protein kinase A, which stimulates the inositol triphosphate receptor (IP3R) in the endoplasmic reticulum. E: the IP_3R activation allows the exit of calcium (Ca^{2+}) from the endoplasmic reticulum into the cytosol, the cytosol increase of Ca^{2+} is ultimately associated with potent inhibition of platelet activation and aggregation. F: dipyridamole can inhibit phosphodiesterase (PDE)-3 and -5, but the concentrations needed to inhibit PDE5 are much higher than those attainable after oral administration. PDE3 and -5 degrade cAMP (more affinity) into AMP and cyclic guanylyl monophosphate (cGMP) into guanosine monophosphate (GMP). AMP and GMP do not exert antiplatelet effects. G: cilostazol is a specific and strong inhibitor of platelet PDE3, and it can inhibit both primary and secondary platelet aggregation. Elevation of cytosolic levels of cAMP and cGMP produces platelet inhibition as in steps D–E.

had vasodilatory properties but caused persistent tachycardia.[11] Subsequent modifications led to the discovery of cilostazol, which preserved the antiplatelet and vasodilator effects but without producing persistent tachycardia.[11] Cilostazol was first marketed in Japan in 1988, and its use extended to the rest of the world in 2000 for treating peripheral artery disease (PAD).[11] Moreover, cilostazol was shown to be effective in preventing stroke recurrence and was approved for this indication in Japan in 2003.[12]

Mechanism of action

Cilostazol's mechanism of action is through inhibition of PDE3 and increase in intracellular cAMP levels (➔ Figure 7.1).[12] PDE3 is predominantly located in platelets, cardiac myocytes, vascular and visceral smooth muscle.[5] PDE3 can hydrolyse cyclic guanosine monophosphate and cAMP, although it has a greater affinity towards cAMP. Increased intracellular concentrations of cAMP promote platelet inhibition.[12]

Clinical evidence

Cilostazol has been studied in several RCTs among patients with PAD, CAD, and stroke, as summarized in ➔ Table 7.2. In 2021, Cochrane reported a systematic review and meta-analysis including 16 double-blinded trials comparing cilostazol and placebo in patients with PAD.[13] Overall, cilostazol effectively increased initial claudication distance and may be associated with increased quality of life. Nevertheless, the certainty of the quality-of-life findings was low. Of note, cilostazol was not associated with a reduction in cardiovascular events but with an increase in side effects, in particular headaches.

Cilostazol has been tested as an antithrombotic drug in patients treated with percutaneous coronary intervention (PCI).[14] In particular, cilostazol was studied in addition to dual antiplatelet therapy (DAPT; aspirin and clopidogrel 75 mg) as part of a triple antiplatelet therapy (TAT) compared to double-dose DAPT (aspirin and clopidogrel 150 mg). TAT, including cilostazol,

Table 7.1 Selected randomized controlled trials of dipyridamole in cardiovascular diseases

Trial	Methods	Key results
Pouleur et al. (1995)[6]	◆ Meta-analysis of RCTs comparing dipyridamole + OAC vs OAC alone for reducing embolization after valve replacement with a mechanical prosthesis ◆ Endpoints: thromboembolic events, bleeding, and mortality	◆ 6 trials, including 1141 patients, were analysed ◆ Dipyridamole + OAC was associated with a significant reduction in thromboembolic events (56%) and mortality (40%) compared to OAC alone ◆ There were no differences in bleeding events
Antithrombotic Trialists' Collaboration (2002)[7]	◆ Collaborative meta-analysis of RCT of antiplatelet therapy for prevention of death, MI, and stroke in high-risk patients ◆ Primary endpoint: serious vascular events defined as the composite of non-fatal MI, non-fatal stroke, or vascular death	◆ 25 trials compared directly (10,404 patients), and 46 trials compared indirectly (19,441 patients) dipyridamole + ASA vs ASA alone ◆ Direct comparisons: there were no significant differences between groups (11.8% vs 12.4%) ◆ Indirect comparison: dipyridamole + ASA was associated with a reduction in vascular events compared to ASA alone (10.7% vs 14.3%)
ESPRIT (2006)[9]	◆ Open-label RCT comparing dipyridamole plus ASA (200 mg and 30–325 mg) vs ASA (30–325 mg) within 6 months of a TIA or minor stroke of presumed arterial origin ◆ Primary endpoint: composite of death from all vascular causes, non-fatal stroke, non-fatal MI, or major bleeding complication	◆ 2739 patients were enrolled with a mean follow-up of 3.5 years ◆ Dipyridamole + ASA was associated with a significant reduction in the primary endpoint (HR 0.80, 95% CI 0.66–0.98) ◆ Patients allocated to dipyridamole + ASA discontinued the medication more frequently than ASA alone
PRoFESS (2008)[10]	◆ Double-blind, 2-by-2 factorial trial RCT comparing dipyridamole + ASA (200/25 mg) vs clopidogrel (75 mg) for preventing recurrent stroke ◆ Primary endpoint: first recurrence of stroke, non-inferiority analysis	◆ 20332 patients were enrolled ◆ Predefined criteria for non-inferiority were not met between dipyridamole + ASA and clopidogrel (HR 1.01, 95% CI 0.92–1.11)

ASA, acetylsalicylic acid; CI, confidence interval; HR, hazard ratio; MI, myocardial infarction; OAC, oral anticoagulation; RCT: randomized controlled trial.

was non-inferior to double-dose DAPT in terms of net clinical outcome. There were no differences in ischaemic or bleeding events between groups. Moreover, cilostazol has been tested for preventing stent restenosis, including with drug-eluting stents. In a pooled analysis of the Drug-Eluting Stenting Followed by Cilostazol Treatment Reduces Late Restenosis (DECLARE) studies, TAT (aspirin, clopidogrel, and cilostazol) reduced the rates of in-stent restenosis in high-risk patients compared with DAPT (aspirin and clopidogrel).[15] The treatment effect was significant in patients treated with sirolimus and zotarolimus-eluting stents but not with paclitaxel-eluting stents.

In Asia, cilostazol has been intensively studied in the field of stroke. The Cilostazol Stroke Prevention Studies (CSPSs) have been the landmark trials in this field. In the CSPS trial, cilostazol was superior to placebo for preventing cerebral infarction recurrence.[16] Subsequently, in the CSPS 2 trial, cilostazol was non-inferior compared to aspirin to prevent recurrent stroke and was associated with fewer bleeding events.[17] In the CSPS.com trial, which was prematurely stopped due to a low enrolment rate, cilostazol combined with either aspirin or clopidogrel reduced stroke recurrence compared to monotherapy with either aspirin or clopidogrel.[18] In the CSPS trials, cilostazol was associated with side effects such as headache, palpitations, and an increase in pulse rate.

Contraindications

Hypersensitivity to cilostazol or any components and heart failure of any severity. Cilostazol and several of its metabolites are inhibitors of PDE3. Several drugs with this pharmacological effect have caused decreased survival compared to placebo in patients with heart failure class III–IV of the New York Heart Association.[19]

Glycoprotein IIb/IIIa inhibitors

GPI development has been closely related to the study of Glanzmann thrombasthenia, an autosomal recessive disorder that manifests as a lifelong moderate to severe bleeding tendency.[3] In the mid-1970s, by studying platelet samples from patients with Glanzmann thrombasthenia, an abnormal platelet GP pattern was observed and subsequently led to the description of GPIIb/IIIa (integrin αIIbβ3).[3] During the 1980s, a patient with Glanzmann thrombasthenia who developed a powerful antibody against GPIIb/IIIa following blood transfusions raised the rationale for a new therapeutic target.[3] In the late 1980s, researchers synthesized a chimeric monoclonal-antibody Fab fragment (c7E3 Fab) that inhibited platelet reactivity in animal models with higher efficacy than aspirin. In 1994, abciximab (c7E3 Fab) was the first GPI introduced into clinical practice. Furthermore, during the 2000s, other GPIs derived from snake venom, eptifibatide and tirofiban, were also introduced into clinical practice.[3] Since 2018, abciximab is no longer supplied by the original drug makers, although generic formulations are available in some parts of the world.[20]

Mechanism of action

The GPIIb/IIIa receptor is an integrin heterodimer that contains a large extracellular region, a transmembrane domain, and a short intracellular cytoplasmic tail. It comprises a heterodimer

Table 7.2 Selected randomized controlled trials of cilostazol in cardiovascular diseases

Trial	Methods	Key results
Brown et al. (2021)[13]	◆ Cochrane systematic review and meta-analysis, including double-blinded RCTs comparing cilostazol vs placebo ◆ Primary outcomes were ICD and QoL	◆ 16 trials (3972 patients) were included, of which 5 also compared with pentoxifylline ◆ Cilostazol was associated with higher ICD than placebo. There was a possible indication of improvement of QoL with cilostazol (low-certainty evidence). There is insufficient evidence about the effectiveness of cilostazol for serious events such as amputation, revascularization, and cardiovascular events ◆ Patients treated with cilostazol reported more frequent headaches as an adverse event
HOST-ASSURE (2013)[14]	◆ Open-label, factorial 2-by-2, RCT comparing TAT with cilostazol 100 mg plus DAPT (aspirin and clopidogrel 75 mg) vs DDAPT (aspirin and clopidogrel 150 mg) ◆ Primary endpoint: net clinical outcome, composite of cardiac death, MI, stroke, and major bleeding at 1 month	◆ 3755 patients were enrolled ◆ TAT met the prespecified margin for non-inferiority for the primary outcome compared to DDAT (1.2% vs 1.4%; P <0.001) ◆ There were no differences in the individual risks of cardiac death, non-fatal MI, ST, stroke, and major bleeding between groups
CSPS (2000)[16]	◆ Double-blinded, placebo-controlled RCT comparing cilostazol 100 mg vs placebo in patients with cerebral infarction within 1–6 months ◆ Primary endpoint: recurrence of cerebral infarction	◆ 1052 patients were enrolled ◆ Cilostazol was associated with a significant relative risk reduction in stroke recurrence compared to placebo (42.3%; 95% CI 10.3–62.9%; P = 0.012) ◆ There was no difference in the rate of bleeding events or significant adverse drug reactions between cilostazol and placebo
CSPS 2 (2010)[17]	◆ Double-blinded, aspirin-controlled, randomized non-inferiority trial comparing cilostazol 100 mg vs ASA 81 mg for 1–5 years in patients aged 20–79 years who had had a cerebral infarction within the previous 26 weeks ◆ Primary endpoint: first occurrence of stroke (cerebral infarction, cerebral haemorrhage, or subarachnoid haemorrhage)	◆ 2757 patients were included ◆ Cilostazol was non-inferior and might be superior to aspirin for the prevention of a stroke after an ischaemic stroke (2.7% vs 3.7%; P = 0.036) and was associated with fewer haemorrhagic events (0.7% vs 1.7%; P <0.001) ◆ Cilostazol was associated with more side effects than aspirin (headache, diarrhoea, palpitations, dizziness, and tachycardia)
CSPS.com (2019)[18]	◆ Open-label RCT comparing monotherapy (aspirin or clopidogrel) vs DAPT (cilostazol plus aspirin or clopidogrel) in patients with high-risk non-cardioembolic ischaemic stroke	◆ Trial was stopped prematurely, 1884 (47%) patients were enrolled ◆ DAPT with cilostazol plus aspirin or clopidogrel reduces ischaemic stroke recurrence when compared to monotherapy (HR 0.49, 95% CI 0.31–0.76; P = 0.001) ◆ There were no differences in severe or life-threatening bleeding events

ASA, acetylsalicylic acid; DAPT, dual antiplatelet therapy; DDAPT, dual DAPT; ICD, initial claudication distance; MI, myocardial infarction; QoL, Quality of Life; RCT, randomized controlled trial; ST, stent thrombosis; TAT, triple antiplatelet therapy.

protein consisting of alpha- and beta-subunits (➔ Figure 7.2).[21] The alpha-subunit is characterized by calcium- or manganese-binding domains and the beta-subunit by binding sites including lysine–glycine–aspartic acid (KGD) or arginine–glycine–aspartic acid (RGD) for attachment of fibrinogen, von Willebrand factor, and prothrombin.[21] GPIIb/IIIa receptor activation, secondary to talin and kindlin-3 interaction with the cytoplasmatic β3 domain, increases the receptor affinity for its ligand in the extracellular domain (inside-out signalling).[21] The activated GPIIb/IIIa receptor interacts with fibrinogen promoting platelet aggregation and platelet plug formation. GPIIb/IIIa receptor interaction with fibrin generates more intracellular signals (outside-in signalling), causing further platelet activation and platelet-plug retraction.[21] Abciximab, a large-sized antibody fragment, irreversibly binds to the β-chain of the receptor, promoting a steric hindrance of access of ligands to their binding pocket.[22] Eptifibatide is a synthetic cyclic heptapeptide with a modification (homo-Arg instead of Lys) that provides a highly specific binding to the GPIIb/IIIa receptor because of the structural resemblance of the KGD sequence.[22] Tirofiban is a non-peptide tyrosine derivative that mimics the RGD integrin recognition sequence, binds to the ligand binding pocket, and competes with them.[22] Eptifibatide and tirofiban acts as reversible competitive antagonists.

Clinical evidence

Over the last three decades, GPIs have been extensively studied in RCTs, as summarized in ➔ Table 7.3. The role of GPIs has substantially changed with the evolution of interventional pharmacology. The introduction of $P2Y_{12}$ receptor inhibitors, particularly the newer-generation agents, characterized by more prompt and potent platelet inhibitory effects (prasugrel and ticagrelor), markedly changed the benefit/risk ratio of GPIs which have gone from being the standard of care among patients undergoing PCI to their use currently being recommended as bail-out strategy in the presence of no-reflow or a thrombotic complication in patients undergoing PCI.[22] RCTs conducted before the advent of $P2Y_{12}$ receptor inhibitors are not discussed here as they are no longer relevant in clinical practice.[22]

In patients with chronic coronary syndromes, the Intracoronary Stenting and Antithrombotic Regimen–Rapid Early Action for

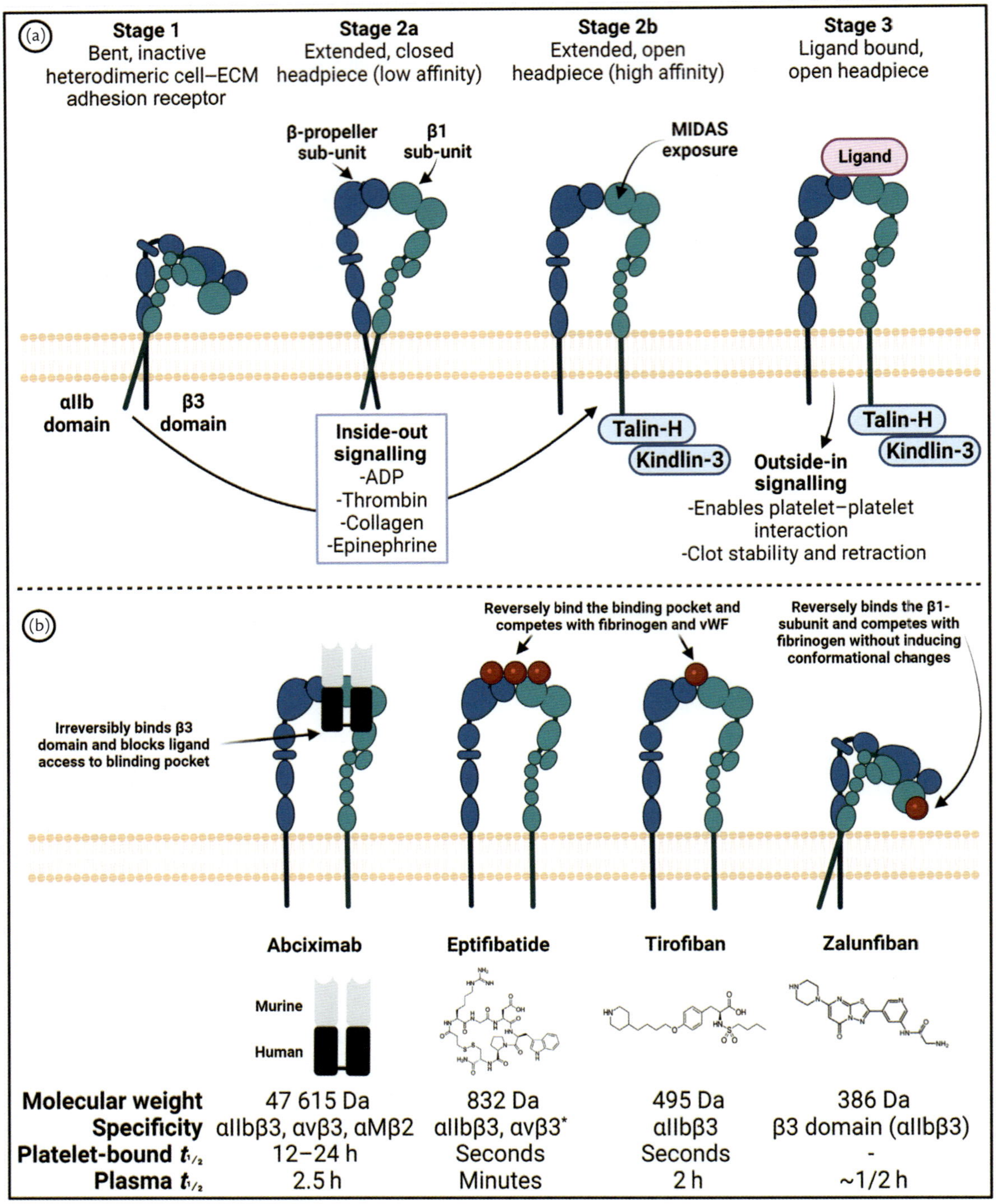

Figure 7.2 Mechanism of platelet inhibition of GP IIb/IIIa inhibitors. (a) the integrin αIIbβ3 receptor is composed of the αIIb and β3 domains. Its main function is cell–extracellular membrane (ECM) adhesion, enabling cell–cell interactions. Platelet activation by means of adenosine diphosphate (ADP), collagen, or epinephrine agonism on their respective receptors promotes a conformational change in the αIIbβ3 (inside-out signalling) from its inactive (stage 1) form to its extended closed (stage 2a) with low affinity for ligands and ultimately to its extended open (stage 2b) with high affinity for ligands. αIIbβ3 ligand can be classified in those with cross-bridging function [fibrinogen and von Willebrand factor (vWF)] and modulate platelet aggregation (fibronectin, vitronectin, thrombospondin, and CD40 ligand). All the ligands express one or more arginine–glycine–aspartic acid (RGD) sequences. Ligand binding to the metal ion-dependent adhesion site (MIDAS) promotes the outside-in signalling, which induces platelet aggregation (stage 3). (b) first-generation glycoprotein inhibitors (GPIs; abciximab, eptifibatide, and tirofiban) are administrated intravenously and can bind the αIIbβ3 receptor in its resting and active form. Some data suggest that they can induce conformational changes in the receptor that may provoke a degree of agonism. Zalunfiban, a second-generation GPI, is administered subcutaneously and binds selectively to the β1-subunit in the β3 domain in resting receptor form (without inducing conformational changes) and competing only with fibrinogen.

Table 7.3 Selected randomized controlled trials of glycoprotein IIb/IIIa inhibitor antagonists in cardiovascular diseases

Trial	Methods	Key results
ISAR-REACT trial (2004)[23]	◆ Double-blinded, placebo-controlled RCT comparing abciximab vs placebo in patients with CAD who underwent PCI and were pretreated with clopidogrel ◆ Primary endpoint: composite of death, MI, and urgent target vessel revascularization at 30 days	◆ 2159 patients were enrolled ◆ Abciximab did not significantly reduce the primary endpoint compared with placebo (RR 1.05; 95% CI 0.69–1.59; P = 0.820) ◆ Abciximab was not associated with an increase in major bleeding compared to placebo but was associated with profound thrombocytopenia (1.0% vs 0.0%; P = 0.002)
ISAR-SWEET (2004)[24]	◆ Double-blinded, placebo-controlled RCT comparing abciximab vs placebo in patients with CAD who underwent PCI and were pretreated with clopidogrel ◆ Primary endpoint: composite of death and MI at 1 year	◆ 701 patients enrolled ◆ Abciximab did not significantly reduce the primary endpoint compared with placebo (RR 0.97; 95% CI 0.58–1.62; P = 0.910) ◆ Abciximab was associated with a reduction of bare-metal stent restenosis and target lesion revascularization compared to placebo, without an increase in major bleeding
ISAR-REACT 2 trial (2006)[26]	◆ Double-blinded, placebo-controlled RCT comparing abciximab vs placebo in patients with NSTE-ACS who underwent PCI and were pretreated with clopidogrel ◆ Primary endpoint: composite of death, MI, or urgent target vessel revascularization at 30 days	◆ 2022 patients enrolled ◆ Among patients with elevated cardiac troponin, abciximab reduced the incidence of the primary endpoint compared to placebo (RR 0.71, 95% CI 0.54–0.95; P = 0.020). There was not a significant reduction among patients without cardiac troponin elevation ◆ There was no significant difference between groups in bleeding events or transfusion of blood products
MATRIX trial (2015)[32]	◆ Open-label, 2-by-2 factorial design RCT comparing UFH ± GPI vs bivalirudin in patients with ACS patients undergoing early invasive management ◆ Co-primary endpoint at 30 days: 1. Composite: death, myocardial infarction, or stroke 2. NACE: major bleeding or MACE	◆ 7213 patients enrolled. In the catheterization laboratory, 165 patients (4.6%) in the bivalirudin group and 933 patients (25.9%) in the UFH were treated with concomitant GPI ◆ UFH ± GPI was not associated with a reduction in MACE (RR 0.94, 95% CI 0.81–1.09; P = 0.440) or NACE compared to bivalirudin (RR 0.89, 95% CI 0.78–1.03; P = 0.120) ◆ Bivalirudin was associated with a reduction in major bleeding compared to UFH ± GPI (RR 0.55, 95% CI 0.39–0.78; P <0.001)
ACUITY Timing Trial (2007)[30]	◆ Open-label RCT comparing routine upstream GPI vs deferred selective GPI in patients with moderate- and high-risk ACS who undergo invasive treatment ◆ Primary endpoint: non-inferiority assessment of death, MI, or unplanned revascularization for ischaemia at 30 days	◆ 9207 patients enrolled ◆ Routine upstream GPI use did not meet the non-inferiority margin compared to deferred selective (RR 1.12; 95% CI 0.97–1.29; P = 0.044 for non-inferiority; P = 0.13 for superiority) ◆ Routine upstream GPI increased major bleeding compared to deferred selective (6.1% vs 4.9%; P = 0.009 for superiority)
EARLY ACS trial (2009)[31]	◆ Double-blinded, placebo-controlled RCT comparing early eptifibatide (≥12 hours before angiography) vs early placebo with delayed eptifibatide (after angiography) in patients with NSTE-ACS assigned to invasive strategy ◆ Primary endpoint: composite of death, MI, recurrent ischaemia requiring urgent revascularization, or thrombotic complication during PCI at 96 hours	◆ 9492 patients enrolled ◆ There was no significant difference in the primary endpoint between early or delayed eptifibatide (OR 0.92; 95% CI 0.80–1.06; P = 0.230) ◆ Early-eptifibatide group had significantly higher rates of bleeding and red cell transfusion
HORIZONS-AMI Trial (2008)[33]	◆ Open-label, 2-by-2 factorial RCT comparing anticoagulation with UFH + GPI vs bivalirudin in patients with STE-ACS who were undergoing primary PCI ◆ Co-primary endpoints at 30 days: 1. NACE: major bleeding or MACE (death, reinfarction, target-vessel revascularization, and stroke) 2. Major bleeding events (protocol-defined)	◆ 3602 patients were enrolled ◆ Bivalirudin significantly reduce NACE compared to UFH + GPI (RR 0.76; 95% CI 0.63–0.92; P = 0.005), owing to a lower rate of major bleeding (RR 0.60; 95% CI 0.46–0.77; P <0.001). However, bivalirudin was associated with a higher rate of acute stent thrombosis (1.3% vs 0.3%; P <0.001) ◆ Bivalirudin significantly reduced all-cause and cardiovascular deaths compared to UFH + GPI
AIDA STEMI trial (2012)[34]	◆ Open-label RCT comparing intracoronary abciximab vs intravenous abciximab bolus, both followed by infusion in patients presenting with STE-ACS ◆ Primary endpoint: composite of all-cause death, recurrent infarction, or new congestive heart failure at 90 days	◆ 2065 patients were enrolled ◆ Intracoronary abciximab did not significantly reduce the incidence of primary endpoint compared to intracoronary abciximab (OR 0.91; 95% CI 0.64–1.28; p = 0.580) ◆ There were no difference between groups in bleeding events

ACS, acute coronary syndrome; CAD, coronary artery disease; GPI, glycoprotein IIb/IIIa inhibitors; MACE, major adverse cardiovascular events; MI, myocardial infarction; OR, odds ratio; NACE, net adverse clinical events; NSTE-ACS, non-ST-segment elevation ACS; RCT, randomized controlled trial; RR, relative risk; STE-ACS; ST-segment elevation ACS, UFH: unfractionated heparin.

Coronary Treatment (ISAR-REACT) study compared abciximab versus placebo in patients who underwent PCI and were pretreated with clopidogrel.[23] Abciximab did not significantly reduce the composite of death, MI, or urgent revascularization compared to placebo and was not associated with an increase in major bleeding. However, abciximab was associated with profound thrombocytopenia. In a dedicated study of diabetic patients with chronic coronary syndromes undergoing PCI with clopidogrel pretreatment, abciximab did not reduce the cumulative incidence of death and MI.[24] Nevertheless, a meta-analysis analysing the safety and efficacy of GPI on the background of stenting and thienopyridines (i.e. ticlopidine and clopidogrel) found that GPIs were associated with a significant reduction of non-fatal MI compared to placebo or standard of care. There were no differences in all-cause death or major bleeding.[25]

In the ISAR-REACT-2 trial, abciximab was compared to placebo in patients with non-ST-segment elevation (NSTE)- acute coronary syndrome (ACS) who underwent PCI and were pretreated with clopidogrel.[26] Among patients with elevated cardiac troponin, abciximab significantly reduced the composite of death, MI, or urgent target vessel revascularization compared to placebo. There was no difference between treatments in patients without elevated cardiac troponin. In the overall cohort, there were no differences between groups in bleeding events or transfusion of blood products. Of note, prasugrel and ticagrelor are currently recommended over clopidogrel in patients with ACS per clinical guidelines.[27] In the Trial to Assess Improvement in Therapeutic Outcomes by Optimizing Platelet Inhibition with Prasugrel (TRITON), and the Platelet Inhibition and Patient Outcomes (PLATO) trials, the benefits in clinical outcomes of prasugrel and ticagrelor over clopidogrel were independent of the concomitant GPI treatment.[28,29] However, these trials were not designed for this purpose and did not allow definite conclusions to be drawn about the benefit of GPIs on top of potent oral $P2Y_{12}$ inhibitors.

Some trials assessed different GPI regimens, such as upstream versus downstream use, to reduce the associated bleeding risk. The Acute Catheterization and Urgent Intervention Triage Strategy (ACUITY) Timing trial compared routine upstream versus deferred selective strategies with abciximab and the Early Glycoprotein IIb/IIIa Inhibition in Non-ST Segment Elevation Acute Coronary Syndrome (EARLY-ACS) trial compared early versus delayed strategies with eptifibatide.[30,31] A routine upstream or early GPI regimen was not associated with an improvement in death or ischaemic outcomes in either of these trials, but significantly increased bleeding events. Later, the Minimizing Adverse Haemorrhagic Events by TRansradial Access Site and Systemic Implementation of angioX (MATRIX) trial compared anticoagulation with unfractionated heparin (UFH) with or without GPI versus bivalirudin in patients with NSTE-ACS and ST-segment elevation (STE)-ACS.[32] Concomitant treatment with GPI was 25.9% in the UFH and 4.6% in the bivalirudin group. There were no significant differences in the co-primary endpoints of major adverse cardiovascular events (MACEs) or net adverse clinical events (NACE). UFH with or without GPI was associated with an increased risk of major bleeding compared to bivalirudin.

The Harmonizing Outcomes with Revascularization and Stents in Acute Myocardial Infarction (HORIZONS-AMI) study compared anticoagulation with UFH plus GPI versus bivalirudin in patients with STE-ACS who were undergoing primary PCI.[33] Bivalirudin significantly reduces NACE compared to UFH plus GPI, owing to a lower rate of major bleeding. In addition, bivalirudin significantly reduced all-cause and cardiovascular death compared to UFH plus GPI. Ultimately, the focus of GPI research moved to the comparison of different administration routes. The Abciximab Intracoronary versus intravenous Drug Application in ST-Elevation Myocardial Infarction (AIDA-STEMI) trial compared the intracoronary abciximab versus intravenous abciximab bolus, both followed by infusion in patients presenting with STE-ACS.[34] Intracoronary abciximab did not reduce the composite of death, recurrent MI, or new congestive heart failure compared to intravenous abciximab bolus, and there were no differences in bleeding outcomes.

Contraindications

- Hypersensitivity to abciximab (including murine proteins), eptifibatide, tirofiban, or any formulation components.
- Active or recent (within 4–6 weeks) haemorrhage or history of bleeding diathesis.
- History of cerebrovascular accident (within 2 years for abciximab or 30 days for eptifibatide) or with significant residual neurological deficit or history of haemorrhagic stroke (eptifibatide).
- Administration of oral anticoagulants within 7 days previously unless prothrombin time is less than or equal to 1.2 times control prothrombin time value (abciximab).
- Thrombocytopenia (<100,000 cells/μL) (abciximab); or history of thrombocytopenia following prior exposure (tirofiban).
- Recent (within 6 weeks) major surgery or trauma.
- Intracranial tumour, arteriovenous malformation, or aneurysm (abciximab).
- Severe uncontrolled hypertension (systolic blood pressure >200 mmHg or diastolic blood pressure >110 mmHg) (abciximab and eptifibatide).
- Presumed or documented history of vasculitis (abciximab).
- Use of dextran before PCI or intent to use dextran during PCI (abciximab).
- Dependency on haemodialysis (eptifibatide).[22]

Protease-activated receptor-1 antagonist

PAR receptors are a subfamily of related G protein-coupled receptors highly expressed in platelets, endothelial cells, myocytes, and neurons.[35] Platelets express PAR-1 and PAR-4, which serve as thrombin receptors. In the 1990s, himbacine, a naturally occurring complex piperdine alkaloid, was studied as a promising drug for Alzheimer's disease.[35] Himbacine's ability to bind the PAR-1 receptor set the foundation for developing the PAR-1 antagonists.[35]

Vorapaxar, a PAR-1 receptor antagonist, showed promising results in *ex vivo* animal platelet inhibition tests and was selected for further clinical development in 2008.[36] Other PAR-1 antagonists were developed later but were never studied in phase III RCTs.[37]

Mechanism of action

PAR-1 receptor activation by thrombin promotes the irreversible cleavage of the extracellular loop of the receptor (➔ Figure 7.3). The new amino terminus becomes a tethered ligand that autoactivates the transmembrane protein after folding back over the receptor.[38] The activation of the G protein-coupled process leads to cytoskeletal response, platelet morphological changes, and decreased cAMP. These intracellular changes enable a modification in the GPIIb/IIIa receptor, allowing it to bind to fibrinogen and von Willebrand factor and stabilize platelet aggregation.[1] Moreover, thrombin-mediated platelet activation releases several platelet activators such as adenosine diphosphate, serotonin, and thromboxane A_2.[1] The activated PAR-1 receptor is rapidly uncoupled from signalling and degraded by lysosomes. PAR-1 antagonists bind to the autoactivation site, avoiding the tethered ligand's interaction with its binding domain and inhibiting the downstream signalling pathways.[38]

Clinical evidence

Vorapaxar has been studied in several RCTs (➔ Table 7.4). In the phase II thrombin receptor antagonist (TRA) PCI trial, vorapaxar was tested using different loading and maintenance doses in patients treated with non-urgent PCI. Vorapaxar was shown to be safe in terms of major and minor bleeding compared to placebo.[39] The Thrombin Receptor Antagonist for Clinical Event Reduction in Acute Coronary Syndrome (TRACER) phase III

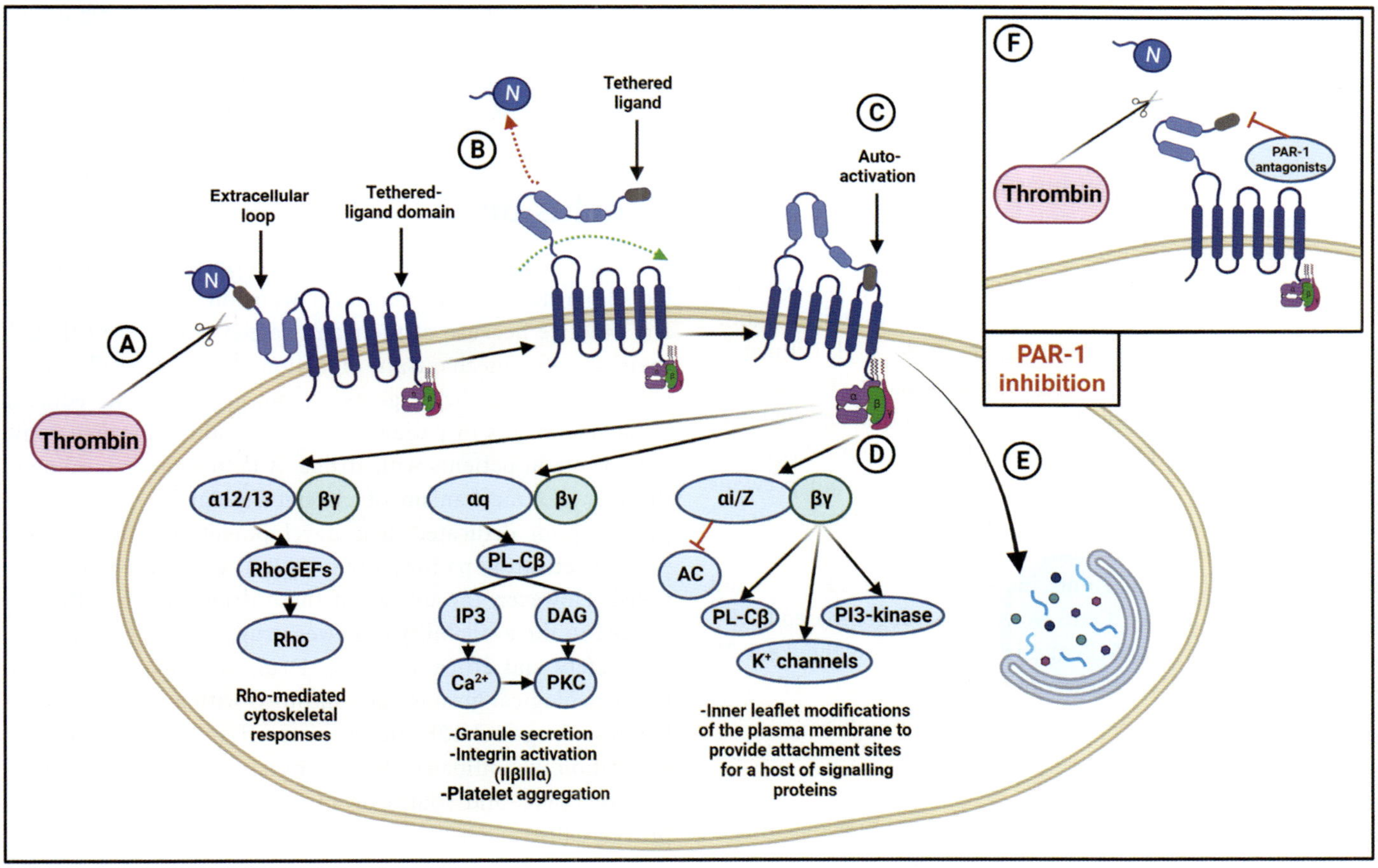

Figure 7.3 Mechanism of platelet inhibition of protease-activated receptors-1 (PAR-1) antagonists. A: PAR-1 is a G protein-coupled receptor for thrombin. Thrombin recognizes and cleaves the N-terminal exodomain of PAR1. B: the N-terminal cleavage (red dashed arrow) unmasks a new amino terminus that functions as a tethered-ligand domain sequence (SFLLRN). C: docking intramolecularly (green dashed arrow) with the body of the receptor (autoactivation) to effect transmembrane signalling. D: PAR-1 can couple to members of the G12/13, Gq, and Gi/Z families. α-subunits of G12/13 bind RhoGEFs (guanine nucleotide exchange factors) which activate small G proteins and promote Rho-mediated cytoskeletal responses that are likely involved in shape change in platelets, permeability, and migration in endothelial cells. Gαq activates phospholipase (PL) Cβ, triggering inositol trisphosphate (IP3) and diacylglycerol (DAG), calcium mobilization, and protein kinase C (PKC) activation, leading to granule secretion, integrin activation, and platelet aggregation. Gαi inhibits adenylyl cyclase (AC, red continuous line). Gβγ subunits can activate phosphoinositide-3 (PI3) kinase, PL-Cβ, and potassium (K^+) channels, leading to modifications in the plasma membrane. In particular, activate cell surface 'sheddases' that liberate ligands for receptor tyrosine kinases, a link between thrombin and receptor tyrosine kinases involved in cell growth and differentiation (pleiotropic effects of PAR1 activation). E: activated PAR-1 receptor is rapidly uncoupled from signalling and degraded by lysosomes. F: PAR-1 antagonists are synthetic peptide of sequence SFLLRN that binds to the autoactivation site and blocks the tethered interaction independently of the receptor cleavage.

Table 7.4 Selected randomized controlled trials of PAR-1 antagonists in cardiovascular diseases.

Trial	Methods	Key results
TRA-PCI (2009)[39]	◆ Double-blinded, placebo-controlled RCT comparing vorapaxar vs placebo (3:1) in patients ≥45 years undergoing non-urgent PCI or coronary angiography with planned PCI. Three oral loading doses (10 mg, 20 mg, or 40 mg) and maintenance doses (0.5 mg, 1.0 mg, or 2.5 mg per day) were used ◆ Primary endpoint: incidence of clinically significant major and minor bleeding	◆ 1030 patients were enrolled (vorapaxar 773 vs placebo 257) ◆ There was no difference in bleeding events after the loading or maintenance dose between vorapaxar and placebo, even when administered concomitantly with aspirin and clopidogrel ◆ Vorapaxar was associated with sustained inhibition of thrombin receptor agonist peptide-induced platelet activation and aggregation
TRACER (2012)[40]	◆ Double-blinded, placebo-controlled RCT comparing vorapaxar (loading dose 40 mg and 2.5 mg maintenance) vs placebo in patients with NSTE-ACS ◆ Primary endpoint: composite of death from cardiovascular causes, MI, stroke, recurrent ischaemia with rehospitalization, or urgent coronary revascularization	◆ 12944 patients were enrolled, follow-up in the trial was terminated early after a safety review, and the median follow-up was 502 days ◆ Vorapaxar was not associated with a significant reduction in the primary endpoint compared to placebo (HR 0.92; 95% CI 0.85–1.01; P = 0.07) but was associated with an increase in severe bleeding, including intracranial haemorrhage (3.39; 95% CI 1.78–6.45; P <0.001)
TRA 2P (2012)[41]	◆ Double-blinded, placebo-controlled RCT comparing vorapaxar (2.5 mg) vs placebo in patients with a history of myocardial infarction, ischaemic stroke, or peripheral arterial disease ◆ Primary endpoint: composite of death from cardiovascular causes, myocardial infarction, or stroke ◆ After 2 years, the DSMB recommended discontinuing the study treatment in patients with a history of stroke	◆ 26449 patients were enrolled ◆ Vorapaxar significantly reduced the primary endpoint compared to placebo (HR 0.87; 95% CI 0.80–0.94; P <0.001) but was associated with an increase in severe bleeding, including intracranial haemorrhage (HR 1.94; 95% CI 1.39–2.70; P <0.001)

DSMB, Data and Safety Monitoring Board; PAR-1, protease-activated receptor-1; PCI, percutaneous coronary intervention; RCT, randomized controlled trial;

trial enrolled over 12,000 patients with NSTE-ACS.[40] The primary efficacy endpoint was the composite of death from cardiovascular causes, MI, stroke, recurrent ischaemia with rehospitalization, or urgent revascularization. The follow-up was terminated early after a safety review. Vorapaxar was associated with a significantly higher rate of severe bleeding, including ICH. Ultimately, the Thrombin Receptor Antagonist in Secondary Prevention of Atherothrombotic Ischemic Events (TRA 2P) trial enrolled over 26,000 patients with a previous history of MI, stroke, or PAD. After 2 years, treatment was discontinued in patients with previous stroke due to the risk of ICH.[41] Vorapaxar significantly reduced the rate of adverse cardiovascular events compared to placebo but increased severe bleeding events, including ICH. In TRA-PCI and TRACER studies, most patients were on clopidogrel-based DAPT as these were PCI and ACS studies. However, in the TRA 2P study, rates of DAPT were lower than in TRA-PCI and TRACER and differed among the qualifying clinical indications.

Contraindications

Vorapaxar is contraindicated in patients with a previous history of stroke, TIA, ICH, or active pathological bleeding.[42]

Conclusion

In the early phases of development of antiplatelet agents, drugs like dipyridamole and cilostazol were introduced into clinical practice because of their antiplatelet effect, even though their specific mechanisms of action were not well understood. Moreover, these agents are not approved for reducing ischaemic events in patients with CAD, although they could have a role in patients with stroke. A better understanding of the complex mechanism of platelet biology opened the opportunity for dedicated drug development targeting specific platelet activation pathways (e.g. PAR-1) and aggregation (e.g. GPIs). However, the uptake of these drugs is currently very limited to the availability of newer drugs with a more favourable safety and efficacy profile. Drug development in these pharmacological groups has continued with a new PAR-1 antagonist drug (PZ-128) under phase II study and a second-generation (zalunfiban) GPI under phase III study. Ultimately, new regimens and routes of administration for current approved GPIs have been tested.

What's new

Dipyridamole

- Dipyridamole plus aspirin was superior for preventing recurrent stroke compared to aspirin alone. However, dipyridamole plus aspirin did not meet the prespecified non-inferiority criteria compared to clopidogrel.

Cilostazol

- In Asians, cilostazol has been found to be superior to placebo and non-inferior to aspirin for the prevention of recurrent stroke. Moreover, dual therapy with cilostazol and aspirin or clopidogrel was superior than monotherapy with aspirin or clopidogrel.

PAR-1 antagonist

- In 2017, the European Medicines Agency marketing authorization for vorapaxar was withdrawn at the request of the marketing authorization holder.
- The atopaxar clinical development programme was halted in phase II RCTs.

Glycoprotein IIb/IIIa inhibitors

- With the introduction of oral $P2Y_{12}$ inhibitors, particularly the newer generation characterized by more prompt and potent effects, GPI use has shifted from being widely used to a bail-out treatment in patients with ACS undergoing PCI with evidence of no-reflow or a thrombotic complication.

Guideline recommendations

Dipyridamole

- In patients with non-cardioembolic ischaemic stroke or TIA, prevention with aspirin only, or dipyridamole plus aspirin, or clopidogrel alone is recommended (class of recommendation I, level of evidence A).[43]
- According to the US Food and Drug Administration, dipyridamole is indicated as an adjunct to coumarin anticoagulants in the prevention of postoperative thromboembolic complications of cardiac valve replacement.[44]

Cilostazol

- Cilostazol decreases walking impairment in patients with PAD, but no formal recommendation is provided.[45]

Vorapaxar

- Vorapaxar is mentioned among pharmacotherapy options indicating that it is associated with a reduction in acute limb ischaemia and peripheral revascularization in patients with PAD, but no formal recommendation is provided.[45]
- According to the US Food and Drug Administration, vorapaxar is indicated for reducing thrombotic cardiovascular events in patients with previous MI or PAD and without a history of stroke, TIA, ICH, or active bleeding.[42]

Glycoprotein IIb/IIIa inhibitors

- In patients with NSTE-ACS and STE-ACS, GPI should be considered for bail-out if there is evidence of no-reflow or a thrombotic complication (class of recommendation IIa, level of evidence C).[46–48]
- In patients with NSTE-ACS, treatment with GPI in patients in whom coronary anatomy is not known is not recommended (class of recommendation III, level of evidence A).[46]
- In patients with NSTE-ACS, UFH (weight-adjusted intravenous bolus during PCI of 70–100 IU/kg, or 50–70 IU/kg in combination with a GPI; activated clotting time (seconds) target range of 250–350 or 200–250 if a GPI is given) is recommended in patients undergoing PCI (class of recommendation I, level of evidence A).[46]

What's next

Dipyridamole

- Preclinical studies have proposed that dipyridamole alone or in combination with statins can reduce ischaemia-reperfusion injury and reducing infarct size. Furthermore, dipyridamole is being tested as a potential treatment for microvascular angina and Takotsubo syndrome.[4]

Cilostazol

- RCTs, including Western patient populations, are needed to confirm the promising result of cilostazol for the prevention of recurrent stroke.[12]

PAR-1 antagonist

- PZ-128, a new lipopeptide pepducin drug, has been tested in phase II trials with promising results.[49] However, it is unclear if phase III testing will occur.

Glycoprotein IIb/IIIa inhibitors

- Zalunfiban (RUC-4), a new second-generation small-molecule platelet GPI designed for subcutaneous injection in patients with STE-ACS has shown promising results and currently is under phase III clinical investigation (NCT04825743).[50]
- Administration routes such intralesional delivery of GPIs have been proposed to maximize efficacy and reduce side effects. Although early RCTs showed promising results, including reduction of infarct size, no large-scale RCTs assessing clinical outcomes have been conducted.[51]

Drug dosing

Dipyridamole

- Thromboembolism prophylaxis in post-cardiac valve replacement: 75–100 mg orally (PO) four times daily as an adjunct to vitamin K antagonist.[44]
- Myocardial perfusion scan: injectable solution of 5 mg/mL is administered at a dose of 0.142 mg/kg/min intravenous infusion over 4 minutes, maximum dose: 70 mg/day.[44]

Cilostazol

- Intermittent claudication, 100 mg PO twice daily.[19]
- 50 mg orally twice daily should be considered during the coadministration of CYP3A4 and CYP2C19 inhibitors.

Vorapaxar

- 2.08 mg PO daily.[42]

Abciximab

- Bolus of 0.25 mg/kg intravenously and 0.125 mcg/kg/min infusion (maximum 10 mcg/min) for 12 hours.[46]

Eptifibatide

- Double bolus of 180 mcg/kg intravenously (given at a 10-minute interval) followed by an infusion of 2.0 mcg/kg/min for up to 18 hours.[46]

- Creatinine clearance (<50 mL/min): double bolus of 180 mcg/kg intravenously (given at a 10-minute interval) followed by an infusion of 1 mcg/kg/min for 18–24 hours.
- End-stage renal disease (i.e. dialysis dependent): contraindicated.

Tirofiban

- In PCI patients: bolus of 25 mcg/kg intravenously over 3 minutes, followed by an infusion of 0.15 mcg/kg/min for up to 18 hours.[46]
- Creatinine clearance (≤60 mL/min): bolus of 25 mcg/kg intravenously for up to 5 minutes, followed by an infusion of 0.075 mcg/kg/min for up to 18 hours.

References

1. Angiolillo DJ, Ueno M, Goto S. Basic principles of platelet biology and clinical implications. Circulation. 2010;74(4):597–607.
2. Picano E. Dipyridamole-echocardiography test: historical background and physiologic basis. Eur Heart J. 1989;10(4):365–76.
3. Coller BS, Shattil SJ. The GPIIb/IIIa (integrin alphaIIbbeta3) odyssey: a technology-driven saga of a receptor with twists, turns, and even a bend. Blood. 2008;112(8):3011–25.
4. Allahham M, Lerman A, Atar D, Birnbaum Y. Why not dipyridamole: a review of current guidelines and re-evaluation of utility in the modern era. Cardiovasc Drugs Ther. 2022;36(3):525–32.
5. Gresele P, Momi S, Falcinelli E. Anti-platelet therapy: phosphodiesterase inhibitors. Br J Clin Pharmacol. 2011;72(4):634–46.
6. Pouleur H, Buyse M. Effects of dipyridamole in combination with anticoagulant therapy on survival and thromboembolic events in patients with prosthetic heart valves. A meta-analysis of the randomized trials. J Thorac Cardiovasc Surg. 1995;110(2):463–72.
7. Antithrombotic Trialists' Collaboration. Collaborative meta-analysis of randomised trials of antiplatelet therapy for prevention of death, myocardial infarction, and stroke in high risk patients. BMJ. 2002; 324(7329):71–86.
8. Group ES, Halkes PH, van Gijn J, Kappelle LJ, Koudstaal PJ, Algra A. Aspirin plus dipyridamole versus aspirin alone after cerebral ischaemia of arterial origin (ESPRIT): randomised controlled trial. Lancet. 2006;367(9523):1665–73.
9. Sacco RL, Diener HC, Yusuf S, et al. Aspirin and extended-release dipyridamole versus clopidogrel for recurrent stroke. N Engl J Med. 2008;359(12):1238–51.
10. Henzlova MJ, Duvall WL, Einstein AJ, Travin MI, Verberne HJ. ASNC imaging guidelines for SPECT nuclear cardiology procedures: stress, protocols, and tracers. J Nucl Cardiol. 2016;23(3):606–39.
11. Nishi T, Kimura Y, Nakagawa K. [Research and development of cilostazol: an antiplatelet agent]. Yakugaku Zasshi. 2000;120(12):1247–60.
12. Kherallah RY, Khawaja M, Olson M, Angiolillo D, Birnbaum Y. Cilostazol: a review of basic mechanisms and clinical uses. Cardiovasc Drugs Ther. 2022;36(4):777–92.
13. Brown T, Forster RB, Cleanthis M, Mikhailidis DP, Stansby G, Stewart M. Cilostazol for intermittent claudication. Cochrane Database Syst Rev. 2021;6:CD003748.
14. Park KW, Kang SH, Park JJ, et al. Adjunctive cilostazol versus double-dose clopidogrel after drug-eluting stent implantation: the HOST-ASSURE randomized trial (Harmonizing Optimal Strategy for Treatment of Coronary Artery Stenosis-Safety & Effectiveness of Drug-Eluting Stents & Anti-platelet Regimen). JACC Cardiovasc Interv. 2013;6(9):932–42.
15. Lee SW, Ahn JM, Han S, et al. Differential impact of cilostazol on restenosis according to implanted stent type (from a pooled analysis of three DECLARE randomized trials). Am J Cardiol. 2013;112(9):1328–34.
16. Gotoh F, Tohgi H, Hirai S, et al. Cilostazol stroke prevention study: a placebo-controlled double-blind trial for secondary prevention of cerebral infarction. J Stroke Cerebrovasc Dis. 2000;9(4):147–57.
17. Shinohara Y, Katayama Y, Uchiyama S, et al. Cilostazol for prevention of secondary stroke (CSPS 2): an aspirin-controlled, double-blind, randomised non-inferiority trial. Lancet Neurol. 2010;9(10):959–68.
18. Toyoda K, Uchiyama S, Yamaguchi T, et al. Dual antiplatelet therapy using cilostazol for secondary prevention in patients with high-risk ischaemic stroke in Japan: a multicentre, open-label, randomised controlled trial. Lancet Neurol. 2019;18(6):539–48.
19. US Food and Drug Administration. Cilostazol FDA label. 1999. Available from: https://www.accessdata.fda.gov/drugsatfda_docs/label/2017/020863s024lbl.pdf
20. US Food and Drug Administration. FDA drug shortages: abciximab. 2002. Available from: https://www.accessdata.fda.gov/scripts/drugshortages/dsp_ActiveIngredientDetails.cfm
21. Du XP, Plow EF, Frelinger AL, 3rd, O'Toole TE, Loftus JC, Ginsberg MH. Ligands 'activate' integrin alpha IIb beta 3 (platelet GPIIb-IIIa). Cell. 1991;65(3):409–16.
22. Capodanno D, Milluzzo RP, Angiolillo DJ. Intravenous antiplatelet therapies (glycoprotein IIb/IIIa receptor inhibitors and cangrelor) in percutaneous coronary intervention: from pharmacology to indications for clinical use. Ther Adv Cardiovasc Dis. 2019;13:1753944719893274.
23. Kastrati A, Mehilli J, Schuhlen H, et al. A clinical trial of abciximab in elective percutaneous coronary intervention after pretreatment with clopidogrel. N Engl J Med. 2004;350(3):232–8.
24. Mehilli J, Kastrati A, Schuhlen H, et al. Randomized clinical trial of abciximab in diabetic patients undergoing elective percutaneous coronary interventions after treatment with a high loading dose of clopidogrel. Circulation. 2004;110(24):3627–35.
25. Winchester DE, Wen X, Brearley WD, Park KE, Anderson RD, Bavry AA. Efficacy and safety of glycoprotein IIb/IIIa inhibitors during elective coronary revascularization: a meta-analysis of randomized trials performed in the era of stents and thienopyridines. J Am Coll Cardiol. 2011;57(10):1190–9.
26. Kastrati A, Mehilli J, Neumann FJ, et al. Abciximab in patients with acute coronary syndromes undergoing percutaneous coronary intervention after clopidogrel pretreatment: the ISAR-REACT 2 randomized trial. JAMA. 2006;295(13):1531–8.
27. Valgimigli M, Bueno H, Byrne RA, et al. 2017 ESC focused update on dual antiplatelet therapy in coronary artery disease developed in collaboration with EACTS: the Task Force for dual antiplatelet therapy in coronary artery disease of the European Society of Cardiology

(ESC) and of the European Association for Cardio-Thoracic Surgery (EACTS). Eur Heart J. 2018;39(3):213–60.
28. Wiviott SD, Braunwald E, McCabe CH, et al. Prasugrel versus clopidogrel in patients with acute coronary syndromes. N Engl J Med. 2007;357(20):2001–15.
29. Wallentin L, Becker RC, Budaj A, et al. Ticagrelor versus clopidogrel in patients with acute coronary syndromes. N Engl J Med. 2009;361(11):1045–57.
30. Stone GW, Bertrand ME, Moses JW, et al. Routine upstream initiation vs deferred selective use of glycoprotein IIb/IIIa inhibitors in acute coronary syndromes: the ACUITY Timing trial. JAMA. 2007;297(6):591–602.
31. Giugliano RP, White JA, Bode C, et al. Early versus delayed, provisional eptifibatide in acute coronary syndromes. N Engl J Med. 2009;360(21):2176–90.
32. Valgimigli M, Frigoli E, Leonardi S, et al. Bivalirudin or unfractionated heparin in acute coronary syndromes. N Engl J Med. 2015;373(11):997–1009.
33. Stone GW, Witzenbichler B, Guagliumi G, et al. Bivalirudin during primary PCI in acute myocardial infarction. N Engl J Med. 2008;358(21):2218–30.
34. Thiele H, Wohrle J, Hambrecht R, et al. Intracoronary versus intravenous bolus abciximab during primary percutaneous coronary intervention in patients with acute ST-elevation myocardial infarction: a randomised trial. Lancet. 2012;379(9819):923–31.
35. Chackalamannil S, Davies RJ, Wang Y, et al. Total synthesis of (+)-himbacine and (+)-himbeline. J Org Chem. 1999;64(6):1932–40.
36. Chackalamannil S, Wang Y, Greenlee WJ, et al. Discovery of a novel, orally active himbacine-based thrombin receptor antagonist (SCH 530348) with potent antiplatelet activity. J Med Chem. 2008;51(11):3061–4.
37. Rollini F, Tello-Montoliu A, Angiolillo DJ. Atopaxar: a review of its mechanism of action and role in patients with coronary artery disease. Future Cardiol. 2012;8(4):503–11.
38. Coughlin SR. Thrombin signalling and protease-activated receptors. Nature. 2000;407(6801):258–64.
39. Becker RC, Moliterno DJ, Jennings LK, et al. Safety and tolerability of SCH 530348 in patients undergoing non-urgent percutaneous coronary intervention: a randomised, double-blind, placebo-controlled phase II study. Lancet. 2009;373(9667):919–28.
40. Tricoci P, Huang Z, Held C, Moliterno DJ, et al. Thrombin-receptor antagonist vorapaxar in acute coronary syndromes. N Engl J Med. 2012;366(1):20–33.
41. Morrow DA, Braunwald E, Bonaca MP, et al. Vorapaxar in the secondary prevention of atherothrombotic events. N Engl J Med. 2012;366(15):1404–13.
42. US Food and Drug Administration. Vorapaxar FDA label. 2014. Available from: https://www.accessdata.fda.gov/drugsatfda_docs/label/2014/204886s000lbl.pdf
43. Visseren FLJ, Mach F, Smulders YM, et al. 2021 ESC Guidelines on cardiovascular disease prevention in clinical practice. Eur Heart J. 2021;42(34):3227–337.
44. US Food and Drug Administration. Dipyridamole FDA label. 2019. Available from: https://www.accessdata.fda.gov/drugsatfda_docs/label/2019/012836s061lbl.pdf
45. Aboyans V, Ricco JB, Bartelink MEL, et al. 2017 ESC Guidelines on the Diagnosis and Treatment of Peripheral Arterial Diseases, in collaboration with the European Society for Vascular Surgery (ESVS): document covering atherosclerotic disease of extracranial carotid and vertebral, mesenteric, renal, upper and lower extremity arteries. Endorsed by: the European Stroke Organization (ESO)The Task Force for the Diagnosis and Treatment of Peripheral Arterial Diseases of the European Society of Cardiology (ESC) and of the European Society for Vascular Surgery (ESVS). Eur Heart J. 2018;39(9):763–816.
46. Collet JP, Thiele H, Barbato E, et al. 2020 ESC Guidelines for the management of acute coronary syndromes in patients presenting without persistent ST-segment elevation. Eur Heart J. 2021;42(14):1289–367.
47. Neumann FJ, Sousa-Uva M, Ahlsson A, et al. 2018 ESC/EACTS Guidelines on myocardial revascularization. Eur Heart J. 2019;40(2):87–165.
48. Ibanez B, James S, Agewall S, et al. 2017 ESC Guidelines for the management of acute myocardial infarction in patients presenting with ST-segment elevation: the Task Force for the management of acute myocardial infarction in patients presenting with ST-segment elevation of the European Society of Cardiology (ESC). Eur Heart J. 2018;39(2):119–77.
49. Kuliopulos A, Gurbel PA, Rade JJ, et al. PAR1 (protease-activated receptor 1) pepducin therapy targeting myocardial necrosis in coronary artery disease and acute coronary syndrome patients undergoing cardiac catheterization: a randomized, placebo-controlled, phase 2 study. Arterioscler thromb Vasc Biol. 2020;40(12):2990–3003.
50. Bor WL, Zheng KL, Tavenier AH, et al. Pharmacokinetics, pharmacodynamics, and tolerability of subcutaneous administration of a novel glycoprotein IIb/IIIa inhibitor, RUC-4, in patients with ST-segment elevation myocardial infarction. EuroIntervention. 2021;17(5):e401–10.
51. Angiolillo DJ, Galli M, Collet JP, Kastrati A, O'Donoghue ML. Antiplatelet therapy after percutaneous coronary intervention. EuroIntervention. 2022;17(17):e1371–96.

CHAPTER 8

Heparins, fondaparinux, hirudin, bivalirudin, argatroban, and danaparoid

Renske H. Olie and Hugo ten Cate

Contents

Summary

Several parenteral anticoagulants are available for thromboprophylaxis as well as for treatment of both venous and arterial thrombosis. In this chapter, the mechanism of action, pharmacology, administration, and monitoring of heparin, low-molecular-weight heparins, fondaparinux, hirudin, bivalirudin, argatroban, and danaparoid are discussed. Indications and adverse effects are summarized, as well as reversal of effect in case of bleeding complications or urgent surgery. Heparin-induced thrombocytopenia is a rare but feared reaction to heparin treatment and requires discontinuation of the drug and alternative treatment with non-heparin anticoagulants such as argatroban, danaparoid or fondaparinux.

Heparin

Mechanism and pharmacology

Heparin refers to 'unfractionated heparin' (UFH), which is the name for a class of glycosaminoglycans purified from animal species (usually bovine or porcine intestinal tissue) of varying molecular weight and molecular composition and with different degree of binding affinity for antithrombin, its main cofactor for anticoagulant activity.[1] Heparin binds to antithrombin through a unique pentasaccharide sequence with high affinity, and in this case changes the conformation of antithrombin, such that the latter accelerates the inactivation of serine proteases including thrombin, but also factors Xa, IXa, and XIa.[2] This way, irreversible complexes between the serine protease inhibitor antithrombin and the serine proteases are formed, heparin then dissociates and stays active. While the pentasaccharide sequence in heparin suffices to accelerate inhibition of factor Xa by antithrombin, inhibition of thrombin requires an oligosaccharide chain of at least 18 saccharides to allow ternary complex formation between heparin, antithrombin, and thrombin. UFH comprises the calcium salt of sulfated oligosaccharides with an apparent molecular weight of 5000–30,000 Da (on average 15,000 Da) and with different affinities for antithrombin; this heterogeneity has an impact on functional activity and clearance of the different molecules.[3] Upon intravenous infusion, the apparent half-life of heparin is dose dependent and increases from about 30 minutes (bolus of 25 units/kg), to 60 minutes (100 units/kg), to 150 minutes for a bolus of 400 units/kg.[4,5] Upon subcutaneous administration, the bioavailability of heparin is about 10% lower than after intravenous infusion and the peak anticoagulant activity appears after 1–2 hours in blood. Clearance of the larger heparin molecules is predominantly through the reticuloendothelial system[6] while the low-molecular-weight heparin (LMWH) fractions are mostly cleared by the kidneys (➔ Low-molecular-weight heparins).

Administration and monitoring

Heparin can be given subcutaneously, mostly for thromboprophylaxis, in fixed or body weight-adjusted doses. Heparin given intravenously is monitored by the activated partial thromboplastin time (aPTT) or the activated clotting time (ACT). Alternatively, heparin may be monitored by an anti-Xa assay, but because of its turnaround time the latter assay is less commonly applied for short-term heparin use. When given for a prolonged period of time (days or longer), the aPTT is preferred, and historically a prolongation of the aPTT by 1.5–2.5 the mean normal reference interval (corresponding to a heparin range of about 0.2–0.8 units/mL) is aimed for. Therapeutic ranges are different for those with venous thromboembolism and for those with acute coronary syndrome (ACS). The limitation of this approach is the variable sensitivity of aPTT reagents and the variable interindividual responsiveness of the aPTT due to patient-associated factors, such as the level of factor VIII. Moreover, some conditions, such as the antiphospholipid syndrome, may be characterized by a prolonged baseline aPTT, which also makes the test unreliable for heparin monitoring. For more accurate estimates of the heparin concentration, a heparin-calibrated anti-Xa assay can be used. Additionally, the aPTT is limited in sensitivity within a range of about 0.1–1.0 units/mL, and in the setting of percutaneous coronary interventions, cardiothoracic surgery, extracorporeal membrane oxygenation (ECMO) or other conditions requiring high heparin doses, the ACT is more suitable to monitor heparin activity (in the range of 1.0–5.0 units/mL), when the aPTT becomes indefinitely prolonged.

Heparin resistance

Heparin resistance is the term used for failure to achieve a specified anticoagulation level despite the use of what is considered to be an adequate dose of heparin.[7] A threshold dose for heparin resistance cannot be specified, although either the need for more than 35,000 units per day, or the requirement of more than 500 units/kg to achieve an ACT of 400–480 seconds (cardiopulmonary bypass surgery), have been used. Factors that underlie heparin resistance include non-specific heparin binding to cells and proteins, acquired antithrombin deficiency (e.g. during sepsis/disseminated intravascular coagulation), platelet interactions—including neutralization of heparin by platelet released platelet factor 4, high levels of coagulation proteins like factor VIII during illness, the use of andexanet alfa as reversal agent for direct oral anticoagulants, and systemic profound prothrombotic coagulopathies including COVID-19. In case of suspected heparin resistance, the anti-Xa level is more informative about the non-clotting-related heparin concentration, particularly in conditions with strong impact on the coagulation test, such as the antiphospholipid syndrome, disseminated intravascular coagulation, or systemic viral infections such as COVID-19. In case of a low level of antithrombin, supplementation of this serum protease inhibitor (serpin) may be considered. Practically, to circumvent the problem, a direct thrombin inhibitor like argatroban (➔ Argatroban) may be used to replace heparin.

Indications and clinical use

Following the introduction of subcutaneous LMWH treatment, the use of heparin is limited to those settings where either LMWHs are not available (too costly), or its implementation is otherwise practically limited. Such settings include extracorporeal systems, like ECMO and cardiopulmonary bypass (CPB) surgery where relatively large amounts of ACT or anti-Xa assay-guided heparin are required to maintain patency of the tubing system. An advantage of heparin over LMWHs is that it can be readily and fully neutralized with protamine (➔ Reversal of effect), which is warranted to limit bleeding risk immediately after CPB because of the very high amounts of heparin given during the bypass procedure. Longer-term heparin infusion can be required in specific settings, such as patients with mechanical valves and thrombosis, antiphospholipid syndrome, a high risk of thrombosis during the periprocedural setting or pregnancy, and the initial phases of anticoagulation in high-risk pulmonary embolism, overt haemodynamic instability, or imminent haemodynamic decompensation in whom primary reperfusion treatment will be necessary. UFH is also recommended for patients with serious renal impairment [creatinine clearance (CrCl) ≤30 mL/min] or severe obesity. Finally, and perhaps most commonly, heparin boluses are given before or during invasive procedures such as percutaneous coronary intervention (PCI), and angiography without a strict need for monitoring or guided by ACT. The routine use of the ACT during PCI is controversial, although its use may be advocated as a check on the heparin administration, comparing pre- and post-heparin ACT values. However, neither low nor high ACT ranges are consistently associated with major clinical outcomes (MACE, bleeding), and the use of ACT as a safeguard to reduce the risk of complications is disputed.[8] Heparin is the preferred agent for PCI in patients with ST-elevation myocardial infarction (STEMI) or non-ST-elevation myocardial infarction (NSTEMI) because of its favourable risk/benefit profile, and also because of its lower cost,[9] and is currently preferred over bivalirudin.[10]

Adverse effects

Except for bleeding, the most serious, but rare adverse effect of heparin is heparin-induced thrombocytopenia (HIT), which is a severe immune-mediated disorder caused by the formation of immunoglobulin G antibodies against ultra-large complexes of heparin and platelet factor 4 (PF4).[11] Larger heparin molecules are more immunogenic than LMWHs, with a minimum of 12 saccharides required for complex formation with PF4. The result of immunoglobin G formation against the heparin–PF4 complex is the formation of immune complexes against FcγRIIa receptors on platelets, subsequent platelet activation, and their clearance from the circulation, resulting in thrombocytopenia. However, platelet activation also elicits a profound prothrombotic phenotype, aggravated due to similar immune-mediated activation of neutrophils and monocytes. This results in thrombosis in venous and arterial vascular beds. The relation with (prior) heparin exposure even in prophylactic doses (or upon exposure to, e.g. heparin locks in intravenous catheters), may trigger HIT, particularly upon repeat exposure to heparin. Thrombocytopenia, with platelet count dropping by more than 30% from baseline, develops gradually over a 4–14-day time course after heparin exposure and may be masked, especially in conditions, such as CPB surgery, where an initial, reversible drop in platelet count is characteristic early after surgery.[12] Without further monitoring of platelets, the occurrence of thrombosis may be the first indication of HIT. The incidence of HIT varies from 0.02% to 1–4% depending on the type of study (population).

The diagnosis of HIT requires clinical suspicion (timing and severity of thrombocytopenia and/or unexpected thrombosis), and should be guided by the 4T scoring system[13] (➔ Table 8.1). The 4T score has a very high negative predictive value (excluding HIT), but a moderate positive predictive power, which requires laboratory confirmation.[14] HIT antibodies can be detected by an immunoglobulin G-specific enzyme-linked immunosorbent assay (ELISA) or a more rapid, but less specific, particle gel assay or chemiluminescence assay, providing a test result in less than 1 hour. The accepted gold standard for the diagnosis of HIT is a functional assay assessing the potency of a patient's serum to trigger serotonin release from aggregating donor platelets in the presence of heparin *in vitro*. However, a negative confirmation assay does not definitively rule out HIT, and the term 'serotonin release assay-negative HIT' has been recently proposed for this situation.[12] Most importantly, for the cardiologist and cardiothoracic surgeon, the suspicion of HIT should trigger immediate contact with the clinical laboratory and consultant haematologists to ensure timely and accurate diagnostics. Timely diagnosis of HIT is critically important, as undetected HIT has a high in-hospital mortality of about 10%. The management of HIT includes the replacement of heparin with an alternative anticoagulant; LMWHs should be avoided as they may cross-react, however the synthetic pentasaccharide fondaparinux may be an option, although not approved for this indication. In case of therapeutic management of thrombosis, a direct thrombin inhibitor is preferred, and argatroban has been approved for treatment of HIT in the US and Europe (➔ Argatroban). Other parenteral options include the off-label use of the thrombin inhibitor bivalirudin (➔ Hirudin and bivalirudin) or the heparinoid danaparoid (➔ Danaparoid). When the platelet count recovers and treatment with oral medication becomes feasible, a vitamin K antagonist (VKA) can be started, although increasingly non-vitamin K antagonist oral anticoagulants (NOACs) are being used, so far without any major adverse events. In patients with demonstrated HIT, it is obvious that the future use of any heparin or LMWHs should be avoided.

Other very rare side effects of heparin are osteoporosis, particularly upon prolonged treatment,[15] and hypoaldosteronism.[16]

Reversal of effect

The effect of heparin can be neutralized with protamine sulfate or hydrochloride, where 1 mg protamine neutralizes 100 units of heparin. Preferably, it must be administered slowly to reduce the risk of hypotension due to mast cell activation, and to minimize allergic reactions in those with a certain sensitivity to protamine, such as those with fish protein allergy or prior vasectomy.[17] Although the aim is to correct heparin 100 IU with 1 mg of protamine, this is not a trivial matter, because the remaining concentration of heparin in blood can only be grossly estimated based on ACT or aPTT measurements; underdosing of protamine may leave too much heparin, while overdosing may paradoxically also enhance bleeding risk, as protamine has intrinsic anticoagulant activities. The optimal protamine dosing schedule still needs to be established.[18] In spite of these shortcomings, protamine is routinely used in cardiothoracic surgery,[19] reduces the risk of major bleeding, and appears to be largely safe with regard to thrombotic complications. Its use for other procedures, such as transcatheter aortic valve implantation surgery, has also been studied and it appears to be beneficial in reducing the risk of bleeding in a safe manner.[20] Other antidotes under clinical investigation to reverse the anticoagulant effects of heparin are the small molecule

Table 8.1 4T scoring system for heparin-induced thrombocytopenia

4Ts category	2 points	1 point	0 points
Thrombocytopenia	Platelet count fall >50% and platelet nadir ≥20	Platelet count 30–50% or platelet nadir 10–19	Platelet count fall <30% or platelet nadir <10
Timing of platelet count fall	Clear onset days 5–10 or platelet fall ≤1 day (prior heparin exposure within 30 days)	Consistent with days 5-10 fall, but not clear (e.g. missing platelet counts); onset after day 10; or fall ≤1 day (prior heparin exposure 30-100 days ago)	Platelet count fall ≤4 days without recent heparin exposure
Thrombosis or other sequelae	New thrombosis (confirmed); skin necrosis; acute systemic reaction after intravenous UFH bolus	Progressive or recurrent thrombosis; non-necrotizing (erythematous) skin lesions; suspected thrombosis (not proven)	None
Other causes of thrombocytopenia	None apparent	Possible	Definite

The 4Ts score is the sum of the values for each of the four categories. Scores of 1–3, 4–5, and 6–8 are considered to correspond to a low, intermediate, and high probability of HIT, respectively. UFH; unfractionated heparin.

ciraparantag[21] and andexanet alfa, a factor Xa decoy that binds to the direct and indirect factor Xa inhibitors.[22]

Low-molecular-weight heparins

Mechanism and pharmacology

LMWHs are produced by depolymerization of UFH. LMWHs and UFH are both glycosaminoglycans. Compared to UFH, the molecules of which range in size from 5000 to 30,000 Da and 45 saccharide units, LMWHs have a lower molecular weight, of 2000–9000 Da, and an average of 15 saccharide units.[23] This lower molecular weight results in the most important pharmacological difference between UFH and LMWHs. LMWHs still potently inhibit factor Xa, while the smaller molecules have less anti-factor IIa activity. Variable LMWH products are available, and the various products have differences in average molecular weight, resulting in differences in the anti-Xa/anti-IIa ratio. This ratio ranges from 4:1 to 1.6:1, compared with 1:1 for UFH. LMWHs exhibit less binding to plasma proteins than UFH, resulting in a more predictable response.[24] Moreover, due to less binding to the endothelium, LWMHs have better bioavailability (almost 100%) compared with UFH. Lastly, LMWHs have a longer half-life compared to UFH, due to reduced binding to macrophages and endothelial cells, allowing once- or twice-daily dosing.[23] Due to these attractive pharmacokinetic properties and their easy practical use, LMWHs have become among the most frequently prescribed in-hospital drugs. The plasma half-life of LMWHs varies from 3 to 6 hours after subcutaneous injection. The clearance of LMWHs is mainly renal, and therapeutic dosages should be adjusted in patients with renal impairment.[25]

Administration and monitoring

LMWHs are administered subcutaneously. There are several available LMWH preparations, which differ according to molecular weight, biological half-life, and the anti-Xa/anti-IIa ratio (➔ Table 8.2). Fixed doses are typically used for thromboprophylaxis whereas for therapeutic treatment, daily dosing depends on type of LMWH, body weight, and estimated glomerular filtration rate. LMWHs are primarily cleared by the kidneys, and accumulation can occur following administration of therapeutic dosages. However, not all preparations accumulate to the same degree, depending on their average molecular weight. A general recommendation is to apply a dose reduction of 25–50% of therapeutic dosages in patients with moderate-to-severe renal insufficiency (i.e. creatinine clearance 15–50 mL/min).[25,26] Because of their predictable anticoagulant effect, regular laboratory monitoring is not deemed necessary. However, anti-Xa activity measurements may be used to monitor the anticoagulant effect in certain situations in which the pharmacokinetics of LMWHs is less well known, such as in renal insufficiency, under- or overweight, pregnancy, or childhood. Peak anti-factor Xa levels should be measured 4 hours after the injection, with a target range of 0.5–1.0 IU/mL (for twice-daily dosing) or 0.85–2.0 IU/mL (for once-daily dosing), depending on the type of LMWH.[25]

Indications and clinical use

LMWHs are used as thromboprophylaxis for patients undergoing major surgeries, but also for hospitalized medical patients with potential risk factors for venous thromboembolism (VTE), with doses dependent on the type of LMWH (➔ Table 8.2). In pregnant patients, LMWHs are prescribed both as thromboprophylaxis and as therapeutic treatment in patients with (a history of) VTE or as substitution of oral anticoagulants during pregnancy. Dosing in pregnant patients should be similar to standard recommendations, although physiological changes during pregnancy such as weight gain and increased volume of distribution may alter LMWH requirements.[27] Periodic measurement of anti-factor Xa levels may help guide dose modification, although not all guidelines consistently support this practice.[28]

In patients with deep vein thrombosis (DVT) or pulmonary embolism, immediate anticoagulation can be achieved with a LMWH. A large meta-analysis reported that fixed-dose LMWHs significantly reduced thrombotic complications, major bleeding, and all-cause mortality compared with adjusted-dose UFH in patients treated for VTE.[29] In cancer patients, LMWHs have been shown to be more effective in preventing VTE recurrence compared with early transition from UFH to VKAs, with no increase

Table 8.2 Comparison of different low-molecular-weight heparins

	Molecular weight (Da)	Anti-Xa/anti-IIa ratio	Half-life (hours)	Regimen
Nadroparin	4300	3.5	3.5	Prophylaxis: 2850–5700 IU daily
				Treatment: 86 IU/kg twice daily
Enoxaparin	4500	3.6	4.5	Prophylaxis: 20–40 mg daily
				Treatment: 1 mg/kg twice daily or 1.5 mg/kg daily
Dalteparin	6000	2.5	4	Prophylaxis: 2500–5000 IU daily
				Treatment: 100 IU/kg twice daily or 200 IU/kg daily
Tinzaparin	6500	1.8	3.5	Prophylaxis: 3500 IU daily
				Treatment: 175 IU/kg daily

in bleeding.[30,31] Therapeutic doses of LMWHs are also frequently used as bridging therapy in patients with high thromboembolic risks during interruption of VKA therapy (i.e. for a surgical procedure) or when the international normalized ratio (INR) is not within therapeutic range. Therapeutic LMWHs need to be stopped at least 24 hours prior to surgery, and can be resumed once normal haemostasis has been achieved (usually 24–48 hours later).[32]

The LMWH enoxaparin is used frequently in the management of ACS patients. Both in STEMI and NSTEMI patients undergoing PCI, an intravenous bolus of 0.5 mg/kg enoxaparin can be considered as peri-interventional anticoagulant treatment in patients pretreated with subcutaneous enoxaparin. In these patients cross-over of UFH and LMWH is not recommended.[9,26,33] The use of anticoagulants is also standard of care during elective PCI, and, based on the results of the STEEPLE trial, enoxaparin can be considered as an alternative for peri-interventional treatment with UFH,[33,34] although now still much less used in this setting compared with UFH.

Adverse effects

The main complication of LMWH use is bleeding. Rates of bleeding depend on the dose used, with lower frequencies at prophylactic levels compared with therapeutic dosing. Local side effects include pain, erythema, ecchymosis, or haematomas at the injection site, but also allergic reactions, pruritus, and urticarial reactions are frequently reported.[35]

Development of HIT is much less frequent than with UFH due to less interaction with platelets, with an approximately tenfold lower incidence compared with UFH.[36] However, the smaller molecules may still interact with PF4 and platelet-activating HIT antibodies, so cross reactivity is frequent.[37] Therefore, patients with a diagnosis or history of HIT should never be treated with a LMWH.

Hepatic side effects include transient elevations in liver function tests. In long-term treatment, the overall risk of osteoporosis seems to be increased, although bone mineral density seems less affected by LMWH than by UFH.[15,25]

Reversal of effect

No specific antidote is available to treat bleeding associated with LMWH treatment. When major bleeding or emergency major surgery requires the immediate reversal of the LMWH anticoagulant effect, protamine can be used. Because the main effect of protamine comes via neutralization of anti-factor IIa activity, the effect of protamine is only about half that when it is to neutralize UFH. Dosing strategies depend on the timing of the last injection of the LMWH. A common recommendation is to administer 1 mg of protamine for every 100 U of anti-factor Xa activity when the last injection took place within the prior 8 hours.[25] Andexanet alfa has been developed as a specific antidote for factor Xa inhibitors. It has been approved by the European Medicines Agency for use in patients treated with a direct factor Xa inhibitor (apixaban or rivaroxaban) when reversal of anticoagulation is needed due to life-threatening or uncontrolled bleeding.[38] Due to lack of data, use of andexanet alfa for reversal of LMWHs is currently not recommended. Ciraparantag is a reversal agent that reverses the effect of LMWHs, but further clinical studies are awaited to assess its therapeutic potential.[21,39]

Pentasaccharides

Mechanism and pharmacology

Heparin binds to antithrombin through a unique sequence of five saccharides (a pentasaccharide), and thereby potentiates the anticoagulant effect of antithrombin manyfold. Heparin is a mixture of polysaccharides of varying length that all share the pentasaccharide sequence. The longer polysaccharide chains (i.e. a saccharide sequence of 12 or more units) are able to bind exosite 2 of thrombin, thereby enhancing the anti-factor IIa effect of antithrombin. LMWH is composed of relatively shorter polysaccharide chains and, as a consequence, binds less to thrombin but is still capable of binding factor Xa. The unique pentasaccharide sequence comprising the minimal antithrombin binding sequence has been chemically synthesized and is commercially available as fondaparinux.[40] Fondaparinux only inhibits factor Xa through antithrombin and not thrombin, due to the fact that the ultrashort saccharide chains cannot bind to thrombin (➔ Figure 8.1).

Fondaparinux is the only drug in this class approved for use in humans. Peak concentrations are reached 2–3 hours after subcutaneous administration, and the mean half-life is 17 hours, enabling once-daily dosing.[25] Idraparinux and idrabiotaparinux are pentasaccharides with longer elimination half-lives than fondaparinux and have been studied in phase III randomized controlled trials, although further development was halted because of bleeding risk and lack of commercial perspective.[41,42]

Administration and monitoring

Fondaparinux is administered with subcutaneous injections. The prophylactic dose is 2.5 mg daily. For therapeutic treatment, daily dosing depends upon body weight; 5 mg for patients less than 50 kg, 7.5 mg for patients 50–100 kg, and 10 mg for patients weighing over 100 kg.[25] A once-daily dose of 2.5 mg is also recommended for treatment of superficial vein thrombosis and for patients with ACS. Fondaparinux is nearly completely dependent on renal clearance, so accumulation can occur with renal dysfunction. Thus, it is contraindicated in patients with severe renal insufficiency (i.e. creatinine clearance <30 mL/min). In patients with moderate renal insufficiency (i.e. creatinine clearance 30–50 mL/min) the prophylactic dose of fondaparinux should be reduced to 1.5 mg once daily, while no data exist on the safety of higher dosages.[25,43] If monitoring is required, fondaparinux levels can be measured with a calibrated anti-factor Xa assay.[43] Fondaparinux has no significant effect on the standard coagulation assays, although therapeutic doses may slightly increase the aPTT.

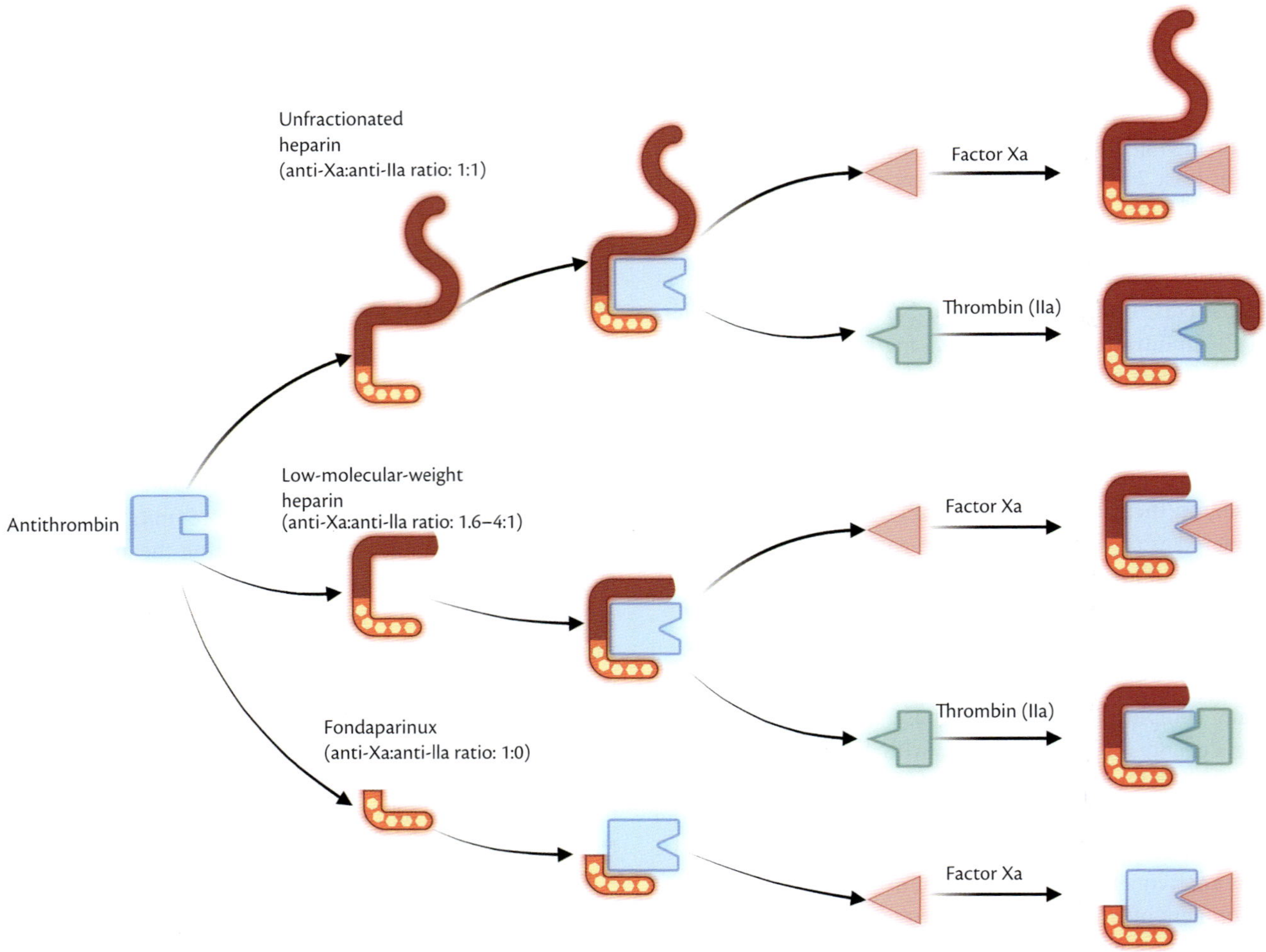

Figure 8.1 Mechanism of action of unfractionated heparin (UFH), low-molecular-weight heparins (LMWHs), and fondaparinux. Binding of UFH, LMWHs, or fondaparinux to antithrombin causes a conformational change that accelerates its interaction with thrombin and/or factor Xa. In contrast to factor Xa inhibition, catalysis of antithrombin-mediated inactivation of thrombin requires the formation of a ternary heparin–antithrombin–thrombin complex, which can only be formed by chains at least 12 saccharide units long. This explains why the shorter polysaccharides of LMWHs have less inhibitory activity against thrombin than UFH. The pentasaccharide fondaparinux only inhibits factor Xa, due to the fact that the ultrashort chains cannot bind thrombin.
Created with BioRender.com.

Indications and clinical use

Since its introduction in 1983, fondaparinux has been widely used in VTE prophylaxis, treatment of superficial venous thrombosis (SVT) and DVT, and in ACS patients. Fondaparinux 2.5 mg can be used for prevention of VTE in major orthopaedic surgery, major abdominal surgery, and hospitalized medical patients.[44]

A study of fondaparinux 2.5 mg once daily for 45 days versus placebo for treatment of SVT showed efficacy in terms of prevention of DVT and pulmonary embolism without any increase in major bleeding.[45] Fondaparinux 7.5 mg is recommended as initial treatment of DVT and pulmonary embolism, and had comparable efficacy to LMWH or UFH with similar bleeding rates.[46,47]

Fondaparinux 2.5 mg is approved for treatment of NSTEMI patients in whom no urgent revascularization procedure is planned. However, when patients undergo cardiac catheterization after an initial conservative treatment phase including fondaparinux treatment, full-dose UFH must be added to prevent thrombus formation when the patient proceeds to PCI, due to increased risk of catheter thrombus formation when fondaparinux is used as the only anticoagulant.[9,48,49] Fondaparinux in the context of primary PCI was associated with potential harm and is not recommended.[50]

Contrary to UFH or LMWH, pentasaccharides do not interact with platelets or PF4. Therefore, patients suspected of having HIT, or who have a history of HIT and require anticoagulation, have been successfully treated with fondaparinux. A fondaparinux-based treatment was shown to be effective in small case series of proven HIT patients,[51,52] although it is not officially approved (i.e. it is 'off label') for this indication.

Adverse effects

Since fondaparinux action is dependent on binding to antithrombin in a 1:1 molar ratio to function with its anti-Xa activity, plasma concentration of antithrombin can be the rate-limiting factor. With low antithrombin levels due to congenital or acquired deficiencies, the effect of fondaparinux can be reduced. *In vitro* studies suggest a 20% or greater reduction in anti-FXa activity with AT levels below 50% of normal.[53] Bleeding is the primary adverse effect of fondaparinux. Bleeding rates are similar to those with LMWHs, and can be exacerbated by impaired renal function.[54]

Reversal of effect

There is no specific antidote for fondaparinux. Protamine does not neutralize the effect of the pentasaccharides. In severe bleeding, recombinant FVIIa has been shown to partially reverse the anticoagulant effect.[43,55] Although andexanet alfa is being studied as a specific antidote for factor Xa inhibitors, reports on its capacity to neutralize the anti-Xa effects of fondaparinux are ambiguous.[56,57] Ciraparantag is a synthetic small molecule currently under development as a reversal agent targeting NOACs, LMWHs, heparin, and fondaparinux.[21,57,58]

Hirudin and bivalirudin

Mechanism and pharmacology

Following the identification of a leech (*Hirudo medicinalis*)-derived compound with anticoagulant properties, its potential to inhibit thrombin was demonstrated, and the structure of the 65-amino-acid-long protein, known as 'hirudin', was characterized. Next, this led to the production of recombinant hirudin, a potent and specific thrombin inhibitor.[10] Lepirudin and desirudin are two structurally identical forms of hirudin except for one amino acid difference in the N-terminal region that were studied in clinical trials. Concerns about bleeding, high costs, and immunogenicity with potential risk of anaphylaxis have limited the use of recombinant hirudin as well as of lepirudin/desirudin, and these products are no longer marketed.

Bivalirudin (originally named Hirulog-1) is a synthetic 20-amino-acid-long polypeptide analogue of hirudin resulting from a bivalent construct of hirugen (a synthetic analogue of the C-terminus of hirudin that partially inhibited thrombin activity) linked to D-Phe–Pro–Arg–Pro via poly-Gly spacers. Upon binding to free or clot-bound thrombin, the Arg–Pro bond in bivalirudin is cleaved, which restores some of thrombin's activity, providing less robust thrombin inhibition than hirudin, which may contribute to a better safety profile of bivalirudin. A half-life (25 minutes) shorter than for hirudin and less immunogenicity made bivalirudin a clinically interesting compound. Only 20% of bivalirudin is cleared by the kidney, the remainder is proteolytically inactivated via non-organ linked pathways.[25,54]

Administration and monitoring

Bivalirudin is given intravenously; the standard dosing protocol recommends a loading dose of 0.75 mg/kg, followed by an infusion of 1.75 mg/kg per hour for 4–12 hours post PCI. Bivalirudin dose-dependently prolongs aPTT, ACT, prothrombin time (PT), and thrombin time.

Indications and clinical use

Advantages of bivalirudin over heparins include the direct antithrombin activity, not requiring antithrombin, stable pharmacokinetics, and lack of inactivation by PF4, as well as absence of interactions with PF4-related antibodies occurring in HIT. Bivalirudin is approved for use in patients with ACS, as well as in PCI, and also in patients with suspected HIT or a history of HIT.[54]

Besides HIT, current indications for bivalirudin include PCI, NSTEMI patients planned for urgent or early intervention, and STEMI patients who undergo PCI. Many studies addressed the benefits of bivalirudin over heparin, but an updated meta-analysis confirmed a lack of benefit and mortality reduction for bivalirudin compared with heparin in ACS patients. In STEMI patients undergoing a primary PCI, current European Society of Cardiology (ESC) 2017 ACS guidelines recommend the use of UFH, with enoxaparin or bivalirudin as alternative, second-line options (class IIA).[26] Similarly, in patients with NSTEMI, bivalirudin is an alternative anticoagulant option for heparin or enoxaparin, while in patients with stable coronary artery disease, bivalirudin is not recommended (unless for heparin replacement in HIT).[9]

Initially, bivalirudin was thought to be safer than heparin in the spectrum of patients with coronary artery disease undergoing PCI, but this benefit may have diminished since the more common use of the radial route of PCI access and the minimal current use of glycoprotein IIb/IIIa antagonists. As bivalirudin is much more expensive than UFH and there are remaining uncertainties about optimal dosing and duration periprocedurally, linked also to concerns about stent thrombosis, the use of bivalirudin for PCI indications is currently limited, and mostly confined to (suspected) HIT as well as for replacement of UFH in high-risk settings like ECMO.[59,60] The use of bivalirudin is not likely to be changed by the recent results of the Bivalirudin With Prolonged Full-Dose Infusion During Primary PCI Versus Heparin Trial (BRIGHT)-4 that compared a strategy of bivalirudin (given during PCI followed by a high-dose infusion for 2–4 hours after PCI) with UFH (given only during PCI) in 6016 patients with STEMI undergoing primary PCI using a randomized open-label design.[61]

Adverse effects

Bleeding is the most important major side effect, but other adverse effects that have been reported include nausea, hypotension, and back pain. Immunogenicity has not been observed yet.

Reversal of effect

In case of bleeding, the infusion must be stopped with the expectation that clotting times will normalize within a few hours given the short half-life of the drug. In case of emergencies and in the absence of a reversal agent, plasmapheresis or haemodialysis may be considered.

Argatroban

Mechanism and pharmacology

Argatroban is the first of a number of direct, active site-targeted small molecules that emerged in 1981, later followed by similarly direct *oral* thrombin inhibitors ximelagatran and dabigatran. Argatroban binds to the active site of thrombin, and has a half-life of 45 minutes after intravenous administration, being cleared through the liver by cytochrome P450 3A4/5 metabolism, and eliminated through the bile. Its effect in blood is measurable by the aPTT and PT.[10,62]

Administration and monitoring

Argatroban is administered as a continuous intravenous infusion starting at 1–2 micrograms/kg, and adjusted based on the aPTT, aiming for a ratio of 1.5–3.0 as compared with baseline.[63] Lower loading and/or infusion doses may be warranted in patients with liver failure or other critical illnesses that may impair effective liver clearance, including congestive heart failure, while renal failure per se does not require dose adjustments.

Indications and clinical use

The primary indication for argatroban is replacement of heparin in patients with HIT-related thromboembolism. As compared with historical controls, the use of argatroban was associated with reduced rates of thromboembolism, death, and a composite of thrombosis, amputation, and mortality without an increased risk of bleeding.[54] More recent studies evaluated argatroban in ischaemic stroke, during cardiac surgery, to prevent mechanical heart valve-associated thromboembolism, and in haemodialysis. A non-randomized trial of short-term argatroban on top of dual antiplatelet therapy (DAPT) in ischaemic stroke patients suggested an acceptable safety profile of this combination, but randomized controlled trials are necessary to support this strategy.[64]

Adverse effects

The primary serious adverse effect is major bleeding that may occur in up to 3% of patients and appears to be in part dependent on the dose and on clearance efficacy. Caution should be exercised upon switching to coumarin derivatives, as both drugs affect the PT, which may require repeated INR testing and argatroban infusion dose adjustment to reduce the risk of excess anticoagulation exposure.

Reversal of effect

There is no antidote for argatroban other than stopping the infusion, upon which clotting times should normalize within 2–4 hours, assuming effective clearance, which may be impaired in situations associated with liver failure.

Danaparoid

Mechanism and pharmacology

Danaparoid is a mixture of glycosaminoglycans containing heparan sulfate (84%), dermatan sulfate (12%), and chondroitin sulfate (4%).[65] Its primary effect is on antithrombin-mediated inactivation of factor Xa, while a secondary effect involves a certain degree of thrombin inhibition through antithrombin and heparin cofactor 2. Danaparoid has an elimination half-life of about 15 hours, mainly via the renal route. Its main indication in the countries where it is registered is replacement of heparin in case of HIT, where the unique mode of action appears to involve replacement of PF4/heparin complexes from the platelet surface.

Administration and monitoring

Danaparoid can be administered subcutaneously for thromboprophylaxis, replacing heparin in case of HIT, and its longer-term use can be monitored with anti-Xa assay. In case of acute HIT, danaparoid is usually given by the intravenous route adjusted for body weight given as a loading dose (2250–3750 anti-Xa units) followed by continuous infusion of doses starting at 400 anti-Xa units/hour for the first 4 hours and then tapered to lower maintenance doses. Monitoring aiming for a plasma anti-Xa level between 0.4 and 0.8 units/mL is not routinely recommended, but should be considered in patients with renal failure (estimated glomerular filtration rate <30 mL/min). Upon stabilization, a switch to subcutaneous danaparoid or another oral drug can be made.

Indications and clinical use

Danaparoid is primarily used for patients with HIT with or without thrombosis, and is an alternative for other agents like argatroban in hospitalized patients. Although the long half-life makes it less suitable for periprocedural use, it has been successfully applied in HIT patients undergoing cardiopulmonary bypass surgery. Danaparoid does not cross the placenta, hence it can be given safely to pregnant patients. In Japan, danaparoid is also used in patients with disseminated intravascular coagulation. Its use in various conditions has been documented in different case series.[66]

Adverse effects

Bleeding is the major side effect, although its prevalence appeared to be lower in HIT patients as compared to lepirudin or warfarin.[67,68] Other adverse effects include bruising, allergic reactions, and persistent thrombocytopenia, with the last of these necessitating control of platelet count in patients with HIT.

Reversal of effect

There is no antidote for danaparoid, and upon discontinuation of the infusion the weaning of the anticoagulant effect may best be monitored by anti-Xa assay, certainly in conditions with renal failure.

Summary and conclusions

Several parenteral anticoagulants are available for thromboprophylaxis as well as treatment of both venous and arterial thrombosis. Properties of these drugs are compared in ➲ Table 8.3. Although the spectrum of oral anticoagulants has expanded in the last decades, several emergency and special indications as described in this chapter will still require the use of parenteral anticoagulants. It is important for clinicians to be familiar with their indications, dosing strategies, adverse effects, and reversal mechanisms.

Table 8.3 Comparison of therapeutic dosing of unfractionated heparin, low-molecular-weight heparins, fondaparinux, bivalirudin, argatroban, and danaparoid

	UFH	LMWH	Fondaparinux	Bivalirudin	Argatroban	Danaparoid
Size	Very large	Large	Small	Small	Very small	Large
Molecular weight (Da)	15,000	5000	1728	2180	527	5500
Thrombin-binding affinity	++	+	None	++	++	+
Route	IV	SC	SC	IV	IV	SC or IV
Dosage	aPTT adjusted	Bodyweight adjusted	2.5–7.5 mg	Loading dose of 0.75 mg/kg; next, infusion of 1.75 mg/kg per hour	Continuous infusion starting at 0.5–2 mcg/kg/min adjusted to prolong the aPTT 1.5–3-fold baseline	IV: loading dose of 2250 U, followed by 400 U/h, stepwise reduced to 200 U/h
Half life	2 h	3–5 h	17–20 h	25 min	45 min	25 h
Reversible	Yes	Partial	No	Partial	Yes	Yes
Clearance	RES and renal	Renal	Renal	20% renal; 80% non-organ pathways	Hepatic (bile)	Renal
Monitoring	aPTT, aXa	aXa	aXa	aPTT, PT, or TT	aPTT	aXa

aXa, antifactor Xa; IV, intravenous; LMWH, low-molecular-weight heparin; PT, prothrombin time; RES, reticuloendothelial system; SC, subcutaneous; TT, thrombin time; UFH, unfractionated heparin.

What's new

- Although most parenteral anticoagulant drugs have been available for several decades, they are still frequently used in a variety of clinical scenarios.
- Parenteral anticoagulation can be indicated for thromboprophylaxis as well as treatment of both arterial and venous thromboembolism.
- In case of HIT, more and more parenteral and oral alternatives have become available, although some alternatives are still off-label.
- Protamine is available as antidote for UFH and (partially) for LMWH. For other parenteral anticoagulants no specific reversal agents are currently available.

Guideline recommendations

Relevant ESC Guideline recommendations for the management of acute coronary syndromes, myocardial revascularization, and cardiac surgery

Recommendation	Class of recommendation	Level of evidence
2020 ESC Guidelines for the management of acute coronary syndromes in patients presenting without persistent ST-segment elevation[9]		
Parenteral anticoagulation is recommended for all patients, in addition to antiplatelet treatment, at the time of diagnosis, and, especially, during revascularization procedures according to both ischaemic and bleeding risks	I	A
UFH (weight-adjusted i.v. bolus during PCI of 70–100 IU/kg, or 50–70 IU/kg in combination with a GP IIb/IIIa inhibitor; activated clotting time target range of 250–350 s, or 200–250 s if a GP IIb/IIIa inhibitor is given) is recommended in patients undergoing PCI	I	A
In cases of medical treatment or logistical constraints for transferring the patient to PCI within the required time frame, fondaparinux is recommended and, in such cases, a single bolus of UFH is recommended at the time of PCI	I	B
Enoxaparin (i.v.) should be considered in patients pre-treated with enoxaparin	IIa	B
Discontinuation of parenteral anticoagulation should be considered immediately after an invasive procedure	IIa	C
Bivalirudin (0.75 mg/kg i.v. bolus, followed by 1.75 mg/kg/h for up to 4 h after the procedure) maybe be considered as an alternative to UFH	IIb	A
Crossover of UFH and LMWH is not recommended	III	B
During PCI, additional parenteral anticoagulation is recommended, irrespective of the timing of last dose of all NOACs and if INR is <2.5 in VKA-treated patients	I	C

Recommendation	Class of recommendation	Level of evidence
2017 ESC Guidelines for the management of acute myocardial infarction in patients presenting with ST-segment elevation: the Task Force for the management of acute myocardial infarction in patients presenting with ST-segment elevation of the European Society of Cardiology (ESC)[26]		
Anticoagulation is recommended for all patients in addition to antiplatelet therapy during primary PCI	I	C
Routine use of UFH is recommended	I	C
In patients with heparin-induced thrombocytopenia, bivalirudin is recommended as the anticoagulant agent during primary PCI	I	C
Routine use of enoxaparin i.v. should be considered	IIa	A
Routine use of bivalirudin should be considered	IIa	A
Fondaparinux is not recommended for primary PCI	III	B
2018 ESC/EACTS Guidelines on myocardial revascularization[33]		
In *stable coronary artery disease patients* undergoing PCI UFH is indicated as the standard anticoagulant (70–100 U/kg)	I	B
In *stable coronary artery disease patients* undergoing PCI enoxaparin (i.v. 0.5 mg/kg) should be considered as an alternative agent	IIa	B
Bivalirudin (0.75 mg/kg bolus, followed by 1.75 mg/kg/h for up to 4 h after the procedure) is indicated in the case of heparin-induced thrombocytopenia	I	C
In *patients with non-ST-elevation acute coronary syndromes* undergoing PCI anticoagulation is recommended for all patients in addition to antiplatelet therapy	I	A
In *patients with non-ST-elevation acute coronary syndromes* undergoing PCI UFH is recommended	I	C
In *patients with non-ST-elevation acute coronary syndromes* undergoing PCI that are on fondaparinux, a single bolus UFH (85 IU/kg, or 60 IU in the case of concomitant use of GP IIb/IIIa receptor inhibitors) is indicated	I	B
In *patients with non-ST-elevation acute coronary syndromes* undergoing PCI, enoxaparin should be considered in patients pre-treated with s.c. enoxaparin	IIa	B
In *patients with non-ST-elevation acute coronary syndromes* undergoing PCI bivalirudin may be considered as an alternative to UFH	IIb	A
In *patients with non-ST-elevation acute coronary syndromes* undergoing PCI crossover of UFH and LMWH is not recommended	III	B
In *patients with ST-elevation myocardial infarction* undergoing PCI anticoagulation is recommended for all patients in addition to antiplatelet therapy during PCI	I	A
In *patients with ST-elevation myocardial infarction* undergoing PCI routine use of UFH is recommended	I	C
In *patients with ST-elevation myocardial infarction* undergoing PCI routine use of enoxaparin should be considered	IIa	A
In *patients with ST-elevation myocardial infarction* undergoing PCI routine use of bivalirudin may be considered	IIb	A
2019 EACTS/EACTA/EBCP guidelines on cardiopulmonary bypass in adult cardiac surgery[19]		
Heparin management. ACT above 480 s during CPB should be considered in CPB with uncoated equipment and cardiotomy suction. The required target ACT is dependent on the type of equipment used	IIa	C
Individualized heparin and protamine management should be considered to reduce postoperative coagulation abnormalities and bleeding complications in cardiac surgery with CPB	IIa	B
Protamine overdosing should be avoided in order to reduce postoperative coagulation abnormalities and bleeding complications in cardiac surgery with CPB	IIa	B
In patients with contraindications to heparin and/or protamine usage and in need of an operation requiring CPB, anticoagulation with bivalirudin should be considered	IIa	B
In patients with contraindications to heparin and/or protamine usage, in need of an operation requiring CPB and significant renal dysfunction, anticoagulation with argatroban may be considered	IIb	C

Collet JP, Thiele H, Barbato E, et al.; ESC Scientific Document Group. 2020 ESC Guidelines for the management of acute coronary syndromes in patients presenting without persistent ST-segment elevation. Eur Heart J. 2021 Apr 7;42(14):1289–1367. doi: 10.1093/eurheartj/ehaa575; and Ibanez B, James S, Agewall S, et al.; ESC Scientific Document Group. 2017 ESC Guidelines for the management of acute myocardial infarction in patients presenting with ST-segment elevation: The Task Force for the management of acute myocardial infarction in patients presenting with ST-segment elevation of the European Society of Cardiology (ESC). Eur Heart J. 2018 Jan 7;39(2):119–177. doi: 10.1093/eurheartj/ehx393; and Neumann FJ, Sousa-Uva M, Ahlsson A, et al.; ESC Scientific Document Group. 2018 ESC/EACTS Guidelines on myocardial revascularization. Eur Heart J. 2019 Jan 7;40(2):87–165. doi: 10.1093/eurheartj/ehy394; and Wahba A, Milojevic M, Boer C, et al; EACTS/EACTA/EBCP Committee Reviewers. 2019 EACTS/EACTA/EBCP guidelines on cardiopulmonary bypass in adult cardiac surgery. Eur J Cardiothorac Surg. 2020 Feb 1;57(2):210-251. doi: 10.1093/ejcts/ezz267.

Relevant guideline recommendations for the management of pulmonary embolism, perioperative management, and heparin-induced thrombocytopenia

2019 ESC Guidelines for the diagnosis and management of acute pulmonary embolism developed in collaboration with the European Respiratory Society (ERS): the Task Force for the diagnosis and management of acute pulmonary embolism of the European Society of Cardiology (ESC)[28]

Recommendation	Class of recommendation	Level of evidence
It is recommended that anticoagulation with UFH, including a weight-adjusted bolus injection, be initiated without delay in patients with high-risk PE	I	C
If anticoagulation is initiated parenterally in a patient without haemodynamic instability, prefer LMWH or fondaparinux over UFH	I	A
A therapeutic, fixed dose of LMWH based on early pregnancy body weight is the recommended therapy for PE in the majority of pregnant women without haemodynamic instability	I	B
Insertion of a spinal or epidural needle is not recommended, unless ≥24 h have passed since the last therapeutic dose of LMWH	III	C
Administration of LMWH is not recommended within 4 h of removal of an epidural catheter	III	C
For patients with PE and cancer, weight-adjusted subcutaneous LMWH should be considered for the first 6 months over VKAs	IIa	A

2022 perioperative management of antithrombotic therapy: an American College of Chest Physicians clinical practice guideline[32]

In patients receiving LMWH bridging for an elective surgery/procedure, we suggest administering the last pre-operative LMWH bridging dose at approximately 24 hours over administering the last dose 10 to 12 hours before a surgery/procedure	Conditional recommendation	Very low certainty
In patient receiving LMWH bridging for an elective surgery/procedure, we suggest administering the first post-operative LMWH bridging dose at least 24 hours after a surgery/procedure over administering it less than 24 hours after a surgery/procedure	Conditional recommendation	Very low certainty

2018 American Society of Hematology guidelines for management of venous thromboembolism: heparin-induced thrombocytopenia (HIT)[69]

In patients with acute HIT complicated with thrombosis (HITT) or acute HIT without thrombosis (isolated HIT) discontinuation of heparin and initiation of a non-heparin anticoagulant is strongly recommended	Strong recommendation	Moderate certainty
When a non-heparin is selected, argatroban, bivalirudin, danaparoid, fondaparinux, or a direct oral anticoagulant (DOAC) are suggested	Conditional recommendation	Very low certainty
In patients with critical illness, increased bleeding risk, or increased potential need for urgent procedures, argatroban or bivalirudin may be preferred because of shorter duration of effect. In patients with moderate or severe hepatic dysfunction it is advisable to avoid argatroban or use a reduced dose	Conditional recommendation	Very low certainty
Fondaparinux and the DOACs are reasonable options in clinically stable patients at average risk of bleeding. In patients with HIT complicated by life- or limb threatening thromboembolism, a parenteral non-heparin anticoagulant may be preferred because few such patients have been treated with a DOAC	Conditional recommendation	Very low certainty

ACT, activated clotting time; CPB, cardiopulmonary bypass; DOAC, direct oral anticoagulant; HIT, heparin-induced thrombocytopenia; i.v., intravenous; LMWH, low-molecular-weight heparin; PCI, percutaneous coronary intervention; PE, pulmonary embolism; s.c., subcutaneous; UFH, unfractionated heparin; VKA; vitamin K antagonist.

Konstantinides SV, Meyer G, Becattini C, et al.; ESC Scientific Document Group. 2019 ESC Guidelines for the diagnosis and management of acute pulmonary embolism developed in collaboration with the European Respiratory Society (ERS). Eur Heart J. 2020 Jan 21;41(4):543–603. doi: 10.1093/eurheartj/ehz405; and Douketis JD, Spyropoulos AC, Murad MH, et al. Perioperative management of antithrombotic therapy: an American College of Chest Physicians clinical practice guideline. Chest. 2022 Nov;162(5):e207–e243. doi: 10.1016/j.chest.2022.07.025; and Lim W, Le Gal G, Bates SM, et al.; American Society of Hematology 2018 guidelines for management of venous thromboembolism: diagnosis of venous thromboembolism. Blood Adv. 2018 Nov 27;2(22):3226–3256. doi: 10.1182/bloodadvances.2018024828.

What's next

- No new parenteral anticoagulants are expected to be introduced in the near future.
- Andexanet alfa and ciraparantag are reversal agents currently being studied as antidotes for several parenteral and oral anticoagulants.

- Regarding HIT, more parenteral and oral alternatives for heparin will become available.

Drug dosing

Drug	Route	Indication	Dosage
Heparin	SC	Prophylaxis	5000 IU twice daily
	SC	Treatment	250 IU/kg twice daily
	IV	Treatment	Loading dose of 5000 IU, followed by continuous infusion 15–25 IU/kg/h, adjusted to prolong aPTT 1.5–2.5-fold
Nadroparin	SC	Prophylaxis	2850–5700 IU daily
		Treatment	86 IU/kg twice daily
Enoxaparin	SC	Prophylaxis	20–40 mg daily
		Treatment	1 mg/kg twice daily or 1.5 mg daily
Dalteparin	SC	Prophylaxis	2500–5000 IU daily
		Treatment	100 IU/kg twice daily or 200 IU/kg daily
Tinzaparin	SC	Prophylaxis	3500 IU daily
		Treatment	175 IU/kg daily
Fondaparinux	SC	Prophylaxis	2.5 once daily
		Treatment SVT or ACS	2.5 mg once daily
		Treatment DVT/PE	<50 kg: 5 mg once daily 50–100 kg 7.5 mg once daily >100 kg 10 mg once daily
Bivalirudin	IV	PCI	Loading dose of 0.75 mg/kg Continuous infusion 1.75 mg/kg/h during PCI, on indication followed by 0.25 mg/kg/h during 4–12 hours post-PCI
Argatroban	IV	HIT	Continuous infusion 0.5–2 mcg/kg/min, adjusted to prolong aPTT 1.5–3-fold from baseline
Danaparoid	SC	Prophylaxis	<90 kg: 750 U twice daily >90 kg: 1250 U twice daily
	IV	HIT	Loading dose of 2250 U, followed by continuous infusion 400 U/h, stepwise reduced to 200 U/h
Protamine sulfate	IV	Reversal of heparin	100 IU per 100 IU heparin administered within the last 3 hours
		Reversal of LMWH	100 IU per 100 IU aXa LMWH administered within the last 8 hours

ACS, acute coronary syndrome; aXa, antifactor Xa; aPTT, activated partial thromboplastin time; DVT, deep venous thrombosis; LMWH, low-molecular-weight heparin; IV, intravenous; LMWH, low-molecular-weight heparin; PCI, percutaneous coronary intervention; SC, subcutaneous; SVT, superficial venous thrombosis; UFH, unfractionated heparin.

References

1. Damus PS, Hicks M, Rosenberg RD. Anticoagulant action of heparin. Nature. 1973;246(5432):355–7.
2. Hirsh J. Heparin. N Engl J Med. 1991;324(22):1565–74.
3. Andersson LO, Barrowcliffe TW, Holmer E, Johnson EA, Soderstrom G. Molecular weight dependency of the heparin potentiated inhibition of thrombin and activated factor X. Effect of heparin neutralization in plasma. Thromb Res. 1979;15(3–4):531–41.
4. Bjornsson TD, Wolfram KM, Kitchell BB. Heparin kinetics determined by three assay methods. Clin Pharmacol Ther. 1982;31(1):104–13.
5. de Swart CA, Nijmeyer B, Roelofs JM, Sixma JJ. Kinetics of intravenously administered heparin in normal humans. Blood. 1982;60(6):1251–8.
6. Estes JW. Clinical pharmacokinetics of heparin. Clin Pharmacokinet. 1980;5(3):204–20.
7. Levy JH, Connors JM. Heparin resistance—clinical perspectives and management strategies. N Engl J Med. 2021;385(9):826–32.
8. Berkowitz O, Halabi M, Goldberg A, et al. Routine fixed-dose heparin vs. ACT-guided heparin administration for elective PCI and its influence on patient in-hospital outcome: a retrospective study. Coron Artery Dis. 2021;32(6):549–53.
9. Collet JP, Thiele H, Barbato E, et al. 2020 ESC Guidelines for the management of acute coronary syndromes in patients presenting without persistent ST-segment elevation. Eur Heart J. 2021;42(14):1289–367.
10. Coppens M, Eikelboom JW, Gustafsson D, Weitz JI, Hirsh J. Translational success stories: development of direct thrombin inhibitors. Circ Res. 2012;111(7):920–9.
11. Greinacher A. Clinical practice. Heparin-induced thrombocytopenia. N Engl J Med. 2015;373(3):252–61.
12. Koster A, Nagler M, Erdoes G, Levy JH. Heparin-induced thrombocytopenia: perioperative diagnosis and management. Anesthesiology. 2022;136(2):336–44.
13. Warkentin TE, Heddle NM. Laboratory diagnosis of immune heparin-induced thrombocytopenia. Curr Hematol Rep. 2003;2(2):148–57.
14. Cuker A, Gimotty PA, Crowther MA, Warkentin TE. Predictive value of the 4Ts scoring system for heparin-induced thrombocytopenia: a systematic review and meta-analysis. Blood. 2012;120(20):4160–7.
15. Signorelli SS, Scuto S, Marino E, Giusti M, Xourafa A, Gaudio A. Anticoagulants and osteoporosis. Int J Mol Sci. 2019;20(21):5275.
16. Bick RL, Frenkel EP. Clinical aspects of heparin-induced thrombocytopenia and thrombosis and other side effects of heparin therapy. Clin Appl Thromb Hemost. 1999;5 Suppl 1:S7–15.
17. Koscielny J, Rutkauskaite E, Sucker C, von Heymann C. How do I reverse oral and parenteral anticoagulants? Hamostaseologie. 2020;40(2):201–13.

18. Hecht P, Besser M, Falter F. Are we able to dose protamine accurately yet? A review of the protamine conundrum. J Extra Corpor Technol. 2020;52(1):63–70.
19. Wahba A, Milojevic M, Boer C, et al. 2019 EACTS/EACTA/EBCP guidelines on cardiopulmonary bypass in adult cardiac surgery. Eur J Cardiothorac Surg. 2020;57(2):210–51.
20. Al-Kassou B, Kandt J, Lohde L, et al. Safety and efficacy of protamine administration for prevention of bleeding complications in patients undergoing TAVR. JACC Cardiovasc Interv. 2020;13(12):1471–80.
21. Ansell J, Laulicht BE, Bakhru SH, et al. Ciraparantag, an anticoagulant reversal drug: mechanism of action, pharmacokinetics, and reversal of anticoagulants. Blood. 2021;137(1):115–25.
22. Lu G. Reversal of heparin-induced anticoagulation by andexanet alfa, a universal antidote for factor Xa inhibitors. Blood. 2015;126(23):2329.
23. Weitz JI. Low-molecular-weight heparins. N Engl J Med. 1997;337(10):688–98.
24. Cosmi B, Fredenburgh JC, Rischke J, Hirsh J, Young E, Weitz JI. Effect of nonspecific binding to plasma proteins on the antithrombin activities of unfractionated heparin, low-molecular-weight heparin, and dermatan sulfate. Circulation. 1997;95(1):118–24.
25. Garcia DA, Baglin TP, Weitz JI, Samama MM. Parenteral anticoagulants: Antithrombotic Therapy and Prevention of Thrombosis, 9th ed: American College of Chest Physicians Evidence-Based Clinical Practice Guidelines. Chest. 2012;141(2 Suppl):e24S–43S.
26. Ibanez B, James S, Agewall S, et al. 2017 ESC Guidelines for the management of acute myocardial infarction in patients presenting with ST-segment elevation: the Task Force for the management of acute myocardial infarction in patients presenting with ST-segment elevation of the European Society of Cardiology (ESC). Eur Heart J. 2018;39(2):119–77.
27. Bates SM. Pregnancy-associated venous thromboembolism: prevention and treatment. Semin Hematol. 2011;48(4):271–84.
28. Konstantinides SV, Meyer G, Becattini C, et al. 2019 ESC Guidelines for the diagnosis and management of acute pulmonary embolism developed in collaboration with the European Respiratory Society (ERS). Eur Heart J. 2020;41(4):543–603.
29. Robertson L, Jones LE. Fixed dose subcutaneous low molecular weight heparins versus adjusted dose unfractionated heparin for the initial treatment of venous thromboembolism. Cochrane Database Syst Rev. 2017;2:CD001100.
30. Lee AY, Levine MN, Baker RI, et al. Low-molecular-weight heparin versus a coumarin for the prevention of recurrent venous thromboembolism in patients with cancer. N Engl J Med. 2003;349(2):146–53.
31. Lee AYY, Kamphuisen PW, Meyer G, et al. Tinzaparin vs warfarin for treatment of acute venous thromboembolism in patients with active cancer: a randomized clinical Trial. JAMA. 2015;314(7):677–86.
32. Douketis JD, Spyropoulos AC, Murad MH, et al. Perioperative management of antithrombotic therapy: an American College of Chest Physicians Clinical Practice Guideline. Chest. 2022;162(5):e207–e43.
33. Neumann FJ, Sousa-Uva M, Ahlsson A, et al. 2018 ESC/EACTS Guidelines on myocardial revascularization. Eur Heart J. 2019;40(2):87–165.
34. Montalescot G, White HD, Gallo R, et al. Enoxaparin versus unfractionated heparin in elective percutaneous coronary intervention. N Engl J Med. 2006;355(10):1006–17.
35. Wutschert R, Piletta P, Bounameaux H. Adverse skin reactions to low molecular weight heparins: frequency, management and prevention. Drug Saf. 1999;20(6):515–25.
36. Warkentin TE, Levine MN, Hirsh J, et al. Heparin-induced thrombocytopenia in patients treated with low-molecular-weight heparin or unfractionated heparin. N Engl J Med. 1995;332(20):1330–5.
37. Prandoni P, Siragusa S, Girolami B, Fabris F, Group BI. The incidence of heparin-induced thrombocytopenia in medical patients treated with low-molecular-weight heparin: a prospective cohort study. Blood. 2005;106(9):3049–54.
38. Connolly SJ, Crowther M, Eikelboom JW, et al. Full study report of andexanet alfa for bleeding associated with factor Xa inhibitors. N Engl J Med. 2019;380(14):1326–35.
39. Ansell JE, Laulicht BE, Bakhru SH, Hoffman M, Steiner SS, Costin JC. Ciraparantag safely and completely reverses the anticoagulant effects of low molecular weight heparin. Thromb Res. 2016;146:113–18.
40. Hemker HC. A century of heparin: past, present and future. J Thromb Haemost. 2016;14(12):2329–38.
41. Buller HR, Gallus AS, Pillion G, Prins MH, Raskob GE, Cassiopea I. Enoxaparin followed by once-weekly idrabiotaparinux versus enoxaparin plus warfarin for patients with acute symptomatic pulmonary embolism: a randomised, double-blind, double-dummy, non-inferiority trial. Lancet. 2012;379(9811):123–9.
42. van Gogh I, Buller HR, Cohen AT, et al. Idraparinux versus standard therapy for venous thromboembolic disease. N Engl J Med. 2007;357(11):1094–104.
43. Nagler M, Haslauer M, Wuillemin WA. Fondaparinux—data on efficacy and safety in special situations. Thromb Res. 2012;129(4):407–17.
44. Geerts WH, Bergqvist D, Pineo GF, et al. Prevention of venous thromboembolism: American College of Chest Physicians Evidence-Based Clinical Practice Guidelines (8th Edition). Chest. 2008;133(6 Suppl):381S–453S.
45. Decousus H, Prandoni P, Mismetti P, et al. Fondaparinux for the treatment of superficial-vein thrombosis in the legs. N Engl J Med. 2010;363(13):1222–32.
46. Buller HR, Davidson BL, Decousus H, et al. Subcutaneous fondaparinux versus intravenous unfractionated heparin in the initial treatment of pulmonary embolism. N Engl J Med. 2003;349(18):1695–702.
47. Buller HR, Davidson BL, Decousus H, et al. Fondaparinux or enoxaparin for the initial treatment of symptomatic deep venous thrombosis: a randomized trial. Ann Intern Med. 2004;140(11):867–73.
48. Group FO-T, Steg PG, Jolly SS, et al. Low-dose vs standard-dose unfractionated heparin for percutaneous coronary intervention in acute coronary syndromes treated with fondaparinux: the FUTURA/OASIS-8 randomized trial. JAMA. 2010;304(12):1339–49.
49. Fifth Organization to Assess Strategies in Acute Ischemic Syndromes Investigators, Yusuf S, Mehta SR, et al. Comparison of fondaparinux and enoxaparin in acute coronary syndromes. N Engl J Med. 2006;354(14):1464–76.
50. Yusuf S, Mehta SR, Chrolavicius S, et al. Effects of fondaparinux on mortality and reinfarction in patients with acute ST-segment elevation myocardial infarction: the OASIS-6 randomized trial. JAMA. 2006;295(13):1519–30.
51. Kelton JG, Arnold DM, Bates SM. Nonheparin anticoagulants for heparin-induced thrombocytopenia. N Engl J Med. 2013;368(8):737–44.
52. Nilius H, Kaufmann J, Cuker A, Nagler M. Comparative effectiveness and safety of anticoagulants for the treatment of heparin-induced thrombocytopenia. Am J Hematol. 2021;96(7):805–15.
53. Jeske WP, Walenga JM, Samama MM, Hoppensteadt D, Mayuga M, Fareed J. Functionality of fondaparinux (pentasaccharide) depends on clinical antithrombin levels. Blood Coagul Fibrinolysis. 2011;22(3):206–10.
54. Crowther MA. Parenteral antithrombotic agents. In: Kitchens CS, Kessler CM, Konkle BA, Streiff MB, Garcia DA, editors. Consultative

Hemostasis and Thrombosis. 4th edition. Philadelphia, PA: Elsevier; 2019: 529–39.
55. Bijsterveld NR, Moons AH, Boekholdt SM, et al. Ability of recombinant factor VIIa to reverse the anticoagulant effect of the pentasaccharide fondaparinux in healthy volunteers. Circulation. 2002;106(20):2550–4.
56. Siddiqui F, Tafur A, Bontekoe E, et al. Assay-based differentiation in the neutralization profile of unfractionated heparin, enoxaparin, and fondaparinux by andexanet alfa. Clin Appl Thromb Hemost. 2020;26:1076029619895120.
57. Lu G, DeGuzman FR, Hollenbach SJ, et al. Reversal of low molecular weight heparin and fondaparinux by a recombinant antidote (r-Antidote, PRT064445). Am Heart Assoc. 2010;122:A12420.
58. Laulicht B. Antidote for new oral anticoagulants: mechanism of action and binding specificity of PER977. J Thromb Haemost. 2013;11(Suppl):1.
59. Koster A, Faraoni D, Levy JH. Argatroban and bivalirudin for perioperative anticoagulation in cardiac surgery. Anesthesiology. 2018;128(2):390–400.
60. Seelhammer TG, Bohman JK, Schulte PJ, Hanson AC, Aganga DO. Comparison of bivalirudin versus heparin for maintenance systemic anticoagulation during adult and pediatric extracorporeal membrane oxygenation. Crit Care Med. 2021;49(9):1481–92.
61. Li Y, Liang Z, Qin L, et al. Bivalirudin plus a high-dose infusion versus heparin monotherapy in patients with ST-segment elevation myocardial infarction undergoing primary percutaneous coronary intervention: a randomised trial. Lancet. 2022;400(10366): 1847–57.
62. McKeage K, Plosker GL. Argatroban. Drugs. 2001;61(4):515–22.
63. Hirsh J, Bauer KA, Donati MB, Gould M, Samama MM, Weitz JI. Parenteral anticoagulants: American College of Chest Physicians Evidence-Based Clinical Practice Guidelines (8th Edition). Chest. 2008;133(6 Suppl):141S–59S.
64. Li XQ, Hou XW, Cui Y, et al. Safety and preliminary efficacy of argatroban plus dual antiplatelet therapy for acute mild to moderate ischemic stroke with large artery atherosclerosis. Brain Behav. 2022:12(7):e2664.
65. Ibbotson T, Perry CM. Danaparoid: a review of its use in thromboembolic and coagulation disorders. Drugs. 2002;62(15): 2283–314.
66. Magnani HN, Gallus A. Heparin-induced thrombocytopenia (HIT). A report of 1,478 clinical outcomes of patients treated with danaparoid (Orgaran) from 1982 to mid-2004. Thromb Haemost. 2006;95(6):967–81.
67. Farner B, Eichler P, Kroll H, Greinacher A. A comparison of danaparoid and lepirudin in heparin-induced thrombocytopenia. Thromb Haemost. 2001;85(6):950–7.
68. Lubenow N, Warkentin TE, Greinacher A, et al. Results of a systematic evaluation of treatment outcomes for heparin-induced thrombocytopenia in patients receiving danaparoid, ancrod, and/or coumarin explain the rapid shift in clinical practice during the 1990s. Thromb Res. 2006;117(5):507–15.
69. Cuker A, Arepally GM, Chong BH, et al. American Society of Hematology 2018 guidelines for management of venous thromboembolism: heparin-induced thrombocytopenia. Blood Adv. 2018;2(22):3360–92.

CHAPTER 9

Vitamin K antagonists

Freek W.A. Verheugt and Marc A. Brouwer

Contents

Summary

Since the 1950s, vitamin K antagonists have been used for the prevention and treatment of venous and arterial thrombotic disorders. They have a narrow therapeutic window. To ensure efficacy and safety, close monitoring of the anticoagulation status is mandatory. Dietary and drug interactions are common. The most frequent side effect is bleeding, but birth defects and skin necrosis may occur as well. Rapid and effective reversal can be achieved with prothrombin complex concentrates. With the advent of direct oral anticoagulants, the use of vitamin K antagonists will diminish, but they currently remain the first choice in anticoagulation-eligible patients with advanced kidney disease, rheumatic heart valve disease, antiphospholipid syndrome, left ventricular thrombus, and in those with mechanical heart valves.

History

Vitamin K was discovered by the Danish biochemist Henrik Dam and the American biochemist Edward Doisy, for which they received the Nobel Prize for Medicine or Physiology in 1943. Dam called it vitamin K from 'Koagulation', the Danish word for coagulation. Vitamin K is essential for blood coagulation, and is administered routinely to each newborn in order to prevent potential vitamin K deficiency, which may lead to severe neonatal bleeding.[1] In the 1940s, coumarin was discovered in the sweet clover (*Melilotus alba* and *M. officinalis*) in Wisconsin meadows, causing fatal bleeding in cattle and sheep. This resulted in the production of vitamin K antagonists (also called coumarins) such as warfarin (after WARF: Wisconsin Alumni Research Foundation).[2] These oral anticoagulants are essential for stroke prevention in high-risk patients with atrial fibrillation,[3] venous thromboembolism,[4] left ventricular thrombus, mechanical heart valves,[5] antiphospholipid syndrome,[5a] and rheumatic mitral valve disease,[6] as recently confirmed in patients with rheumatic mitral stenosis.[7] They can also be used for secondary prevention in patients with stable coronary artery disease.[8,9] It is very likely that Dam and Doisy were not aware of their clinically most important discovery.

Pharmacology

Vitamin K antagonists act through interference with the vitamin K-dependent production of coagulation factors II, VII, IX, and X, which are produced by the liver (➔ Figure 9.1).[8] In the liver, proteins C and S—natural anticoagulants—are also produced in a biologically less active form after vitamin K antagonist treatment. Because of their respective half-lives, there is an initial procoagulant effect in the 24 hours after initiation of vitamin K antagonists, which is related to their effect on anticoagulants protein C and protein S (see below). This explains why, in case of initiation of vitamin K antagonists, heparin has to be co-administered when patients are in a high thrombotic state (pulmonary embolism, deep venous thrombosis, acute coronary syndrome). Absorption of vitamin K antagonists from the gastrointestinal tract is rapid, with a high bioavailability. The drugs are bound to plasma proteins, with subsequent accumulation and metabolization in the liver. Accordingly, dietary aspects related to increased or decreased intake of the fat-soluble vitamin K, gastrointestinal malabsorption, and hepatic dysfunction are factors that can interfere with the response to oral anticoagulation therapy.

Absorption, bioavailability, distribution, and elimination

Vitamin K antagonists can be given orally, intravenously, or rectally. When given through the gastrointestinal route the absorption is almost 100% and their peak plasma levels are reached within 6–8 hours.[10] There is almost complete binding to plasma proteins, and the drugs are metabolized through the cytochrome P450 (CYP)-2C9 enzyme pathway. Half-life varies widely—between 24 and 60 hours with a mean of 40 hours[10]—making the duration of action of vitamin K antagonists between 2 and 5 days. The inactive metabolites are excreted through stools and urine.

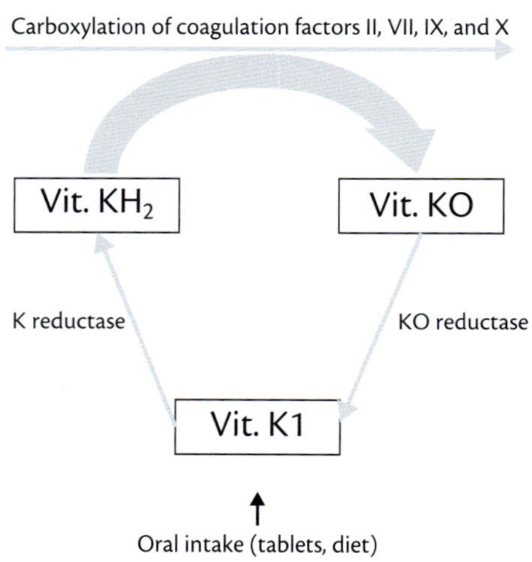

Figure 9.1 Mechanism of action of vitamin K antagonists.[8] Coumarins inhibit the conversion of oxidized vitamin K epoxide (Vit. KO) to its reduced form (Vit. KH$_2$) by interfering with two reductases: KO-reductase and K-reductase. Subsequent insufficient γ-carboxylation results in coagulation factors with impaired biological function. Most of the coumarin impact is exerted through inhibition of the coumarin-sensitive KO-reductase, whereas K-reductase is relatively coumarin resistant. Thus, both diet and the administration of vitamin K (Vit. K1) are factors interfering with the carboxylation of coagulation factors II, VII, IX and X.

Various forms of vitamin K antagonists

There is a wide variety of vitamin K antagonists used worldwide. In the US, warfarin is the most often-used agent, whereas acenocoumarol, phenprocoumon, and phenindione are also commonly used in Europe and in the rest of the world. Acenocoumarol and phenindione have the shortest half-life (half a day) followed by warfarin and phenprocoumon (up to 4 days).[11]

Dosing and therapeutic window

A narrow therapeutic window and interference with food and concomitant medications are the two major drawbacks of vitamin K antagonists. The usual dose of warfarin and acenocoumarol is 2–5 mg daily. The prothrombin time (PT) is used to indicate an optimal therapeutic window, that is, the delicate balance between anticoagulation status and the risk of bleeding. The PT responds to reduction of the vitamin K-dependent procoagulant coagulation factors II, VII, and X, that are reduced by vitamin K antagonists at a rate proportionate to their respective half-lives. Because of the large variation in PT assays, an international normalized ratio (INR) has been developed using the International Sensitivity Index of the thromboplastin time used at the local laboratory to perform the PT measurement.[12] The INR is calculated as the ratio of the patient's PT divided by the mean normal institutional PT.

When initiating warfarin or acenocoumarol, a starting dose is indicated. In case of warfarin, 5–10 mg are given, followed by INR checks after 2–3 days and then twice weekly until a therapeutic and stable INR level has been reached, which may take up to 4 weeks. In the young individual, 10 mg can be considered, while starting doses of 2.5 mg may be appropriate in the elderly and/or frail patient.[13,14] For acenocoumarol the recommended starting dose is 6 mg, and this may be reduced to 2–4 mg. In view of its different pharmacokinetics, initial treatment with phenprocoumon requires a loading dose followed by a markedly lower maintenance dose.[15–17] In patients with a high thrombotic state (pulmonary embolism, deep venous thrombosis, acute coronary syndrome), a lower starting dose may mitigate the initial procoagulant reaction. Depending on local availability of laboratories, regular INR checks should be done monthly. Self-monitoring of INR was introduced in the late 1980s[18] and approved in the early 2000s after randomized trials showed an acceptable time in therapeutic range of INR with self-testing compared with laboratory tests.[19,20] Target INR intervals vary with the clinical indication for which oral anticoagulation is administered. These indications and target INR intervals are specified in the respective chapters in this book [see chapters on atrial fibrillation (➔ Chapter 20), venous thromboembolism (➔ Chapter 21), and mechanical heart valves (➔ Chapter 17)].

Genetic variability of the response to vitamin K antagonists

Among other factors, polymorphisms of both CYP2C9 and vitamin K epoxide reductase complex (VKORC) can be responsible for variability in the response to vitamin K antagonists. Variants of CYP2C9 influence the pharmacokinetics of vitamin K antagonists, whereas VKORC variants affect their pharmacodynamics. Both polymorphisms have various ethnic frequencies, and usually lead to reduced dose requirements of vitamin K antagonists to achieve a therapeutic level of INR. In east Asian populations, target INR levels are different, with a downward adjustment compared to the rest of the world.[10] Pharmacogenetic-based dosing of vitamin K antagonists has been evaluated in randomized trials comparing it with clinical algorithms, and these studies showed conflicting results with regard to time in therapeutic range in the short term.[21,22] So far, this has not resulted in the adoption of pharmacogenetic-based dosing of vitamin K antagonists in routine clinical practice.

Dietary interactions

Food may contain large quantities of vitamin K[23] which interfere with the inhibition of vitamin K-dependent coagulation factors (➔ Figure 9.1), resulting in the need for higher doses of vitamin K antagonists to achieve an optimal time in therapeutic range. Examples include vegetables such as broccoli, cauliflower, and avocado. Alcohol use may enhance warfarin breakdown, also resulting in a higher need for warfarin dosing.[12] In contrast, a chronic high intake of alcohol may impair liver function and, thus, a lower dose of vitamin K antagonists is needed to avoid toxicity.

Drug interactions

There is a plethora of drugs interacting with the efficacy and safety of vitamin K antagonists.[25] They are summarized in ➔ Boxes 9.1 and 9.2.[24] When patients are treated with one of these agents, closer INR monitoring is indicated. As a rule of thumb, initiating antibiotic therapy should always trigger the prescriber's attention to a closer monitoring. For the cardiologist, awareness of concomitant use of amiodarone is required, as this prolongs the INR. With regard to the concomitant use of antiplatelet therapy, the indication deserves careful consideration and treatment should be restricted to cases with an estimated favourable risk/benefit ratio.[13]

Side effects

Bleeding

By far the most important and frequent side effect of vitamin K antagonists is bleeding, since these drugs interfere with coagulation factors of both the intrinsic (factor IX) and extrinsic (factor VII) pathways of the coagulation cascade. Major bleeding is seen in up to 20% of patients within 4 years, and about a third of these

Box 9.1 Agents potentiating vitamin K antagonists

Antibiotics

- Ciprofloxacin.
- Cotrimoxazole.
- Erythromycin.
- Fluconazole.
- Isoniazid.
- Itraconazole.
- Metronidazole.
- Miconazole.
- Tetracycline.

Cardiologic agents

- Amiodarone.
- Aspirin.
- Clofibrate.
- Propafenone.
- Propranolol.
- Quinidine.
- Simvastatin.

Anti-inflammatory/analgesic drugs

- Acetaminophen.
- Dextropropoxyphene.
- Phenylbutazone.
- Piroxicam.

Other agents

- Anabolic steroids.
- Chloral hydrate.
- Cimetidine.
- Disulfiram.
- Influenza vaccines.
- Omeprazole.
- Phenytoin.
- Tamoxifen.

Box 9.2 Agents inhibiting vitamin K antagonists

Antibiotics

- Dicloxacillin.
- Griseofulvin.
- Nafcillin.
- Rifampicin.

Other agents

- Azathioprine.
- Barbiturates.
- Carbamazepine.
- Chlordiazepoxide.
- Cholestyramine.
- Ciclosporin.
- Trazodone.

bleeding events are observed in the first month of treatment.[25] In 3% of patients, fatal bleeding events occur within 4 years: gastrointestinal and intracranial bleeding account for most cases. In the current era, major vitamin K antagonist-related gastrointestinal bleeding is observed in around 2% and intracranial bleeding in less than 1% of patients per year.[26]

Skin necrosis

The natural fibrinolysis factors protein C and protein S are also vitamin K dependent and, thus, will be reduced by vitamin K antagonists. The half-times of these factors are shorter than for factors II, IX, and X. In the initial phase of vitamin K antagonist treatment, the effect of these fibrinolytic factors may dominate and impair natural fibrinolysis, which can result in skin necrosis 3–10 days after treatment has started. In particular, patients with heterozygous protein C or protein S deficiency may be victims of this rare side effect. Very rarely, patients without these deficiencies develop this type of skin necrosis.[27]

Birth defects

The use of vitamin K antagonists is associated with embryopathy during pregnancy in 0.6–10% of cases. Parenteral anticoagulation during the first trimester almost completely eliminates the risk. For uncomplicated pregnancy European guidelines recommend vitamin K antagonists in a low dose (low-dose vitamin K antagonist: warfarin <5 mg/day, phenprocoumon <3 mg/day, or acenocoumarol <2 mg/day) during the second and third trimesters until the 36th week of gestation.[28]

Reversal

In cases of urgent surgery to be performed in patients on vitamin K antagonists, prothrombin complex concentrate or full plasma should be administered immediately, which bypass the effect of vitamin K antagonists. Within 30 minutes the INR is reduced in the majority of patients when prothrombin complex concentrate had been used, while it takes about 24 hours for a reversal with plasma.[29] As the effect of these interventions fades with the halve lives of the respective coagulation factors, administration of (parenteral) vitamin K should also be considered. The same results can be obtained in patients facing major bleeding on vitamin K antagonists.[30]

Periprocedural management

Although the indications for bridging of anticoagulant therapy have become much more stringent, bridging still applies in numerous situations and should be carefully managed according to prevailing guidelines and local protocols, especially in case of prosthetic mechanical heart valves.[31–33] In short, vitamin K antagonists have to be discontinued 3–5 days before the procedure, with low-molecular-weight heparin or unfractionated heparin as a bridging agent. A key aspect to prevent bleeding after the postoperative initiation of vitamin K antagonists is to avoid a loading dose, and to resume the prescription schedule as followed during the outpatient preoperative period.

Summary

Vitamin K antagonist therapy has dominated treatment for atrial fibrillation, deep venous thrombosis, and pulmonary embolism for many years. Although the direct oral anticoagulants are now the preferred agents for these indications, there are still many patients on vitamin K antagonist treatment (e.g. those with advanced kidney disease). Specific groups of interest where a vitamin K antagonist is still the first-choice anticoagulant agent are patients with prosthetic mechanical heart valves, rheumatic mitral valve stenosis, left ventricular thrombus, and the antiphospholipid syndrome. Although the use of vitamin K antagonists will gradually decrease over time, which is likely to affect familiarity with their use among prescribers, this class of drugs is here to stay in the aforementioned indications. This underscores the importance of continuing education and research to maintain and improve knowledge of their specific characteristics.

References

1. Sankar MJ, Chandrasekaran A, Kumar P, Thukral A, Agarwal R, Paul VK. Vitamin K prophylaxis. Vitamin K prophylaxis for prevention of vitamin K deficiency bleeding: a systematic review. J Perinatol. 2016;36 Suppl 1:S29–35.
2. Link KP. The discovery of dicumarol and its sequels. Circulation. 1959;19:97–107.
3. Hart RG, Pearce LA, Aguilar MI. Meta-analysis: antithrombotic therapy to prevent stroke in patients who have nonvalvular atrial fibrillation. Ann Intern Med. 2007;146:857–67.
4. Van Es N, Coppens M, Schulman S, Middeldorp S, Büller HR. Direct oral anticoagulants compared with vitamin K antagonists for acute venous thromboembolism: evidence from phase 3 trials. Blood. 2014;124:1968–75.
5. Vahanian A, Beyersdorf F, Praz F, et al. 2021 ESC/EACTS Guidelines for the management of valvular heart disease. Eur Heart J. 2022;43:561–632.

5a. Khairani CD, Bejjani A, Piazza G, et al. Direct oral anticoagulants vs vitamin K antagonists in patients with antiphospholipid syndromes: meta-analysis of randomized trials. J Am Coll Cardiol. 2023;81(1):16–30.

6. Hindricks G, Potpara T, Dagres N, et al. 2020 ESC Guidelines for the diagnosis and management of atrial fibrillation developed in collaboration with the European Association of Cardio-Thoracic Surgery (EACTS). Eur Heart J. 2020;42:373–498.
7. Connolly SJ, Karthikeyan G, Ntsekhe, A, et al. Rivaroxaban in rheumatic heart disease-associated atrial fibrillation. N Engl J Med. 2022:387:978–88.
8. Brouwer MA, Verheugt FWA. Oral anticoagulation for acute coronary syndromes. Circulation. 2002;105:1270–4.
9. Verheugt FWA. Return of oral anticoagulation in chronic stable coronary disease. Circulation. 2018;137:1655–7.
10. Brunton LL, Lazo JS, Parker KL, editors. Goodman & Gilman's The Pharmacological Basis of Therapeutics. 11th edition, pp. 862–3. New York: McGraw-Hill; 2005.
11. De Caterina R, Husted S, Wallentin L, et al. Vitamin K antagonists in heart disease: current status and perspectives (Section III). Position paper of the ESC Working Group on Thrombosis—Task Force on Anticoagulants in Heart Disease. Thromb Haemost. 2013;110:1087–107.
12. Hirsh J, Fuster V, Ansell J, Halperin J. American Heart Association/American College of Cardiology Foundation guide to warfarin therapy. Circulation. 2003;107:1692–711.
13. Ageno W, Gallus AS, Wittkowsky A, Crowther M, Hylek EM, Palareti G. Oral anticoagulant therapy: Antithrombotic Therapy and Prevention of Thrombosis, 9th ed: American College of Chest Physicians Evidence-Based Clinical Practice Guidelines. Chest. 2012;141(2 Suppl):e44S–88S.
14. Holbrook A, Schulman S, Witt DM, et al. Evidence-based management of anticoagulant therapy: Antithrombotic Therapy and Prevention of Thrombosis, 9th ed: American College of Chest Physicians Evidence-Based Clinical Practice Guidelines. Chest. 2012;141(2 Suppl):e152S–84S.
15. Van Geest-Daalderop JH, Hutten BA, Péquériaux NC, Levi M, Sturk A. Improvement in the regulation of the vitamin K antagonist acenocoumarol after a standard initial dose regimen: prospective validation of a prescription model. J Thromb Thrombolysis. 2009; 27:207–14.
16. Heaf J, Guldager B. Algorithm for short-term prescription of phenprocoumon. Haemostasis. 1990;20(1):21–30.
17. Good AC, Henz S. A clinical algorithm to predict the loading dose of phenprocoumon. Thromb Res. 2007;120(6):921–5.
18. Lucas FV, Duncan A, Jay R, et al. A novel whole blood capillary technique for measuring prothrombin time. Am J Clin Pathol. 1987;88:442–6.
19. Watzke HH, Forberg E, Svolba G, et al. A prospective controlled trial comparing weekly self-testing and self-dosing with the standard management of patients on stable oral anticoagulation. Thromb Haemost. 2000;83: 661–5.
20. Cromheecke ME, Levi M, Colly LP, et al. Oral anticoagulation self management and management by a specialist anticoagulation clinic: a randomized cross-over comparison. Lancet. 2000;356:97–102.
21. Pirmohamed M, Burnside G, Eriksson N, et al. A randomized trial of genotype-guided dosing of warfarin. N Engl J Med. 2013;369:2294–303.
22. Kimmel SE, French B, Kasner SE, et al. A pharmacogenetic versus a clinical algorithm for warfarin dosing. N Engl J Med. 2013;369:2283–92.
23. Booth SL, Charnley JM, Sadowski JA, et al. Dietary vitamin K1 and stability of oral anticoagulation: proposal of a diet with a constant vitamin K1 content. Thromb Haemost. 1997;77:504–9.
24. Wells PS, Holbrook AM, Crowther NR, Hirsh J. Interactions of warfarin with drugs and food. Ann Intern Med. 1994;121:676–83.
25. Landefeld CS, Goldman L. Major bleeding in outpatients treated with warfarin: incidence and prediction by factors known at the start of outpatient therapy. Am J Med. 1989;87:144–52.
26. Carnicelli AP, Hong H, Connolly SJ, Eikelboom J, et al. Direct oral anticoagulants versus warfarin in patients with atrial fibrillation: patient-level network meta-analyses of randomized clinical trials with interaction testing by age and sex. Circulation. 2022;145:242–55.
27. Stewart AJ, Penman ID, Cook MK, Ludlam CA. Warfarin-induced skin necrosis. Postgrad Med J. 1999;75:233–5.
28. Regitz-Zagrosek V, Roos-Hesselink JW, Bauersachs J, et al. 2018 ESC Guidelines for the management of cardiovascular diseases during pregnancy. Eur Heart J. 2018;39:3165–241.
29. Goldstein JN, Refaai MA, Milling TJ, et al. Four-factor prothrombin complex concentrate versus plasma for rapid vitamin K antagonist reversal in patients needing urgent surgical or invasive interventions: a phase 3b, open-label, non-inferiority, randomised trial. Lancet. 2015;385:2077–87.
30. Sarode R, Milling TJ, Refaai MA, et al. Efficacy and safety of a 4-factor prothrombin complex concentrate in patients on vitamin K antagonists presenting with major bleeding: a randomized, plasma-controlled, phase IIIb study. Circulation. 2013;128:1234–43.
31. Singh M, Sporn ZA, Schaff HV, Pellikka PA. ACC/AHA versus ESC guidelines on prosthetic heart valve management: JACC guideline comparison. J Am Coll Cardiol. 2019;73:1707–18.
32. Doherty JU, Gluckman TJ, Hucker WJ, et al. 2017 ACC expert consensus decision pathway for periprocedural management of anticoagulation in patients with nonvalvular atrial fibrillation: a report of the American College of Cardiology Clinical Expert Consensus Document Task Force. J Am Coll Cardiol. 2017;69:871–98.
33. Rechenmacher SJ, Fang JC. Bridging anticoagulation: primum non nocere. J Am Coll Cardiol. 2015;66:1392–403.

CHAPTER 10

Dabigatran

Alexander P. Benz and Stefan H. Hohnloser

Contents

Summary

Dabigatran is a direct oral anticoagulant that acts through specific and reversible inhibition of thrombin. It has been developed as a fixed-dose, modern alternative to vitamin K antagonists such as warfarin. Dabigatran does not require frequent blood testing or dose adjustments. The main indication for dabigatran is the prevention of stroke and systemic embolism in patients with atrial fibrillation and risk factors for stroke. Furthermore, there is high-quality evidence supporting its use in patients with atrial fibrillation undergoing percutaneous coronary intervention or catheter ablation. Dabigatran has also received approval for the prevention of venous thromboembolism after major orthopaedic surgery and recurrent venous thromboembolism, and the treatment of venous thromboembolism. Dabigatran is contraindicated in patients with severe renal impairment (creatinine clearance <30 mL/min), and in patients with moderate-to-severe mitral stenosis or with a mechanical heart valve prosthesis. Idarucizumab is a monoclonal antibody fragment that specifically reverses the anticoagulant activity of dabigatran.

Dabigatran: pharmacology

Dabigatran etexilate is the prodrug of dabigatran. Following oral administration, dabigatran etexilate is rapidly hydrolysed by serum esterase to the active moiety (➔ Figure 10.1). Dabigatran is a non-peptidic, potent small molecule which specifically and reversibly inhibits both free and clot-bound thrombin by binding to its active site (➔ Figure 10.2).[1,2]

The effect of dabigatran commences immediately, with maximal anticoagulant effect achieved within 2–3 hours from intake. The resulting half-life of dabigatran is 12–14 hours. There is a close correlation between dabigatran plasma concentration and the degree of anticoagulant effect.[1]

Renal excretion of dabigatran is the predominant elimination pathway, with about 80% excreted unchanged in the urine.[2,3] Dabigatran is not metabolized by cytochrome P450 drug enzymes, and the compound does not induce or inhibit the cytochrome P450 system. Dabigatran has low plasma protein binding (35%), implying that displacement interactions are unlikely to meaningfully affect its pharmacokinetics and pharmacodynamics.[1]

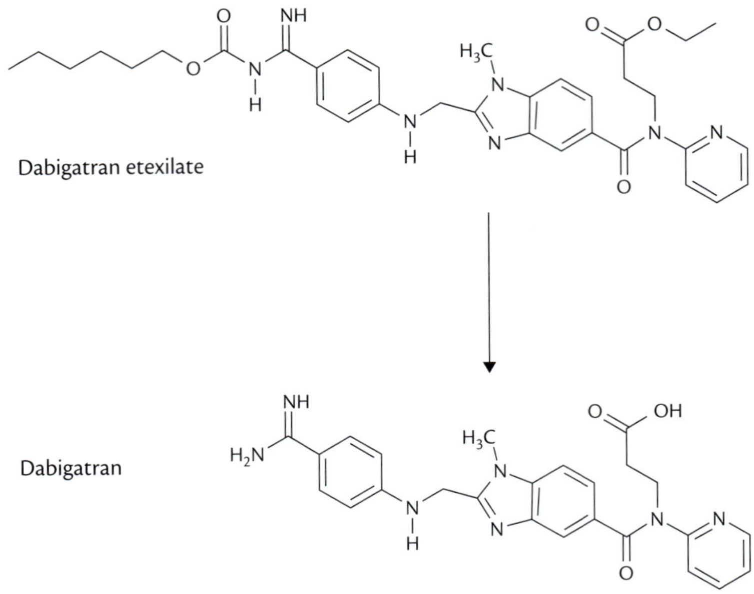

Figure 10.1 Dabigatran etexilate and dabigatran.
Reproduced from Ebner T, Wagner K, Wienen W. Dabigatran acylglucuronide, the major human metabolite of dabigatran: in vitro formation, stability, and pharmacological activity. Drug Metab Dispos. 2010 Sep;38(9):1567–75. doi: 10.1124/dmd.110.033696.

Given this profile, consideration of renal function is of paramount importance when prescribing the drug. It is recommended to calculate the creatinine clearance (CrCl) using the Cockcroft–Gault formula prior to commencing dabigatran therapy, and in regular time intervals during long-term treatment.[4] In Europe, dabigatran is contraindicated in patients with severe renal impairment (CrCl <30 mL/min).[1,4,5]

Oral administration of dabigatran produces a predictable pharmacodynamic effect.[1] Accordingly, the drug has been tested for various indications in fixed doses, without routine coagulation monitoring or dose adjustments. Clinically, dabigatran was first tested in a phase II trial involving patients with atrial fibrillation (AF) as well as in large studies for the prevention of venous thromboembolism (VTE) in patients undergoing total knee or hip replacement.[6–8] In the studies involving orthopaedic surgery patients, dabigatran at doses of 150 mg twice daily and of 220 mg once daily was found to have an excellent efficacy and safety profile. In most subsequent studies, particularly in patients with AF, doses of 150 mg twice daily and 110 mg twice daily underwent further investigation.

Dabigatran for the prevention of stroke and systemic embolism in patients with atrial fibrillation

RE-LY: the pivotal phase III trial of dabigatran in patients with atrial fibrillation

For decades, vitamin K antagonists (VKAs) such as warfarin had been the standard of care for the prevention of stroke and systemic embolism in patients with AF.[9] The efficacy and safety of dabigatran in this population were evaluated in the Randomized Evaluation of Long-Term Anticoagulation Therapy (RE-LY) trial.[10–12] This non-inferiority trial randomized 18,113 patients with AF in 1:1:1 fashion to warfarin [with a target international

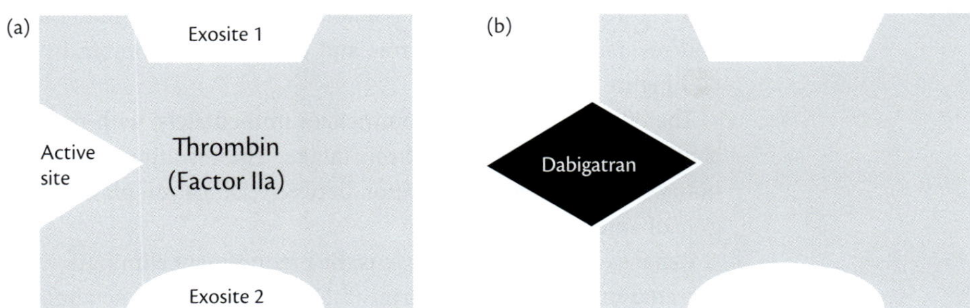

Figure 10.2 Dabigatran is a direct thrombin inhibitor. (a) Thrombin (factor II) contains an active site and two exosites. (b) Dabigatran specifically and reversibly inhibits both free and clot-bound thrombin by binding to its active site.
Source data from Lee CJ, Ansell JE. Direct thrombin inhibitors. Br J Clin Pharmacol. 2011 Oct;72(4):581–92. doi: 10.1111/j.1365-2125.2011.03916.x. Erratum in: Br J Clin Pharmacol. 2011 Oct;72(4):718. Dosage error in article text.

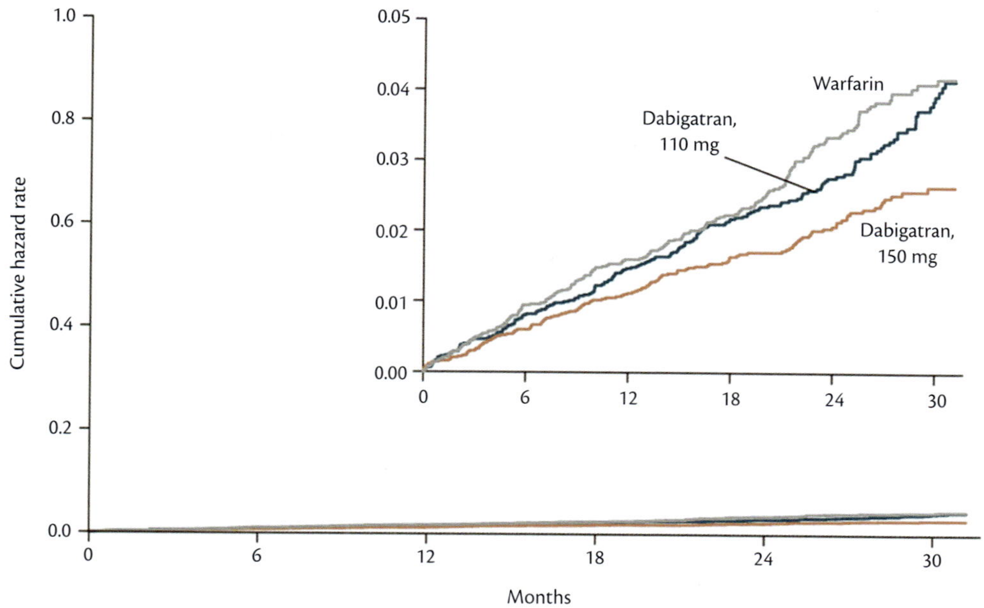

No. at risk

Warfarin	6022	5862	5718	4593	2890	1322
Dabigatran, 110 mg	6015	5862	5710	4593	2945	1385
Dabigatran, 150 mg	6076	5939	5779	4682	3044	1429

Figure 10.3 Stroke or systemic embolism in RE-LY. Warfarin versus dabigatran 110 mg twice daily versus dabigatran 150 mg twice daily in patients with atrial fibrillation and risk factors for stroke.

Reproduced from Connolly SJ, Ezekowitz MD, Yusuf S, et al.; RE-LY Steering Committee and Investigators. Dabigatran versus warfarin in patients with atrial fibrillation. N Engl J Med. 2009 Sep 17;361(12):1139–51. doi: 10.1056/NEJMoa0905561 with permission from Massachusetts Medical Society.

normalized ratio (INR) 2.0–3.0, with an achieved median 64% time in the therapeutic range], dabigatran 110 mg twice daily, or dabigatran 150 mg twice daily. Study participants had AF, at least one additional risk factor for stroke, and a CrCl of at least 30 mL/min. RE-LY was open-label as to whether patients had been randomized to warfarin or dabigatran, but double-blind with respect to the dose of dabigatran. Outcomes were centrally adjudicated by experts blinded to treatment allocation. The primary efficacy outcome was a composite of all-cause stroke or systemic embolism.[10] During a median follow-up duration of 2.0 years, the rate of the primary efficacy outcome was 1.71%/year in the warfarin group, compared with 1.54%/year in the dabigatran 110 mg group [relative risk (RR) with dabigatran 0.90, 95% confidence interval (CI) 0.74–1.10; P <0.001 for non-inferiority, P = 0.29 for superiority] and 1.11%/year in the dabigatran 150 mg group (RR 0.65, 95% CI 0.52–0.81; P <0.001 for superiority) (➔ Figure 10.3).[11,12]

Haemorrhagic stroke occurred at a rate of 0.38%/year in the warfarin group, as compared to 0.12% and 0.10%/year in the dabigatran 110 mg and 150 mg groups, respectively, corresponding to relative risk reductions of 69% and 74% in haemorrhagic stroke with dabigatran (P <0.001 for both comparisons).[11,12] Patients who had been treated with a VKA prior to study enrolment and anticoagulation-naïve patients derived similar benefit from dabigatran.[13] Mortality rates were 4.13%/year in the warfarin group, 3.75%/year with dabigatran 110 mg (RR with dabigatran 0.91, 95% CI 0.80–1.03; P = 0.13), and 3.64%/year with dabigatran 150 mg (RR 0.88, 95% CI 0.77–1.00; P = 0.051).[11,12]

Rates of the primary safety outcome major bleeding were 3.57%/year in the warfarin group, 2.87%/year in the dabigatran 110 mg group (P = 0.003), and 3.32%/year in the dabigatran 150 mg group (P = 0.31) (➔ Figure 10.4).[11,12,14]

Intracranial bleeding, including intracerebral, subarachnoidal, and subdural haematoma, occurred less frequently in the dabigatran groups than in the warfarin group (RR with dabigatran 110 mg 0.30, 95% CI 0.19–0.45; RR with dabigatran 150 mg 0.41, 95% CI 0.28–0.60; P <0.001 for superiority for both) (➔ Figure 10.5).[11,12,14]

Major gastrointestinal bleeding was more common with dabigatran 150 mg than with warfarin (RR 1.50, 95% CI 1.19–1.89; P <0.001). The rate of permanent study drug discontinuation at the end of the study was higher in both dabigatran groups (21%) compared to the warfarin group (17%), mainly due to dyspepsia, nausea, or diarrhoea.[11,12]

Based on these findings, dabigatran received approval for the prevention of stroke and systemic embolism in patients with AF. In Europe, both dabigatran 150 mg and 110 mg twice daily are available.

In a dedicated RE-LY substudy, dabigatran-associated bleeding risk was further scrutinized. This detailed analysis of all bleeding events revealed a significant treatment-by-age interaction. Dabigatran 110 mg twice daily compared with warfarin reduced major bleeding in patients aged less than 75 years (1.89% vs 3.04%/year), but carried a similar risk for major bleeding in those aged 75 years and older (4.43% vs 4.37%/year) (P-value for

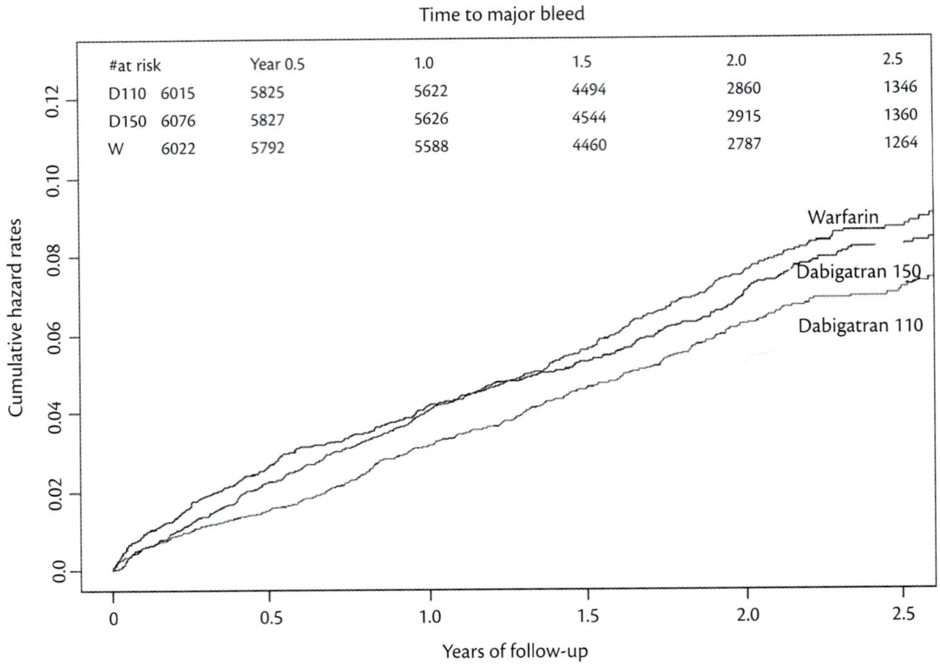

Figure 10.4 Major bleeding in RE-LY. Warfarin versus dabigatran 110 mg twice daily versus dabigatran 150 mg twice daily in patients with atrial fibrillation and risk factors for stroke.

Reproduced from Eikelboom JW, Wallentin L, Connolly SJ, et al. Risk of bleeding with 2 doses of dabigatran compared with warfarin in older and younger patients with atrial fibrillation: an analysis of the randomized evaluation of long-term anticoagulant therapy (RE-LY) trial. Circulation. 2011 May 31;123(21):2363–72. doi: 10.1161/CIRCULATIONAHA.110.004747 with permission from Wolters Kluwer.

interaction <0.001).[14] Dabigatran 150 mg twice daily compared with warfarin reduced major bleeding in individuals aged less than 75 years (2.12% vs 3.04%/year), but showed a strong trend towards an increase in major bleeding in patients aged 75 years and older (5.10% vs 4.37%/year) (P-value for interaction <0.001). Notably, this interaction with age was evident for major extra-cranial bleeding but not for intracranial bleeding. Irrespective of age, both doses of dabigatran reduced the risk of intracranial

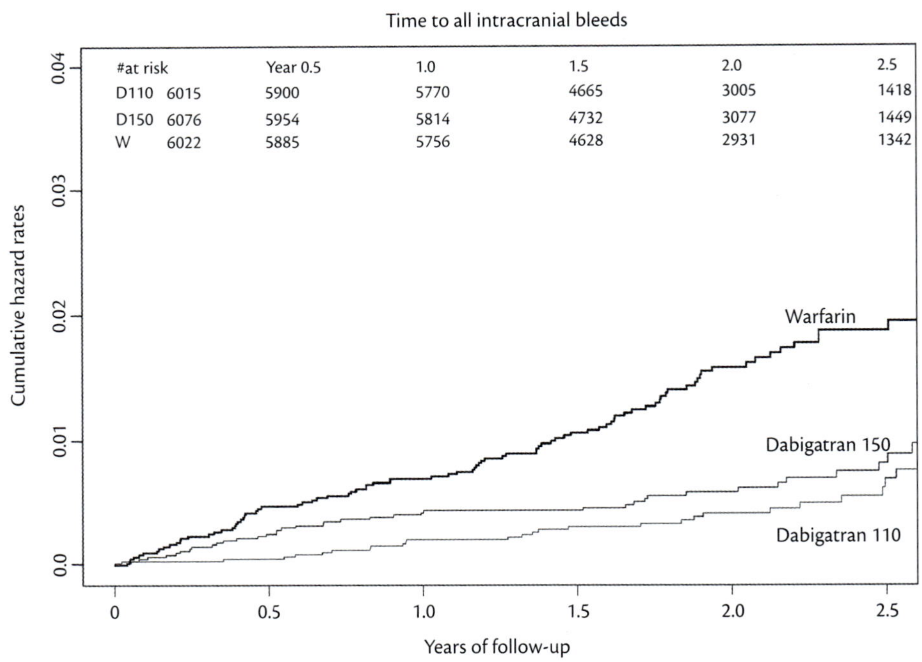

Figure 10.5 Intracranial haemorrhage in RE-LY. Warfarin versus dabigatran 110 mg twice daily versus dabigatran 150 mg twice daily in patients with atrial fibrillation and risk factors for stroke.

Reproduced from Eikelboom JW, Wallentin L, Connolly SJ, et al. Risk of bleeding with 2 doses of dabigatran compared with warfarin in older and younger patients with atrial fibrillation: an analysis of the randomized evaluation of long-term anticoagulant therapy (RE-LY) trial. Circulation. 2011 May 31;123(21):2363–72. doi: 10.1161/CIRCULATIONAHA.110.004747 with permission from Wolters Kluwer.

bleeding compared with warfarin. Based on these findings, European guidelines recommend that patients over 75–80 years of age should preferably be treated with dabigatran 110 mg twice daily.[4,5,14] In contrast, this dose did not receive approval by the US Food and Drug Administration.[15]

RELY-ABLE: long-term open-label extension following RE-LY

Following conclusion of RE-LY, the Long-term Multicenter Extension of Dabigatran Treatment in Patients with Atrial Fibrillation (RELY-ABLE) trial was conducted to collect data on long-term efficacy and safety of dabigatran.[16] Patients who had been randomly assigned to dabigatran were eligible for RELY-ABLE if they had not permanently discontinued study medication at the time of their final RE-LY study visit. Maintaining blinding to dose, 5851 patients continued dabigatran as received during RE-LY and were followed for an additional median of 2.3 years. Rates of all-cause stroke or systemic embolism were 1.60% and 1.46%/year in patients on dabigatran 110 mg and 150 mg twice daily, respectively [hazard ratio (HR) with dabigatran 150 mg 0.91, 95% CI 0.69–1.20]. Corresponding rates of major bleeding were 2.99% and 3.74%/year, and rates of haemorrhagic stroke were 0.14% and 0.13%/year, respectively. Mortality occurred at rates of 3.10% and 3.02%/year in patients on dabigatran 110 and 150 mg twice daily, respectively.[16]

Real-world data on dabigatran to complement findings from RE-LY

In general, the efficacy and safety of a novel therapy may not necessarily be the same in a clinical trial setting and in routine practice because of differences in the patient populations (e.g. due to specific eligibility criteria of randomized trials), intensity of follow-up in experienced study centres, or variation in care.[17,18] Extrapolating findings from trials to general practice is especially challenging for antithrombotic drugs as they are often primarily used as long-term preventive medications that do not address symptoms. Medication adherence, for instance, is substantially lower in observational studies than in clinical trials.[19] Therefore, observational analyses of real-world data on the use of direct oral anticoagulants and warfarin complement the results from randomized controlled trials.[18–24]

Many real-word studies specifically focused on safety issues associated with direct oral anticoagulants supported the main findings of the RE-LY trial. In one of the largest of these studies, investigators analysed insurance data of patients with AF treated with warfarin, dabigatran, apixaban, or rivaroxaban in the US between 2010 and 2015.[20] Using propensity score matching, they found that dabigatran as compared to warfarin was associated with a reduction in major bleeding (including intracranial haemorrhage, gastrointestinal bleeding, or bleeding from other sites) (HR 0.79, 95% CI 0.67–0.94; P <0.01) and intracranial haemorrhage (HR 0.36, 95% CI 0.23–0.56; P <0.001).[20]

Another example is a report based on insurance data of 45,361 newly anticoagulated AF patients started on warfarin (34.1%), apixaban (16.4%), rivaroxaban (39.2%), or dabigatran (10.3%).[21] Compared to propensity score-matched warfarin initiation, new use of dabigatran was associated with a lower risk of bleeding requiring hospitalization (HR 0.69, 95% CI 0.50–0.96).

Recently, investigators performed a comparative review of the data from major phase III clinical trials and real-world evidence from large-scale phase IV studies assessing the efficacy and safety of direct oral anticoagulants versus VKA in patients with AF.[24] These data suggest that dabigatran has similar efficacy as warfarin but a better safety profile (➔ Table 10.1). Compared with warfarin, dabigatran was associated with a lower risk of intracranial haemorrhage (HR 0.42, 95% CI 0.37–0.49; P <0.001). There was a trend for an association with a decrease in major bleeding (HR 0.83, 95% CI 0.65–1.05; P = 0.12).

In summary, the available real-world evidence supporting the use of dabigatran for stroke prevention in AF is consistent with the findings from the pivotal RE-LY trial.

RE-DUAL PCI: dabigatran in patients with atrial fibrillation undergoing percutaneous coronary intervention

Coronary artery disease and AF often coexist, particularly in elderly patients. It has been estimated that approximately 5–15% of patients with AF will undergo percutaneous coronary intervention (PCI), either in the setting of an acute coronary syndrome or due to symptomatic progressive coronary artery disease.[25] Dual antiplatelet therapy (i.e. aspirin plus a $P2Y_{12}$ inhibitor) is indicated for prevention of cardiovascular events after PCI, including stent thrombosis. But antiplatelet therapy is clearly inferior to oral anticoagulation for stroke prevention in AF.[26–28] Therefore, past editions of guidelines had recommended a combination of anticoagulation and dual antiplatelet therapy (so-called triple therapy) for various periods of time following PCI in AF patients.[25,29] However, triple therapy, particularly including a VKA, is associated with high rates of major bleeding, especially in combination with a potent $P2Y_{12}$ inhibitor.[30,31] Hence, there was a need to develop strategies which would allow the time period of triple therapy to be shortened or, ultimately, to avoid triple therapy altogether while effectively protecting patients from thrombotic complications. Until 2021, four dedicated studies were performed testing the efficacy and safety of each of the four available direct oral anticoagulants (DOACs) in AF patients presenting with an acute coronary syndrome or undergoing elective PCI.[32–35]

The respective study involving dabigatran was the Randomized Evaluation of Dual Antithrombotic Therapy with Dabigatran versus Triple Therapy with Warfarin in Patients with Nonvalvular Atrial Fibrillation Undergoing Percutaneous Coronary Intervention (RE-DUAL PCI) trial, designed to compare a dual dabigatran versus triple VKA antithrombotic strategy.[33,36] In this open-label, non-inferiority trial, 2725 patients with AF who had undergone PCI were randomly assigned in a 1:1:1 ratio to warfarin triple therapy [warfarin plus a $P2Y_{12}$ inhibitor (clopidogrel or ticagrelor) for at least 12 months, and aspirin for 1–3 months]

Table 10.1 Dabigatran versus warfarin in observational real-world studies and in the pivotal RE-LY trial

	Real-world data studies[24] (observational)	RE-LY trial[11,12] (randomized)	
Event / Dose (mg)	**Dabigatran (dose-adjusted)**	**Dabigatran 110 mg twice daily**	**Dabigatran 150 mg twice daily**
Stroke or systemic embolism	*No statistical difference*	*No statistical difference*	*Reduction*
	HR 0.93, 95% CI 0.77–1.14; P = 0.21	RR 0.90, 95% CI 0.74–1.10; P = 0.29	RR 0.65, 95% CI 0.52–0.81; P <0.001
Ischaemic stroke	*No statistical difference*	*No statistical difference*	*Reduction*
	HR 0.96, 95% CI 0.80–1.16; P = 0.69	RR 1.11, 95% CI 0.88–1.39; 0.35	RR 0.76, 95% CI 0.59–0.97; P = 0.03
Myocardial infarction	*No statistical difference*	*No statistical difference*	*No statistical difference*
	HR 0.96, 95% CI 0.77–1.21; P = 0.74	RR 1.29, 95% CI 0.96–1.75; P = 0.09	RR 1.27, 95% CI 0.94–1.71; P = 0.12
All-cause mortality	*Reduction*	*No statistical difference*	*No statistical difference*
	HR 0.63, 95% CI 0.52–0.76; P <0.001	RR 0.91, 95% CI 0.80–1.03, P = 0.13	RR 0.88, 95% CI 0.77–1.00; P = 0.051
Major bleeding	*No statistical difference*	*Reduction*	*No statistical difference*
	HR 0.83, 95% CI 0.65–1.05; P = 0.12	RR 0.80, 95% CI 0.70–0.93; P = 0.003	RR 0.93, 95% CI 0.81–1.07; P = 0.31
Intracranial haemorrhage	*Reduction*	*Reduction*	*Reduction*
	HR 0.42, 95% CI 0.37–0.49; P <0.001	RR 0.30, 95% CI 0.19–0.45; P <0.001	RR 0.41, 95% CI 0.28–0.60; P <0.001
Major gastrointestinal bleeding	*Increase*	*No statistical difference*	*Increase*
	HR 1.20, 95% CI 1.06–1.36; P = 0.003	RR 1.08, 95% CI 0.85–1.38; P = 0.52	RR 1.48, 95% CI 1.18–1.85; P = 0.001

CI, confidence interval; HR, hazard ratio; RR, relative risk.

Source data from Domek M, Gumprecht J, Ding WY, Lip GYH, Lane DA. Practice-derived data on non-vitamin K antagonist oral anticoagulant therapy to complement observations from randomized trials. Eur Heart J Suppl. 2020;22(Suppl I):I1–12. doi: 10.1093/eurheartj/suaa100.

or dual antithrombotic therapy with dabigatran [110 mg or 150 mg twice daily, plus a $P2Y_{12}$ inhibitor (clopidogrel or ticagrelor) for at least 12 months, without aspirin]. The primary endpoint was a composite of major or clinically relevant non-major bleeding as assessed by an adjudication committee blinded to treatment allocation.[36]

The main indication for PCI was acute coronary syndrome in 50.5% of study participants, 82.6% received at least one drug-eluting stent, and the most commonly used $P2Y_{12}$ inhibitor was clopidogrel (12.0% ticagrelor). During a mean follow-up duration of 14 months, the incidence of the primary endpoint was 15.4% in the 110 mg dual therapy group versus 26.9% in the warfarin triple therapy group (HR with dabigatran 110 mg 0.52, 95% CI 0.42–0.63; P <0.001 for non-inferiority; P <0.001 for superiority) and 20.2% in the 150 mg dual therapy group as compared with 25.7% in the corresponding warfarin triple therapy group (HR with dabigatran 150 mg 0.72, 95% CI 0.58–0.88; P <0.001 for non-inferiority) (➔ Figure 10.6). Thus, both dabigatran dual antithrombotic regimens led to large absolute risk reductions in the primary endpoint compared to warfarin triple therapy.[33] Both dabigatran dual antithrombotic groups combined were non-inferior to warfarin triple therapy with respect to a composite efficacy endpoint of thromboembolic events, unplanned revascularization, or death (13.7% vs 13.4%, HR with dabigatran 110/150 mg 1.04, 95% CI 0.84–1.29; P = 0.005 for non-inferiority).[33]

As with the RE-LY trial, there are numerous secondary publications from the RE-DUAL PCI trial. One of these predefined subanalyses concerned the indication for PCI and the choice of the $P2Y_{12}$ inhibitor.[37] There was consistent benefit with respect to the RE-DUAL PCI primary endpoint of major or clinically relevant non-major bleeding with both dabigatran dual antithrombotic therapies versus warfarin triple therapy in all four studied subgroups (acute coronary syndrome and elective PCI, clopidogrel and ticagrelor, all P-values for interaction >0.10).[37] Furthermore, there were no statistically significant interactions across these subgroups with respect to a composite outcome of thrombotic complications, unplanned revascularization, or death. There was, however, a significant interaction with indication for PCI with respect to stent thrombosis in the dabigatran 110 mg dual therapy versus warfarin triple therapy comparison (acute coronary syndrome: 2.4% vs 0.6%, elective PCI: 0.6% vs 1.0%, P-value for interaction 0.07).

A second substudy focused on early and late benefits and risks of dabigatran versus warfarin combined antithrombotic therapy.[38] Both dabigatran dual antithrombotic strategies yielded early net clinical benefit in the first month following randomization. This was due to a larger reduction in bleeding than increase in thrombotic events with dabigatran 110 mg dual therapy, and a reduction in bleeding without an increase in thrombotic events with dabigatran 150 mg dual therapy. In landmark analyses following cessation of aspirin in patients assigned to warfarin triple therapy (30 days for patients receiving a bare metal stent, 90 days for those receiving a drug-eluting stent), dabigatran 110 mg dual therapy continued to reduce

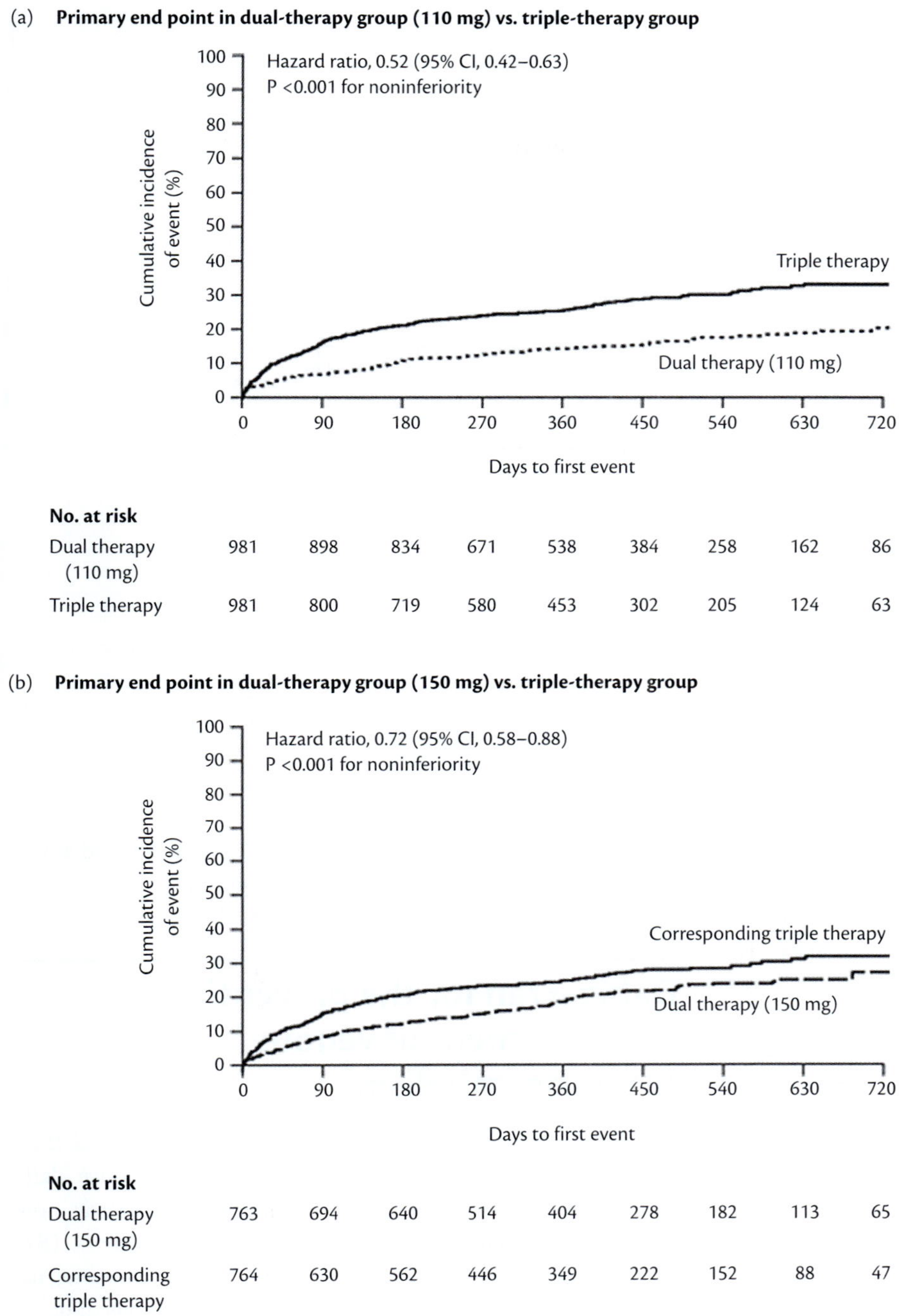

Figure 10.6 Major or clinically relevant non-major bleeding in RE-DUAL PCI. Warfarin triple therapy versus dabigatran 110 mg dual antithrombotic therapy, warfarin triple therapy versus dabigatran 150 mg dual antithrombotic therapy in patients with atrial fibrillation who had undergone percutaneous coronary intervention.

Reproduced from Cannon CP, Bhatt DL, Oldgren J, et al.; RE-DUAL PCI Steering Committee and Investigators. Dual Antithrombotic Therapy with Dabigatran after PCI in Atrial Fibrillation. N Engl J Med. 2017 Oct 19;377(16):1513–1524. doi: 10.1056/NEJMoa1708454 with permission from Massachusetts Medical Society.

bleeding, and dabigatran 150 mg and warfarin dual therapies yielded similar rates of bleeding.[38]

RE-CIRCUIT: uninterrupted dabigatran in patients undergoing catheter ablation for atrial fibrillation

Catheter ablation is a widely used procedure aimed at restoration of sinus rhythm in symptomatic patients with AF. The most hazardous complications of AF ablation include periprocedural stroke and cardiac tamponade. Systemic anticoagulation reduces the risk of thrombotic cerebrovascular events before, during, and after ablation but carries a risk of bleeding. Based on the results of the COMPARE trial, uninterrupted VKA therapy around the time of catheter ablation had become the standard of care.[39] Given its overall efficacy and safety profile, a randomized, open-label trial of dabigatran versus warfarin in

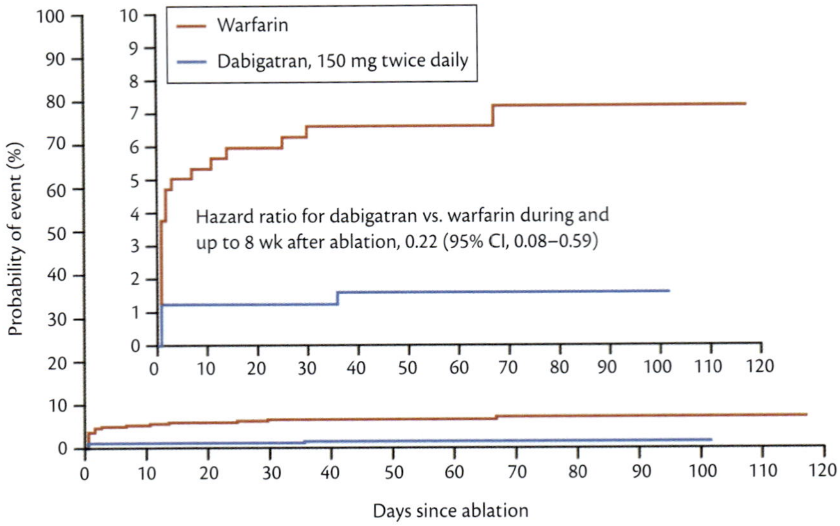

No. at risk													
Dabigatran	317	313	311	311	306	305	297	83	4	2	1	0	0
Warfarin	318	301	297	296	295	295	278	85	13	5	3	1	0

Figure 10.7 Major bleeding in RE-CIRCUIT. Warfarin versus dabigatran 150 mg twice daily in patients with atrial fibrillation undergoing catheter ablation of atrial fibrillation.

Reproduced from Calkins H, Willems S, Gerstenfeld EP, et al.; RE-CIRCUIT Investigators. Uninterrupted Dabigatran versus Warfarin for Ablation in Atrial Fibrillation. N Engl J Med. 2017 Apr 27;376(17):1627–1636. doi: 10.1056/NEJMoa1701005 with permission from Massachusetts Medical Society.

patients undergoing catheter ablation for AF was initiated. In the Randomized Evaluation of Dabigatran Etexilate Compared to Warfarin in Pulmonary Vein Ablation: Assessment of Uninterrupted Periprocedural Anticoagulation Strategy (RE-CIRCUIT) trial, patients scheduled for AF ablation were randomly assigned to receive dabigatran 150 mg twice daily or warfarin (target INR 2.0–3.0) for 4–8 weeks of uninterrupted anticoagulation prior to ablation.[40] Anticoagulation was continued during and for at least 8 weeks after the procedure. The primary endpoint was major bleeding. A total of 635 patients were enrolled and underwent catheter ablation. At 8 weeks following catheter ablation, the incidence of major bleeding was lower in the dabigatran group than in the warfarin group (1.6% vs 6.9%, absolute risk difference −5.3%, 95% CI −8.4 to −2.2; P <0.001) (➔ Figure 10.7). Cardiac tamponade occurred less frequently in patients randomized to dabigatran (one vs six events). Thrombotic events were extremely rare in both groups (no strokes or systemic embolism events, zero vs one transient ischaemic attack).

In summary, the RE-CIRCUIT trial demonstrated the superiority of uninterrupted dabigatran over uninterrupted warfarin therapy in patients undergoing catheter ablation for AF.[40]

Dabigatran use in patients with moderate-to-severe mitral stenosis

Because patients with AF who had moderate-to-severe mitral stenosis had been excluded from the pivotal trials of warfarin therapy, they were also ineligible for inclusion in the pivotal trials of DOAC therapy, including RE-LY.[9,11,41] Current guidelines continue to only recommend VKAs in such patients, and advise against the use of DOACs, including dabigatran.[4,5]

Dabigatran for the prevention and treatment of venous thromboembolism

Dabigatran has also been evaluated in large randomized trials involving VTE. Compared to enoxaparin 40 mg once daily, dabigatran at doses of 220 mg or 150 mg once daily was non-inferior in reducing VTE after total knee replacement (RE-MODEL), total hip replacement (RE-NOVATE), and total hip arthroplasty (RE-NOVATE II), without increasing bleeding.[7,8,42] Dabigatran 220 mg and 150 mg once daily, however, were inferior to enoxaparin 30 mg twice daily in reducing VTE in patients undergoing unilateral total knee arthroplasty (RE-MOBILIZE).[43] Dabigatran 150 mg twice daily was non-inferior to warfarin (RE-MEDY) and superior to placebo (RE-SONATE) in reducing recurrence of VTE in patients who had received initial anticoagulation for at least 90 days.[44] Furthermore, dabigatran was shown to be non-inferior to warfarin for the treatment of acute VTE after initial treatment with parenteral anticoagulation for at least 5 days, without increasing major bleeding while providing a reduction in total bleeding (RE-COVER, RE-COVER II).[45,46]

Based on these findings, dabigatran received approval for the prevention of VTE in patients undergoing total hip or knee replacement, for the prevention of recurrent VTE as well as the treatment of VTE.

RE-ALIGN: dabigatran use in patients with a mechanical heart valve prosthesis

Patients with a mechanical heart valve prosthesis require long-term oral anticoagulation to prevent thrombotic complications inherent to the thrombogenicity of the device. VKAs such as warfarin are approved for this indication. However, all direct oral anticoagulants, including dabigatran, are contraindicated in this setting. This is based on findings from the Randomized, Phase II Study to Evaluate the Safety and Pharmacokinetics of Oral Dabigatran Etexilate in Patients after Heart Valve Replacement (RE-ALIGN).[47,48] Patients who had undergone implantation of a mechanical heart valve prosthesis in the aortic or mitral position (within the past 7 days, or at least 3 months earlier) were randomized in a 2:1 ratio to receive dabigatran or warfarin. Dabigatran dosage was based on renal function, and was adjusted to ensure a through plasma level of 50 ng/mL or greater. The target INR in patients randomized to warfarin was 2.0–3.0 or 2.5–3.5, depending on the estimated risk for thrombotic complications. The primary endpoint was the trough plasma level of dabigatran.[47] After 252 patients were enrolled (168 randomized to dabigatran, 84 randomized to warfarin), the trial was terminated prematurely. An interim unblinded review of safety data by the Data Safety and Monitoring Board had shown an excess of both thrombotic [ischaemic stroke: nine (5%) vs zero patients, valve thrombosis without symptoms: five (3%) vs zero patients) and bleeding events in patients randomized to receive dabigatran (major bleeding: seven (4%) vs two patients (2%)].[48]

These findings resulted in a Drug Safety Warning issued by the US Food and Drug Administration, advising against the use of dabigatran in patients with a mechanical heart valve prosthesis.[49]

MANAGE trial: dabigatran in patients with myocardial injury after non-cardiac surgery

Myocardial injury after non-cardiac surgery (MINS) is associated with adverse clinical outcomes. The Management of Myocardial Injury After Noncardiac Surgery Trial (MANAGE) tested the hypothesis that dabigatran would reduce a composite primary efficacy outcome of vascular mortality and non-fatal myocardial infarction, non-haemorrhagic stroke, peripheral arterial thrombosis, amputation, or symptomatic VTE in patients with MINS.[50] A total of 1754 patients who had undergone non-cardiac surgery and who had MINS within the preceding 35 days were randomized to receive dabigatran 110 mg twice daily or placebo. MINS represented myocardial infarction according to standard criteria (20% of study participants) or isolated ischaemic troponin elevation (80%). During a mean follow-up duration of 16 months, 97 patients (11%) randomized to dabigatran and 133 patients (15%) randomized to placebo had a primary efficacy outcome event (HR with dabigatran 0.72, 95% CI 0.55–0.93; P = 0.012). Dabigatran did not increase a composite of life-threatening, major, or critical organ bleeding (3% vs 4%, HR 0.92, 95% CI 0.55–1.53; P = 0.78). Overall rates of concomitant use of at least one antiplatelet drug and a statin during follow-up were 74% and 69%, respectively. The rate of early permanent discontinuation of study drug was high in both groups (46% and 43%, respectively).[50]

Despite the encouraging results from this trial, the optimal management of patients experiencing MINS remains uncertain.[51]

RE-SPECT ESUS: dabigatran in patients with embolic stroke of unknown source

An embolic stroke of unknown source (ESUS) has been defined as a non-lacunar brain infarct without proximal arterial stenosis or cardioembolism warranting anticoagulation. ESUS accounts for a large proportion of cryptogenic ischaemic stroke.[52] Oral anticoagulation has been hypothesized to reduce ESUS. In The Randomized, Double-Blind, Evaluation in Secondary Stroke Prevention Comparing the Efficacy and Safety of the Oral Thrombin Inhibitor Dabigatran Etexilate versus Acetylsalicylic Acid in Patients with Embolic Stroke of Undetermined Source (RE-SPECT ESUS) trial, 5390 patients with a history of ESUS were randomized to receive dabigatran 150 mg twice daily (110 mg twice daily in patients ≥75 years of age or with a CrCl 30–50 mL/min) or aspirin.[53] The primary efficacy outcome was recurrent stroke. During a median follow-up duration of 19 months, 177 patients (6.6%) randomized to dabigatran and 207 patients (7.7%) randomized to aspirin had a recurrent stroke (HR with dabigatran 0.84, 95% CI 0.68–1.03; P = 0.10). There was no statistically significant difference in major bleeding (HR 1.19, 95% CI 0.85–1.66), but more clinically relevant non-major bleeding in patients randomized to dabigatran (HR 1.73, 95% CI 1.17–2.54).[53]

Based on these findings, routine use of dabigatran in unselected patients with ESUS cannot be recommended.

Dabigatran-specific anticoagulation reversal with idarucizumab

Dabigatran is at least as effective as warfarin in reducing stroke or systemic embolism in patients with AF and the prevention and treatment of VTE, while showing lower or similar rates of major bleeding. Nonetheless, there still is a risk of bleeding with dabigatran therapy and some patients may require reversal of anticoagulant activity.

Accordingly, idarucizumab was developed as a specific reversal agent of dabigatran.[54,55] It is a humanized antibody fragment with structural features similar to those of thrombin, but with an affinity for dabigatran that is approximately 350 times greater. By binding to dabigatran, idarucizumab prevents it

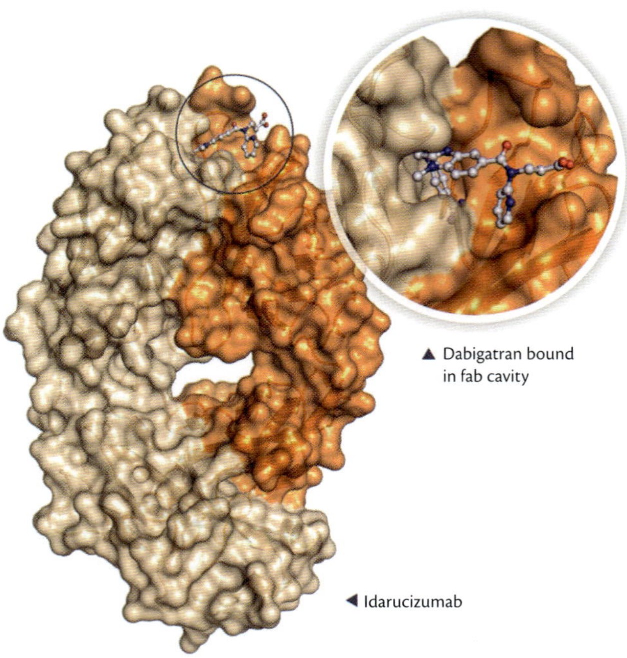

Figure 10.8 Idarucizumab. Idarucizumab specifically reverses the anticoagulant effect of dabigatran by binding to dabigatran, preventing it from binding to thrombin.

Reproduced from Eikelboom JW, Quinlan DJ, van Ryn J, Weitz JI. Idarucizumab: the antidote for reversal of dabigatran. Circulation. 2015 Dec 22;132(25):2412–22. doi: 10.1161/CIRCULATIONAHA.115.019628 with permission from Wolters Kluwer.

from binding to thrombin and thereby neutralizes its anticoagulant effect (➔ Figure 10.8). Idarucizumab lacks a thrombin-like catalytic triad and had no detectable activity in functional clotting and platelet aggregation tests.[55] Preclinical studies in rats have shown that a single bolus of idarucizumab completely reversed the anticoagulant activity of dabigatran within minutes of injection.[55]

The compound was tested in a randomized, placebo-controlled, double-blind, proof-of-concept phase I study in 47 healthy volunteers who received dabigatran for 4 days, followed by an infusion of between 1 g and 5 g of idarucizumab.[56] Idarucizumab immediately and completely reversed dabigatran-mediated anticoagulation in a dose-dependent manner.[56] Subsequently, the prospective, open-label, single-arm Reversal Effects of Idarucizumab on Active Dabigatran (RE-VERSE AD) cohort study was conducted to determine whether idarucizumab reverses the anticoagulant effect of dabigatran in emergency situations.[57–59] A total of 503 patients were enrolled. Of those, 301 had uncontrolled bleeding (group A) and 202 were about to undergo an urgent procedure (group B).[58,59] The primary study endpoint was the maximum percentage reversal of dabigatran's anticoagulant effect within 4 hours after the administration idarucizumab, determined by the diluted thrombin time or ecarin clotting time. The median maximum percentage reversal of dabigatran was 100% (95% CI 100–100%), with a median time to bleeding cessation of 2.5 hours in group A. In group B, the median time to the initiation of the intended procedure was 1.6 hours, with periprocedural haemostasis assessed as normal in 93.4% of patients. At 90 days of follow-up, 6.3% of patients in group A and 7.4% in group B had experienced a thrombotic event.[59]

Thus, idarucizumab is a rapidly and durably acting specific reversal agent for patients with life-threatening or uncontrolled bleeding, or patients who require an urgent procedure during treatment with dabigatran.

What's new

- Available in Europe since 2008, dabigatran is a DOAC acting through specific and reversible inhibition of thrombin.
- The main indication for dabigatran is the prevention of stroke and systemic embolism in patients with AF.
- High-quality evidence supports its use in patients with AF undergoing PCI or catheter ablation.
- Dabigatran has also received approval for the prevention and treatment of VTE.
- Dabigatran is contraindicated in patients with severe renal impairment (CrCl <30 mL/min), and in patients with moderate-to-severe mitral stenosis or a mechanical heart valve prosthesis.
- Available since 2015, idarucizumab is a specific reversal agent of the anticoagulant effects of dabigatran.

Guideline recommendations (2020 ESC Guidelines for the diagnosis and management of atrial fibrillation)

- For stroke prevention in AF patients who are eligible for oral anticoagulation (OAC), DOACs are recommended in preference to VKAs (excluding patients with mechanical heart valves or moderate-to-severe mitral stenosis) (class I, level A).
- OAC is recommended for stroke prevention in AF patients with a CHA_2DS_2-VASc score of 2 or greater in men or 3 or greater in women (class I, level A).
- In AF patients [with an indication for concomitant antiplatelet therapy and who are] eligible for DOACs, it is recommended to use a DOAC in preference to a VKA in combination with antiplatelet therapy (class I, level A).
- For patients with AF and an indication for concomitant antiplatelet therapy [...] [who are] at high bleeding risk (HAS-BLED ≥3), dabigatran 110 mg twice daily should be considered in preference to dabigatran 150 mg twice daily for the duration of concomitant single or dual antiplatelet therapy, to mitigate bleeding risk (class IIa, level B).
- For patients undergoing AF catheter ablation who have been therapeutically anticoagulated with dabigatran, performance of the ablation procedure without OAC interruption is recommended (class I, level A).
- DOACs are contraindicated in patients with a prosthetic mechanical valve (class III, level B).
- Use of DOACs is not recommended in patients with AF and moderate-to-severe mitral stenosis (class III, level C).

What's next

- The DOACs, including dabigatran, are expected to become broadly available as generic drugs in the near future.
- This may lead to more widespread use of DOACs in low- and middle-income countries.
- The next generation of oral anticoagulants (such as factor XIa and XII inhibitors, see ➔ Chapter 12) is currently under investigation in large clinical trials.

Drug dosing

Dabigatran

- Prevention of stroke and systemic embolism in patients with AF (long-term treatment):
  - Standard dose: dabigatran 150 mg twice daily.
  - Lower dose: dabigatran 110 mg twice daily in patients aged 80 years and older, with concomitant use of verapamil, or at increased bleeding risk.
  - *Note:* the dabigatran 110 mg twice daily regimen is not approved in the US.
- Primary prevention of venous thromboembolism:
  - After total knee replacement: 1 × dabigatran 110 mg 1–4 hours postoperatively, followed by 220 mg once daily for 10 days.
  - In patients after total hip replacement: 1 × dabigatran 110 mg 1–4 hours postoperatively, followed by 220 mg once daily for 28–35 days.
  - *Note:* dose reduction (1 × dabigatran 75 mg, followed by 150 mg once daily) in patients with CrCl 30–50 mL/min, concomitant therapy with verapamil (and CrCl 30–50 mL/min), amiodarone or quinidine, or patients aged 75 years or older.
- Treatment of venous thromboembolism, and prevention of recurrent venous thromboembolism (usually for ≥3 months):
  - Dabigatran 150 mg twice daily, after pretreatment with parenteral anticoagulation for at least 5 days.
  - *Note:* dose reduction to 110 mg twice daily is recommended in patients aged 80 years or older, or those with concomitant therapy with verapamil. There are other factors (e.g. renal function, high bleeding risk) which may warrant a dose reduction of dabigatran.

Idarucizumab (specific dabigatran reversal agent)

- Patients treated with dabigatran, when rapid reversal of its anticoagulant effects is required for emergency surgery/urgent procedures or in life-threatening or uncontrolled bleeding:
  - 5 g intravenously in two consecutive infusions of 2.5. g intravenously over 5–10 minutes each (or as a bolus).

References

1. van Ryn J, Stangier J, Haertter S, et al. Dabigatran etexilate—a novel, reversible, oral direct thrombin inhibitor: interpretation of coagulation assays and reversal of anticoagulant activity. Thromb Haemost. 2010;103(6):1116–27.
2. Huisman MV, Lip GY, Diener HC, Brueckmann M, van Ryn J, Clemens A. Dabigatran etexilate for stroke prevention in patients with atrial fibrillation: resolving uncertainties in routine practice. Thromb Haemost. 2012;107(5):838–47.
3. Blech S, Ebner T, Ludwig-Schwellinger E, Stangier J, Roth W. The metabolism and disposition of the oral direct thrombin inhibitor, dabigatran, in humans. Drug Metab Dispos. 2008;36(2):386–99.
4. Steffel J, Collins R, Antz M, et al. 2021 European Heart Rhythm Association Practical guide on the use of non-vitamin k antagonist oral anticoagulants in patients with atrial fibrillation. Europace. 2021;23(10):1612–76.
5. Hindricks G, Potpara T, Dagres N, et al. 2020 ESC Guidelines for the diagnosis and management of atrial fibrillation developed in collaboration with the European Association for Cardio-Thoracic Surgery (EACTS): the Task Force for the diagnosis and management of atrial fibrillation of the European Society of Cardiology (ESC) Developed with the special contribution of the European Heart Rhythm Association (EHRA) of the ESC. Eur Heart J. 2021;42(5):373–498.
6. Ezekowitz MD, Reilly PA, Nehmiz G, et al. Dabigatran with or without concomitant aspirin compared with warfarin alone in patients with nonvalvular atrial fibrillation (PETRO Study). Am J Cardiol. 2007;100(9):1419–26.
7. Eriksson BI, Dahl OE, Rosencher N, et al. Oral dabigatran etexilate vs. subcutaneous enoxaparin for the prevention of venous thromboembolism after total knee replacement: the RE-MODEL randomized trial. J Thromb Haemost. 2007;5(11):2178–85.
8. Eriksson BI, Dahl OE, Rosencher N, et al. Dabigatran etexilate versus enoxaparin for prevention of venous thromboembolism after total hip replacement: a randomised, double-blind, non-inferiority trial. Lancet. 2007;370(9591):949–56.
9. Hart RG, Pearce LA, Aguilar MI. Meta-analysis: antithrombotic therapy to prevent stroke in patients who have nonvalvular atrial fibrillation. Ann Intern Med. 2007;146(12):857–67.
10. Ezekowitz MD, Connolly S, Parekh A, et al. Rationale and design of RE-LY: randomized evaluation of long-term anticoagulant therapy, warfarin, compared with dabigatran. Am Heart J. 2009;157(5):805–10.
11. Connolly SJ, Ezekowitz MD, Yusuf S, et al. Dabigatran versus warfarin in patients with atrial fibrillation. N Engl J Med. 2009;361(12):1139–51.
12. Connolly SJ, Ezekowitz MD, Yusuf S, Reilly PA, Wallentin L. Newly identified events in the RE-LY trial. N Engl J Med. 2010;363(19):1875–6.
13. Ezekowitz MD, Wallentin L, Connolly SJ, et al. Dabigatran and warfarin in vitamin K antagonist-naive and -experienced cohorts with atrial fibrillation. Circulation. 2010;122(22):2246–53.
14. Eikelboom JW, Wallentin L, Connolly SJ, et al. Risk of bleeding with 2 doses of dabigatran compared with warfarin in older and younger patients with atrial fibrillation: an analysis of the randomized

evaluation of long-term anticoagulant therapy (RE-LY) trial. Circulation. 2011;123(21):2363–72.

15. Beasley BN, Unger EF, Temple R. Anticoagulant options—why the FDA approved a higher but not a lower dose of dabigatran. N Engl J Med. 2011;364(19):1788–90.
16. Connolly SJ, Wallentin L, Ezekowitz MD, et al. The long-term multicenter observational study of dabigatran treatment in patients with atrial fibrillation (RELY-ABLE) study. Circulation. 2013;128(3):237–43.
17. Erath JW, Hohnloser SH. Anticoagulation in atrial fibrillation: current evidence and guideline recommendations. Herz. 2018;43(1):2–10.
18. Gorst-Rasmussen A, Skjøth F, Larsen TB, Rasmussen LH, Lip GY, Lane DA. Dabigatran adherence in atrial fibrillation patients during the first year after diagnosis: a nationwide cohort study. J Thromb Haemost. 2015;13(4):495–504.
19. Steinberg BA, Holmes DN, Piccini JP, et al. Early adoption of dabigatran and its dosing in US patients with atrial fibrillation: results from the outcomes registry for better informed treatment of atrial fibrillation. J Am Heart Assoc. 2013;2(6):e000535.
20. Yao X, Abraham NS, Sangaralingham LR, et al. Effectiveness and safety of dabigatran, rivaroxaban, and apixaban versus warfarin in nonvalvular atrial fibrillation. J Am Heart Assoc. 2016;5(6):e003725.
21. Lip GY, Keshishian A, Kamble S, et al. Real-world comparison of major bleeding risk among non-valvular atrial fibrillation patients initiated on apixaban, dabigatran, rivaroxaban, or warfarin. A propensity score matched analysis. Thromb Haemost. 2016;116(5):975–86.
22. Deitelzweig S, Farmer C, Luo X, et al. Risk of major bleeding in patients with non-valvular atrial fibrillation treated with oral anticoagulants: a systematic review of real-world observational studies. Curr Med Res Opin. 2017;33(9):1583–94.
23. Hohnloser SH, Basic E, Nabauer M. Comparative risk of major bleeding with new oral anticoagulants (NOACs) and phenprocoumon in patients with atrial fibrillation: a post-marketing surveillance study. Clin Res Cardiol. 2017;106(8):618–28.
24. Domek M, Gumprecht J, Ding WY, Lip GYH, Lane DA. Practice-derived data on non-vitamin K antagonist oral anticoagulant therapy to complement observations from randomized trials. Eur Heart J Suppl. 2020;22(Suppl I):I1–12.
25. Lip GY, Windecker S, Huber K, et al. Management of antithrombotic therapy in atrial fibrillation patients presenting with acute coronary syndrome and/or undergoing percutaneous coronary or valve interventions: a joint consensus document of the European Society of Cardiology Working Group on Thrombosis, European Heart Rhythm Association (EHRA), European Association of Percutaneous Cardiovascular Interventions (EAPCI) and European Association of Acute Cardiac Care (ACCA) endorsed by the Heart Rhythm Society (HRS) and Asia-Pacific Heart Rhythm Society (APHRS). Eur Heart J. 2014;35(45):3155–79.
26. Connolly S, Pogue J, Hart R, et al. Clopidogrel plus aspirin versus oral anticoagulation for atrial fibrillation in the Atrial fibrillation Clopidogrel Trial with Irbesartan for prevention of Vascular Events (ACTIVE W): a randomised controlled trial. Lancet. 2006;367(9526):1903–12.
27. Mant J, Hobbs FD, Fletcher K, et al. Warfarin versus aspirin for stroke prevention in an elderly community population with atrial fibrillation (the Birmingham Atrial Fibrillation Treatment of the Aged Study, BAFTA): a randomised controlled trial. Lancet. 2007;370(9586):493–503.
28. Connolly SJ, Eikelboom J, Joyner C, et al. Apixaban in patients with atrial fibrillation. N Engl J Med. 2011;364(9):806–17.
29. Kirchhof P, Benussi S, Kotecha D, et al. 2016 ESC Guidelines for the management of atrial fibrillation developed in collaboration with EACTS. Eur Heart J. 2016;37(38):2893–962.
30. Dewilde WJ, Oirbans T, Verheugt FW, et al. Use of clopidogrel with or without aspirin in patients taking oral anticoagulant therapy and undergoing percutaneous coronary intervention: an open-label, randomised, controlled trial. Lancet. 2013;381(9872):1107–15.
31. Jackson LR 2nd, Ju C, Zettler M, et al. Outcomes of patients with acute myocardial infarction undergoing percutaneous coronary intervention receiving an oral anticoagulant and dual antiplatelet therapy: a comparison of clopidogrel versus prasugrel from the TRANSLATE-ACS study. JACC Cardiovasc Interv. 2015;8(14):1880–9.
32. Gibson CM, Mehran R, Bode C, et al. Prevention of bleeding in patients with atrial fibrillation undergoing PCI. N Engl J Med. 2016;375(25):2423–34.
33. Cannon CP, Bhatt DL, Oldgren J, et al. Dual antithrombotic therapy with dabigatran after PCI in atrial fibrillation. N Engl J Med. 2017;377(16):1513–24.
34. Lopes RD, Heizer G, Aronson R, et al. Antithrombotic therapy after acute coronary syndrome or PCI in atrial fibrillation. N Engl J Med. 2019;380(16):1509–24.
35. Vranckx P, Valgimigli M, Eckardt L, et al. Edoxaban-based versus vitamin K antagonist-based antithrombotic regimen after successful coronary stenting in patients with atrial fibrillation (ENTRUST-AF PCI): a randomised, open-label, phase 3b trial. Lancet. 2019;394(10206):1335–43.
36. Cannon CP, Gropper S, Bhatt DL, et al. Design and rationale of the RE-DUAL PCI trial: a prospective, randomized, phase 3b study comparing the safety and efficacy of dual antithrombotic therapy with dabigatran etexilate versus warfarin triple therapy in patients with nonvalvular atrial fibrillation who have undergone percutaneous coronary intervention with stenting. Clin Cardiol. 2016;39(10):555–64.
37. Oldgren J, Steg PG, Hohnloser SH, et al. Dabigatran dual therapy with ticagrelor or clopidogrel after percutaneous coronary intervention in atrial fibrillation patients with or without acute coronary syndrome: a subgroup analysis from the RE-DUAL PCI trial. Eur Heart J. 2019;40(19):1553–62.
38. Peterson BE, Bhatt DL, Gabriel Steg P, et al. Evaluation of dual versus triple therapy by landmark analysis in the RE-DUAL PCI trial. JACC Cardiovasc Interv. 2021;14(7):768–80.
39. Di Biase L, Burkhardt JD, Santangeli P, et al. Periprocedural stroke and bleeding complications in patients undergoing catheter ablation of atrial fibrillation with different anticoagulation management: results from the Role of Coumadin in Preventing Thromboembolism in Atrial Fibrillation (AF) Patients Undergoing Catheter Ablation (COMPARE) randomized trial. Circulation. 2014;129(25):2638–44.
40. Calkins H, Willems S, Gerstenfeld EP, et al. Uninterrupted dabigatran versus warfarin for ablation in atrial fibrillation. N Engl J Med. 2017;376(17):1627–36.
41. Ruff CT, Giugliano RP, Braunwald E, et al. Comparison of the efficacy and safety of new oral anticoagulants with warfarin in patients with atrial fibrillation: a meta-analysis of randomised trials. Lancet. 2014;383(9921):955–62.
42. Eriksson BI, Dahl OE, Huo MH, et al. Oral dabigatran versus enoxaparin for thromboprophylaxis after primary total hip arthroplasty (RE-NOVATE II*). A randomised, double-blind, non-inferiority trial. Thromb Haemost. 2011;105(4):721–9.
43. Ginsberg JS, Davidson BL, Comp PC, et al. Oral thrombin inhibitor dabigatran etexilate vs North American enoxaparin regimen for prevention of venous thromboembolism after knee arthroplasty surgery. J Arthroplasty. 2009;24(1):1–9.

44. Schulman S, Kearon C, Kakkar AK, et al. Extended use of dabigatran, warfarin, or placebo in venous thromboembolism. N Engl J Med. 2013;368(8):709–18.
45. Schulman S, Kearon C, Kakkar AK, et al. Dabigatran versus warfarin in the treatment of acute venous thromboembolism. N Engl J Med. 2009;361(24):2342–52.
46. Schulman S, Kakkar AK, Goldhaber SZ, et al. Treatment of acute venous thromboembolism with dabigatran or warfarin and pooled analysis. Circulation. 2014;129(7):764–72.
47. Van de Werf F, Brueckmann M, Connolly SJ, et al. A comparison of dabigatran etexilate with warfarin in patients with mechanical heart valves: the randomized, phase II study to evaluate the safety and pharmacokinetics of oral dabigatran etexilate in patients after heart valve replacement (RE-ALIGN). Am Heart J. 2012;163(6):931–7.e1.
48. Eikelboom JW, Connolly SJ, Brueckmann M, et al. Dabigatran versus warfarin in patients with mechanical heart valves. N Engl J Med. 2013;369(13):1206–14.
49. US Food and Drug Administration. FDA Drug Safety Communication: Pradaxa (dabigatran etexilate mesylate) should not be used in patients with mechanical prosthetic heart valves. February 2018. Available at: https://www.fda.gov/drugs/drug-safety-and-availability/fda-drug-safety-communication-pradaxa-dabigatran-etexilate-mesylate-should-not-be-used-patients
50. Devereaux PJ, Duceppe E, Guyatt G, et al. Dabigatran in patients with myocardial injury after non-cardiac surgery (MANAGE): an international, randomised, placebo-controlled trial. Lancet. 2018;391(10137):2325–34.
51. Ruetzler K, Smilowitz NR, Berger JS, et al. Diagnosis and management of patients with myocardial injury after noncardiac surgery: a scientific statement from the american heart association. Circulation. 2021;144(19):e287–305.
52. Hart RG, Diener HC, Coutts SB, et al. Embolic strokes of undetermined source: the case for a new clinical construct. Lancet Neurol. 2014;13(4):429–38.
53. Diener HC, Sacco RL, Easton JD, et al. Dabigatran for prevention of stroke after embolic stroke of undetermined source. N Engl J Med. 2019;380(20):1906–17.
54. Lauw MN, Coppens M, Eikelboom JW. Recent advances in antidotes for direct oral anticoagulants: their arrival is imminent. Can J Cardiol. 2014;30(4):381–4.
55. Schiele F, van Ryn J, Canada K, et al. A specific antidote for dabigatran: functional and structural characterization. Blood. 2013;121(18):3554–62.
56. Glund S, Stangier J, Schmohl M, et al. Safety, tolerability, and efficacy of idarucizumab for the reversal of the anticoagulant effect of dabigatran in healthy male volunteers: a randomised, placebo-controlled, double-blind phase 1 trial. Lancet. 2015;386(9994):680–90.
57. Pollack CV Jr, Reilly PA, Bernstein R, et al. Design and rationale for RE-VERSE AD: a phase 3 study of idarucizumab, a specific reversal agent for dabigatran. Thromb Haemost. 2015;114(1):198–205.
58. Pollack CV Jr, Reilly PA, Eikelboom J, et al. Idarucizumab for dabigatran reversal. N Engl J Med. 2015;373(6):511–20.
59. Pollack CV Jr, Reilly PA, van Ryn J, et al. Idarucizumab for dabigatran reversal—full cohort analysis. N Engl J Med. 2017;377(5):431–41.

CHAPTER 11

Oral factor Xa inhibitors

Agneta Siegbahn, Peter J. Svensson, Håkan Wallén, and Lars Wallentin

Contents

Summary

Oral factor Xa (FXa) inhibitors exert their antithrombotic effects and increase the risk of bleeding by their effects on the coagulation system. The oral direct FXa inhibitors are highly potent, reversible active-site inhibitors of FXa with good bioavailability, rapid onset, and used in a daily standard dose without laboratory monitoring. Dose adjustment is needed in relation to renal function. Three FXa inhibitors are registered for clinical use in the European Union for the prevention and treatment of venous thromboembolism and for the prevention of stroke in atrial fibrillation—rivaroxaban, apixaban, and edoxaban. The FXa inhibitors provide similar or better protection against venous thromboembolism and stroke than warfarin. In patients with atrial fibrillation there is improved long-term survival as compared with warfarin. Simultaneously, there is a much lower risk of intracranial bleeding and, with apixaban and edoxaban, also a lower risk of all bleeding than with warfarin. The treatment is cost-effective and preferred by most patients.

Factor Xa and its inhibition in the coagulation system

The coagulation system

Oral factor (F)-Xa inhibitors exert their antithrombotic effects and increase the risk of bleeding by their effects on the coagulation system. Blood coagulation is essential to maintain vascular integrity at injury sites, so-called haemostasis, but also contributes to thrombus formation in arterial and venous vessels resulting in myocardial infarction, ischaemic stroke, and deep vein thrombosis. Today the coagulation process is best understood by the 'cell-based model' in which the interactions of the coagulation proteins with cell membranes are mandatory.[1] The cell-based model includes three phases of coagulation: initiation, amplification, and propagation phases,[1] see ➔ Figure 11.1.

Upon vascular injury, tissue factor (TF) is exposed to the blood and its ligand, coagulation FVII. In the initiation phase, binding of FVII to TF leads to autoactivation of FVII to FVIIa and formation of the binary complex TF/FVIIa, and subsequent initiation of the coagulation process. TF is a 47 kDa transmembrane glycoprotein and is normally not expressed in cells that are in contact with the flowing blood and the

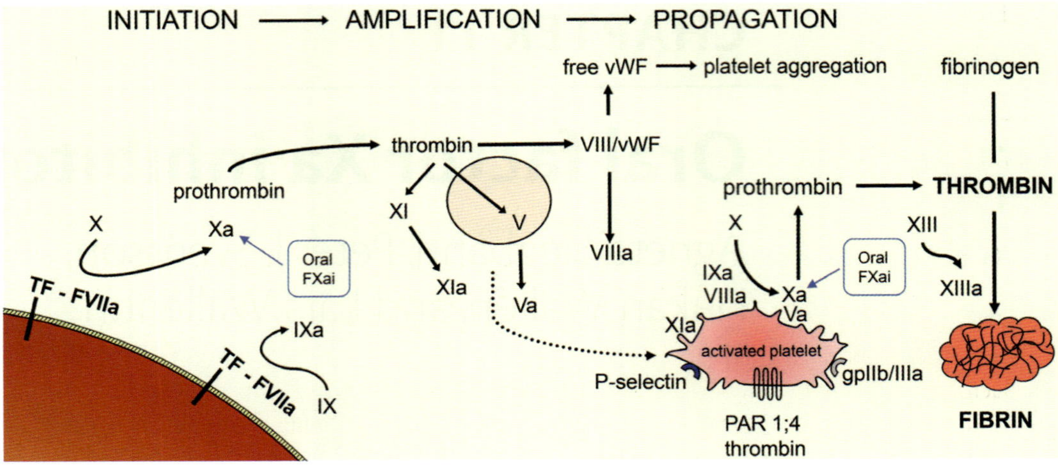

Figure 11.1 The cell-based coagulation model and oral FXa inhibitors' site of action. VWF, von Willebrand factor.
Image courtesy of A. Siegbahn and M. Åberg.

distribution functions as a haemostatic envelope. Sub-endothelial cells (e.g. smooth muscle cells, fibroblasts, and pericytes) and cells surrounding blood vessels have a constitutive TF expression. Predominantly non-coagulant TF exists on the cell surface. The regulation mechanisms of TF from its inactive form to the coagulation active form are not fully understood but are influenced by expression of negatively charged phosphatidylserine on the cell membrane and by involvement of protein disulfide isomerase (PDI).[2] Upon disruption of vascular integrity, circulating platelets adhere immediately to the injured vessel wall mediated by cross binding of the von Willebrand factor and the platelets and collagen, which leads to activation of the platelets and release of their granule contents and extracellular vesicles (e.g. microparticles and exosomes). Moreover, platelets aggregate by binding to each other by cross binding of fibrinogen to the platelet receptor glycoprotein IIb/IIIa forming a platelet plug. The TF/FVIIa complex activates coagulation FIX and coagulation FX at the site of injury triggering production of small amounts of thrombin, which contributes to further platelet activation with procoagulant phospholipids on the cell membrane. In the amplification phase, thrombin generates a local increase of activated FV, FVIII, and FXI on the platelet surface and further activation of the platelets, and the process then proceeds on the activated platelet surfaces rich in phosphatidylserine. Finally, in the propagation phase, the activated FIX/FVIIIa complex provides FXa, which associates with FVa forming the prothrombinase complex (prothrombin, FVa, and FXa) and a burst of thrombin is generated leading to cleavage of fibrinogen to fibrin and formation of the fibrin meshwork. Thrombin also activates FXIII (a fibrin stabilizing factor) which links and stabilizes the fibrin polymers and the retention of red blood cells to the blood clot forming a stable thrombus.

Regulation of the coagulation process

To keep the coagulation process tightly regulated at various stages there are a number of inhibitors that prevent inappropriate activation. The protease inhibitor tissue factor pathway inhibitor (TFPI) acts on the TF-dependent initiation phase by blocking FVIIa and FXa activity.[3] In a heparan sulfate-dependent reaction, antithrombin inhibits thrombin and FXa. The healthy endothelium express thrombomodulin which binds circulating thrombin and changes its specificity to prevent platelet activation and fibrin generation. The thrombin/thrombomodulin complex activates protein C which in complex with protein S inactivates FVa and FVIIIa and thereby regulates the amplification phase.[4] Finally, the fibrin meshwork is degraded in the fibrinolytic process by the proteolytic enzyme plasmin. Plasmin limits the thrombus expansion and removes the clot when the wound is healed.

Oral factor Xa inhibitory anticoagulants

The activated serine protease FXa is an attractive target for non-vitamin K oral anticoagulants (NOACs) based on its central role in the coagulation process. Serine proteases of the coagulation system act on their cognate protein substrates with marked and distinctive specificity[5] and the oral target-specific FXa inhibitors, developed during 1990–2010, were based on the knowledge of the crystal structure of FXa and the sequence specificity of the substrate cleavage site.[6] In the initiation phase of coagulation FXa is responsible for cleavage of prothrombin to thrombin. The substrate specificity by FXa also depends on interaction with the cell membrane and the prothrombinase complex in the amplification and propagation phases of coagulation. The prothrombinase reaction with coagulant-activated FX induces a burst of thrombin and each molecule of FXa assembled in the prothrombinase complex generates more than 1000 thrombin molecules.[7] The oral direct FXa inhibitors are highly potent, reversible active-site inhibitors of human FXa.[8,9] They are low-molecular-weight active compounds with good bioavailability and therefore have a rapid onset. These oral FXa inhibitors are all binding in an L-shaped fashion in the active site of FXa and they inhibit free FXa, FXa within the prothrombinase complex, and clot-bound FXa.[10,11] Unlike indirect FXa inhibitors, such as heparin, low-molecular-weight heparin (LMWH), and fondaparinux, they do not require antithrombin for the inhibition of FXa. The oral direct FXa inhibitors have no effect on platelet function, but have indirect effects through the inhibition of thrombin which is the major platelet activator.

Clinical pharmacology of oral factor Xa inhibitors

Of the numerous FXa inhibitors tested, only a few have succeeded all the way to approval for clinical use. Clinical development of some FXa inhibitors, like razaxaban,[12] otamixaban,[13] and darexaban,[14] were halted following phase II/III studies due to various reasons, such as increased bleeding, insufficient efficacy for the clinical indication tested, or due to prioritizations within the pharmaceutical industry. There are presently three FXa inhibitors registered for clinical use in the European Union (EU)—rivaroxaban, apixaban, and edoxaban. A fourth FXa inhibitor, betrixaban, is also approved for clinical use in the US. The posology of the FXa inhibitors for approved indications is summarized in Table 11.1.

Rivaroxaban

Rivaroxaban has a molecular weight of 436 g/mol, and an inhibition constant (K_i) for FXa of 0.4 nM (at 25 °C).[15] The drug is primarily absorbed in the lower parts of the ventricle and proximal parts of the small intestine. The absorption is dose limited and at higher doses (>10 mg) the drug should be taken with food as the oral bioavailability then approaches 100%. The plasma drug concentration reaches its peak (C_{max}) at 2–4 hours after dose intake, the drug is highly bound to plasma proteins (92–95%), and the distribution volume at steady state (Vd_{ss}) is approximately 50 L (0.7 L/kg). The drug is, due to its high protein binding, not dialysable. Rivaroxaban is cleared directly by renal excretion to 35%, whereas 65% of the absorbed drug is metabolized, partly via the cytochrome P450 (CYP) system and partly by non-CYP

Table 11.1 Posology of FXa inhibitors

Indication	Rivaroxaban	Apixaban	Edoxaban	Betrixaban
Thromboprophylaxis in orthopaedic surgery	10 mg OD	2.5 mg BID	No indication	No indication
Thromboprophylaxis in hospitalized for acute medical illness	No indication	No indication	No indication	Only approved in the US: 160 mg followed by 80 BID, if concomitant P-gp inhibitors Or CrCl 15–30: 80 mg followed by 40 mg OD; CrCl <15: not recommended
Venous thromboembolism: treatment and prevention of recurrent thromboembolism	15 mg BID first 3 weeks, followed by 20 mg OD; 10 mg OD if extended treatment (>6 months)	10 mg BID first week, followed by 5 mg BID; 2.5 mg BID if extended treatment (>6 months) CrCl 15–30: used with caution CrCl <15: not recommended	60 mg OD after ≥5 days parenteral anticoagulation, 30 mg OD if: CrCl 15–50 Or Concomitant strong Pgp inhibitor[a] or body weight ≤60 kg; CrCl <15: not recommended	No indication
Non-valvular atrial fibrillation	20 mg OD, CrCl 15–50: 15 mg OD CrCl <15: not recommended	5 mg BID, 2.5 mg BID if ≥2 of following: age ≥80 years, weight ≤60 kg, s-creatinine ≥133 mmol/L (>1.5 mg/dL) CrCl 15–30: 2.5 mg BID CrCl <15: not recommended in EU	60 mg OD Dose reduction as in venous thromboembolism CrCl <15: not recommended	No indication
Acute coronary syndrome, stabilized patients	2.5 mg BID, in combination with single or dual antiplatelet treatment	No indication	No indication	No indication
Chronic coronary artery disease and/or peripheral artery disease	2.5 mg BID, in combination with single antiplatelet treatment	No indication	No indication	No indication

BID, twice daily; OD, once daily.

In patients with moderate–severe liver function (corresponding to Child–Pugh score B or C, or liver disease otherwise associated with disturbances in haemostasis) treatment is not recommended with any of the FXa inhibitors.

[a] Dronedarone, erythromycin, ciclosporin, ketoconazole.

dependent mechanisms. Unchanged rivaroxaban is the major drug component in human plasma, and there are no active metabolites. Rivaroxaban is a substrate for the efflux transporter protein permeability-glycoprotein (P-gp) which, together with CYP-dependent metabolism, renders the drug sensitive to some drug–drug interactions. The terminal half-life of rivaroxaban is 5–9 hours in young and 11–13 hours in elderly subjects. Renal function is the clinical characteristic with highest impact on rivaroxaban clearance and to a great extent explains the age-related effect observed on drug exposure.

Apixaban

Apixaban has a molecular weight of 460 g/mol, and a K_i of 0.08 nM at 25 °C[16] and 0.25 nM at 37 °C.[17] The oral availability is around 50% and not influenced by food intake. Apixaban reaches its peak concentration in plasma 3–4 hours after drug ingestion and the plasma protein binding is around 87%. The Vd_{ss} is 21 L (0.3 L/kg) and the unchanged form of apixaban is the predominant drug form in plasma. Apixaban is eliminated via multiple routes. Around 27% is renally excreted, and the drug is metabolized mainly by phase I non-CYP450-dependent enzymes and partly via CYP3A4, and to a minor degree also via other CYP450 enzymes. Apixaban is a substrate of P-gp, and some parent drug is excreted via direct intestinal excretion and in the bile. There are no active metabolites found in the circulation, and the elimination half-life is around 8–15 hours in healthy individuals.[18] Drug exposure increases with progressive renal impairment and a 55% increase in exposure [area under the curve (AUC)] has been estimated when creatinine clearance (CrCl) is around 15 mL/min.[16] The drug should therefore be used with caution in patients with CrCl of 15–30 mL/min. Haemodialysis has been found to reduce apixaban exposure (AUC) by 4–14%[19,20] and is thus ineffective to reduce circulating apixaban. Notably, apixaban is not approved for use in patients with end-stage renal disease in Europe and is not to be used in patients with CrCl less than 15 mL/min, whereas the US Food and Drug Administration (FDA) has approved apixaban for treatment of atrial fibrillation in patients with end-stage renal disease on haemodialysis.

Edoxaban

Edoxaban has a molecular weight of 548 g/mol and a K_i for FXa of 0.56 nM (at 30°C).[21] The drug was the last of the oral FXa inhibitors to be approved for clinical use in the EU. Edoxaban has an oral bioavailability of approximately 62%, and food increases the bioavailability to some degree but without affecting drug exposure to any clinically significant extent. Peak plasma levels of edoxaban are reached within 1–2 hours after drug intake, and the Vd_{ss} is 107 L (1.5 L/kg). Unchanged edoxaban is the predominant form circulating in plasma, and the plasma protein binding in plasma is approximately 55%. Edoxaban is metabolized through CYP-independent and CYP-dependent (CYP3A4) mechanisms. It has three active metabolites which, in subjects with normal renal function, do not reach more than 10% of the exposure of the unchanged compound. The drug is a substrate for P-gp, and the elimination half-life of edoxaban is around 10–14 hours. Approximately 50% of the drug is renally cleared. In severe renal impairment (CrCl <30 mL/min), total drug exposure (plasma AUC) was 72% higher than in subjects with normal renal function. Haemodialysis reduces total edoxaban exposure by less than 9% and is thus not effective in reducing circulating edoxaban. In patients with a high CrCl (>95 mL/min) drug exposure is reduced and a trend towards lower efficacy of edoxaban has been observed in patients with increased CrCl.[22] Therefore, edoxaban should be used with caution in patients with high CrCl.

Betrixaban

Betrixaban has a molecular weight of 452 g/mol. The drug is rapidly absorbed and has an oral bioavailability of 34%. Peak plasma concentrations are obtained within 3–4 hours. The absorption is influenced by food; drug exposure is reduced by 50–60% if administered together with either high-fat or low-fat meals. The protein binding is 60% and the distribution volume is high, around 2100 L (32 L/kg). The elimination half-life is approximately 37 hours. Betrixaban is mainly metabolized by CYP-independent hydrolysis, and 85% of the drug is excreted through the hepatobiliary system. Around 11% is excreted renally. Betrixaban is a substrate for P-gp.[23] The dose of betrixaban should be reduced in patients with CrCl between 15 and 30 mL/min, and the drug should not be used if CrCl is below 15 mL/min or in patients with moderate or severe liver impairment (Bevyxxa®, package insert; Portola Pharmaceuticals). Betrixaban is not approved for clinical use in the EU (Dexxience, assessment report, European Medicines Agency (EMA) 2018). It was the EMA's opinion that betrixaban did not demonstrate sufficient efficacy and safety in the pivotal study that was submitted for assessment to the EMA.[24] The drug is approved in the US for thromboprophylaxis of venous thromboembolism (VTE) in patients hospitalized with acute medical illness (Bevyxxa®, package insert; Portola Pharmaceuticals).

Monitoring of factor Xa inhibitors

One advantage of FXa inhibitors is that there is no need for routine drug monitoring, as is a requirement in the treatment with vitamin K antagonists. FXa inhibitors are all developed for fixed dose treatment, where dose adjustments are made according to a few simple patient characteristics which differ slightly between the FXa inhibitors (➔ Table 11.1). However, there are a few clinical situations where determination of drug plasma concentrations or anti-Xa activity may aid in clinical decision-making. These situations include, for example, acute major bleeding, need for urgent surgery, suspected pharmacokinetic drug–drug interactions, or in patients with progressive renal failure or extreme body weight. Interpretation of drug concentration data should be done together with coagulation specialists or experts from centres where concentration determinations are performed. Information regarding sampling in relation to last dose is essential in non-emergency situations. Maximal effects of the drug will occur when peak plasma levels are attained, which is usually 2–4 hours after drug intake (➔ Table 11.2). Plasma levels should normally

Table 11.2 Clinical pharmacology of FXa inhibitors

	Rivaroxaban	Apixaban	Edoxaban	Betrixaban[a]
Oral bioavailability (%)	70–100% (inversely dose dependent; almost complete with food)	50%	60%	35% (food may reduce exposure by 40–60%)
C_{max} (hours)	2–4	3–4	1–2	3–4
$T_{½}$ (terminal; hours)	5–9 (young subjects) 11–13 (elderly)	8–15	10–14	~37 (pharmacodynamic $T_{½}$ ~20)
Plasma protein binding (%)	95	87	55	60
Volume of distribution (L)	50	21	107	~2000
Clearance non-renal/renal	65%/35%	73%/27%	50%/50%	~90%/~10%
CYP substrate	CYP3A4 (18%)	CYP3A4 (25%)	CYP3A4 (<5%), 2 active metabolites—low circulating concentrations	Metabolized by non-CYP enzymes (hydrolysis), 85% excreted unchanged by hepato-biliary route
P-gp substrate	Yes	Yes	Yes	Yes
Expected plasma levels ng/mL, trough (peak levels); 5–95% percentiles (AF patient data[b])	12–137 (178–343)	34–230 (69–321)	12–43 (101–288)	8[c] (34[c])

Data are estimates from various sources of the literature (including SPC on EMA website).

[a] Not approved in the EU, but by FDA on indication prophylaxis of VTE in acute medically ill patients with risk factors for VTE. Data from APEX study protocol.[24]

[b] EHRA guidelines 2021 Steffel et al.[25].

[c] Geometric mean, 80 mg once daily healthy subjects, steady state, data from EMA assessment report on Dexxience, 26 July 2018.

be in the range of concentrations observed in larger patient populations (➔ Table 11.2). Of note, standard coagulation tests are not reliable, although they are often influenced by FXa inhibitors, especially at high plasma drug levels.[25]

Drug–drug interactions

Pharmacodynamic interactions

Pharmacodynamic drug interactions of FXa inhibitors mainly include interactions with drugs that inhibit platelet function and therefore increase the risk of bleeding.[26] Important drugs in this respect are non-steroidal anti-inflammatory drugs, and platelet inhibitors used in the treatment of coronary artery disease, acting through inhibition of cyclooxygenase or blocking platelet $P2Y_{12}$-receptors, but also selective serotonin reuptake inhibitors.[26] The latter type of drugs inhibit platelet function by depleting platelet stores of serotonin, a platelet secretagogue which acts as a second-line reinforcer of platelet activation.[27] From a bleeding perspective, pharmacodynamic interactions may quantitatively be even more important than pharmacokinetic interactions, as combining FXa inhibitors and antiplatelet agents is common (up to one-third of patients in large atrial fibrillation trials) and is associated with a significantly increased risk of bleeding.[28]

Pharmacokinetic interactions

Rivaroxaban, apixaban, edoxaban, and betrixaban are all substrates for the P-gp efflux transporter and drugs that interfere with P-pg may therefore interact with these FXa inhibitors.[29] Rivaroxaban and apixaban are also metabolized by the enzymes belonging to the CYP system, mainly CYP3A4 enzyme, which makes these drugs vulnerable for interaction with other drugs influencing this enzyme.[29] Interpretation of pharmacokinetic drug–drug interaction data is, however, a challenging area. Such data often come from pharmacokinetic studies in healthy volunteers, observational studies, or subgroup analyses of larger clinical studies, and the evidence grade may be variable. Furthermore, inherent characteristics of the actual patient (e.g. renal failure or polypharmacy) may also influence the significance of the interaction. Drug monitoring with measurement of plasma concentrations of the FXa inhibitors may be a possibility. However, such analyses may not be widespread, there are no established therapeutic ranges, and there are at present no evidence-based guidelines on how to adjust doses based on the determined plasma concentration. If possible, it may be advisable to choose another drug, or in some cases switch to warfarin where dosing can be made according to international normalized ratio (INR) measurements.

To help the clinician, there are comprehensive recommendations to follow, such as the European Heart Rhythm Association guideline,[25] where important pharmacokinetic interactions are listed. It is also recommended that the clinician when faced with a possible interaction performs database searches and scrutinizes the literature for new data.

Factor Xa inhibitors for venous thromboembolism

VTE is a multicausal disease influenced by a variety of acquired and inherited risk factors with annual incidence of 1–2 cases per 1000 in the population. VTE, comprising both deep vein thrombosis and pulmonary embolism, is a chronic illness that affects nearly 10 million people every year worldwide.[30] VTE is the third most common cardiovascular disease and is associated with significant morbidity ranging from painful leg swelling, chest pain, and shortness of breath to death. Long-term complications include recurrent VTE, post-pulmonary embolism syndrome, chronic thromboembolic pulmonary hypertension, and post-thrombotic syndrome.

Anticoagulation with LMWH and vitamin K antagonists has been the standard of care for treatment and prevention of VTE. However, after the introduction of NOACs, these have replaced LMWH and vitamin K antagonists in guidelines for most indications of VTE treatment.

The clinical development of these direct-acting oral anticoagulants is following the well-tested strategy of dose-ranging and registration studies in major orthopaedic surgery, prior to development in arterial or other venous indications.[31,32]

Factor Xa inhibition for symptomatic venous thromboembolism

There are four pivotal studies on oral FXa inhibitors in the treatment of acute venous thrombosis.[33–36] The four studies had similar design and the main endpoint was recurrent venous thrombosis. The principal safety outcome was major or clinically relevant non-major bleeding or a composite endpoint of those two. The comparator to the oral FXa inhibitors was a conventional therapy of LMWH and warfarin.

In the Apixaban for the Initial Management of Pulmonary Embolism and Deep-Vein Thrombosis as First-Line Therapy (AMPLIFY) trial,[33] recurrent VTE occurred in 2.3% of patients in the apixaban group, as compared with 2.7% in the conventional therapy group. Major bleeding occurred in 0.6% of patients who received apixaban and in 1.8% of those who received conventional therapy. The composite outcome of major bleeding and clinically relevant non-major bleeding occurred in 4.3% of the patients in the apixaban group, as compared with 9.7% of those in the conventional therapy group.

In the Hokusai-VTE study,[35] VTE recurrence occurred in 3.2% in the edoxaban group compared with 3.5% in the warfarin group. The safety outcome occurred in 8.5% in the edoxaban group and 10.3% in the conventional therapy group.

In the EINSTEIN–PE study,[36] recurrent VTE occurred in the rivaroxaban group in 2.1% of the patients compared with 1.8% in the conventional therapy group. The principal safety outcome occurred in 10.3% of patients in the rivaroxaban group and 11.4% of those in the conventional therapy group. Major bleeding was observed in 1.1% in the rivaroxaban group and 2.2% in the conventional therapy group.

Finally, in the EINSTEIN study,[34] rivaroxaban met the primary efficacy, recurrent VTE in 2.1% compared with 3.1% in the conventional therapy group. The safety outcome occurred in 8.1% of the patients in each treatment group.

Indirect comparisons in meta-analysis indicated similar reductions in the risk of VTE or VTE-related death for all FXa inhibitors.[37] For patients with transient risk factors associated with VTE the recommendation is 3–6 months of therapy with oral anticoagulation. For patients with no obvious risk factor associated with VTE the recommendation is extended therapy if no contraindication is identified.[37,38] (for information on thrombophilia, see ➔ Chapter 23). Reductions in major or clinically relevant non-major bleeding for initial or long-term treatment suggest that apixaban compared with the other FXa inhibitors could have a more favourable profile in indirect comparisons.[37] However, no direct comparison for the primary effect or bleeding outcomes is available.

Guide for use of oral Xa inhibitors in the treatment of venous thromboembolism

See ➔ Table 11.1.

Apixaban

Apixaban is started without initial parenteral therapy but requires a higher dose (10 mg twice daily) for 7 days, followed by the standard treatment dose of 5 mg twice daily. In contrast to treatment for atrial fibrillation, no dose adjustment is performed in deep venous thrombosis treatment in the presence of renal insufficiency. However, in patients with a CrCl of 15–29 mL/min, apixaban should be used with caution, and is not recommended with a CrCl less than 15 mL/min. A lower dose of 2.5 mg twice daily can be used for extended therapy.

Edoxaban

Edoxaban requires at least 5 days of parenteral anticoagulation with LMWH before starting oral dosing at 60 mg once daily, reduced to 30 mg once daily if CrCl is 15–50 mL/min.

Rivaroxaban

Rivaroxaban is started without initial parenteral therapy but requires a higher dose (15 mg twice daily) for 3 weeks, followed by the standard treatment dose of 20 mg once daily. In contrast to atrial fibrillation, no fixed dose adjustment is required for patients with a CrCl of 15–49 mL/min and a dose of either 20 or 15 mg once daily can be selected, respectively, depending on the risk of bleeding or thromboembolism. A rivaroxaban dose of 20 or 15 mg should be taken with food, which improves its bioavailability. A lower dose of 10 mg once daily can be used for extended therapy.

Factor Xa inhibition for venous thromboembolism in medical patients

VTE in acute medically ill patients is one of the leading causes of morbidity and mortality. Recent clinical trials of extended-duration thromboprophylaxis with enoxaparin, rivaroxaban, and apixaban in acute medically ill patients did not demonstrate a net clinical benefit compared with in-hospital thromboprophylaxis, and were shown to be associated with higher risks of major bleeding. Betrixaban is a new FXa inhibitor with a specific pharmacokinetic profile.[39] Betrixaban is currently only approved for the indication of extended thromboprophylaxis in acute medical illness in the US based on the APEX trial.[24,39] The recommended dose of betrixaban is an initial single dose of 160 mg starting on day 1, followed by 80 mg once daily taken for 35–42 days at the same time each day with food.

Factor Xa inhibition in children with venous thromboembolism

In a large pivotal multicentre randomized trial, children with documented acute VTE (0–17 years) were, after 5–9 days with heparin treatment, randomized to standard anticoagulants or rivaroxaban.[40] Five hundred patients were enrolled in the study. For patients on rivaroxaban or standard therapy the primary efficacy outcome (recurrent VTE) was 1% versus 3% and the safety outcome of major or clinically relevant non-major bleeding was 3% versus 2%, respectively. The conclusion of the study was that in children with acute VTE, treatment with rivaroxaban compared with standard therapy had a low recurrence rate without increased risk of bleeding.[40] Rivaroxaban is therefore approved for treatment of VTE in children by both the FDA and EMA.

Factor Xa inhibition for treatment of cancer-associated venous thromboembolism

The four pivotal clinical trials addressing direct oral anticoagulants in treatment of acute VTE associated with cancer were analysed in a recently published systematic review and meta-analysis.[41] The four studies included 2894 patients comparing apixaban, edoxaban, and rivaroxaban with dalteparin. Recurrent VTE occurred in 5.2% versus 8.2% in oral FXa inhibitors versus LMWH, respectively. Major bleeding occurred in 4.3% versus 3.3% in oral FXa inhibitors versus LMWH, respectively. The conclusion of the study was that in patients with cancer-associated VTE, oral FXa inhibitors reduced the risk of recurrence without higher likelihood for risk of bleeding.[41] International guidelines therefore state that direct oral FXa inhibitors could be an alternative to LMWH in treatments of cancer-associated VTE.

Factor Xa inhibitors for stroke prevention in atrial fibrillation

Atrial fibrillation is the most common cardiac arrhythmia, and affects around 3% of the population in middle- and high-income countries with an ageing population. The occurrence of atrial fibrillation increases to around 10% above 70 years of age. Atrial fibrillation is associated with formation of thrombi in the fibrillating atrium leading to an increased risk of thromboembolic stroke and peripheral embolic events.[42–44] In the 1990s, seven clinical trials, randomizing patients with atrial fibrillation to vitamin K antagonist versus placebo, showed a median of 65% relative reduction of the risk of stroke and systemic embolism. Also, platelet inhibition with aspirin was tested for stroke prevention in atrial fibrillation although with more limited efficacy as compared with vitamin K antagonists in randomized head-to-head trials. Treatment with vitamin K antagonists has been the treatment of choice for stroke prevention in patients with atrial fibrillation and a raised risk of stroke since the 1990s. However, treatment with vitamin K antagonists is cumbersome and demanding for the patient as it requires regular laboratory monitoring of the level of anticoagulation by INR and adjustment of the dose in order to maintain the optimal target range of INR between 2.0 and 3.0. Therefore, there was an urgent need for alternative oral anticoagulant treatments that could be used in an oral fixed dose without laboratory monitoring and preferably associated with a better stroke prevention, less side effects of major bleeding, lower risk of intracranial bleeding, and lower mortality.

The development of NOACs in the form of direct thrombin inhibitors or direct FXa inhibitors in the beginning of the 2000s provided a major opportunity for improving and facilitating anticoagulant treatment in atrial fibrillation. The pivotal trials on the efficacy and safety of the direct FXa inhibitors for stroke prevention in atrial fibrillation were performed between 2006 and 2015. Based on these trials, the direct-acting oral anticoagulants are now preferred over vitamin K antagonists for stroke prevention in atrial fibrillation.[42–44] Three FXa inhibitors (rivaroxaban, apixaban, and edoxaban) today have worldwide approval for stroke prevention in patients with atrial fibrillation and a raised risk of stroke. The approval and the current treatment guidelines were based on the efficacy and safety results from the three large randomized clinical trials comparing FXa inhibitor with warfarin (ROCKET AF, ARISTOTLE, and ENGAGE AF-TIMI 48).[45–48] Apixaban has also been compared with aspirin alone in patients with atrial fibrillation and a raised risk of stroke unsuitable for or unwilling to receive vitamin K antagonist treatment in the AVERROES trial.[49] The key characteristics of these pivotal trials and their patient populations and results are summarized in ➔ Figure 11.2. The details of the study designs have all been published.[50–53] Several study-level meta-analyses based on published aggregate data from the pivotal trials[54–56] as well as one individual level meta-analysis are publicly available.[57]

The AVERROES trial enrolled 5599 adult patients (age ≥50 years) with $CHADS_2$ score of at least 1 who were either unsuitable for or unwilling to receive warfarin.[58] They were randomized to double-blind, double-dummy, treatment with either aspirin (81–324 mg daily) or apixaban 5 mg twice daily with dose reduction to 2.5 mg twice daily at (1) age 80 years or older, (2) body weight of 60 kg or less, or (3) serum creatinine level of at least 1.5 mg/dL (133 mmol/L). The primary efficacy endpoint was the composite of stroke or systemic embolism and the primary safety endpoint major bleeding, as defined by the International Society on Thrombosis and Haemostasis.[59] All primary events were adjudicated by an independent clinical adverse events committee. The AVERROES trial was designed to test for superiority of apixaban over aspirin for stroke prevention. The trial had to be prematurely terminated as the first planned interim analysis, after a median follow-up of 13 months, showed a clear benefit in favour of apixaban.

Endpoint	Study	Levels	N	N Cases	HR [95% CI]	P (superiority)	P (non-inferiority)
Stroke/SE	AVERROES	Apixaban vs Aspirin	2808/2791	51/113	0.45 [0.32,0.62]	<0.001	
	ARISTOTLE	Apixaban vs Warfarin	9120/9081	212/265	0.79 [0.66,0.95]	0.010	<0.001
	ROCKET	Rivaroxaban vs Warfarin	7081/7090	269/306	0.88 [0.75,1 .03]	0.120	<0.001
	ENGAGE	Edoxaban Low vs Warfarin	7034/7036	253/232	1.07 [0.87,1.31]	0.440	0.005
	ENGAGE	Edoxaban High vs Warfarin	7035/7036	182/232	0.79 [0.63,0.99]	0.020	<0.001
Ischaemic stroke	AVERROES	Apixaban vs Aspirin	2808/2791	35/93	0.37 [0.25,0.55]	<0.001	
	ARISTOTLE	Apixaban vs Warfarin	9120/9081	162/175	0.92 [0.74,1.13]	0.420	
	ROCKET	Rivaroxaban vs Warfarin	7082/7061	149/161	0.94 [0.75,1.17]	0.581	
	ENGAGE	Edoxaban Low vs Warfarin	7035/7036	333/235	1.41 [1.19,1.67]	<0.001	
	ENGAGE	Edoxaban High vs Warfarin	7034/7036	236/235	1.00 [0.83,1.19]	0.970	
Intracranial beeding	AVERROES	Apixaban vs Aspirin	2808/2791	11/13	0.85 [0.38,1.90]	0.690	
	ARISTOTLE	Apixaban vs Warfarin	9088/9052	52/122	0.42 [0.30,0.58]	<0.001	
	ROCKET	Rivaroxaban vs Warfarin	7111/7125	55/84	0.67 [0.47,0.93]	0.020	
	ENGAGE	Edoxaban Low vs Warfarin	7002/7012	41/132	0.30 [0.21,0.43]	<0.001	
	ENGAGE	Edoxaban High vs Warfarin	7012/7012	61/132	0.47 [0.34,0.63]	<0.001	
Major bleeding	AVERROES	Apixaban vs Aspirin	2808/2791	44/39	1.13 [0.74,1.75]	0.570	
	ARISTOTLE	Apixaban vs Warfarin	9088/9052	327/462	0.69 [0.60,0.80]	<0.001	
	ROCKET	Rivaroxaban vs Warfarin	7111/7125	395/386	1.04 [0.90,1.20]	0.580	
	ENGAGE	Edoxaban Low vs Warfarin	7002/7012	254/524	0.47 [0.41,0.55]	<0.001	
	ENGAGE	Edoxaban High vs Warfarin	7012/7012	418/524	0.80 [0.71,0.91]	<0.001	
Total death	AVERROES	Apixaban vs Aspirin	2808/2791	111/40	0.79 [0.62,1.02]	0.070	
	ARISTOTLE	Apixaban vs Warfarin	9120/9081	603/669	0.89 [0.80,1.00]	0.0470	
	ROCKET	Rivaroxaban vs Warfarin	7082/7061	208/250	0.85 [0.70,1.02]	0.073	
	ENGAGE	Edoxaban Low vs Warfarin	7035/7036	737/839	0.87 [0.70,0.96]	0.006	
	ENGAGE	Edoxaban High vs Warfarin	7034/7036	773/839	0.92 [0.83,1.01]	0.080	

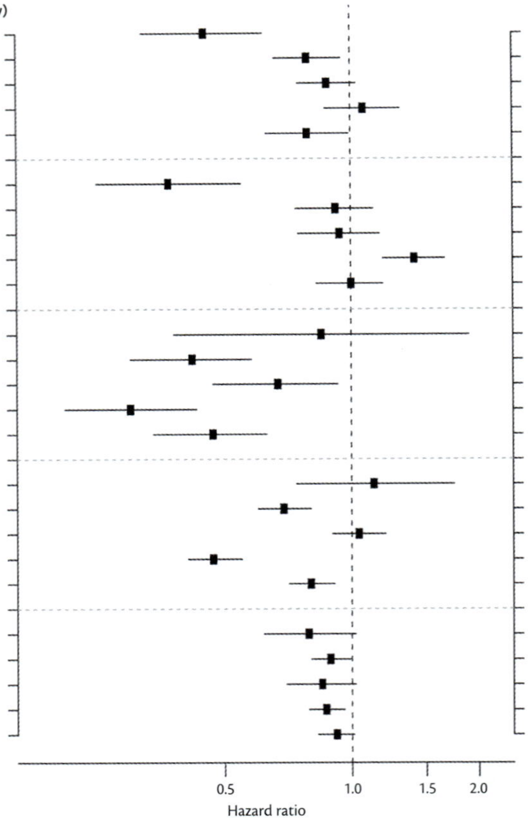

Figure 11.2 Efficacy and safety outcomes of factor Xa inhibitors in comparison to aspirin or warfarin in the five pivotal trials leading to regulatory approval for stroke prevention in patients with atrial fibrillation and an increased risk of stroke. FXa inhibition with apixaban versus aspirin in atrial fibrillation. CI, confidence interval; HR, hazard ratio.

The final results with apixaban versus aspirin showed a 55% relative reduction in stroke and systemic embolism mainly based on a 63% relative reduction in ischaemic stroke. There was no significant difference in intracranial or major bleeding. There was a trend with a 21% relative reduction in total death with apixaban versus aspirin. It should be remembered that the power to obtain significant findings concerning secondary events became lower because of the early termination.

These AVERROES results clearly established that patients with atrial fibrillation and an increased risk of stroke should be treated with oral anticoagulation and not with aspirin because of the substantial net benefit with a more than halving in the risk of stroke without any increase in the risk of major bleeding. Patients with atrial fibrillation who are still using aspirin for stroke prevention should be recommended to switch to prophylactic treatment with oral anticoagulation (e.g. apixaban).

Factor Xa inhibition versus warfarin in atrial fibrillation

The three clinical trials evaluating FXa inhibition versus warfarin (ROCKET AF, ARISTOTLE, and ENGAGE AF-TIMI 48) have included 53,570 (= 14,264 + 18,201 + 21,105, respectively) adult patients with a confirmed history of atrial fibrillation or atrial flutter and a raised risk for stroke, and excluded patients with poor renal function or a history of recent stroke or high-risk bleeding. The rivaroxaban (ROCKET-AF) and apixaban (ARISTOTLE) trials randomized patients to either FXa inhibitor or warfarin. The edoxaban (ENGAGE AF-TIMI 48) trial randomized patients to higher-dose or lower-dose FXa inhibitors, using the third group assigned to warfarin as a common comparator. All trials used a double-blind/double-dummy design with warfarin/placebo dose adjustments based on regular INR/sham INR control in all patients.[46–48]

In ROCKET AF,[46] the rivaroxaban arm dose was 20 mg once daily although patients with estimated CrCl of 30–49 mL/min/1.73 m^2 received a dose of 15 mg once daily. In ARISTOTLE,[47] the apixaban dose was 5 mg twice daily with dose reduction to 2.5 mg twice daily at two of the following prespecified criteria: (1) age 80 years or older, (2) body weight of 60 kg or less, or (3) serum creatinine level of at least 1.5 mg/dL (133 mmol/L). In ENGAGE AF-TIMI 48,[48] the higher dose of edoxaban was 60 mg once daily and the lower dose 30 mg once daily. This was the only trial allowing dose reduction (halving of the dose) both at screening and during follow-up when meeting the following prespecified criteria: (1) estimated Cr/Cl of 30–50 mL/min, (2) body weight 60 kg of less, or (3) the concomitant use of verapamil or quinidine (potent P-gp inhibitors). The primary efficacy endpoint in all trials was the composite of stroke or systemic embolism. In the ARISTOTLE and ENGAGE AF-TIMI 48 trials, the primary safety endpoint was major bleeding as defined by the International Society on Thrombosis and Haemostasis[59] while in ROCKET it was the composite of major and clinically relevant non-major bleeding. In all trials the primary efficacy and safety endpoints were adjudicated by an independent clinical adverse events committee. All trials were designed and powered to test for non-inferiority of FXa inhibitor compared with warfarin for stroke prevention as the primary efficacy endpoint. The median follow-up was 22 months in the ROCKET-AF and ARISTOTLE trials and 33 months in the ENGAGE-TIMI 48 trial.

The final results showed that all three FXa inhibitors were non-inferior to warfarin concerning stroke and systemic embolism. In addition, in the respective trials apixaban and edoxaban (60 mg) provided a significant 21% relative reduction in the composite of stroke and systemic embolism. This was mainly caused by a reduction in haemorrhagic stroke as there was no difference in ischaemic stroke in any trial comparing FXa inhibition with warfarin. However, the lower 30 mg daily dose of edoxaban was associated with a higher rate of ischaemic stroke than warfarin. All three FXa inhibitors lowered the risk of intracranial bleeding where there was a 33% relative reduction with rivaroxaban and a more than 50% relative reduction with apixaban and edoxaban. Major bleeding showed a 20% relative reduction with edoxaban 60 mg, 31% relative reduction with apixaban, and 43% relative reduction with edoxaban 30 mg as compared with warfarin. With rivaroxaban there was an increase in gastrointestinal bleeding and accordingly no significant difference in total major bleeding. Concerning total mortality there was a trend to reduction in all FXa inhibitor trials versus warfarin. A meta-analysis including patients from all the trials accordingly showed a significant reduction in total mortality with FXa inhibition as compared with warfarin in patients with atrial fibrillation and an increased risk of stroke.[57] Finally, there was no difference in compliance and adherence with FXa inhibitors and warfarin in the pivotal trials. In the real-life setting, the experiences show a better adherence with FXa inhibition than vitamin K antagonist despite the much less frequent monitoring needed during FXa inhibitor treatment. During the trials there was no significant difference in outcomes between the patients who had severe bleeding on a FXa inhibitor as compared with warfarin despite the lack of an antidote for anti-Xa inhibition during the trials. At present, rapid reversal of the anti Xa inhibitor effect can be accomplished by a specific FXa-antidote, which also lowers the risk of bleeding during surgical procedures and trauma.[60]

These results comparing FXa inhibitors with warfarin clearly established that patients with atrial fibrillation and an increased risk of stroke should preferably be treated with FXa inhibition and not with warfarin because of a substantial net benefit with at least similar protection against stroke, lower risk of intracranial bleeding, and better survival. When using apixaban or edoxaban 60 mg there is also a lower risk of total major bleeding. However, the lower edoxaban 30 mg dose is not recommended and not approved as it is associated with less protection against ischaemic stroke, which is the primary indication for oral anticoagulation in patients with atrial fibrillation. In addition to the improved cardiovascular outcomes, treatment with an oral FXa inhibitor is more convenient as it is given as a daily standard dose without any need for laboratory testing and as there are very few interactions with food or pharmaceutical agents. Furthermore, as FXa inhibitor treatment has a fairly short half-life, temporary cessation for surgical interventions is considerably shorter and safer than warfarin.

Since the presentation of these milestone results from the pivotal trials, a multitude of substudies on different subgroups have been presented. Overall, these studies show a robust consistency of the relative differences of the primary efficacy and safety results across almost all evaluated subgroups, procedures, co-medications, and clinical settings. Some uncertainties might remain in small parts of the populations, such as extremes of body weight, extremes of renal function, certain co-medications, etc. Ancillary studies have later been performed confirming the convenience, safety, and time saving of oral FXa inhibition at cardioversion and other elective cardiac procedures. Several trials have elucidated that, in patients with atrial fibrillation undergoing coronary stenting procedures, it is preferable to use a combination with only one rather the two platelet inhibitors for prevention of recurrences of coronary events.[61]

Factor Xa inhibitors for protection against ischaemic events in atherosclerotic vascular disease

In patients with atherosclerotic vascular disease there is often an indication for platelet inhibition with aspirin and/or a $P2Y_{12}$ inhibitor. The combination of platelet inhibition and oral anticoagulation is associated with a higher risk of bleeding than with either treatment alone. Combinations with more than one platelet inhibitor should generally be avoided because of a more pronounced risk of bleeding. So far only direct FXa inhibition with a low dose of rivaroxaban twice daily has been proven to provide incremental protection against ischaemic events in comparison with aspirin alone in patients with atherosclerotic cardiovascular disease. In the ATLAS-ACS-2-TIMI51 trial,[62] 15,526 patients with acute coronary syndrome treated with dual antiplatelet treatment were randomized to rivaroxaban 2.5–5.0 mg versus placebo twice daily. In this setting rivaroxaban was associated with a 16% relative and 1.8% absolute reduction in the risk of the composite endpoint of cardiovascular death, myocardial infarction, or stroke, but with a 1.5% absolute increase in major bleeding including intracranial haemorrhage. In the COMPASS trial,[63] 27,395 patients with stable atherosclerotic vascular disease were randomized to receive rivaroxaban (2.5 mg twice daily) plus aspirin (100 mg once daily), rivaroxaban (5 mg twice daily), or aspirin (100 mg once daily). The study was stopped for superiority of the rivaroxaban-plus-aspirin group after a mean follow-up of 23 months when there was a 24% relative and 1.3% absolute reduction in cardiovascular death, myocardial infarction, or stroke, and a 0.7% absolute reduction in total mortality at the cost of a

1.2% absolute increase in major bleeding in comparison to aspirin alone. There was no significant advantage of rivaroxaban alone versus aspirin alone concerning ischaemic events but a higher rate of major bleeding. The results were consistent in patients with coronary artery disease[64] and peripheral arterial disease,[65] where there also was a reduction in ischaemic limb events.

What's new

- Safe and effective in a daily standard dose without laboratory monitoring.
- No interaction with food and few interactions with other medications.
- Adherence and compliance similar or better than with warfarin.

Guideline recommendations

- Similar or better protection against stroke in atrial fibrillation than warfarin and much better protection than aspirin.
- Similar or better protection against venous thromboembolism than warfarin.
- Much lower risk of intracranial bleeding than warfarin (similar to aspirin).
- Improved long-term survival in atrial fibrillation as compared with warfarin or aspirin.
- Lower risk of major bleeding than warfarin (similar to aspirin) with apixaban or edoxaban.
- Combination with more than one platelet inhibitor should be avoided to reduce the risk of bleeding.
- Practical advantages and similar safety and efficacy at cardioversion and interventional procedures in patients with atrial fibrillation.
- Cost-effective, more convenient, and preferred by patients as compared with warfarin.

What's next

- Evaluation of new indications and combinations.
- Evaluation of dosing and duration at different comorbidities and procedures.
- Comparisons with FXIa inhibitors concerning efficacy and safety.

Drug dosing

- See ➔ Table 11.1 for dosing of different compounds in different settings.
- Dose adjustment needed in relation to renal function (test every year or at severe disease).
- Antidote for rapid reversal of anticoagulation available at urgent surgery or trauma.

References

1. Hoffman M, Monroe DM, 3rd. A cell-based model of hemostasis. Thromb Haemost. 2001;85(6):958–65.
2. Langer F, Ruf W. Synergies of phosphatidylserine and protein disulfide isomerase in tissue factor activation. Thromb Haemost. 2014;111(4):590–7.
3. Wood JP, Ellery PE, Maroney SA, Mast AE. Biology of tissue factor pathway inhibitor. Blood. 2014;123(19):2934–43.
4. Esmon CT. Regulation of blood coagulation. Biochim Biophys Acta. 2000;1477(1–2):349–60.
5. Krishnaswamy S. Exosite-driven substrate specificity and function in coagulation. J Thromb Haemost. 2005;3(1):54–67.
6. Nar H. The role of structural information in the discovery of direct thrombin and factor Xa inhibitors. Trends Pharmacol Sci. 2012;33(5):279–88.
7. Mann KG, Brummel K, Butenas S. What is all that thrombin for? J Thromb Haemost. 2003;1(7):1504–14.
8. Chaudhary R, Sharma T, Garg J, et al. Direct oral anticoagulants: a review on the current role and scope of reversal agents. J Thromb Thrombolysis. 2020;49(2):271–86.
9. Yeh CH, Fredenburgh JC, Weitz JI. Oral direct factor Xa inhibitors. Circ Res. 2012;111(8):1069–78.
10. Jiang X, Crain EJ, Luettgen JM, Schumacher WA, Wong PC. Apixaban, an oral direct factor Xa inhibitor, inhibits human clot-bound factor Xa activity in vitro. Thromb Haemost. 2009;101(4):780–2.
11. Steinberg BA, Becker RC. Structure-function relationships of factor Xa inhibitors: implications for the practicing clinician. J Thromb Thrombolysis. 2014;37(2):234–41.
12. Lassen M, Davidson BL, Gallus A, Pineo G, Ansell J, Deitchman D. A phase II randomized, double-blind, five-arm, parallel-group, dose-response study of a new oral directly-acting factor Xa inhibitor, Razaxaban, for the prevention of deep vein thrombosis in knee replacement surgery—on behalf of the Razaxaban investigators. Blood. 2003;102:Abstract 41.
13. Steg PG, Mehta SR, Pollack CV Jr, et al. Anticoagulation with otamixaban and ischemic events in non-ST-segment elevation acute coronary syndromes: the TAO randomized clinical trial. JAMA. 2013;310(11):1145–55.
14. Lip GY, Halperin JL, Petersen P, Rodgers GM, Pall D, Renfurm RW. A phase II, double-blind, randomized, parallel group, dose-finding study of the safety and tolerability of darexaban compared with warfarin in patients with non-valvular atrial fibrillation: the oral factor Xa inhibitor for prophylaxis of stroke in atrial fibrillation study 2 (OPAL-2). J Thromb Haemost. 2015;13(8):1405–13.
15. Perzborn E, Strassburger J, Wilmen A, et al. In vitro and in vivo studies of the novel antithrombotic agent BAY 59–7939--an oral, direct factor Xa inhibitor. J Thromb Haemost. 2005;3(3):514–21.
16. Byon W, Garonzik S, Boyd RA, Frost CE. Apixaban: a clinical pharmacokinetic and pharmacodynamic review. Clin Pharmacokinet. 2019;58(10):1265–79.
17. Luettgen JM, Knabb RM, He K, Pinto DJ, Rendina AR. Apixaban inhibition of factor Xa: microscopic rate constants and inhibition mechanism in purified protein systems and in human plasma. J Enzyme Inhib Med Chem. 2011;26(4):514–26.
18. Frost C, Wang J, Nepal S, et al. Apixaban, an oral, direct factor Xa inhibitor: single dose safety, pharmacokinetics, pharmacodynamics and food effect in healthy subjects. Br J Clin Pharmacol. 2013;75(2):476–87.

19. Mavrakanas TA, Samer CF, Nessim SJ, Frisch G, Lipman ML. Apixaban pharmacokinetics at steady state in hemodialysis patients. J Am Soc Nephrol. 2017;28(7):2241–8.
20. Wang X, Tirucherai G, Marbury TC, et al. Pharmacokinetics, pharmacodynamics, and safety of apixaban in subjects with end-stage renal disease on hemodialysis. J Clin Pharmacol. 2016;56(5):628–36.
21. Furugohri T, Isobe K, Honda Y, et al. DU-176b, a potent and orally active factor Xa inhibitor: in vitro and in vivo pharmacological profiles. J Thromb Haemost. 2008;6(9):1542–9.
22. Bohula EA, Giugliano RP, Ruff CT, et al. Impact of renal function on outcomes with edoxaban in the ENGAGE AF-TIMI 48 trial. Circulation. 2016;134(1):24–36.
23. Chan NC, Hirsh J, Ginsberg JS, Eikelboom JW. Betrixaban (PRT054021): pharmacology, dose selection and clinical studies. Future Cardiol. 2014;10(1):43–52.
24. Cohen AT, Harrington RA, Goldhaber SZ, et al. Extended thromboprophylaxis with betrixaban in acutely ill medical patients. N Engl J Med. 2016;375(6):534–44.
25. Steffel J, Collins R, Antz M, et al. 2021 European Heart Rhythm Association practical guide on the use of non-vitamin K antagonist oral anticoagulants in patients with atrial fibrillation. Europace. 2021;23(10):1612–76.
26. Vazquez SR. Drug-drug interactions in an era of multiple anticoagulants: a focus on clinically relevant drug interactions. Blood. 2018;132(21):2230–9.
27. Hoirisch-Clapauch S, Nardi AE, Gris JC, Brenner B. Are the antiplatelet and profibrinolytic properties of selective serotonin-reuptake inhibitors relevant to their brain effects? Thromb Res. 2014;134(1):11–6.
28. Kumar S, Danik SB, Altman RK, et al. Non-vitamin K antagonist oral anticoagulants and antiplatelet therapy for stroke prevention in patients with atrial fibrillation: a meta-analysis of randomized controlled trials. Cardiol Rev. 2016;24(5):218–23.
29. Wiggins BS, Dixon DL, Neyens RR, Page RL, 2nd, Gluckman TJ. Select drug-drug interactions with direct oral anticoagulants: JACC review topic of the week. J Am Coll Cardiol. 2020;75(11):1341–50.
30. Khan F, Tritschler T, Kahn SR, Rodger MA. Venous thromboembolism. Lancet. 2021;398(10294):64–77.
31. Eriksson BI, Quinlan DJ, Eikelboom JW. Novel oral factor Xa and thrombin inhibitors in the management of thromboembolism. Annu Rev Med. 2011;62:41–57.
32. Quinlan DJ, Eriksson BI. Novel oral anticoagulants for thromboprophylaxis after orthopaedic surgery. Best Pract Res Clin Haematol. 2013;26(2):171–82.
33. Agnelli G, Buller HR, Cohen A, et al. Oral apixaban for the treatment of acute venous thromboembolism. N Engl J Med. 2013;369(9):799–808.
34. Bauersachs R, Berkowitz SD, Brenner B, et al. Oral rivaroxaban for symptomatic venous thromboembolism. N Engl J Med. 2010;363(26):2499–510.
35. Büller HR, Décousus H, Grosso MA, et al. Edoxaban versus warfarin for the treatment of symptomatic venous thromboembolism. N Engl J Med. 2013;369(15):1406–15.
36. Büller HR, Prins MH, Lensin AW, et al. Oral rivaroxaban for the treatment of symptomatic pulmonary embolism. N Engl J Med. 2012;366(14):1287–97.
37. Cohen AT, Hamilton M, Mitchell SA, et al. Comparison of the novel oral anticoagulants apixaban, dabigatran, edoxaban, and rivaroxaban in the initial and long-term treatment and prevention of venous thromboembolism: systematic review and network meta-analysis. PLoS One. 2015;10(12):e0144856.
38. Stevens SM, Woller SC, Baumann Kreuziger L, et al. Executive summary: antithrombotic therapy for VTE disease: second update of the CHEST Guideline and Expert Panel Report. Chest. 2021;160(6):2247–59.
39. Huisman MV, Klok FA. Pharmacological properties of betrixaban. Eur Heart J Suppl. 2018;20(Suppl E):E12–5.
40. Male C, Lensing AWA, Palumbo JS, et al. Rivaroxaban compared with standard anticoagulants for the treatment of acute venous thromboembolism in children: a randomised, controlled, phase 3 trial. Lancet Haematol. 2020;7(1):e18–27.
41. Giustozzi M, Agnelli G, Del Toro-Cervera J, et al. Direct oral anticoagulants for the treatment of acute venous thromboembolism associated with cancer: a systematic review and meta-analysis. Thromb Haemost. 2020;120(7):1128–36.
42. January CT, Wann LS, Alpert JS, et al. 2014 AHA/ACC/HRS guideline for the management of patients with atrial fibrillation: executive summary: a report of the American College of Cardiology/American Heart Association Task Force on practice guidelines and the Heart Rhythm Society. Circulation. 2014;130(23):2071–104.
43. Kirchhof P, Benussi S, Kotecha D, et al. 2016 ESC Guidelines for the management of atrial fibrillation developed in collaboration with EACTS. Eur Heart J. 2016;37(38):2893–962.
44. Steffel J, Verhamme P, Potpara TS, et al. The 2018 European Heart Rhythm Association Practical guide on the use of non-vitamin K antagonist oral anticoagulants in patients with atrial fibrillation. Eur Heart J. 2018;39(16):1330–93.
45. Connolly SJ, Ezekowitz MD, Yusuf S, et al. Dabigatran versus warfarin in patients with atrial fibrillation. N Engl J Med. 2009;361(12):1139–51.
46. Patel MR, Mahaffey KW, Garg J, et al. Rivaroxaban versus warfarin in nonvalvular atrial fibrillation. N Engl J Med. 2011;365(10):883–91.
47. Granger CB, Alexander JH, McMurray JJ, et al. Apixaban versus warfarin in patients with atrial fibrillation. N Engl J Med. 2011;365(11):981–92.
48. Giugliano RP, Ruff CT, Braunwald E, et al. Edoxaban versus warfarin in patients with atrial fibrillation. N Engl J Med. 2013;369(22):2093–104.
49. Connolly SJ, Eikelboom J, Joyner C, et al. Apixaban in patients with atrial fibrillation. N Engl J Med. 2011;364(9):806–17.
50. Ezekowitz MD, Connolly S, Parekh A, et al. Rationale and design of RE-LY: randomized evaluation of long-term anticoagulant therapy, warfarin, compared with dabigatran. Am Heart J. 2009;157(5):805–10.
51. ROCKET AF Study Investigators. Rivaroxaban-once daily, oral, direct factor Xa inhibition compared with vitamin K antagonism for prevention of stroke and Embolism Trial in Atrial Fibrillation: rationale and design of the ROCKET AF study. Am Heart J. 2010;159(3):340–7.e1.
52. Lopes RD, Alexander JH, Al-Khatib SM, et al. Apixaban for reduction in stroke and other thromboembolic events in atrial fibrillation (ARISTOTLE) trial: design and rationale. Am Heart J. 2010;159(3):331–9.
53. Ruff CT, Giugliano RP, Antman EM, et al. Evaluation of the novel factor Xa inhibitor edoxaban compared with warfarin in patients with atrial fibrillation: design and rationale for the Effective aNticoaGulation with factor xA next GEneration in Atrial Fibrillation-Thrombolysis In Myocardial Infarction study 48 (ENGAGE AF-TIMI 48). Am Heart J. 2010;160(4):635–41.
54. Ruff CT, Giugliano RP, Braunwald E, et al. Comparison of the efficacy and safety of new oral anticoagulants with warfarin in patients with atrial fibrillation: a meta-analysis of randomised trials. Lancet. 2014;383(9921):955–62.

55. Pan KL, Singer DE, Ovbiagele B, Wu YL, Ahmed MA, Lee M. Effects of non-vitamin K antagonist oral anticoagulants versus warfarin in patients with atrial fibrillation and valvular heart disease: a systematic review and meta-analysis. J Am Heart Assoc. 2017;6(7):e005835.
56. Savarese G, Giugliano RP, Rosano GM, et al. Efficacy and safety of novel oral anticoagulants in patients with atrial fibrillation and heart failure: a meta-analysis. JACC Heart Fail. 2016;4(11):870–80.
57. Carnicelli AP, Hong H, Connolly SJ, et al. Direct oral anticoagulants versus warfarin in patients with atrial fibrillation: patient-level network meta-analyses of randomized clinical trials with interaction testing by age and sex. Circulation. 2022;145(4):242–55.
58. Eikelboom JW, O'Donnell M, Yusuf S, et al. Rationale and design of AVERROES: apixaban versus acetylsalicylic acid to prevent stroke in atrial fibrillation patients who have failed or are unsuitable for vitamin K antagonist treatment. Am Heart J. 2010;159(3):348–53.e1.
59. Schulman S, Kearon C, Subcommittee on Control of Anticoagulation of the Scientific and Standardization Committee of the International Society on Thrombosis and Haemostasis. Definition of major bleeding in clinical investigations of antihemostatic medicinal products in non-surgical patients. J Thromb Haemost. 2005;3(4):692–4.
60. Connolly SJ, Milling TJ Jr, Eikelboom JW, et al. Andexanet alfa for acute major bleeding associated with factor Xa inhibitors. N Engl J Med. 2016;375(12):1131–41.
61. Alexander JH, Lopes RD, James S, et al. Apixaban with antiplatelet therapy after acute coronary syndrome. N Engl J Med. 2011;365(8):699–708.
62. Mega JL, Braunwald E, Wiviott SD, et al. Rivaroxaban in patients with a recent acute coronary syndrome. N Engl J Med. 2012;366(1):9–19.
63. Eikelboom JW, Connolly SJ, Bosch J, et al. Rivaroxaban with or without aspirin in stable cardiovascular disease. N Engl J Med. 2017;377(14):1319–30.
64. Connolly SJ, Eikelboom JW, Bosch J, et al. Rivaroxaban with or without aspirin in patients with stable coronary artery disease: an international, randomised, double-blind, placebo-controlled trial. Lancet. 2018;391(10117):205–18.
65. Anand SS, Bosch J, Eikelboom JW, et al. Rivaroxaban with or without aspirin in patients with stable peripheral or carotid artery disease: an international, randomised, double-blind, placebo-controlled trial. Lancet. 2018;391(10117):219–29.

CHAPTER 12

Forthcoming oral factor XIa and factor XIIa inhibitors

James C. Fredenburgh and Jeffrey I. Weitz

Contents

Summary

Oral anticoagulants are a mainstay for the prevention and treatment of arterial and venous thrombosis. Direct oral anticoagulants (DOACs) have replaced vitamin K antagonists for many indications. Currently available DOACs include dabigatran, which inhibits thrombin, and apixaban, edoxaban, and rivaroxaban, which inhibit factor (F)-Xa. A new class of DOACs is under development. These new DOACs, which include asundexian and milvexian, inhibit FXIa, which is positioned in the intrinsic pathway of coagulation. Anticoagulants that target FXIa have the potential to be safer than the current DOACs because there is emerging evidence that FXI is essential for thrombosis but mostly dispensable for haemostasis. In addition to the oral inhibitors of FXIa, parenteral inhibitors also are under development. These include fesomersen, an antisense oligonucleotide that reduces the hepatic synthesis of FXI, abelacimab, an antibody that binds FXI and blocks its activation, and osocimab, an FXIa inhibitory antibody. FXII inhibitors, which may be even safer than those that target FXI, are at an earlier stage of development. Focusing on these new agents, this chapter (1) describes the unmet needs in oral anticoagulation therapy, (2) explains why FXI and FXII are promising targets for new oral anticoagulants, (3) reviews the clinical data with the new agents, and (4) provides perspective on the opportunities and challenges for oral FXIa and FXIIa inhibitors.

Introduction

Oral anticoagulants are a cornerstone for the prevention and treatment of arterial and venous thrombosis. The currently available direct oral anticoagulants (DOACs), which came to the market in 2010, have taken over from the vitamin K antagonists (VKAs) for many indications because they are at least as effective for stroke prevention in patients with atrial fibrillation (AF) and treatment of venous thromboembolism (VTE), and are associated with a lower risk of serious bleeding, particularly intracranial haemorrhage.[1,2] Furthermore, DOACs are more convenient to administer than VKAs because they can be given in fixed doses without the need for routine coagulation monitoring. With the current DOACs now firmly entrenched and with their uptake increasing with the introduction of generic versions, never have the hurdles for the development of new oral anticoagulants been higher.

Whereas VKAs and current DOACs target the distal end of the coagulation system, newer agents targeting upstream factors in the contact pathway are under development. Thus, two oral factor (F)-XIa inhibitors are under evaluation in phase III programmes, and efforts to develop oral FXIIa inhibitors are continuing. Focusing on these new agents, this chapter (1) describes the unmet needs in oral anticoagulation therapy, (2) explains why FXI and FXII are promising targets for new oral anticoagulants, (3) reviews the clinical data available thus far with the new agents, and (4) provides perspective on the opportunities and challenges for oral FXIa and FXIIa inhibitors.

Unmet needs in oral anticoagulation therapy

The goal of anticoagulation therapy is to attenuate thrombosis with minimal disruption of haemostasis. Although the current DOACs come closer to this goal than VKAs, bleeding is not eliminated with the current DOACs. Thus, even with the current DOACs, the annual rate of major bleeding in patients with AF is 2–3%, while the annual rate of intracranial bleeding is 0.3–0.5%.[1] The fear of bleeding explains at least in part why at least one-third of patients with AF fail to receive anticoagulant prophylaxis and among those given anticoagulation therapy,[3] up to 50% are inappropriately treated with lower doses of the current DOACs.[4] Therefore, there remains a need for safer anticoagulants. FXI and FXII are the targets for these new agents.

Factor XI and factor XII as targets

The current DOACs target FXa or thrombin, which are enzymes in the common pathway of coagulation that are essential for fibrin formation. Because they attenuate fibrin formation, the current DOACs are effective for the prevention and treatment of thrombosis. However, fibrin is a major component of physiological haemostatic plugs as well as pathological thrombi. Therefore, it is not surprising that current DOACs are associated with a risk of bleeding. To circumvent inhibition of enzymes in the common pathway, upstream factors in the contact and intrinsic pathways are being examined as new targets for anticoagulation. The focus on FXII and FXI stemmed from studies in animals that suggest that these factors are important in thrombosis but are dispensable for haemostasis. Consequently, by uncoupling thrombosis and haemostasis, inhibitors of FXII and FXI have the potential to be safer than the current DOACs.

FXII or FXI inhibitors can uncouple thrombosis and haemostasis because even though thrombin generation and fibrin formation are hallmarks of both processes, the pathways for thrombin generation and the sites of thrombus formation differ.[5] Thrombosis involves the formation of an intravascular thrombus that blocks blood flow in arteries or veins. In contrast, haemostasis is a predominantly extravascular process that culminates in the formation of a haemostatic plug that stops the leakage of blood from a damaged blood vessel (➔ Figure 12.1).

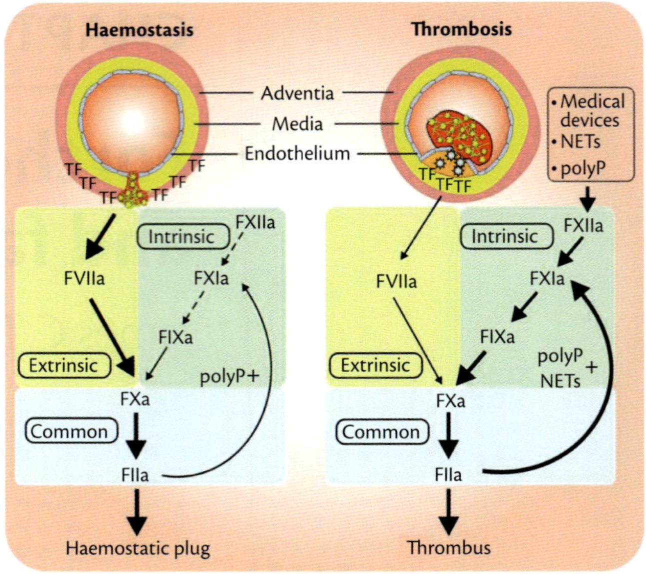

Figure 12.1 Separating haemostasis from thrombosis. Blood vessels are surrounded by a haemostatic envelope of tissue factor (TF) in the adventitia. Haemostasis is triggered when the adventitia is breached by vessel injury. The high concentrations of TF surrounding the vessel initiate explosive thrombin generation via the extrinsic pathway (yellow) leading to the formation of a haemostatic plug that seals the leak. FXII is dispensable for haemostasis and feedback activation of FXI by thrombin is of minor importance for amplification of thrombin generation. Thrombosis is initiated by lower concentrations of TF exposed at the site of atherosclerotic plaque rupture or on activated monocytes or microvesicles. The initial small amounts of thrombin produced in the common pathway (blue) feed back to activate FXI when stimulated by polyphosphates (polyP) or neutrophil extracellular traps (NETs). These polyanions and blood contacting medical devices can also bind to FXII and induce its autoactivation. FXIIa then activates FXI to trigger the generation of thrombin via the intrinsic pathway (green).

Reproduced from Fredenburgh JC, Weitz JI. Factor XI as a Target for New Anticoagulants. Hamostaseologie. 2021 Apr;41(2):104–110. doi: 10.1055/a-1384-3715 with permission from Thieme.

Thrombosis is usually triggered by tissue factor (TF) exposed on disrupted atherosclerotic plaques or expressed on leucocytes or extracellular vesicles tethered to the activated endothelium. TF binds circulating FVII or FVIIa and the TF–FVIIa complex activates FX to FXa, which then converts a limited amount of prothrombin into thrombin. This small amount of thrombin initiates fibrin formation and, along with FXa, provides positive feedback by activating the key cofactor proteins, FV and FVIII. The TF–FVIIa complex also activates FIX, and the resultant FIXa, together with its cofactor FVIIIa, amplifies FXa and thrombin generation. Once the thrombus expands beyond the site of injury, the TF–FVIIa complex can no longer sustain thrombus growth. Instead, back activation of FXI by thrombin drives further thrombin generation and thrombus expansion.

FXI can be activated by FXIIa as well as by thrombin. FXII is activated when the blood contacts medical devices such as central venous catheters, mechanical heart valves, or dialysis membranes, and the resultant FXIIa can initiate thrombosis by activating FXI and inducing thrombin generation. In addition to its activation by medical devices, FXII can be activated by naturally occurring polyanions such as neutrophil extracellular traps, inorganic polyphosphate released from activated platelets, or DNA or RNA released from dead or dying cells. The contribution of these polyanions to thrombosis in humans, however, is uncertain.

In contrast to thrombosis where there is intravascular thrombus formation, haemostasis is a predominantly extravascular event that is initiated when the TF surrounding blood vessels is exposed to blood by outside-in damage to the vessel wall. The high concentrations of TF in the haemostatic envelope trigger explosive thrombin generation. FXII activation is not part of this process, which explains why subjects with congenital FXII deficiency do not experience excessive bleeding. Likewise, FXI is mostly dispensable for haemostasis because feedback activation of FXI by thrombin is rarely needed to sustain the formation of the haemostatic plug. Consequently, spontaneous bleeding is rare in patients with congenital FXI deficiency and correlates poorly with FXI levels. Furthermore, when bleeding occurs, it is usually mild, and bleeding after surgery is often localized to the oropharynx or the urinary tract where there is abundant fibrinolytic activity. The spontaneous bleeds into muscles or joints, and the life-threatening intracranial or gastrointestinal bleeding that are characteristics of haemophilia A or B, do not occur with FXI deficiency. Therefore, although essential for thrombosis, FXI is mostly dispensable for haemostasis. The observations of absent to mild bleeding diatheses associated with deficiencies of FXII and FXI are central to development of anticoagulants targeting these factors.

Factor XI or factor XII, which is the better target?

The pros and cons of FXI and FXII as targets are listed in ➔ Table 12.1. FXII is a safer target than FXI because congenital FXII deficiency is not associated with bleeding, whereas FXI deficiency is associated with a mild bleeding diathesis. Nonetheless, most of the attention has focused on FXI inhibition because of concerns about the contribution of FXII to thrombosis initiated by TF and because of the weak epidemiological data linking FXII with thrombosis.

FXII is an important driver of clotting on blood-contacting medical devices or extracorporeal circuits because thrombosis on artificial surfaces is initiated by FXII activation. If thrombosis is triggered by TF, however, feedback activation of FXI by thrombin would bypass inhibition of FXII, thereby rendering FXII inhibitors ineffective. In contrast, regardless of whether thrombosis is driven by contact of the blood with medical devices or by TF, FXI plays a central part because of its activation by both FXIIa and thrombin. Therefore, FXI appears to be a more important modulator of thrombosis than FXI.

Epidemiological, Mendelian randomization, and genome-wide association studies reveal links between FXI levels and thrombosis, whereas no such link exists for FXII.[6–8] In epidemiological studies, congenital FXI deficiency is protective against VTE, ischaemic stroke, and, at least in one study, myocardial infarction (MI).[9–11] In contrast, FXII deficiency is not protective, and may even be associated with an increased risk of VTE. Mendelian randomization studies suggest that subjects with higher FXI levels are more prone to ischaemic stroke and VTE than those with normal FXI levels, whereas those with lower FXI are at reduced risk. Furthermore, the extent of elevation in FXI levels correlates with stroke risk in women taking oral contraceptives. Whereas FXI levels correlate with the risk of thrombosis, there is a poor correlation with the risk of bleeding.[12,13] Although bleeding is not an issue with FXII deficiency, FXII levels are not associated with the risk of thrombotic disorders,[14] and there are some reports of increased thrombosis in patients with congenital FXII deficiency.[6] Therefore, epidemiological studies support the role of FXI in thrombosis, but not FXII. Consequently, FXI has emerged as the preferred target for new anticoagulants.

Clinical evaluation of new anticoagulants usually starts in patients undergoing elective hip or knee replacement surgery because of their risk of postoperative deep vein thrombosis that can be efficiently detected on venography. The first-generation antisense oligonucleotide,[15] osocimab, a monoclonal antibody that inhibits FXIa,[16] abelacimab,[17] an antibody that binds to FXI and prevents its activation by FXIIa or thrombin, and milvexian, an oral FXIa inhibitor,[18] have been compared with enoxaparin in such patients in phase II proof-of-concept studies. Exploratory meta-analyses using postoperative VTE and clinically relevant bleeding (the composite of major and clinically relevant non-major bleeding) for the efficacy and safety analysis, respectively, reported a 40–50% reduction in VTE with FXI inhibition compared with enoxaparin and a 59% reduction in bleeding.[19]

Table 12.1 Relative advantages and disadvantages of factor XII or factor XI as targets for new anticoagulants

	Factor XII	Factor XI
Epidemiological data	Weak	Strong
Risk of bleeding	None	Low
Level of evidence for role in thrombosis	Preclinical	Phase II and early phase III
Potential for bypassing inhibition	Thrombin-mediated activation of FXI could bypass FXII inhibition	None
Potential for off-target effects	May modulate inflammation by inhibiting kinin generation	Unlikely

Source data from Fredenburgh JC, Weitz JI. Factor XI as a target for new anticoagulants. Hamostaseologie. 2021;41(2):104–110. doi: 10.1055/a-1384-3715.

Once proof of concept was shown, attention shifted from thromboprophylaxis to indications with greater unmet needs. In separate, phase II studies, fesomersen, a second-generation ligand-conjugated antisense oligonucleotide targeting FXI, and osocimab were compared with a placebo in patients with end-stage kidney disease undergoing haemodialysis, a population at high risk for atherothrombotic complications and bleeding. Although the results have not been reported, both studies went to completion, and fesomersen was reported to be safe and well tolerated. Therefore, phase II studies with parenteral FXI inhibitors support the concept that FXI inhibition is both effective and safe, thereby setting the stage for trials with oral FXI inhibitors.

Oral factor XIa inhibitors

The oral FXIa inhibitors in the most advanced stage of development are asundexian (BAY 2433334)[20] and milvexian (BMS-986177/JNJ-70033093).[21,22] Both are small molecules that bind reversibly to the active site of FXIa and inhibit its activity. As illustrated in ➔ Table 12.2, asundexian and milvexian are rapidly absorbed after oral administration, and have half-lives that permit once- or twice-daily oral dosing. The specificity of asundexian and milvexian for FXIa is highlighted by the fact that they prolong the activated partial thromboplastin time in a dose-dependent manner but have no effect on the prothrombin time. Asundexian and milvexian are both moving forward into phase III based on the results of the phase II trials (➔ Table 12.3). Details of the trials with the oral agents targeting FXIa are outlined below.

Asundexian

PACIFIC-AF

The Safety of the Oral Factor XIa Inhibitor Asundexian Compared with Apixaban in Patients with Atrial Fibrillation (PACIFIC-AF)[23] randomized, double-blind, double-dummy, phase II trial enrolled 862 patients with AF who were 45 years of age or older and were at increased bleeding risk. Participants were randomized to receive asundexian at doses of 20 mg or 50 mg once daily, or apixaban 5 mg twice daily with a dose reduction to 2.5 mg twice daily according to the usual criteria. The primary outcome of the trial was the composite of major or clinically relevant non-major bleeds, based on the International Society on Thrombosis and Haemostasis (ISTH) criteria.

Of a total of 753 patients included in the final analysis, 249 and 254 received the 20 mg and 50 mg doses of asundexian, respectively, and 250 received apixaban. With the 20 mg asundexian dose there was 90% and 81% inhibition of FXIa activity at peak and trough, respectively, whereas with the 50 mg dose there was 94% and 92% FXIa inhibition at peak and trough, respectively. There were no major bleeds with asundexian or apixaban. Clinically relevant non-major bleeds occurred in three patients in the 20 mg asundexian group, one patient in the 50 mg asundexian group, and six patients in the apixaban group yielding incidence ratios of 0.50 for asundexian 20 mg [90% confidence interval (CI) 0.09–0.97], 0.16 for asundexian 50 mg (90% CI 0.01–0.99), and 0.33 for both asundexian doses (90% CI 0.09–0.97). Adverse events occurred in 47% of patients in each asundexian group and in 49% of patients in the apixaban group. The study was underpowered for efficacy; the efficacy outcome, a composite of ischaemic stroke, systemic embolism, MI, or cardiovascular death occurred in two, four, and three patients in the asundexian 20 mg, asundexian 50 mg, and apixaban groups, respectively. Therefore, at doses of 20 mg or 50 mg once daily, asundexian was associated with less bleeding than apixaban.

Table 12.2 Pharmacological properties of asundexian and milvexian

Characteristic	Asundexian	Milvexian
Molecular weight (Da)	593	626
Tmax (hours)	2–4	2–4
Food effect	Minimal	Modest
Half-life (hours)	14–17	8–14
Renal elimination (%)	14	18
Dose-proportional exposure	Yes	Yes
CYP3A4 interaction	No	Yes

CYP, cytochrome P450; Da, Dalton; Tmax, time to maximal concentration.

PACIFIC-AMI

The goal of the Proper Dosing and Safety of the Oral FXIa Inhibitor BAY 2433334 in Patients Following an Acute Heart Attack (PACIFIC-AMI)[24] double-blind phase II trial was to assess the safety and efficacy of three doses of asundexian compared with a placebo in patients with acute MI who were treated with dual antiplatelet therapy. A total of 1601 patients were randomized in a 1:1:1:1 manner to either asundexian 50 mg once daily (n = 402), asundexian 20 mg once daily (n = 401), asundexian 10 mg once daily (n = 397), or placebo (n = 401). All patients were on aspirin (81 mg once daily) and a $P2Y_{12}$ inhibitor; ticagrelor or prasugrel was used by 80% of the patients. Over 99% of patients underwent a percutaneous coronary intervention for their index event, which was an ST-elevation MI in 52% and non-ST-elevation MI in the remainder.

Asundexian inhibited FXIa in a dose-dependent manner, and there was over 90% inhibition with the 50 mg asundexian dose. The primary safety outcome, Bleeding Academic Research Consortium (BARC) 2, 3, or 5 bleeding at 6 months, occurred in 10.5%, 8.1%, and 7.6% of patients in the asundexian 50 mg, 20 mg, and 10 mg groups, respectively, and in 9.0% of those in the placebo group. Two patients in the asundexian 50 mg group and one in the placebo group had an intracerebral haemorrhage. The primary efficacy outcome, a composite of cardiovascular death, MI, stroke, and stent thrombosis, occurred in 5.5%, 6.0%, and 6.8% of patients in the asundexian 50 mg, 20 mg, and 10 mg groups, respectively, and in 5.5% of those in the placebo group. Therefore, asundexian in addition to dual antiplatelet therapy among patients undergoing percutaneous coronary intervention for MI did not significantly increase bleeding compared with the placebo. Recurrent ischaemic events were infrequent, but there

Table 12.3 Summary of phase II trials with asundexian and milvexian

Trial	N	Eligibility	Experimental	Control	Efficacy		Safety	
					Definition (composite)	**Result**	**Definition (composite)**	**Result**
PACIFIC-AF	755	Age ≥45 years, AF, CHA_2DS_2-VASc score ≥2 if male or ≥3 if female, increased bleeding risk	Asundexian 20 or 50 mg OD	Apixaban 5 mg BD (2.5 mg BD if criteria met for dose reduction)	Ischaemic stroke, systemic embolism, MI, or CV death	Asundexian 20 mg OD: 2 events, asundexian 50 mg OD: 4 events, vs apixaban: 3 events	ISTH major or clinically relevant non-major bleeding	Asundexian 20 mg OD: 1.2%, asundexian 50 mg OD: 0.4%, vs apixaban: 2.4%
PACIFIC-Stroke	1808	Age ≥45 years, non-cardioembolic ischaemic stroke, to be treated with antiplatelet therapy, able to have MRI	Asundexian 10, 20, or 50 mg OD	Placebo	Ischaemic stroke or covert infarction detected by MRI	Asundexian 10 mg OD: 19%, asundexian 20 mg OD: 22%, asundexian 50 mg OD: 20%, vs placebo 19%	ISTH major or clinically relevant non-major bleeding	Asundexian 10 mg OD: 4%, asundexian 20 mg OD: 3%, asundexian 50 mg OD: 4%, vs placebo 2%
PACIFIC-MI	1601	Within 5 days of acute MI	Asundexian 10, 20, or 50 mg OD	Placebo	CV death, MI, stroke, stent thrombosis	Asundexian 10 mg OD: 6.8%, asundexian 20 mg OD: 6.0%, asundexian 50 mg OD: 5.5%, vs placebo 5.5%	BARC 2, 3, or 5 bleeding	Asundexian 10 mg OD: 7.6%, asundexian 20 mg OD: 8.1%, asundexian 50 mg OD: 10.5%, vs placebo: 9.0%
AXIOMATIC-SSP	2366	Non-cardio-embolic ischaemic stroke or TIA	Milvexian 25 mg OD or 25, 50, 100 or 200 mg BD	Placebo	Ischaemic stroke or covert infarction detected by MRI	Milvexian 25 mg OD: 16.2%, milvexian 25 mg BD: 18.5%, milvexian 50 mg BD: 14.1%, milvexian 100 mg BD: 14.8%, milvexian 200 mg BD: 16.4%, placebo: 16.6%	BARC 3 or 5 bleeding	Milvexian 25 mg OD: 0.6%, milvexian 25 mg BD: 0.6%, milvexian 50 mg BD: 1.5%, milvexian 100 mg BD: 1.6%, milvexian 200 mg BD: 1.5%, vs placebo: 0.6%

AF, atrial fibrillation; BARC, Bleeding Academic Research Consortium; BD, twice daily; CV, cardiovascular; ISTH, International Society on Thrombosis and Haemostasis; MI, myocardial infarction; MRI, magnetic resonance imaging; OD, once daily; TIA, transient ischaemic attack.
Source date from Weitz JI, Eikelboom JW. What is the future of factor XI inhibitors? Circulation. 2022;146(25):1899–902.

was no significant difference between the rates with asundexian and placebo.

PACIFIC-Stroke

The Factor XIa Inhibition with Asundexian After Acute Non-cardioembolic Ischemic Stroke (PACIFIC-Stroke) trial[25] was undertaken to assess the safety and efficacy of three once-daily doses of asundexian compared with a placebo in patients with non-cardioembolic ischaemic stroke who were enrolled within 48 hours from symptom onset. A total of 1808 patients were randomized in a double-blind 1:1:1:1 manner to either asundexian 50 mg (n = 447), asundexian 20 mg (n = 450), asundexian 10 mg (n = 455), or placebo (n = 456). Treatments were given for 6 months.

The primary efficacy outcome, the composite of ischaemic stroke or covert stroke on repeat imaging at 6 months, occurred in 20.1%, 22.0%, and 18.9% in the asundexian 50 mg, 20 mg, and 10 mg treatment groups, respectively, and in 19.1% of those given placebo. The principal safety outcome, the composite of major or clinically relevant non-major bleeding, occurred in 4.3%, 3.1%, and 4.3% in the asundexian 50 mg, 20 mg, and 10 mg treatment groups, respectively, and in 2.4% of those given placebo. In a post hoc analysis, recurrent ischaemic stroke or transient ischaemic attack (TIA) occurred in 5.4%, 6.2%, and 7.7% in the asundexian 50 mg, 20 mg, and 10 mg treatment groups, respectively, and in 8.3% of those given placebo. The hazard ratio for asundexian 50 mg versus placebo was 0.64 (95% CI 0.41–0.98). Rates of haemorrhagic transformation in the 50 mg, 20 mg, and 10 mg asundexian groups were 1.4%, 1.1%, and 0.4%, respectively. There were no haemorrhagic transformations in the placebo group.

Therefore, asundexian was not associated with an increase in bleeding. Although asundexian did not reduce the composite of covert brain infarction or ischaemic stroke compared with placebo, there appeared to be a reduction in recurrent symptomatic ischaemic stroke or TIA in the asundexian 50 mg group compared with placebo, particularly among patients with atherosclerosis.

Milvexian

AXIOMATIC TKR

The goal of the Antithrombotic Treatment with Factor XIa Inhibition to Optimize Management of Acute Thromboembolic Events in Total Knee Replacement (AXIOMATIC TKR)[18] proof-of-principle study was to demonstrate that milvexian has antithrombotic activity. A total of 1242 patients undergoing knee arthroplasty were randomized to one of seven postoperative regimens of milvexian (25 mg, 50 mg, 100 mg, or 200 mg twice daily or 25 mg, 50 mg, or 200 mg once daily) or enoxaparin (40 mg once daily). The primary efficacy outcome was VTE, the composite of fatal or non-fatal pulmonary and symptomatic or asymptomatic deep vein thrombosis. With twice-daily dosing, VTE occurred in 27 of 129 patients (21%) taking 25 mg, in 14 of 124 (11%) taking 50 mg, in 12 of 134 (9%) taking 100 mg, and in 10 of 131 (8%) taking 200 mg, while with once-daily dosing, VTE occurred in 7 of 28 (25%) taking 25 mg, in 30 of 127 (24%) taking 50 mg, and in 8 of 123 (7%) taking 200 mg. In those given enoxaparin, VTE occurred in 54 of 252 patients (21%). The dose–response relationship with twice-daily milvexian was significant (one-sided P <0.001), and the 12% incidence of VTE with twice-daily milvexian was significantly lower than the prespecified benchmark of 30%. Consequently, the two prespecified criteria for efficacy were met. The incidences of bleeding of any severity were 4% with milvexian and enoxaparin; the incidence of clinically relevant bleeding (the composite of major and clinically relevant non-major bleeding) was 1% with milvexian and 2% with enoxaparin. Serious adverse events were reported in 2% and 4% of patients in the milvexian and enoxaparin groups, respectively.

AXIOMATIC SSP

The goal of the Antithrombotic Treatment with Factor XIa Inhibition to Optimize Management of Acute Thromboembolic Events for Secondary Stroke Prevention (AXIOMATIC SSP)[26] double-blind trial was to assess the safety and efficacy of five doses of milvexian compared with a placebo in patients with non-cardioembolic ischaemic stroke or TIA on the background of atherosclerotic disease who presented within 48 hours of symptom onset. A total of 2295 patients were randomized in a 1:1:1:1:1:2 manner to either milvexian 25 mg once daily (n = 325), milvexian 25 mg twice daily (n = 313), milvexian 50 mg twice daily (n = 325), milvexian 100 mg twice daily (n = 306), milvexian 200 mg twice daily (n = 344), or a placebo (n = 682). All patients also received clopidogrel (75 mg once daily) and aspirin (100 mg once daily) for 21 days, followed by aspirin alone for 90 days; dual antiplatelet therapy was continued for 21 days and then switched to aspirin 100 mg daily thereafter.

The incidence of the primary efficacy outcome, the composite of symptomatic ischaemic stroke and covert brain infarction on repeat brain imaging at 90 days, did not differ between milvexian and placebo. Symptomatic ischaemic stroke or TIA occurred in 4.6%, 3.8%, 4.0%, 3.5%, and 7.7% of patients in the milvexian 25 mg once-daily, 25 mg twice-daily, 50 mg twice-daily, 100 mg twice-daily, and 200 mg twice-daily groups, respectively, and in 5.5% of those in the placebo group. All BARC bleeding occurred in 0.8%, 8.6%, 12.3%, 13.1%, and 10.2%, of patients in the milvexian 25 mg once-daily, 25 mg twice-daily, 50 mg twice-daily, 100 mg twice-daily, and 200 mg twice-daily groups, respectively, and in 7.9% of those given placebo. There were no fatal bleeds and symptomatic intracranial haemorrhage was rare. Therefore, milvexian was not associated with a reduction in the incidence of recurrent symptomatic ischaemic stroke or covert brain infarction at 90 days compared with placebo, but a post hoc analysis suggested that there was a reduction in recurrent symptomatic ischaemic stroke. Milvexian was not associated with a significant increase in bleeding compared with a placebo.

Conclusions and future directions

The evidence from available phase II trials suggests that, unlike the current DOACs, drugs that target FXI reduce thrombosis without a dose-dependent increase in bleeding, thereby raising the potential for a more favourable benefit/risk profile. Large phase III trials are needed to determine whether asundexian and milvexian can prevent stroke without increasing bleeding in AF. This is a high bar to achieve because numerous post-marketing studies[27,28] confirm the efficacy and safety of currently available DOACs for this indication, particularly apixaban.

Asundexian and milvexian may reduce recurrence in patients with non-cardioembolic stroke, but choosing the right dose requires a balance between efficacy and safety. Capitalizing on the benefits of dual pathway inhibition with aspirin and low-dose rivaroxaban seen in the Anti-Xa Therapy to Lower Cardiovascular Events in Addition to Standard Therapy in Subjects with Acute Coronary Syndrome–Thrombolysis in Myocardial Infarction 46 (ATLAS ACS–TIMI 46)[29] and Cardiovascular Outcomes for People Using Anticoagulation Strategies (COMPASS)[30] trials, extended treatment with an FXI inhibitor after an acute coronary syndrome may safely reduce recurrent ischaemic events, but large trials will be needed to show this. Abelacimab is being evaluated in patients with AF (ClinicalTrials.gov Identifier: NCT04755283) and cancer-associated VTE (ClinicalTrials.gov Identifiers: NCT05171049 and NCT05171075), trials that may identify a role for parenteral FXI inhibitors. Therefore, the future of FXI inhibitors appears bright, but the promise of uncoupling thrombosis from haemostasis requires confirmation in large phase III trials.

What's new

- Currently available DOACs target factor FXa or thrombin.
- Asundexian and milvexian are new DOACs that target FXIa.
- FXIa inhibitors may be safer than the currently available DOACs.

What's next

- Phase III trials with asundexian and milvexian are underway.
- Asundexian and milvexian will be compared with apixaban for stroke prevention in AF in the OCEANIC-AF and LIBREXIA-AF trials, respectively.
- Asundexian and milvexian will be compared with placebo for stroke prevention in the OCEANIC-Stroke and LIBREXIA-stroke trials, respectively.
- Milvexian will be compared with placebo for prevention of thrombotic events after acute coronary syndrome in the LIBREXIA-ACS trial.

References

1. Ruff CT, Giugliano RP, Braunwald E, et al. Comparison of the efficacy and safety of new oral anticoagulants with warfarin in patients with atrial fibrillation: a meta-analysis of randomised trials. *Lancet*. 2014;383(9921):955–62.
2. van Es N, Coppens M, Schulman S, et al. Direct oral anticoagulants compared with vitamin K antagonists for acute venous thromboembolism: evidence from phase 3 trials. *Blood*. 2014;124(12):1968–75.
3. Ogilvie IM, Newton N, Welner SA, et al. Underuse of oral anticoagulants in atrial fibrillation: a systematic review. *Am J Med*. 2010;123(7):638–45.e4.
4. Sanghai S, Wong C, Wang Z, et al. Rates of potentially inappropriate dosing of direct-acting oral anticoagulants and associations with geriatric conditions among older patients with atrial fibrillation: the SAGE-AF study. *J Am Heart Assoc*. 2020;9(6):e014108.
5. Hsu C, Hutt E, Bloomfield DM, et al. Factor XI inhibition to uncouple thrombosis from hemostasis: JACC review topic of the week. *J Am Coll Cardiol*. 2021;78(6):625–31.
6. Key NS. Epidemiologic and clinical data linking factors XI and XII to thrombosis. *Hematology Am Soc Hematol Educ Program*. 2014;2014(1):66–70.
7. Gill D, Georgakis MK, Laffan M, et al. Genetically determined FXI (factor XI) levels and risk of stroke. *Stroke*. 2018;49(11):2761–3.
8. Yuan S, Burgess S, Laffan M, et al. Genetically proxied inhibition of coagulation factors and risk of cardiovascular disease: a Mendelian randomization study. *J Am Heart Assoc*. 2021;10(8):e019644.
9. Preis M, Hirsch J, Kotler A, et al. Factor XI deficiency is associated with decreased risk for cardiovascular and venous thromboembolism events. *Blood*. 2017;129(9):1210–15.
10. Salomon O, Steinberg DM, Koren-Morag N, et al. Reduced incidence of ischemic stroke in patients with severe factor XI deficiency. *Blood*. 2008;111(8):4113–17.
11. Salomon O, Steinberg DM, Zucker M, et al. Patients with severe factor XI deficiency have a reduced incidence of deep-vein thrombosis. *Thromb Haemost*. 2011;105(2):269–73.
12. Peyvandi F, Palla R, Menegatti M, et al. Coagulation factor activity and clinical bleeding severity in rare bleeding disorders: results from the European Network of Rare Bleeding Disorders. *J Thromb Haemost*. 2012;10(4):615–21.
13. Bolton-Maggs PH, Patterson DA, Wensley RT, et al. Definition of the bleeding tendency in factor XI-deficient kindreds—a clinical and laboratory study. *Thromb Haemost*. 1995;73(2):194–202.
14. Girolami A, Cosi E, Santarossa C, et al. Thrombotic events in asymptomatic FXII deficiency versus symptomatic FXI deficiency: surprising observations. *Acta Haematol*. 2016;136(2):118–22.
15. Buller HR, Bethune C, Bhanot S, et al. Factor XI antisense oligonucleotide for prevention of venous thrombosis. *N Engl J Med*. 2015;372(3):232–40.
16. Weitz JI, Bauersachs R, Becker B, et al. Effect of osocimab in preventing venous thromboembolism among patients undergoing knee arthroplasty: the FOXTROT randomized clinical trial. *JAMA*. 2020;323(2):130–9.
17. Verhamme P, Yi BA, Segers A, et al. Abelacimab for prevention of venous thromboembolism. *N Engl J Med*. 2021;385(7):609–17.
18. Weitz JI, Strony J, Ageno W, et al. Milvexian for the prevention of venous thromboembolism. *N Engl J Med*. 2021;385(23):2161–72.
19. Nopp S, Kraemmer D, Ay C. Factor XI inhibitors for prevention and treatment of venous thromboembolism: a review on the rationale and update on current evidence. *Front Cardiovasc Med*. 2022;9:903029.
20. Kubitza D, Heckmann M, Distler J, et al. Pharmacokinetics, pharmacodynamics and safety of BAY 2433334, a novel activated factor XI inhibitor, in healthy volunteers: a randomized phase 1 multiple-dose study. *Br J Clin Pharmacol*. 2022;88(7):3447–62.
21. Wong PC, Crain EJ, Bozarth JM, et al. Milvexian, an orally bioavailable, small-molecule, reversible, direct inhibitor of factor XIa: in vitro studies and in vivo evaluation in experimental thrombosis in rabbits. *J Thromb Haemost*. 2022;20(2):399–408.
22. Perera V, Wang Z, Luettgen J, et al. First-in-human study of milvexian, an oral, direct, small molecule factor XIa inhibitor. *Clin Transl Sci*. 2022;15(2):330–42.
23. Piccini JP, Caso V, Connolly SJ, et al. Safety of the oral factor XIa inhibitor asundexian compared with apixaban in patients with atrial fibrillation (PACIFIC-AF): a multicentre, randomised, double-blind, double-dummy, dose-finding phase 2 study. *Lancet*. 2022;399(10333):1383–90.
24. Rao SV, Kirsch B, Bhatt DL, et al. A multicenter, phase 2, randomized, placebo-controlled, double-blind, parallel-group, dose-finding trial of the oral factor XIa inhibitor asundexian to prevent adverse cardiovascular outcomes after acute myocardial infarction. *Circulation*. 2022;146(16):1196–206.
25. Shoamanesh A, Mundl H, Smith EE, et al. Factor XIa inhibition with asundexian after acute non-cardioembolic ischaemic stroke (PACIFIC-Stroke): an international, randomised, double-blind, placebo-controlled, phase 2b trial. *Lancet*. 2022;400(10357):997–1007.
26. Sharma M, Molina CA, Hankey GJ. Efficacy and safety of the FXIa inhibitor milvexian for secondary stroke prevention: final results of the AXIOMATIC-SSP dose-finding randomized trial. European Society of Cardiology Congress. Barcelona, Spain. 2022.
27. Hutto D, Siontis GCM, Noseworthy PA, et al. On-treatment follow-up in real-world studies of direct oral anticoagulants in atrial fibrillation: association with treatment effects. *Int J Cardiol Heart Vasc*. 2022;40:101024.
28. Menichelli D, Del Sole F, Di Rocco A, et al. Real-world safety and efficacy of direct oral anticoagulants in atrial fibrillation: a systematic review and meta-analysis of 605 771 patients. *Eur Heart J Cardiovasc Pharmacother*. 2021;7(Fi1):f11–19.
29. Mega JL, Braunwald E, Wiviott SD, et al. Rivaroxaban in patients with a recent acute coronary syndrome. *N Engl J Med*. 2012;366(1):9–19.
30. Eikelboom JW, Connolly SJ, Bosch J, et al. Rivaroxaban with or without aspirin in stable cardiovascular disease. *N Engl J Med*. 2017;377(14):1319–30.

CHAPTER 13

Thrombolytic therapy and ancillary antithrombotic therapies

Peter R. Sinnaeve and Frans Van de Werf

Contents

Summary

Fibrinolytic therapy is still necessary to treat ST-elevation myocardial infarction patients in many centres worldwide because of limited access to catheterization facilities. In contemporary practice, fibrinolysis is given as a bolus combined with anticoagulation and antiplatelets, followed by an early catheterization in a strategy termed the 'pharmacoinvasive approach'. In this strategy, ST-segment resolution is checked at 60–90 minutes after fibrinolysis. Patients without signs of reperfusion are immediately taken to the catheterization laboratory, while stable, successfully reperfused patients receive a 'scheduled' catheterization between 2 and 24 hours after thrombolysis. The advantage of this approach is that unnecessary percutaneous coronary intervention procedures can be avoided in the very early phase after lysis when the risk of prothrombotic and bleeding complications is higher. The optimal dose of bolus fibrinolysis in pharmacoinvasive strategies remains unclear and is currently being prospectively studied.

Introduction

Fibrinolytic agents continue to be relevant in the 21st century. In ST-elevation myocardial infarction (STEMI), primary percutaneous coronary intervention (PCI), performed in a timely manner by an experienced team, is superior to fibrinolysis, as it achieves higher patency rates and carries a lower risk of intracranial bleeding complications (➔ Chapter 16). Still, pharmacological reperfusion can be given earlier, is less costly, widely available, and less dependent on operator experience. Because of limited access to catheterization facilities as well as organizational challenges to perform a primary PCI within 2 hours, fibrinolytic therapy is still necessary or even the only option to treat STEMI in many centres worldwide. The most recent European Society of Cardiology (ESC) survey indeed shows that fibrinolysis is still used in about one out of five STEMI patients, although the percentage is highly dependent on the location, with a rate of only 1% fibrinolysis in Western Europe, over 8% in Northern Europe or 10% in Eastern Europe, to more than 40% in Northern Africa.[1] Fibrinolytic agents are also used in patients with mechanical valve thrombosis and have been evaluated in out-of-hospital cardiac arrest. They also remain essential in treatment strategies for stroke and pulmonary emboli, which are discussed in ➔ Chapters 18 and 21. In this chapter, the different fibrinolytic agents are discussed, as well as their indications and practical use in combination with antiplatelets and anticoagulation.

Fibrinolytic therapy—mechanism

The goal of fibrinolytic therapy is to dissolve the fibrin network of a thrombus to restore blood flow in an occluded blood vessel. The thrombus can be dissolved by activating the endogenous fibrinolytic system using intravenous plasminogen-activating agents. Plasminogen activators convert the proenzyme plasminogen to plasmin, which then degrades fibrin, a major constituent of clots (➔ Figure 13.1). Fibrinolytic agents can be categorized as fibrin-selective versus non-selective agents, depending on whether they dissolve clots in the absence of systemic plasminogen activation. Fibrin-selective fibrinolytic drugs, such as alteplase or its derivatives but also staphylokinase, digest the clot without activating systemic plasminogen. In contrast, non-fibrin-selective agents, such as streptokinase or urokinase, activate both systemic and clot-bound plasminogen (➔ Figure 13.2). Fibrin-selective drugs are more efficient in dissolving thrombi and they do not deplete systemic coagulation factors. However, this potential asset can increase the risk of rethrombosis and reocclusion. Consequently, concomitant anticoagulant treatment is required in patients receiving fibrin-specific fibrinolytics, while this is still a matter of debate with non-fibrin-selective agents.

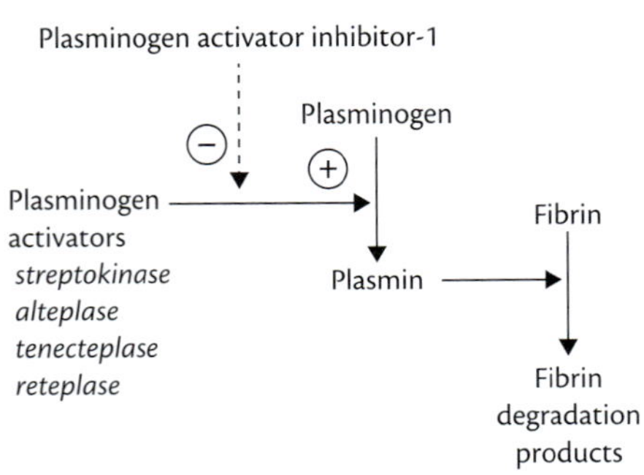

Figure 13.1 Mechanism of action of plasminogen activators.

Several circulating factors suppress the activation of plasminogen, especially plasminogen activator inhibitor 1 (PAI-1), while active plasmin can also be inhibited by alpha-2-antiplasmin. Resistance or lack of resistance to PAI-1 affects the potency of the different fibrinolytic agents, making PAI-1 a major determinant of the resistance of clots to lysis by fibrinolytic agents.

Fibrinolytic therapy—indications and contraindications

ST-elevation myocardial infarction

Administration of fibrinolytic drugs should be considered in patients with typical chest pain and/or other infarct-related symptoms and presenting with typical ST-segment elevation on electrocardiography. Treatment needs to be initiated as soon as possible, preferably within the first hours after symptom onset, when the clot is still fresh and more amenable to lysis. Although administering fibrinolytic agents up to 12 hours after the onset of symptoms may still be beneficial in terms of outcome, every minute that reperfusion is postponed will inevitably lead to more extensive necrosis. Treatment delay is associated with less successful ST-segment resolution and subsequent higher long-term mortality rates.[2] Fibrinolytic therapy is *not* recommended for non-ST-segment elevation myocardial infarction (NSTEMI) or unstable angina. Non-ST-segment elevation acute coronary syndromes are more likely to be caused by platelet-rich thrombi that include only small amounts of fibrin and are therefore not an ideal target for lytic agents.

Fibrinolytic therapy does suffer from several limitations when used in STEMI patients. Fibrinolytics need between 45 and 60 minutes to recanalize the infarct-related artery, and complete epicardial patency [i.e. Thrombolysis in Myocardial Infarction (TIMI) grade 3 flow] is only achieved in 60% of patients. Reocclusion due to prothrombotic side effects is also common, occurring in 5–15% of successfully recanalized arteries. To prevent reocclusion, antithrombotic agents are hence given concomitantly with (selective) fibrinolytic agents, and further invasive

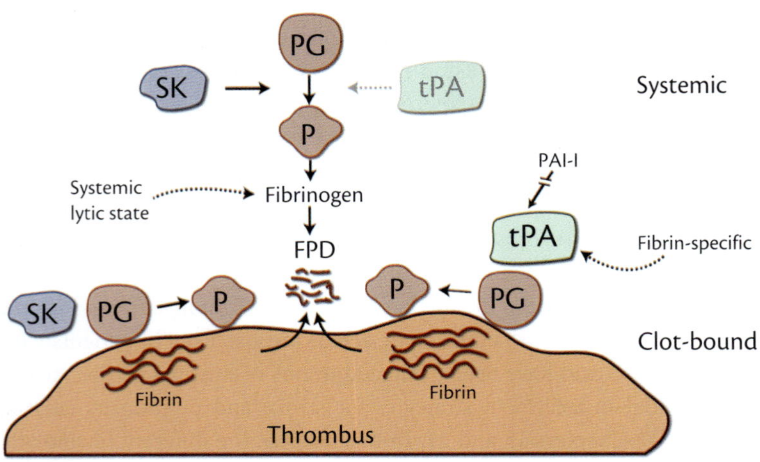

Figure 13.2 Fibrin-specific versus non-fibrin-specific fibrinolytics. FPD, fibrin degradation products; P, plasmin; PAI-1, plasminogen activator inhibitor 1; PG, plasminogen; SK, streptokinase; t-PA, tissue-type plasminogen activator.

management should be planned. Furthermore, even when blood flow to the infarct-related artery is restored, microcirculatory reperfusion might be insufficient ('no-reflow' phenomenon, see below). Finally, bleeding complications, especially intracranial haemorrhages (ICHs), continue to be a concern in high-risk patients. Therefore, contraindications to fibrinolysis include a previous history of stroke or recent major surgery (➔ Table 13.1). In these patients, a primary PCI should be offered, even if this would be performed beyond the delay time of 120 minutes from first medical contact.

Standard contemporary thrombolytic strategies for STEMI consist of a fibrinolytic agent administered via bolus, in combination with both aspirin and clopidogrel, and enoxaparin, followed by early coronary angiography. Bolus fibrinolytics are easier to prepare and administer, which reduces the risk of dosing error, but also shortens treatment delays and facilitates prehospital treatment. The organization of a primary PCI in a STEMI patient who does not present directly to a PCI-capable facility is complex and challenging. This implies that transporting a STEMI patient for a primary PCI inherently comes at the cost of a system-related delay compared to immediate administration of a fibrinolytic. It is clear that the longer this delay, the smaller the advantage of a primary PCI becomes.[3] When the system delay from electrocardiogram diagnosis to wire-crossing is expected to exceed 120 minutes, fibrinolysis is the preferred method of reperfusion, and should be administered within 10 minutes after the diagnosis. The ESC Guidelines hence recommend administering a bolus fibrinolytic (in the ambulance or non-PCI hospital) and transferring the patient immediately to the nearest PCI-capable center.[4]

Prosthetic valve thrombosis

Thrombosis of a prosthetic heart valve is a potentially life-threatening condition. It occurs mainly in mechanical valves, but should be ruled out via imaging in patients with any type of prosthetic valve presenting with an embolic event or unexplained dyspnoea. Fibrinolysis should be considered in critically ill patients with clear obstructive mechanical valve thrombosis, when urgent surgery is not an option or contraindicated.[5] Compared to surgery, fibrinolysis carries a higher risk of bleeding, thromboembolic events, and recurrent valve thrombosis.[6] In patients with non-obstructive prosthetic valve thrombosis, fibrinolysis should only be considered if there is evidence of thromboembolism on imaging and the thrombus is either large (≥10 mm) or persists despite adequate anticoagulation.[7] Usually, alteplase is chosen as fibrinolytic agent [10 mg bolus followed by a 90-minute infusion of 90 mg, in combination with unfractionated heparin (UFH)].

Fibrinolytic agents

See ➔ Table 13.2.

Streptokinase

Streptokinase is a non-fibrinogen-specific fibrinolytic that indirectly activates plasminogen (➔ Box 13.1). Because it is produced by haemolytic streptococci, patients who receive streptokinase invariably develop antistreptococcal antibodies, precluding re-administration. In addition, pre-existing anti-streptokinase antibodies may reduce fibrinolytic activity and consequently impede reperfusion in patients with acute myocardial infarction. Although newer fibrin-specific fibrinolytics have theoretical advantages, streptokinase remains widely used in part because of its low cost. The first trial to show a significant reduction in mortality with a fibrinolytic agent was the landmark GISSI-1 trial.[8] In this study, patients with a STEMI presenting within 12 hours of symptom onset were randomized to either streptokinase or standard non-fibrinolytic therapy. No concomitant antithrombotic was required. In-hospital mortality was 10.7% in patients treated with intravenous streptokinase versus 13.1% in control patients, representing 23 lives saved per 1000 patients treated. This difference remained significant after 10 years of follow-up.

Alteplase

Alteplase is a single-chain recombinant tissue-type plasminogen activator (tPA) molecule (➔ Box 13.1). Due to its short half-life, alteplase requires a continuous infusion. It has considerably greater fibrin specificity than streptokinase, but still induces systemic fibrinogen depletion to some extent. Because the reocclusion rate with alteplase given alone is almost twice as high than with non-fibrin specific drugs, concomitant antithrombin treatment is required.

The question whether alteplase is superior to streptokinase in terms of mortality reduction was answered in the first GUSTO-1 trial.[9] In this trial that included over 40,000 patients,

Table 13.1 Contraindications for fibrinolysis

Relative	Absolute
Transient ischaemic attack <6 months	Previous haemorrhagic stroke at any time or non-haemorrhagic stroke <6 months
Refractory hypertension	Central nervous system malformation or neoplasm
Prolonged cardiopulmonary resuscitation	Active (uncontrolled) bleeding
Current use of anticoagulants	Gastrointestinal bleeding within last month
Recent bleeding	Known bleeding disorder
Pregnancy	Aortic dissection
Thrombocytopenia	

Table 13.2 Lytic agents and their characteristics

	Fibrin specificity	Half-life (minutes)	PAI-1 resistance
Streptokinase	–	18–23	–
Urokinase	–	9	–
Alteplase	↑	3–4	–
Reteplase	↓	15–18	–
Tenecteplase	↑↑	20–24	↑
Staphylokinase (PEG)	↑↑↑	13	–

Box 13.1 Dosing regimens of frequently used fibrinolytic agents (intravenous doses)

Streptokinase

- STEMI: 1.5 million IU over1 hour.
- PE: 250,000 U over 30 minutes, 100,000 U/hour over 24 hours.

Alteplase

- STEMI:
  - 15 mg bolus.
  - 90-minute infusion:
    1. 0.75 mg/kg over 30 minutes (max. 50 mg).
    2. 0.50 mg/kg over next hour (max. 35 mg).
    3. Total dose max. 100 mg.
- Prosthetic valve thrombosis: 10 mg bolus followed by a 90-minute infusion of 90 mg.
- PE: 100 mg over 2 hours.
- AIS: 0.9 mg/kg intravenously; max. 90 mg; 10% as an initial intravenous bolus over 1 minute and the remainder infused over 60 minutes.

Reteplase

- A 10 U bolus, followed by second 10 U bolus 30 minutes later.

Tenecteplase

- STEMI or PE: weight-adjusted single bolus:
  - 30 mg if <60 kg.
  - 35 mg if 60–69 kg.
  - 40 mg if 70–79 kg.
  - 45 mg if 80–89 kg.
  - 50 mg if 90 kg or greater.
  - Half-dose if age over 75 years.
- AIS: 0.25 mg/kg, max. 25 mg.

a 'front-loaded' 90-minute dosing regimen of alteplase was used. The 30-day mortality was 6.3% in patients receiving alteplase compared to 7.4% in patients treated with streptokinase ($P = 0.001$). This 1% lower 30-day mortality with alteplase over streptokinase could be explained by a significantly higher TIMI flow grade 3 at 90 minutes.[10]

Alteplase is effective for the treatment of patients with pulmonary emboli (PE) and acute ischaemic stroke (AIS) as well. In the pivotal NINDS trial, alteplase (0.9 mg/kg with 10% given as a bolus, the remainder over 60 minutes) was given to ischaemic stroke patients within 3 hours of symptom onset.[11] Alteplase treatment led to significantly improved neurological outcomes at 3-month follow-up. Although the dose has remained unchanged, subsequent studies have extended the treatment window to 4.5 hours. Alteplase for AIS works best on small emboli, and on aggregate only achieves sufficient patency in less than half of patients. Furthermore, it carries a significant risk of symptomatic haemorrhagic conversion of the brain lesion.[12]

Reteplase

Reteplase (recombinant tPA), a second-generation fibrinolytic agent, was a first attempt to improve on the shortcomings of alteplase. It is a mutant of alteplase in which the finger domain, the kringle-1 domain, and epidermal growth factor domains were removed, resulting in decreased plasma clearance. In contrast with alteplase, which requires a continuous infusion, reteplase can be given as a double bolus. The removal of the finger domain reduces fibrin specificity to some extent, although inactivation by PAI-1 remains similar as with alteplase. Phase II trials with reteplase consistently showed higher patency rates, as assessed by TIMI-3 flow rates, with reteplase than with alteplase.

In the GUSTO-III trial, which was designed as a superiority trial, 15,059 patients were randomized to double-bolus reteplase (10 MU), given 30 minutes apart, or front-loaded alteplase.[13] Mortality at 30 days was similar for both treatment arms (7.47% vs 7.24%, respectively), as was the incidence of haemorrhagic stroke or other major bleeding complications. Similar mortality rates were maintained for both treatment groups at 1-year follow-up. Thus, higher TIMI-3 rates at 90 minutes with reteplase, as seen in earlier pilot studies, were not associated with lower short-term mortality rates. This might be explained in part by increased platelet activation and surface receptor expression with reteplase compared to alteplase.[14]

Tenecteplase

Tenecteplase (TNK-tPA) is also derived from alteplase. Mutations at three places (T103, N117, KHRR296-299) increase the plasma half-life, increase fibrin binding and specificity, and increase resistance to PAI-1 (➔ Box 13.1). Its slower clearance allows convenient single-bolus administration. The efficiency of tenecteplase to activate plasminogen is reduced in the presence of fibrinogen and fibrin degradation products, while efficiency in the presence of fibrin remains equivalent, explaining its improved fibrin specificity. Tenecteplase has also higher thrombolytic potency than its parent molecule or recombinant tPA. Consequently, tenecteplase leads to faster recanalization compared to alteplase.[15]

In the ASSENT-2 trial, 16,949 patients were randomized to single-bolus tenecteplase or weight-adjusted front-loaded alteplase.[16] Specifically designed as an equivalency trial, this study showed that tenecteplase and alteplase had equivalent 30-day mortality [6.18% vs 6.15%, respectively; relative risk 1.004, 90% confidence interval (CI) 0.917–1.104]. Although the rates of ICH were similar for tenecteplase (0.93%) and alteplase (0.94%), female patients, elderly patients aged over 75 years, and patients weighing less than 67 kg tended to have lower rates of ICH after treatment with tenecteplase.[17] Non-cerebral bleeding complications occurred less frequently in the tenecteplase group. Differences were even more apparent in high-risk women. Thus, increased fibrin specificity of tenecteplase may induce both a better outcome and fewer bleeding complications, especially in high-risk patients. Based on findings from the STREAM trial (➔ Fibrinolysis and the planning of percutaneous coronary intervention in STEMI), a half-dose bolus tenecteplase is now recommended for STEMI patients above the age of 75.[18]

Tenecteplase was also compared to alteplase in patients presenting with an AIS within 4.5 hours after symptom onset, and scheduled for invasive management with early thrombectomy. A total of 202 patients were randomized to receive standard dose alteplase (0.9 mg/kg) or bolus tenecteplase (0.25 mg/kg, maximum 25 mg).[19] Tenecteplase before thrombectomy was associated with a higher rate of reperfusion but also better functional outcomes at 90 days. A second study could not demonstrate a benefit of a 0.4 mg/kg bolus over the 0.25 mg/kg bolus in patients with a large vessel occlusion, and the risk of haemorrhagic conversion appeared to be more than three times higher.[20]

The largest trial evaluating fibrinolysis for PE, the PEITHO trial, was carried out with tenecteplase in 1006 normotensive patients presenting with intermediate- to high-risk PE (i.e. with right ventricular dysfunction and evidence of myocardial injury).[21] They were treated with weight-adjusted single-bolus tenecteplase or placebo, both in the presence of UFH. The primary endpoint, a composite of all-cause death or haemodynamic decompensation within 7 days after randomization, was lower after tenecteplase (2.6%) than placebo (5.6%) [odds ratio (OR) 0.44, 95% CI 0.23–0.87; P = 0.02]. This benefit was mainly driven by a reduction in haemodynamic decompensation, as mortality rates were similar in both groups. Major extracranial bleeding complications, however, were significantly higher after tenecteplase (6.3% vs 1.2% after placebo; P <0.001), as was the risk of haemorrhagic stroke (2.0% vs 0.2%). In essence, the benefit of fibrinolysis in haemodynamically stable PE patients at intermediate to high risk is largely offset by an increased risk of major bleeding, and should only be used with caution in this population. The use of fibrinolytic agents in acute PE has also been thought to help to improve longer-term outcome and to prevent subsequent complications such as the development of chronic thromboembolic pulmonary hypertension. Data from the PEITHO trial, however, did not show a reduction of mortality, right ventricular dysfunction, or symptoms such as residual dyspnoea after a median follow-up duration of 38 months.[22] A few small studies have also studied the effect of fibrinolysis delivered directly to the pulmonary artery via a catheter-directed approach, but the benefit of such a strategy needs confirmation from larger trials.[23,24]

Antithrombotic co-therapy in fibrinolysis

Aspirin

The landmark Second International Study of Infarct Survival (ISIS-2) study clearly showed a benefit of adding aspirin to streptokinase. A total of 17,187 patients with a myocardial infarction received 1.5 MU streptokinase, or 160 mg aspirin daily for 1 month, both treatments, or neither.[25] Treatment with aspirin or streptokinase alone resulted in a significant reduction in mortality (23% and 24%, respectively), an effect that was additive, as shown by a 43% reduction in the combination group. Reinfarction rate was higher when streptokinase was used alone, an effect that was abolished when aspirin was added. A retrospective analysis from the CHARISMA trial suggests that a 75–81 mg maintenance dose of aspirin is associated with the most optimal benefit/bleeding ratio (➔ Table 13.3).[26]

Table 13.3 Antiplatelets and anticoagulation doses with fibrinolysis

Antiplatelet therapy	*Aspirin*: 150–325 mg chewable, non-enteric coated (75–81 mg daily lifelong) *Clopidogrel*: 300 mg (75 mg if <75 years) loading dose, 75 mg daily for 1 year *Ticagrelor*: 180 mg loading dose at the time of PCI, 90 mg twice daily for 1 year
Anticoagulation	*Enoxaparin* Bolus 30 mg IV, 1 mg/kg SC (>75 years no bolus) 1 mg/kg per 12 hours (max. 100 mg for first two doses) (0.75 mg/kg if >75 year) Or *Fondaparinux* (with streptokinase) Bolus 2.5 mg IV 2.5 mg SC per day up to 8 days or discharge Or *UFH* 60 U/kg (max. 4000 U) 12 U/kg per hour (max. 1000 U/hour) 50–70 seconds first measurement at 3 hours

$P2Y_{12}$ inhibitors

Despite the use of aspirin in lytic-treated STEMI patients, reocclusion and reinfarction after successful pharmacological reperfusion continues to be a problem. The Clopidogrel as Adjunctive Reperfusion Therapy (CLARITY) trial examined whether addition of a second oral antiplatelet agent on top of aspirin, the $P2Y_{12}$ receptor inhibitor clopidogrel (300 mg bolus followed by 75 mg daily), was associated with higher rates of infarct-related artery patency in patients treated with a fibrinolytic agent [27]. At angiographic follow-up at least 2 days after fibrinolytic therapy, patients receiving clopidogrel had significantly better TIMI flow grade rates (➔ Figure 13.3). Clopidogrel appeared to improve patency rates by preventing reocclusion rather than through facilitating early reperfusion.[28] No increased risk of bleeding complications with clopidogrel was observed. Since no patients over 75 years of age were included in CLARITY, however, it remains uncertain whether dual antiplatelet therapy is safe in elderly patients treated with fibrinolysis. As a consequence, a loading dose of only 75 mg clopidogrel is given to lytic-treated patients aged over 75 years. Clopidogrel also improved outcome after a PCI in CLARITY, regardless of the duration of pretreatment or whether patients received additional glycoprotein IIb/IIIa inhibitors.[29] These results suggest that adding clopidogrel early to fibrinolysis obviates the need for additional glycoprotein IIb/IIIa inhibitors at the time of PCI.

Ticagrelor is a more potent and less variable $P2Y_{12}$ inhibitor than clopidogrel. While it improves outcome at 1 year compared to clopidogrel in acute coronary syndrome patients, it also

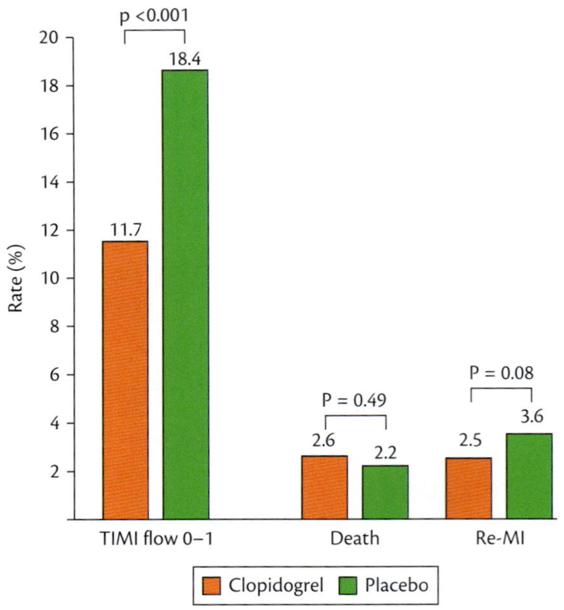

Figure 13.3 TIMI flow grade rates at angiographic follow-up at least 2 days after fibrinolytic therapy and outcomes before angiography.

increases bleeding risk.[30] It has therefore not been evaluated in combination with fibrinolysis in the acute phase. Ticagrelor was nevertheless compared to clopidogrel *after* fibrinolytic therapy in the TREAT trial.[31] In this trial, 3799 predominantly clopidogrel-pretreated STEMI patients younger than 75 years were randomized to ticagrelor (180 mg loading dose, 90 mg twice daily thereafter) or clopidogrel (300/600 mg loading dose, 75 mg once daily thereafter) about 11 hours after receiving fibrinolysis. Major bleeding complications were rare and not significantly different at 30 days between the two $P2Y_{12}$ inhibitors. At 1 year, there appeared to be no benefit of ticagrelor in reducing cardiovascular events, but there were more minor bleeding complications related to ticagrelor.[32] In an observational study, pharmacoinvasively (PI)-treated patients who were switched to ticagrelor at the time of PCI had a 54% lower risk of the composite of death, reinfarction, or stroke at 1 year compared to patients who remained on clopidogrel.[33] As there appeared to be no excess risk of major bleeding or ICH in this study, these data suggest that a switch from clopidogrel to ticagrelor at the time of PCI may be safe and beneficial in PI-treated STEMI patients.

Unfractionated heparin

Since the publication of GUSTO-I, intravenous UFH has been the standard adjunctive antithrombotic therapy with fibrin-specific fibrinolytics for STEMI patients. Even though intravenous UFH does not improve early patency rates, patency after alteplase is enhanced by UFH at later time points because it reduces the likelihood of reocclusion.[34] The use of UFH suffers from several drawbacks: the effectiveness of UFH is highly variable, due to low bioavailability and variable clearance, and its anticoagulant effect has to be monitored. UFH is also relatively ineffective in inhibiting clot-associated thrombin and factor Xa, and does not reduce thrombin generation associated with fibrinolysis. This can result in rebound activation of the coagulation cascade after cessation of an infusion, increasing the risk of reocclusion. In the PEITHO trial, tenecteplase was also accompanied by UFH in patients with PE, targeting an activated partial thromboplastin time of 2–2.5 times the upper limit (corresponding to a factor Xa inhibition level of 0.3–0.7 IU/mL).[21]

Low-molecular-weight heparin

Low-molecular-weight heparin (LMWH) offers several advantages over conventional UFH, including greater bioavailability, better resistance to inhibition by activated platelets, lower incidence of heparin-induced thrombocytopenia, and increased anti-factor Xa activity. LMWH has a more stable and predictable anticoagulant response that eliminates the need for monitoring of activated partial thromboplastin time. Also, a better anti-Xa:IIa ratio than that of UFH more efficiently promotes the inhibition of thrombin generation. Furthermore, subcutaneous administration and a longer half-life greatly facilitate administration when compared to UFH. Studies have shown a reduction in reinfarction rates and enhanced late patency with the use of LMWH in acute coronary syndromes.[35]

In the ASSENT-3 study, enoxaparin, UFH, and abciximab were compared in combination with tenecteplase.[36] A total of 6095 STEMI patients received either full-dose weight-adjusted single-bolus tenecteplase with weight-adjusted enoxaparin (30 mg intravenous bolus followed by 1 mg/kg immediately and every 12 hours subcutaneous for 7 days) or UFH, or half-dose tenecteplase with abciximab and weight-adjusted low-dose UFH. Enoxaparin and full-dose tenecteplase significantly reduced the risk for ischaemic complications at 30 days. A significant improvement in the primary efficacy and safety endpoint was seen with tenecteplase and enoxaparin when compared to tenecteplase and UFH, but 30-day and 1-year mortality rates were similar in the three groups.[37] Enoxaparin in combination with tenecteplase was also evaluated in the prehospital setting in the ASSENT-3 PLUS trial.[38] A non-significant reduction in ischaemic complications with enoxaparin was observed, at the expense of an increase in ICH in elderly patients (>75 years). Using an age-adjusted dose (no bolus and 75% of the maintenance dose), however, enoxaparin still increased the risk of major bleeding but not the risk of ICH after fibrinolytic therapy, while still reducing the risk of ischaemic complications in the ExTRACT-TIMI 25 study.[39] Meta-analyses of trials comparing LMWH to UFH confirm that LMWHs reduce the risk of death and reinfarction, but are associated with a higher risk of major bleeding complications (OR 1.45, 95% CI 1.24–1.91).[40,41] The 2017 ESC STEMI guidelines recommend either enoxaparin (class I, level of evidence A) or UFH (class I, level of evidence B) in lytic-treated patients.[4]

Factor Xa inhibitor

Fondaparinux, a synthetic pentasaccharide, is a selective antithrombin-dependent factor Xa inhibitor. Fondaparinux is associated with less biological variability or immunogenic reactivity. As with LMWH, fondaparinux does not need monitoring of its anticoagulant effect. Also, in contrast with UFH or LMWH, fondaparinux does not bind to platelet factor 4 and thus reduces the risk of platelet activation. In the OASIS-6 trial, fondaparinux was compared with UFH or placebo in 12,092 patients with STEMI. Lytic therapy was used in 45% of patients, most of them receiving a non-fibrin-specific agent. In these patients, fondaparinux was associated with a significant 21% lower risk of death or myocardial infarction when compared to standard UFH or placebo.[42] Moreover, the risk of bleeding, including ICH, was considerably lower with fondaparinux, irrespective of the type of fibrinolytic agent. ESC Guidelines recommend fondaparinux as adjunctive therapy to streptokinase only.[4]

Glycoprotein IIb/IIIa inhibitors

The addition of glycoprotein IIb/IIIa inhibitors to fibrinolytic regimens might also overcome some of the drawbacks of fibrinolysis. The combination of half-dose lytic and a glycoprotein IIb/IIIa inhibitor was shown to induce less systemic plasminogen activation and to reverse the platelet activating effect of fibrinolytic drugs. This results in a reduction in angiographically evident thrombus, which is thought to improve epicardial and tissue perfusion. The efficacy and safety of abciximab in combination with reduced-dose fibrinolysis was evaluated in the GUSTO-V and ASSENT-3 studies, both without clopidogrel preloading.[36,43] In the GUSTO-V trial, an open-label non-inferiority trial, 16,588 patients were randomized to either reteplase or half-dose reteplase with weight-adjusted abciximab. Thirty-day mortality rates were 5.9% for reteplase and 5.6% for the combined reteplase–abciximab group, thus fulfilling the criteria for non-inferiority. The overall risk of bleeding, however, was significantly higher with reteplase and abciximab than with reteplase alone. ICH rates in patients above 75 years of age was almost twice as high in the combination treatment arm. In the ASSENT-3 study, a significant decrease in ischaemic complications with abciximab was also offset by an increase in bleeding complications. Although ICH rates were very similar in the three treatment arms, major and minor bleeding complications, thrombocytopenia, and transfusion rates were more frequent in the half-dose tenecteplase plus abciximab arm. Like in the GUSTO-V trial, patients older than 75 years experienced significantly more bleeding complications. Taken together, combination therapy with half-dose fibrinolytic and abciximab results in a reduction in ischaemic complications after acute myocardial infarction (in the absence of concomitant clopidogrel), but this benefit is offset by an increased risk of bleeding complications, particularly in the elderly. Abciximab is not available anymore, although small molecule glycoprotein IIb/IIIa inhibitors can still be used for bail-out use during PCI.

Direct thrombin inhibitors

In contrast with UFH, which only inhibits fluid-phase thrombin, direct thrombin inhibitors inhibit both fibrin-bound and fluid-phase thrombin. Because inadequately inactivated thrombin at the site of the thrombus is in part responsible for the procoagulant side effect of fibrinolysis, direct inhibition of thrombin might reduce the occurrence of ischaemic complications after reperfusion. There is no evidence of the safety/benefit balance of bivalirudin with fibrin-selective fibrinolytic agents. In the HERO-2 trial, 17,073 patients with STEMI were randomized to streptokinase and UFH or streptokinase and bivalirudin.[44] Mortality at 30 days was not different for both regimens: 10.5% for bivalirudin and 10.9% for UFH. On the other hand, reinfarction rate within 96 hours was significantly lower in the bivalirudin group (1.6% vs 2.3% for UFH), suggesting that early and more efficient inhibition of thrombin can inhibit reocclusion. Mild to moderate bleeding complications were higher in the bivalirudin group, but ICH occurred infrequently in both groups.

Prehospital fibrinolysis for STEMI

Time lost between symptom onset and treatment initiation remains a crucial contributor to treatment delay in STEMI, regardless of the mode of reperfusion. Bolus fibrinolytic agents undoubtedly facilitate prehospital reperfusion protocols. The combination of single-bolus tenecteplase plus enoxaparin, which emerged as a convenient and attractive therapy in the ASSENT-3 study, was investigated in the prehospital setting in the ASSENT-3 PLUS trial. A total of 1639 patients with acute myocardial infarction received prehospital tenecteplase.[38] A time gain of 47 minutes was observed, increasing the fraction of patients treated within 2 hours of symptom onset from 29% in ASSENT-3 to 52% in ASSENT-3 PLUS. Early treatment (<2 hours) was associated with a lower 30-day mortality [4.4% vs 6.2 (2–4 hours) and 10.4% (4–6 hours)]. A meta-analysis of six trials including 6434 patients showed that the time gained with prehospital treatment resulted in a significant 17% mortality reduction compared to in-hospital fibrinolysis[45]. In later studies, time to fibrinolysis was significantly shorter with prehospital fibrinolysis, when compared with regular in-hospital lytic, resulting in improved outcome.[46]

The question whether prehospital fibrinolysis compares favourably to transport to a centre with interventional facilities for primary PCI was addressed in the CAPTIM trial.[47] Primary PCI was *not* found to be superior to prehospital fibrinolysis in terms of outcome, even at 5-year follow-up. It is important to note that 26% of the patients randomized to prehospital fibrinolysis subsequently underwent rescue PCI in the tertiary care hospital, which might have contributed to the favourable outcomes in the prehospital group. Also, prehospital fibrinolysis was associated with a mortality reduction in patients randomized within 2 hours of symptom onset.[48] A meta-analysis suggests that outcome after prehospital fibrinolysis is at least comparable to that with primary PCI, and that prehospital fibrinolysis prevents the evolution to cardiogenic shock but increases the risk of haemorrhagic stroke.[49] Taken together, prehospital fibrinolysis allows the initiation of reperfusion therapy as soon as possible after symptom onset and appears to be at least as effective as primary PCI, especially in patients presenting early.[50]

Fibrinolysis and the planning of percutaneous coronary intervention in STEMI

Primary PCI is superior to fibrinolysis in randomized trials.[51] Although the efficacy of primary PCI is less dependent on the time elapsed between symptom onset and treatment initiation than fibrinolysis, longer symptom onset-to-balloon delays also lead to worse outcome in primary PCI (➔ Chapter 16). Unfortunately, for patients presenting to a centre without catheterization facilities, much time is often lost between diagnosis and PCI in daily practice due to transport to the PCI centre, and few eligible patients are treated with fibrinolysis before transfer.[52] Interestingly, up to 20% of patients with STEMI appear to have spontaneous epicardial reperfusion to some degree before the intervention in primary PCI studies, which is an independent predictor of outcome.[53] Patients with reperfusion before the procedure also have better preserved left ventricular function, and less progression to heart failure and cardiogenic shock.[54,55] Therefore, the next logical step in treatment for STEMI is to combine the advantages of both primary PCI and fibrinolysis.

In essence, there are two strategies for combining fibrinolysis and an early PCI. The first is to take *all* lytic-treated patients immediately to the catheterization laboratory for an urgent angiography and/or PCI, an approach called 'facilitated PCI'. The second is to first assess ST-segment resolution at 60–90 minutes after fibrinolysis, and schedule the catheterization based on the presence of reperfusion, an approach termed the 'pharmacoinvasive' (PI) approach. With a PI approach, unstable patients or those without signs of reperfusion are immediately taken to the catheterization laboratory, while stable, successfully reperfused patients receive a 'scheduled' catheterization between 2 and 24 hours after thrombolysis. The advantage of this approach is that unnecessary PCI procedures can be avoided in the very early phase after lysis when the risk of prothrombotic and bleeding complications is higher. While studies such as TRANSFER-AMI and CARESS-in-AMI showed that transferring patients who were treated with fibrinolysis at a centre without PCI capability had improved outcomes if they were transferred for angiography within 6 hours versus standard care (➔ Figure 13.4),[56,57] results from the large ASSENT-4 PCI outcome trial indeed suggest that a systematically planned PCI *within the first 2 hours* after fibrinolysis is harmful.[58]

Since ASSENT-4 PCI, several PI studies have tried to address the shortcomings of facilitated PCI. In STREAM, 1892 STEMI patients who presented within 3 hours after symptom onset and who were unable to undergo a PCI within 1 hour were randomized to bolus tenecteplase or primary PCI.[59] Tenecteplase was reduced to half-dose bolus in patients above 75 years of age after an amendment. In the lytic-treated patients, a catheterization was planned between 6 and 24 hours after randomization, and a clopidogrel loading dose of 300 mg was given unless the patient was 75 years or older. An urgent catheterization was only performed if fibrinolysis was unsuccessful within 90 minutes; this appeared to be necessary in 36% of patients. The remainder of the lytic-treated patients underwent a catheterization at a median of 17 hours after randomization. At 30 days, the primary endpoint of death, shock, congestive heart failure, or reinfarction occurred in 12.4% of the patients in the fibrinolysis arm, compared to 14.3% in the primary PCI arm ($P = 0.21$). After reducing the fibrinolytic therapy to half a bolus in patients aged 75 years or older, the number of ICHs was low and similar in both treatment arms (0.5% vs 0.3% after primary PCI), while halving the dose did not appear to affect ischaemic outcomes. A PI strategy of half-dose bolus tenecteplase followed by planned angiography between 6 and 24 hours is currently being compared to transport for primary PCI in STEMI patients aged 60 years or older who are unable to undergo primary PCI within 1 hour (STREAM-2).[60]

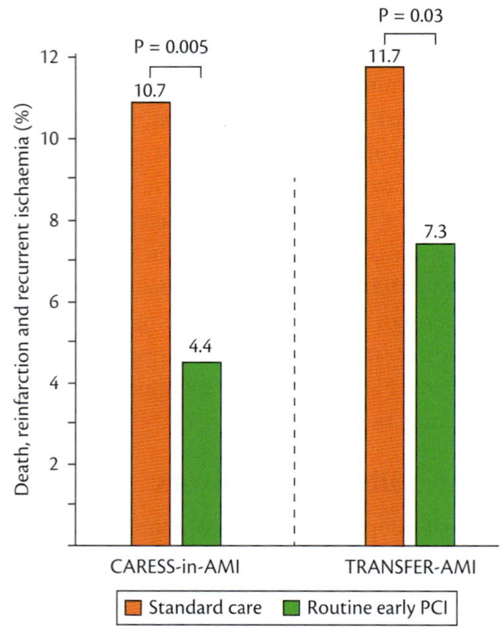

Figure 13.4 Outcomes after routine early PCI versus standard care in CARESS-in-AMI and TRANSFER-AMI.

Other contemporary trials have compared similar reperfusion strategies as well. In a large and comprehensive meta-analysis including 31 trials, fibrinolysis was compared to fibrinolysis followed by routine early PCI or primary PCI alone.[61] Patients undergoing routine early PCI were further categorized as undergoing either 'facilitated PCI' when the median time interval between lysis and PCI was less than 2 hours, or a PI approach when this interval exceeded 2 hours. Compared to fibrinolysis 'only', primary PCI (OR 0.73, 95% CI 0.61–0.89) as well as PI management (OR 0.79, 95% CI 0.59–1.08) but not facilitated PCI (OR 0.90, 95% CI 0.66–1.24) was associated with a lower mortality risk. When compared head to head, a PI approach appeared to be associated with a superior efficacy and safety than facilitated PCI. Taken together, when primary PCI is not available, fibrinolysis with routine early PCI is superior to fibrinolysis alone. It also clearly indicates that a PI strategy (i.e. PCI between 2 and 24 hours) is better than facilitated PCI (i.e. PCI within 2 hours after lysis).

Intracoronary fibrinolysis during primary percutaneous coronary intervention

Several early thrombolytic strategies in the 1970s and 1980s aimed at intracoronary administration of fibrinolytic drugs, in part to reduce systemic bleeding complications.[62,63] The logistic challenge associated with routine intracoronary administration of fibrinolytics quickly redirected focus to the intravenous route. In recent years, however, the intracoronary route attracted renewed attention as a treatment for microvascular obstruction. The pathophysiological mechanisms leading to microvascular obstruction are complex, but distal embolization of fibrin-rich microthrombi during PCI is thought to play an important role. In this respect, fibrinolysis before a primary PCI could theoretically help to prevent no-reflow. A subanalysis of ASSENT-4 PCI, however, showed that thrombus burden was higher when fibrinolysis preceded the PCI.[64] This was likely due to the prothrombotic state triggered by fibrinolysis in the absence of potent antiplatelet therapy. The next logical step was to administer a low dose of a fibrinolytic agent directly into the culprit coronary artery, in addition to conventional dual antiplatelet therapy. A small pilot trial (n = 41) in 2007 showed that low-dose intracoronary streptokinase (250 kU) did lead to improved indices of myocardial reperfusion.[65] Unfortunately, this did not translate into improved left ventricular function.

More recent PI studies with intracoronary fibrinolysis in addition to primary PCI did not demonstrate a benefit.[66,67] The largest study to date, T-TIME, randomized patients within 6 hours of a STEMI due to a proximal/mid occlusion of a major coronary artery to placebo (n = 151) versus low-dose intracoronary alteplase [10 mg (n = 144) or 20 mg (n = 145)].[66] The primary endpoint, the amount of microvascular obstruction on magnetic resonance imaging at days 2–7 after enrolment, was not different between the three treatment groups. A subanalysis even suggests that low-dose intracoronary alteplase was harmful in patients with an ischaemic time of more than 4 hours.[68] A second study reported an increased risk of subacute stent thrombosis and poorer reperfusion after intracoronary reduced-dose tenecteplase.[67] Taken together, the systematic use of intracoronary (low-dose) fibrinolysis as an adjunct to primary PCI cannot be recommended.[69] Intracoronary fibrinolysis might still be an option in case of high thrombus burden in selected cases, especially when thrombectomy fails.[70]

What's new

- A PI strategy with bolus fibrinolysis is now the preferred strategy for patients not able to undergo immediate primary PCI.
- A switch from clopidogrel to ticagrelor at the time of PCI is safe and may be beneficial in PI-treated STEMI patients.
- The systematic use of intracoronary (low-dose) fibrinolysis as an adjunct to primary PCI cannot be recommended.

Guideline recommendations

Recommendation	Class	Level of evidence
A primary PCI strategy is recommended over fibrinolysis within indicated time frames	I	A
If timely primary PCI cannot be performed after STEMI diagnosis, fibrinolytic therapy is recommended within 12 h of symptom onset in patients without contraindications	I	A
When fibrinolysis is the reperfusion strategy, it is recommended to initiate this treatment as soon as possible after STEMI diagnosis, preferably in the prehospital setting	I	A
A fibrin-specific agent (i.e. tenecteplase, alteplase, or reteplase) is recommended	I	B
A half-dose of tenecteplase should be considered in patients ≥75 years of age	IIa	B
Transfer to a PCI-capable centre following fibrinolysis is indicated in all patients immediately after fibrinolysis	I	A
Rescue PCI is indicated immediately when fibrinolysis has failed (<50% ST-segment resolution at 60–90 minutes) or at any time in the presence of haemodynamic or electrical instability, or worsening ischaemia	I	A
Emergency angiography and PCI if needed is indicated in the case of recurrent ischaemia or evidence of reocclusion after initial successful fibrinolysis	I	B
Emergency angiography and PCI if indicated is recommended in patients with heart failure/shock	I	A
Intervals	**Time targets**	
Maximum time from STEMI diagnosis to bolus or infusion start of fibrinolysis in patients unable to meet primary PCI target times	≤10 minutes	
Time delay from start of fibrinolysis to evaluation of its efficacy	60–90 minutes	
Time delay from start of fibrinolysis to angiography (if fibrinolysis is successful)	2–24 hours	

Source data from Ibanez B, James S, Agewall S, Antunes MJ, Bucciarelli-Ducci C, Bueno H, Caforio ALP, Crea F, Goudevenos JA, Halvorsen S, et al. 2017 ESC Guidelines for the management of acute myocardial infarction in patients presenting with ST-segment elevation: the Task Force for the management of acute myocardial infarction in patients presenting with ST-segment elevation of the European Society of Cardiology (ESC). Eur Heart J. 2018;39:119–77. doi: 10.1093/eurheartj/ehx393.

What's next

- Half-dose tenecteplase reduces the risk of intracranial bleeding in STEMI patients above 75 years of age. Whether it is also effective compared to primary PCI is being studied in the STREAM-2 trial in patients above 60 years of age.
- The upfront use of a loading dose of ticagrelor with fibrinolytic agents needs further study.
- Intracoronary fibrinolysis might be an option in case of high thrombus burden during primary PCI, especially when thrombectomy fails, but needs prospective study.

References

1. Zeymer U, Ludman P, Danchin N, et al. Reperfusion therapies and in-hospital outcomes for ST-elevation myocardial infarction in Europe: the ACVC-EAPCI EORP STEMI Registry of the European Society of Cardiology. Eur Heart J. 2021;42:4536–49. doi: 10.1093/eurheartj/ehab342
2. Nallamothu B, Fox KA, Kennelly BM, et al. Relationship of treatment delays and mortality in patients undergoing fibrinolysis and primary percutaneous coronary intervention. The Global Registry of Acute Coronary Events. Heart. 2007;93:1552–5. doi: 10.1136/hrt.2006.112847
3. Gershlick AH, Westerhout CM, Armstrong PW, et al. Impact of a pharmacoinvasive strategy when delays to primary PCI are prolonged. Heart. 2015;101:692–8. doi: 10.1136/heartjnl-2014-306686
4. Ibanez B, James S, Agewall S, et al. 2017 ESC Guidelines for the management of acute myocardial infarction in patients presenting with ST-segment elevation: the Task Force for the management of acute myocardial infarction in patients presenting with ST-segment elevation of the European Society of Cardiology (ESC). Eur Heart J. 2018;39:119–77. doi: 10.1093/eurheartj/ehx393
5. Keuleers S, Herijgers P, Herregods MC, et al. Comparison of thrombolysis versus surgery as a first line therapy for prosthetic heart valve thrombosis. Am J Cardiol. 2011;107:275–9. doi: 10.1016/j.amjcard.2010.09.013
6. Karthikeyan G, Senguttuvan NB, Joseph J, Devasenapathy N, Bahl VK, Airan B. Urgent surgery compared with fibrinolytic therapy for the treatment of left-sided prosthetic heart valve thrombosis: a systematic review and meta-analysis of observational studies. Eur Heart J. 2013;34:1557–66. doi: 10.1093/eurheartj/ehs486
7. Vahanian A, Beyersdorf F, Praz F, et al. 2021 ESC/EACTS Guidelines for the management of valvular heart disease. Eur Heart J. 2022;43:561–632. doi: 10.1093/eurheartj/ehab395
8. Gruppo Italiano per lo Studio della Streptochinasi nell'Infarto Miocardico (GISSI). Effectiveness of intravenous thrombolytic treatment in acute myocardial infarction. Lancet. 1986;1:397–402.
9. GUSTO investigators. An international randomized trial comparing four thrombolytic strategies for acute myocardial infarction. N Engl J Med. 1993;329:673–82. doi: 10.1056/nejm199309023291001
10. GUSTO Angiographic Investigators. The effects of tissue plasminogen activator, streptokinase, or both on coronary-artery patency, ventricular function, and survival after acute myocardial infarction. N Engl J Med. 1993;329:1615–22. doi: 10.1056/nejm199311253292204
11. National Institute of Neurological Disorders and Stroke rt-PA Stroke Study Group. Tissue plasminogen activator for acute ischemic stroke. N Engl J Med. 1995;333:1581–7. doi: 10.1056/nejm199512143332401
12. Thiebaut AM, Gauberti M, Ali C, et al. The role of plasminogen activators in stroke treatment: fibrinolysis and beyond. Lancet Neurol. 2018;17:1121–32. doi: 10.1016/s1474-4422(18)30323-5
13. Global Use of Strategies to Open Occluded Coronary Arteries (GUSTO III) Investigators. A comparison of reteplase with alteplase for acute myocardial infarction. N Engl J Med. 1997;337:1118–23. doi: 10.1056/nejm199710163371603
14. Gurbel PA, Serebruany VL, Shustov AR, et al. Effects of reteplase and alteplase on platelet aggregation and major receptor expression during the first 24 hours of acute myocardial infarction treatment. GUSTO-III Investigators. Global Use of Strategies to Open Occluded Coronary Arteries. J Am Coll Cardiol. 1998;31:1466–73. doi: 10.1016/s0735-1097(98)00172-7
15. Cannon CP, Gibson CM, McCabe CH, et al. TNK-tissue plasminogen activator compared with front-loaded alteplase in acute myocardial infarction: results of the TIMI 10B trial. Thrombolysis in Myocardial Infarction (TIMI) 10B Investigators. Circulation. 1998;98:2805–14. doi: 10.1161/01.cir.98.25.2805
16. Van De Werf F, Adgey J, Ardissino D, et al. Single-bolus tenecteplase compared with front-loaded alteplase in acute myocardial infarction: the ASSENT-2 double-blind randomised trial. Lancet. 1999;354:716–22. doi: 10.1016/s0140-6736(99)07403-6
17. Van de Werf F, Barron HV, Armstrong PW, et al. Incidence and predictors of bleeding events after fibrinolytic therapy with fibrin-specific agents: a comparison of TNK-tPA and rt-PA. Eur Heart J. 2001;22:2253–61. doi: 10.1053/euhj.2001.2686
18. Armstrong PW, Zheng Y, Westerhout CM, et al. Reduced dose tenecteplase and outcomes in elderly ST-segment elevation myocardial infarction patients: insights from the STrategic Reperfusion Early After Myocardial infarction trial. Am Heart J. 2015;169:890–8.e891. doi: 10.1016/j.ahj.2015.03.011
19. Campbell BCV, Mitchell PJ, Churilov L, et al. Tenecteplase versus alteplase before thrombectomy for ischemic stroke. N Engl J Med. 2018;378:1573–82. doi: 10.1056/NEJMoa1716405
20. Campbell BCV, Mitchell PJ, Churilov L, et al. Effect of intravenous tenecteplase dose on cerebral reperfusion before thrombectomy in patients with large vessel occlusion ischemic stroke: the EXTEND-IA TNK Part 2 randomized clinical trial. JAMA. 2020;323:1257–65. doi: 10.1001/jama.2020.1511
21. Meyer G, Vicaut E, Danays T, et al. Fibrinolysis for patients with intermediate-risk pulmonary embolism. N Engl J Med. 2014;370:1402–11. doi: 10.1056/NEJMoa1302097
22. Konstantinides SV, Vicaut E, Danays T, et al. Impact of thrombolytic therapy on the long-term outcome of intermediate-risk pulmonary embolism. J Am Coll Cardiol. 2017;69:1536–44. doi: 10.1016/j.jacc.2016.12.039
23. Piazza G, Hohlfelder B, Jaff MR, et al. A prospective, single-arm, multicenter trial of ultrasound-facilitated, catheter-directed, low-dose fibrinolysis for acute massive and submassive pulmonary embolism: the SEATTLE II Study. JACC Cardiovasc Interv. 2015;8:1382–92. doi: 10.1016/j.jcin.2015.04.020
24. Kucher N, Boekstegers P, Müller OJ, et al. Randomized, controlled trial of ultrasound-assisted catheter-directed thrombolysis for acute intermediate-risk pulmonary embolism. Circulation. 2014;129:479–86. doi: 10.1161/circulationaha.113.005544
25. ISIS-1 (First International Study of Infarct Survival) Collaborative Group. Mechanisms for the early mortality reduction produced by beta-blockade started early in acute myocardial infarction: ISIS-1. Lancet. 1988;1:921–3.
26. Steinhubl SR, Bhatt DL, Brennan DM, et al. Aspirin to prevent cardiovascular disease: the association of aspirin dose and clopidogrel with thrombosis and bleeding. Ann Intern Med. 2009;150:379–86. doi: 10.7326/0003-4819-150-6-200903170-00006
27. Sabatine MS, Cannon CP, Gibson CM, et al. Addition of clopidogrel to aspirin and fibrinolytic therapy for myocardial infarction with ST-segment elevation. N Engl J Med. 2005;352:1179–89. doi: 10.1056/NEJMoa050522
28. Scirica BM, Sabatine MS, Morrow DA, et al. The role of clopidogrel in early and sustained arterial patency after fibrinolysis for ST-segment elevation myocardial infarction: the ECG CLARITY-TIMI 28 Study. J Am Coll Cardiol. 2006;48:37–42. doi: 10.1016/j.jacc.2006.02.052
29. Sabatine MS, Cannon CP, Gibson CM, et al. Effect of clopidogrel pretreatment before percutaneous coronary intervention in patients with ST-elevation myocardial infarction treated with fibrinolytics: the PCI-CLARITY study. JAMA. 2005;294:1224–32. doi: 10.1001/jama.294.10.1224

30. Wallentin L, Becker RC, Budaj A, et al. Ticagrelor versus clopidogrel in patients with acute coronary syndromes. N Engl J Med. 2009;361:1045–57. doi: 10.1056/NEJMoa0904327
31. Berwanger O, Nicolau JC, Carvalho AC, et al. Ticagrelor vs clopidogrel after fibrinolytic therapy in patients with ST-elevation myocardial infarction: a randomized clinical trial. JAMA Cardiol. 2018;3:391–9. doi: 10.1001/jamacardio.2018.0612
32. Berwanger O, Lopes RD, Moia DDF, et al. Ticagrelor versus clopidogrel in patients with stemi treated with fibrinolysis: TREAT trial. J Am Coll Cardiol. 2019;73:2819–28. doi: 10.1016/j.jacc.2019.03.011
33. Welsh RC, Shavadia JS, Zheng Y, Tyrrell BD, Leung R, Bainey KR. Ticagrelor or clopidogrel dual antiplatelet therapy following a pharmacoinvasive strategy in ST-segment elevation myocardial infarction. Clinical cardiology. 2021;44:1543–50. doi: 10.1002/clc.23716
34. Mahaffey KW, Granger CB, Collins R, et al. Overview of randomized trials of intravenous heparin in patients with acute myocardial infarction treated with thrombolytic therapy. Am J Cardiol. 1996;77:551–6. doi: 10.1016/s0002-9149(97)89305-8
35. Antman EM, Louwerenburg HW, Baars HF, et al. Enoxaparin as adjunctive antithrombin therapy for ST-elevation myocardial infarction: results of the ENTIRE-Thrombolysis in Myocardial Infarction (TIMI) 23 Trial. Circulation. 2002;105:1642–49. doi: 10.1161/01.cir.0000013402.34759.46
36. Efficacy and safety of tenecteplase in combination with enoxaparin, abciximab, or unfractionated heparin: the ASSENT-3 randomised trial in acute myocardial infarction. Lancet. 2001;358:605–13. doi: 10.1016/s0140-6736(01)05775-0
37. Sinnaeve PR, Alexander JH, Bogaerts K, et al. Efficacy of tenecteplase in combination with enoxaparin, abciximab, or unfractionated heparin: one-year follow-up results of the Assessment of the Safety of a New Thrombolytic-3 (ASSENT-3) randomized trial in acute myocardial infarction. Am Heart J. 2004;147:993.
38. Wallentin L, Goldstein P, Armstrong PW, et al. Efficacy and safety of tenecteplase in combination with the low-molecular-weight heparin enoxaparin or unfractionated heparin in the prehospital setting: the Assessment of the Safety and Efficacy of a New Thrombolytic Regimen (ASSENT)-3 PLUS randomized trial in acute myocardial infarction. Circulation. 2003;108:135–42. doi: 10.1161/01.Cir.0000081659.72985.A8
39. Antman EM, Morrow DA, McCabe CH, et al. Enoxaparin versus unfractionated heparin with fibrinolysis for ST-elevation myocardial infarction. N Engl J Med. 2006;354:1477–88. doi: 10.1056/NEJMoa060898
40. Eikelboom JW, Quinlan DJ, Mehta SR, Turpie AG, Menown IB, Yusuf S. Unfractionated and low-molecular-weight heparin as adjuncts to thrombolysis in aspirin-treated patients with ST-elevation acute myocardial infarction: a meta-analysis of the randomized trials. Circulation. 2005;112:3855–67. doi: 10.1161/circulationaha.105.573550
41. Murphy SA, Gibson CM, Morrow DA, et al. Efficacy and safety of the low-molecular weight heparin enoxaparin compared with unfractionated heparin across the acute coronary syndrome spectrum: a meta-analysis. Eur Heart J. 2007;28:2077–86. doi: 10.1093/eurheartj/ehm224
42. Peters RJ, Joyner C, Bassand JP, et al. The role of fondaparinux as an adjunct to thrombolytic therapy in acute myocardial infarction: a subgroup analysis of the OASIS-6 trial. Eur Heart J. 2008;29:324–31. doi: 10.1093/eurheartj/ehm616
43. Topol EJ. Reperfusion therapy for acute myocardial infarction with fibrinolytic therapy or combination reduced fibrinolytic therapy and platelet glycoprotein IIb/IIIa inhibition: the GUSTO V randomised trial. Lancet. 2001;357:1905–14. doi: 10.1016/s0140-6736(00)05059-5
44. White H. Thrombin-specific anticoagulation with bivalirudin versus heparin in patients receiving fibrinolytic therapy for acute myocardial infarction: the HERO-2 randomised trial. Lancet. 2001;358:1855–63. doi: 10.1016/s0140-6736(01)06887-8
45. Morrison LJ, Verbeek PR, McDonald AC, Sawadsky BV, Cook DJ. Mortality and prehospital thrombolysis for acute myocardial infarction: a meta-analysis. JAMA. 2000;283:2686–92. doi: 10.1001/jama.283.20.2686
46. Danchin N, Blanchard D, Steg PG, et al. Impact of prehospital thrombolysis for acute myocardial infarction on 1-year outcome: results from the French Nationwide USIC 2000 Registry. Circulation. 2004;110:1909–15. doi: 10.1161/01.Cir.0000143144.82338.36
47. Bonnefoy E, Lapostolle F, Leizorovicz A, et al. Primary angioplasty versus prehospital fibrinolysis in acute myocardial infarction: a randomised study. Lancet. 2002;360:825–9. doi: 10.1016/s0140-6736(02)09963-4
48. Steg PG, Bonnefoy E, Chabaud S, et al. Impact of time to treatment on mortality after prehospital fibrinolysis or primary angioplasty: data from the CAPTIM randomized clinical trial. Circulation. 2003;108:2851–6. doi: 10.1161/01.Cir.0000103122.10021.F2
49. Roule V, Ardouin P, Blanchart K, et al. Prehospital fibrinolysis versus primary percutaneous coronary intervention in ST-elevation myocardial infarction: a systematic review and meta-analysis of randomized controlled trials. Crit Care. 2016;20:359. doi: 10.1186/s13054-016-1530-z
50. Solhpour A, Chang KW, Arain SA, et al. Comparison of 30-day mortality and myocardial scar indices for patients treated with prehospital reduced dose fibrinolytic followed by percutaneous coronary intervention versus percutaneous coronary intervention alone for treatment of ST-elevation myocardial infarction. Catheter Cardiovasc Interv. 2016;88:709–15. doi: 10.1002/ccd.26523
51. Keeley EC, Boura JA, Grines CL. Primary angioplasty versus intravenous thrombolytic therapy for acute myocardial infarction: a quantitative review of 23 randomised trials. Lancet. 2003;361:13–20. doi: 10.1016/s0140-6736(03)12113-7
52. Vora AN, Holmes DN, Rokos I, et al. Fibrinolysis use among patients requiring interhospital transfer for ST-segment elevation myocardial infarction care: a report from the US National Cardiovascular Data Registry. JAMA Intern Med. 2015;175:207–15. doi: 10.1001/jamainternmed.2014.6573
53. De Luca G, Ernst N, Zijlstra F, et al. Preprocedural TIMI flow and mortality in patients with acute myocardial infarction treated by primary angioplasty. J Am Coll Cardiol. 2004;43:1363–7. doi: 10.1016/j.jacc.2003.11.042
54. Gibson CM, Cannon CP, Murphy SA, Marble SJ, Barron HV, Braunwald E. Relationship of the TIMI myocardial perfusion grades, flow grades, frame count, and percutaneous coronary intervention to long-term outcomes after thrombolytic administration in acute myocardial infarction. Circulation. 2002;105:1909–13. doi: 10.1161/01.cir.0000014683.52177.b5
55. Stone GW, Cox D, Garcia E, et al. Normal flow (TIMI-3) before mechanical reperfusion therapy is an independent determinant of survival in acute myocardial infarction: analysis from the primary angioplasty in myocardial infarction trials. Circulation. 2001;104:636–41. doi: 10.1161/hc3101.093701
56. Di Mario C, Dudek D, Piscione F, et al. Immediate angioplasty versus standard therapy with rescue angioplasty after thrombolysis in the Combined Abciximab REteplase Stent Study in Acute Myocardial Infarction (CARESS-in-AMI): an open, prospective, randomised, multicentre trial. Lancet. 2008;371:559–68. doi: 10.1016/s0140-6736(08)60268-8

57. Cantor WJ, Fitchett D, Borgundvaag B, et al. Routine early angioplasty after fibrinolysis for acute myocardial infarction. N Engl J Med. 2009;360:2705–18. doi: 10.1056/NEJMoa0808276
58. Assessment of the Safety and Efficacy of a New Treatment Strategy with Percutaneous Coronary Intervention (ASSENT-4 PCI) investigators. Primary versus tenecteplase-facilitated percutaneous coronary intervention in patients with ST-segment elevation acute myocardial infarction (ASSENT-4 PCI): randomised trial. Lancet. 2006;367:569–78. doi: 10.1016/s0140-6736(06)68147-6
59. Armstrong PW, Gershlick AH, Goldstein P, et al. Fibrinolysis or primary PCI in ST-segment elevation myocardial infarction. N Engl J Med. 2013;368:1379–87. doi: 10.1056/NEJMoa1301092
60. Armstrong PW, Bogaerts K, Welsh R, et al. The Second Strategic Reperfusion Early After Myocardial Infarction (STREAM-2) study optimizing pharmacoinvasive reperfusion strategy in older ST-elevation myocardial infarction patients. Am Heart J. 2020;226:140–6. doi: 10.1016/j.ahj.2020.04.029
61. Fazel R, Joseph TI, Sankardas MA, et al. Comparison of reperfusion strategies for ST-segment-elevation myocardial infarction: a multivariate network meta-analysis. J Am Heart Assoc. 2020;9:e015186. doi: 10.1161/jaha.119.015186
62. Kennedy JW, Ritchie JL, Davis KB, Fritz JK. Western Washington randomized trial of intracoronary streptokinase in acute myocardial infarction. N Engl J Med. 1983;309:1477–82. doi: 10.1056/nejm198312153092402
63. Rentrop KP, Blanke H, Karsch KR, Kreuzer H. Initial experience with transluminal recanalization of the recently occluded infarct-related coronary artery in acute myocardial infarction—comparison with conventionally treated patients. Clinical cardiology. 1979;2:92–105. doi: 10.1002/clc.4960020203
64. Zalewski J, Bogaerts K, Desmet W, et al. Intraluminal thrombus in facilitated versus primary percutaneous coronary intervention: an angiographic substudy of the ASSENT-4 PCI (Assessment of the Safety and Efficacy of a New Treatment Strategy with Percutaneous Coronary Intervention) trial. J Am Coll Cardiol. 2011;57:1867–73. doi: 10.1016/j.jacc.2010.10.061
65. Sezer M, Oflaz H, Gören T, et al. Intracoronary streptokinase after primary percutaneous coronary intervention. N Engl J Med. 2007;356:1823–34. doi: 10.1056/NEJMoa054374
66. McCartney PJ, Eteiba H, Maznyczka AM, et al. Effect of low-dose intracoronary alteplase during primary percutaneous coronary intervention on microvascular obstruction in patients with acute myocardial infarction: a randomized clinical trial. JAMA. 2019;321:56–68. doi: 10.1001/jama.2018.19802
67. Morales-Ponce FJ, Lozano-Cid FJ, Martinez-Romero P, et al. Intracoronary tenecteplase versus abciximab as adjunctive treatment during primary percutaneous coronary intervention in patients with anterior myocardial infarction. EuroIntervention. 2019;14:1668–75. doi: 10.4244/eij-d-18-00885
68. McCartney PJ, Maznyczka AM, Eteiba H, et al. Low-dose alteplase during primary percutaneous coronary intervention according to ischemic time. J Am Coll Cardiol. 2020;75:1406–21. doi: 10.1016/j.jacc.2020.01.041
69. Dauerman HL. Darkness on the edge of thrombolysis. J Am Coll Cardiol. 2020;75:1422–25. doi: 10.1016/j.jacc.2020.02.007
70. Noma S, Miyachi H, Fukuizumi I, et al. Adjunctive catheter-directed thrombolysis during primary PCI for ST-segment elevation myocardial infarction with high thrombus burden. J Clin Med. 2022;11:262. doi: 10.3390/jcm11010262

SECTION 3

Therapeutic strategies

CHAPTER 14

Antithrombotic strategies in primary cardiovascular prevention

Erica Michelotti, Paul M. Ridker, and Raffaele De Caterina

Contents

Summary

Antithrombotic strategies in primary cardiovascular prevention essentially revolve around the use of aspirin. This chapter provides an update and guidance for the use of aspirin in patients without previous clinical evidence of vascular disease. In contrast to secondary prevention, aspirin in primary prevention is widely debated in part because early trials predated the statin era. Furthermore, because prevention of cardiovascular outcomes demonstrated in several trials was counterbalanced by increased risk for bleeding, a net clinical benefit has not clearly been shown in pooled estimates. Using data from the most recent trials, and performing a meta-regression of benefits and risks associated with aspirin use as related to the 10-year risk of major adverse cardiovascular events (MACEs), a tailored approach to aspirin prescription in primary prevention is proposed. In patients aged less than 70 years with optimal risk factor control, individual cardiovascular risk should be carefully evaluated, while also considering bleeding risk and patient preferences. Absolute MACE reduction appears superior to the hazard of haemorrhagic events in patients at intermediate–high cardiovascular risk without a prohibitive bleeding risk, and this category of individuals, as well as those with documented evidence of subclinical carotid, coronary, or peripheral atherosclerotic vascular disease, appear to be a proper target population. Treatment of other cardiovascular risk factors, such as high cholesterol, should, however, be prioritized prior to aspirin administration, and this should be accompanied, especially in the elderly, by the concurrent administration of gastroprotective agents.

Introduction

The use of antithrombotic drugs in primary cardiovascular prevention, before the occurrence of clinical manifestations of atherosclerotic cardiovascular disease, essentially revolves around the use of aspirin. Aspirin was first synthesized in Bayer's laboratories at the end of 19th century to obtain an anti-inflammatory drug better tolerated than salicylates, at that time mostly used against rheumatic fever.[1] Currently, aspirin is the most widely used antithrombotic drug for prevention of recurrences and treatment of cardio- and cerebrovascular diseases.[1] Its pharmacodynamic effect (as detailed in ➔ Chapter 5) results largely from inhibition of platelet cyclooxygenase (COX)-1 by serin 530 acetylation, leading to inhibition of thromboxane (TX) A_2 synthesis.[2] As knowledge has grown as an antiplatelet drug, aspirin has become a cornerstone for acute coronary syndrome treatment and prevention.[3,4] Nowadays, the European Society of Cardiology (ESC),[5,6] as well as the American College of Cardiology (ACC)/American Heart Association (AHA) Guidelines[7] recommend aspirin primary prevention only in selected patient categories, thought to be at high or very high cardiovascular risk. Caution in aspirin use in this setting derives from randomized clinical trials in which the benefit in reducing acute atherothrombotic events was counterbalanced by increased bleeding, and because several early trials predated the statin era. A recent analysis of the characteristics of the populations studied in these trials concluded that prescription among individuals with intermediate–low cardiovascular risk requires an individualized approach as the bleeding risk induced by aspirin is in the same order of magnitude as the benefits in reducing atherothrombotic events.[8] Considering new evidence recently accrued on aspirin treatment for primary prevention in patients at intermediate cardiovascular risk, a proper identification of this patient category is needed, and will be the focus of this chapter.

Aspirin in primary prevention

Aspirin therapy is firmly established and widely recommended in clinical practice in patients with acute or chronic coronary syndromes,[9] previous transient ischaemic attack (TIA)/stroke,[10] and symptomatic peripheral arterial disease[11] (➔ Table 14.1). Prescription patterns are much less consolidated—and the scientific basis for aspirin use in primary prevention much weaker—in the primary prevention setting[12–14] because major adverse cardiovascular event (MACE) reduction becomes comparable with the excess risk of bleeding related to aspirin use.[15,16] Although several clinical trials of aspirin versus placebo have been published for over 30 years[17–32] (reviewed in reference 33), a clear consensus regarding use in primary prevention is lacking. The heterogeneity of guideline recommendations[5,6,9,11,24] (➔ Table 14.2) derives from the small absolute benefit in most healthy subjects (one to two cardiovascular events avoided every 1000 patients treated per year), counterbalanced by a similarly increased bleeding risk. Some recommendations plainly do not suggest aspirin use in primary prevention, whereas others recommend aspirin treatment in high cardiovascular risk subjects. To maximize the benefit in patients without clinically manifest cardiovascular disease, it is important to identify subjects at high cardiovascular risk and, at the same time, low bleeding risk. We here discuss evidence from the latest trials published in the past 4 years and provide the rationale for a decision strategy based on this double-edged risk stratification. We propose an algorithm that can be used in clinical practice to assist physicians in deciding whether an individual patient should consider use of aspirin in primary prevention.

Table 14.1 Recommendations from guidelines on secondary cardiovascular prevention

Guideline, year (reference)	Recommendation	Class	LOE
ESC Guidelines on cardiovascular disease prevention in clinical practice, 2021[6]	Aspirin 75–100 mg daily is recommended for secondary prevention of CVD	I	A
ESC Guidelines for the diagnosis and management of chronic coronary syndromes, 2019[9]	Aspirin 75–100 mg daily is recommended in patients with a previous MI or revascularization	I	A
ESC Guidelines for the diagnosis and management of chronic coronary syndromes, 2019[9]	Aspirin 75–100 mg daily is recommended following stenting	I	A
ESC Guidelines on cardiovascular disease prevention in clinical practice, 2021[6]	In patients with non-cardioembolic ischaemic stroke or TIA, prevention with aspirin only, or dipyridamole plus aspirin, or clopidogrel alone is recommended	I	A
ESC/ESH Guidelines for the management of arterial hypertension, 2018[34]	Antiplatelet therapy, in particular low-dose aspirin, is recommended for secondary prevention in hypertensive patients	I	A
ESC Guidelines on diabetes, pre-diabetes, and cardiovascular diseases, 2019[5]	Aspirin at a dose of 75–160 mg/day is recommended as secondary prevention in patients with DM	I	A
AHA/ACCF secondary prevention and risk reduction therapy for patients with coronary and other atherosclerotic vascular disease, 2011[7]	Aspirin 75–162 mg daily is recommended in all patients with coronary artery disease unless contraindicated	I	A
AHA/ACC Guidelines for the diagnosis and management of patients with stable ischemic heart disease, 2012[7]	Treatment with aspirin 75–162 mg daily should be continued indefinitely in the absence of contraindications in patients with stable ischaemic heart disease	I	A
AHA/ACC Guidelines on the management of patients with lower extremity peripheral artery disease, 2016[7]	Antiplatelet therapy with aspirin alone (range 75–325 mg per day) or clopidogrel alone (75 mg per day) is recommended to reduce MI, stroke, and vascular death in patients with symptomatic peripheral arterial disease	I	A

ACC, American College of Cardiology; ACCF, American College of Cardiology Foundation; AHA, American Heart Association; CVD, cardiovascular disease; DM, diabetes mellitus; ESC, European Society of Cardiology; ESH, European Society of Hypertension; LOE, level of evidence; MI, myocardial infarction; TIA, transient ischaemic attack.

Table 14.2 Recommendations from guidelines on primary cardiovascular prevention

Guideline, year (reference)	Recommendation	Class	LOE
ESC Guidelines on cardiovascular disease prevention in clinical practice, 2021[6]	In patients with DM at high or very high CVD risk, low-dose aspirin may be considered for primary prevention in the absence of clear contraindications	IIb	A
ESC Guidelines on cardiovascular disease prevention in clinical practice, 2021[6]	Antiplatelet therapy is not recommended in individuals with low/moderate CV risk due to the increased risk of major bleeding	III	A
ESC Guidelines on diabetes, pre-diabetes, and cardiovascular diseases, 2019[5]	In patients with DM at moderate CV risk, aspirin for primary prevention is not recommended	III	B
ESC Guidelines on the diagnosis and treatment of peripheral arterial diseases, 2017[11]	In patients with asymptomatic >50% carotid artery stenosis, long-term antiplatelet therapy (commonly low-dose aspirin) should be considered when the bleeding risk is low	IIa	C
ESC Guidelines on the diagnosis and treatment of peripheral arterial diseases, 2017[11]	Because of a lack of proven benefit, antiplatelet therapy is not routinely indicated in patients with isolated asymptomatic LEAD	III	A
ESC/ESH Guidelines for the management of arterial hypertension, 2018[34]	Aspirin is not recommended for primary prevention in hypertensive patients without CVD	III	A
ESC Guidelines for the diagnosis and management of chronic coronary syndromes, 2019[9]	Aspirin 75–100 mg daily may be considered in patients without a history of MI or revascularization, but with definitive evidence of CAD on imaging	IIb	C
ACC/AHA Guidelines on the Primary Prevention of Cardiovascular Disease, 2019[7]	Low-dose aspirin (75–100 mg orally daily) might be considered for the primary prevention of ASCVD among select adults 40–70 years of age who are at higher ASCVD risk but not at increased bleeding risk	IIb	A
ACC/AHA Guidelines on the Primary Prevention of Cardiovascular Disease, 2019[7]	Low-dose aspirin (75–100 mg orally daily) should not be administered on a routine basis for the primary prevention of ASCVD among adults > 70 years of age	III	B
ACC/AHA Guidelines on the Primary Prevention of Cardiovascular Disease, 2019[7]	Low-dose aspirin (75–100 mg orally daily) should not be administered for the primary prevention of ASCVD among adults of any age who are at increased risk of bleeding	III	C

ACC, American College of Cardiology; AHA, American Heart Association; ASCVD atherosclerotic cardiovascular disease; CAD, coronary artery disease; CV, cardiovascular; CVD, cardiovascular disease; DM, diabetes mellitus; ESC, European Society of Cardiology; ESH, European Society of Hypertension; LEAD, lower extremities artery disease; LOE, level of evidence; MI, myocardial infarction.

The 2018 'big three': the ASPREE, ARRIVE, and ASCEND trials

In 2018, knowledge on aspirin use for primary prevention was enhanced by three large studies that evaluated treatment with low-dose aspirin—100 mg once daily—(as discussed in ➔ Chapter 5) versus placebo in various populations: healthy elderly patients in the Aspirin in Reducing Events in the Elderly (ASPREE) trial,[24] individuals at moderate cardiovascular risk in the Aspirin to Reduce Risk of Initial Vascular Events (ARRIVE) trial,[34] and diabetic patients without history of cardiovascular disease in the A Study of Cardiovascular Events in Diabetes (ASCEND) trial.[26]

ASPREE

ASPREE randomly allocated 19,114 healthy elderly people (age ≥70 years) at low bleeding risk to enteric-coated aspirin (100 mg daily) or to placebo. The primary endpoint was a composite of death, dementia, or persistent physical disability. The study was interrupted for futility after a follow-up of 4.7 years because of the lack of benefit in terms of disability-free survival in the aspirin group [hazard ratio (HR) 1.01, 95% confidence interval (CI) 0.92–1.11]. The secondary endpoint, consisting of non-fatal myocardial infarction, cardiovascular death, non-fatal stroke, and hospitalization for heart failure, was also not appreciably influenced by aspirin therapy (HR 0.95, 95% CI 0.83–1.08). Moreover, statistically significant increases in major bleeding (HR 1.38, 95% CI 1.18–1.62; P <0.001), haemorrhagic stroke and extra- as well as intracranial bleeding were observed in the aspirin group, with a significant rise in all-cause mortality (HR 1.14, 95% CI 1.01–1.29), mainly due to cancer. This latter finding is not in line with previous data reporting a possible role of aspirin in gastrointestinal cancer prevention, in particular colorectal cancer.[35]

ARRIVE

ARRIVE randomly allocated 12,546 patients at supposedly moderate cardiovascular risk (target: 10-year MACE risk between 10% and 20%) to 100 mg enteric-coated aspirin daily or placebo. The primary endpoint was a composite of myocardial infarction, stroke, cardiovascular death, stable angina, or TIA. There were no differences in the primary endpoint after 60 months of follow-up (HR 0.96, 95% CI 0.81–1.13; P = 0.60) and mild gastrointestinal bleeds were more frequent in the aspirin group (HR 2.11, 95% CI 1.36–3.28; P <0.001). Although this trial was initially designed for population at moderate cardiovascular risk, the MACE rate was substantially lower (4%) than expected, undermining the original study aims and possibly explaining the negative results in term of risk/benefit ratio.

ASCEND

ASCEND randomly allocated 15,480 patients with diabetes without known history of cardiovascular disease to 100 mg aspirin or placebo. After a mean follow-up of 7.4 years, the primary endpoint of myocardial infarction, non-haemorrhagic stroke, TIA, or cardiovascular death was reduced by 12% in the aspirin group (HR 0.88, 95% CI 0.79–0.97; P = 0.01). At the same time, aspirin therapy was associated with an increased risk of major bleeding (HR 1.29, 95% CI 1.09–1.52; P = 0.003), predominantly due to gastrointestinal and extracranial events. Subgroup analyses did not show specific categories with enhanced benefit, even in subjects at higher cardiovascular risk. Similar to the ARRIVE trial, in this study global cardiovascular risk was low to moderate: only 17.2% of subjects had a 10-year MACE risk greater than 20%.

The latest novelty: TIPS-3

The International Polycap Study 3 (TIPS-3) was published in 2020 and investigated the effects of aspirin administration for primary prevention in patients at truly intermediate cardiovascular risk.[36]

TIPS-3 was a multicentre, randomized, double-blind, placebo-controlled trial with a 2 × 2 × 2 factorial randomization design, including 5713 participants without clinically manifest cardiovascular disease. The first comparison regarded patients treated with a daily polypill (containing simvastatin 40 mg, atenolol 100 mg, hydrochlorothiazide 25 mg, and ramipril 10 mg) or placebo. The second comparison was on the effect of aspirin 75 mg once daily alone versus placebo. The third comparison was on the combination of all the polypill components plus aspirin versus double placebo. A fourth comparison studied the effects of vitamin D (60,000 IU per month) versus placebo on bone fractures and falls rate. Not including aspirin, we will not discuss the first and last comparisons. The median follow-up was 4.4 years. The primary endpoint in the group of patients treated with the polypill plus aspirin was a composite of cardiovascular death, stroke, myocardial infarction, heart failure, resuscitated cardiac arrest, and arterial revascularization. The primary endpoint in patients on aspirin therapy alone was a composite of cardiovascular death, myocardial infarction, and stroke; cancer prevention was also evaluated in this study arm. Safety outcomes included major bleeding according to International Society of Thrombosis and Haemostasis criteria.

- *Aspirin versus placebo.* A non-significant 14% reduction in the primary endpoint was observed in the aspirin group compared with placebo (HR 0.86, 95% CI 0.67–1.10). The incidence of stroke was the only primary endpoint component with a considerable reduction (HR 0.58, 95% CI 0.35–0.98). Although cancer incidence was reduced by 17% in the aspirin group (HR 0.83, 95% CI 0.54–1.27), this result was not statistically significant. The incidence of major bleeding [relative risk (RR) 1.10, 95% CI 0.59–2.05; P = 0.76], minor bleeding (RR 1.21, 95% CI 0.60–2.45; P = 0.59), and gastrointestinal bleeding (RR 1.20, 95% CI 0.52–2.77; P = 0.67) were non-significantly increased with aspirin.
- *Polypill plus aspirin versus double placebo.* A 31% reduction in the primary endpoint was observed in the polypill plus aspirin group (HR 0.69, 95% CI 0.50–0.97), compared with the double placebo. Notably, only stroke reduction among the individual components of the primary endpoint was statistically significant (HR 0.42, 95% CI 0.20–0.89). Minor bleeding (RR 1.66, 95% CI 0.60–4.55; P = 0.33) and gastrointestinal bleeding (RR 2.98, 95% CI 0.31–28.65; P = 0.34) were more common in the polypill plus aspirin group, but not to a statistically significant extent. Surprisingly, major bleeding was numerically more frequent in the double placebo group (RR 0.75, 95% CI 0.32–1.77; P = 0.50).

Differently from previous clinical trials, the TIPS-3 study investigated a population at true intermediate cardiovascular risk (mean INTERHEART risk score 17.9). In this setting, MACE reduction with the combined therapy (polypill plus low-dose aspirin) occurred without a significant excess of major bleeding, pointing to a net clinical benefit. Two points are worth considering: one is the appropriate choice of the target population, better than in previous—no matter how numerically larger—studies; the other is the synergy of multiple risk factor prevention, with the simultaneous administration of antithrombotic, antihypertensive, and lipid-lowering drugs.

Problems related to selection of appropriate patient category

The disappointing performance of aspirin treatment in the overall primary prevention setting may be explained by an inaccurate selection of the proper patient category: it is crucial for an appropriate favourable outcome for the identification of subjects at intermediate–high cardiovascular risk, defined as patients with an expected rate of MACE greater than 10/100 patients at 10 years[36] and low bleeding risk. The analysis of results of randomized clinical trials allows series of factors to be found that can affect the efficacy and safety of aspirin therapy, and, if taken into proper consideration, lead to a correct use of this important antiplatelet drug.

Poor performance of current cardiovascular risk stratification methods

Currently used scores for cardiovascular risk stratification are based on demographic and clinical parameters (age, sex, smoking habits, blood pressure, cholesterol, and cholesterol subfractions levels),[37] which are often only moderately associated with the global cardiovascular risk in healthy subjects. Such risk factors classify most subjects as low risk (MACE risk <10/100 patients at 10 years).[33] Also the geographic area where subjects are screened for this purpose appears to play a role, probably for its relationship with non-measured poorer or better life habits, and should therefore also be considered.[6] A comprehensive evaluation should consider the important risk modifiers for silent, subclinical, atherosclerotic vascular disease. The coronary artery calcium (CAC) score is a specific index of coronary atherosclerosis in asymptomatic patients,[38] especially when its value exceeds 100 Agatston units.[39,40] The presence of carotid artery plaques identified at carotid ultrasound considerably increases cardiovascular risk, although—apparently—with a lower impact on risk than CAC score.[41,42] Finally, evidence of asymptomatic peripheral arterial disease diagnosed by an ankle–brachial index (ABI) of 0.90 or less, is associated with a doubling in the risk of coronary events, as well as cardiovascular and all-cause mortality.[43] Despite the exposure to radiation and contrast medium, computed tomography (CT) coronary angiography can also provide information about the extent and possibly the phenotype of coronary plaques and on the overall coronary atherosclerotic burden.[44] As such, CAC score, carotid ultrasound, ABI measurement, and, possibly, CT coronary angiography can be used to improve cardiovascular risk estimation in primary prevention, refining assessments based on risk charts, and reclassifying a considerable proportion of patients.

Particular patient categories

Essential thrombocythaemia and obesity

Once-daily aspirin administration is thought to provide a complete TXA_2-mediated platelet inactivation up to 24 hours by irreversible COX-1 inhibition and the lack of sufficient *de novo* TX biosynthesis near the end of the dosing interval in most healthy subjects.[45] However, enzymatic synthesis can be accelerated by anomalous megakaryocytopoiesis, such as that occurring in essential thrombocythaemia,[46] and/or in the presence of reduced COX-1 acetylation due to an impaired aspirin bioavailability in obese patients.[47] In such conditions, more frequent (e.g. every 12 hours) aspirin administration may be required, even maintaining the same daily aspirin dose. Efficacy and safety of a twice-daily aspirin administration (in this case 100 mg twice daily for practical reasons) have recently been proven in the Aspirin Regimens in Essential Thrombocythemia (ARES) trial for patients with essential thrombocythaemia.[48] A randomized phase III clinical trial [Aspirin Twice a Day in Patients With Diabetes and Acute Coronary Syndrome (ANDAMAN)] is investigating the effects of a twice-daily aspirin regimen on ischaemic event reduction in obese and diabetic patients after an acute coronary syndrome.

High bleeding risk patients: proton pump inhibitor therapy

Due to effects on primary haemostasis, the main risk related to aspirin therapy, even at low doses, consists of increased bleeding, mostly mucosal bleeding, as it occurs for all antiplatelet agents. Observational studies[49] and a meta-analysis of randomized trials in patients at high cardiovascular risk[50] showed a doubling in major extracranial haemorrhages in subjects on low-dose aspirin treatment, mainly related to upper gastrointestinal bleeding. This risk increases with patient age (in particular ≥70 years), concomitant use of non-steroidal anti-inflammatory drugs, or history of previous gastrointestinal bleeding. This was fully confirmed in ASPREE,[24] ARRIVE,[20] and ASCEND.[26] The increase in gastrointestinal bleeding risk related to antiplatelet treatment may not have the same prognostic impact as intracranial haemorrhage, since intracranial haemorrhage is often fatal and hard to prevent or treat. The incidence of fatal and intracranial haemorrhagic events was low in both the aspirin and the control groups, but in ASPREE, a statistically significant increase also in intracranial bleeding was observed, probably because of the population age (mean age 74 years vs 64 and 63 years in the ARRIVE and ASCEND trials, respectively). Although not preventing intracranial bleeding, which is rare in absolute terms, but more common in elderly patients, proton pump inhibitors are an important and effective tool to reduce gastrointestinal bleeding in patients on aspirin therapy and with a high risk of haemorrhagic events.[51,52] Despite this concept being widely acknowledged, only a quarter of subjects included in the most recent clinical trials were on proton pump inhibitor therapy. In the COMPASS trial,[53] pantoprazole administration led to a major reduction in upper gastrointestinal haemorrhage in patients treated with antithrombotic drugs (low-dose aspirin, rivaroxaban, or both) compared with subjects on a placebo. Clinical judgement about the risk of cardiovascular and gastrointestinal bleeding may be supported by a dedicated risk calculator, as proposed by Lanas et al.[54]

Patients with colorectal cancer history: the potential chemopreventive effect of aspirin.

A beneficial effect of aspirin has been hypothesized, with some supporting data, in cancer prevention. This effect may appear after the regular aspirin (even at low doses) administration for at least a decade and seems to be mainly, but not exclusively, related to gastrointestinal cancer prevention.[18] Therefore, before prescribing aspirin therapy in the context of primary prevention, physicians should also evaluate and factor in the family history of gastrointestinal cancer.[55] However, the preventive role in cancer prevention of aspirin is not yet firmly established, and further trials with longer follow-up duration are also needed to clarify the real mechanism.[35]

Low number of patients at high cardiovascular risk and low bleeding risk

In the most recent studies, probably because of a greater attention to lifestyle (regular physical activity, body weight control, smoking cessation) and a more intensive use of cardioactive drugs (antihypertensive and lipid-lowering drugs), the number of ischaemic events has been lower than what could be expected according to previous risk scores. Furthermore, in contemporary preventive clinics, statins are commonly introduced as an initial intervention, further lowering absolute event rates. This clinical practice is increasingly being pursued because of the few adverse events associated with statin administration and the wide benefit derived from it, including in primary prevention.[56]

Notably, such scores had been introduced even more than 10 years before the start of the recent randomized trials. In balancing the advantage of MACE reduction with the added risk of extracranial (and also—to a limited extent—intracranial) bleeding, a recent analysis has shown that only 3% of examined individuals would have a net clinical benefit.[33] These data may explain the low percentage of patients at high cardiovascular risk enrolled in clinical trials: with the maintenance of the same reduction in relative risk, a lower absolute risk of cardiovascular events has, as a consequence, a lower absolute benefit. The TIPS-3 trial showed that MACE reduction is predominantly guided by the combination of antiplatelet therapy and the treatment of cardiovascular risk factors, instead of the isolated aspirin administration in patients at intermediate cardiovascular risk.[36] As reported above, in this trial aspirin alone did not achieve statistical significance in term of cardiovascular events reduction, but its association with angiotensin-converting enzyme inhibitors, diuretics, beta-blockers, and statins within the polypill proved to be statistically effective in reducing atherothrombotic events compared with the double placebo administration. These results confirm finding from previous trials, such as JUPITER[57] and HOPE-3,[58] showing synergy between aspirin and other cardioactive drugs.

Towards the identification of the proper patient category to treat

Concurrently, the literature discourages withdrawal of aspirin therapy in subjects already on treatment for at least 1 year, in the context of both secondary, but also primary prevention.[59] Notably, a Swedish study enrolled more than 600,000 patients aged over 40 years, without active cancer and with antiplatelet therapy adherence of at least 80% in the last year. After a median follow-up of 3 years, a 28% increase in cardiovascular events after aspirin withdrawal (not justified by surgery or bleeding) was observed (HR 1.28, 95% CI 1.22–1.34). The increased incidence of atherothrombotic events was mainly concentrated in the first month after therapy discontinuation, and the difference between the two groups (antiplatelet therapy withdrawal vs continuation) remained stable during the follow-up period. Experimental studies have suggested a rebound effect after aspirin withdrawal, involving increased TXA_2 levels derived from a possible prothrombotic effect of residual low aspirin levels[60–62]: this process could continuously be present in patients with poor treatment adherence. This mechanism is supported by the lack of increase in cardiovascular events in patients who continued to be on other antiplatelet and/or anticoagulant drugs at the time of aspirin discontinuation.

In 2014, an ESC Working Group on Thrombosis Expert document proposed a therapeutic algorithm based on risk stratification.[63] The authors recommended not to prescribe aspirin in primary prevention in patients with 10-year MACE risk of less than 10%, and to consider its administration in case of cardiovascular risk ranging from 10% to 20%, especially in subjects at low bleeding risk. In this category of patients, a family history of gastrointestinal cancer could further enhance the indication for treatment. Finally, a clear recommendation was issued for patients with 10-year MACE risk greater than 20%. This algorithm was developed after comparing clinical benefit and bleeding risk, according to the 10-year MACE risk calculated in the control group. The benefit of aspirin in terms of reduction of thromboembolic events increased progressively with the increased risk of MACE, while the risk of major bleeding increased less steeply in the various groups of subjects included in the clinical trials. The conclusion was that the reduction in atherothrombotic events was balanced by an equal risk of bleeding in patients at the lowest cardiovascular risk, whereas the net clinical benefit from aspirin administration became apparent in subjects at higher risk. The authors identified 10% and 20% 10-year MACE risks as the cut-off values for treatment decisions, with an area of uncertainty between these thresholds. Furthermore, it was proposed to consider patients' bleeding risk and the potential for aspirin in preventing gastrointestinal cancer. At this time, in subjects aged less than 70 years, it is still appropriate to maintain a 10-year MACE risk of 20% as a threshold for aspirin treatment in primary prevention for two main reasons: first, it coincides with the risk observed in clinical practice in the context of secondary prevention, as shown in the COMPASS trial,[53] in which aspirin was the standard of care; second, this cut-off value approximates the risk of patients with significant atherosclerosis, proved by an ABI less than 0.9,[64] the presence of carotid plaques,[65] or a CAC score greater than 100 Agatston units.[39,40] The same trends in risk of atherothrombotic events and haemorrhagic events as a function of the 10-year risk for MACE risk are observed in an updated meta-regression that includes ASPREE,[24] ARRIVE,[20] ASCEND,[26] and TIPS-3[36] (➔ Figure 14.1). Notably, the first three studies enrolled subjects with a 10-year MACE risk of 10% or less (8.3% in ASPREE, 10.2% in ASCEND, and 6.8% in ARRIVE), whereas TIPS-3 included patients at intermediate cardiovascular risk (12%). When compared with the results of our previous 2014 meta-regression,[63] the integration of these new data shows a reduction in the relationship between MACE and baseline cardiovascular risk, while still maintaining statistical significance ($r = 0.618$; $P = 0.024$). In addition, the slope of the regression line relating major bleeding with cardiovascular risk was also found to be lower compared with the previous meta-regression, attaining statistical significance with the regression line of atherothrombotic events (coincidence test, $P < 0.001$). The separation of the regression lines, depicting the net clinical benefit, tends to increase as a function of cardiovascular risk: this finding results from the relative stability of the bleeding regression line with minimal slope, even in patients at higher cardiovascular risk (➔ Figure 14.1). This evidence confirms the indication for aspirin administration in primary prevention in individuals at high cardiovascular risk and low bleeding risk, and supports its 'possible' use even in intermediate-risk patients.

A new decision-making algorithm for aspirin therapy in primary prevention is therefore proposed (➔ Figure 14.2), quite similar to that proposed in the 2019 ACC/AHA guidelines on cardiovascular prevention.[7] This algorithm suggests prophylactic aspirin administration in patients aged less than 70 years with optimal risk factor control, ultimately also obtained by a proper use of antihypertensive and lipid-lowering drugs.[36]

Evolution of risk estimation charts

Until 2020, the use of the Atherosclerotic Cardiovascular Disease Score,[66] designed for estimating the risk of cardiovascular disease

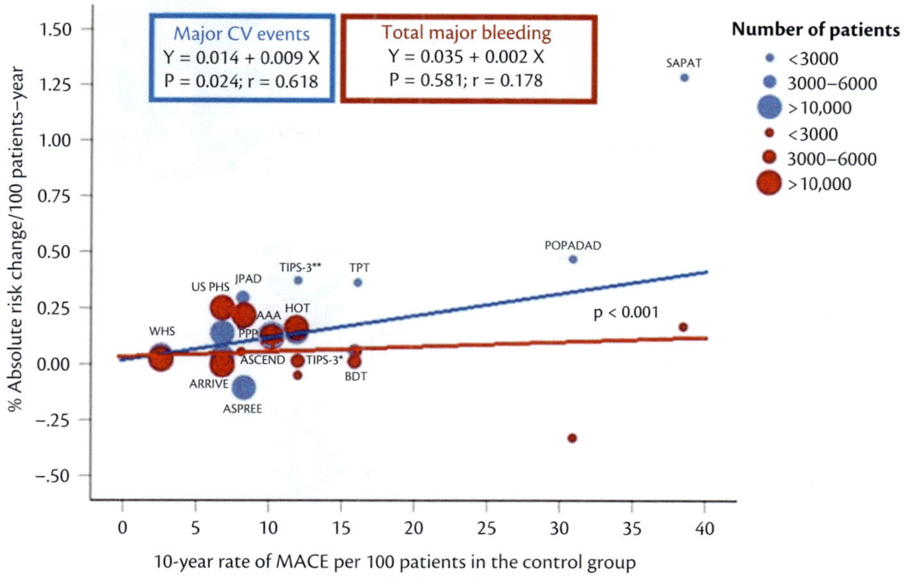

Figure 14.1 Relationships between antithrombotic benefit and risk of major bleeding and absolute cardiovascular (CV) risk associated with aspirin use in primary prevention. This linear meta-regression reports the effect of aspirin as a function of baseline cardiovascular risk. The blue-coloured line represents major cardiovascular events (cardiovascular death, non-fatal myocardial infarction, and non-fatal stroke). The red-coloured line represents total major haemorrhagic events. The independent variable is the 10-year risk of major cardiovascular events in the control groups of each randomized clinical trial. On the y-axis the difference in absolute risk per 100 subjects per year is shown: for major cardiovascular events it is calculated as the risk/years of follow-up per 100 of control group minus the risk/years of follow-up per 100 of aspirin group; for total major bleeding it is calculated as the risk/years of follow-up per 100 of aspirin group minus the risk/years of follow-up per 100 of control group. The weight of each study is proportional to the number of subjects included. Each study is represented by two circles (blue for risk of major cardiovascular events and red for risk of total major bleeding), the size of which is proportional to the sample size. For the TIPS-3 trial, the two comparison groups were considered separately (TIPS-3*: aspirin vs placebo; TIPS**: aspirin + polypill vs double placebo) and were, therefore, graphically represented by means of four circles. AAA, Aspirin for Asymptomatic Atherosclerosis[25]; ARRIVE, Aspirin to Reduce Risk of Initial Vascular Events[20]; ASCEND, A Study of Cardiovascular Events In Diabetes[26]; ASPREE, Aspirin in Reducing Events in the Elderly[24]; BDT, British Doctors Trial[32]; HOT, Hypertension Optimal Treatment[30]; JPAD, Japanese Primary Prevention of Atherosclerosis With Aspirin for Diabetes[27]; MACE, major adverse cardiovascular event; POPADAD, Prevention of Progression of Arterial Disease and Diabetes[28]; PPP, Primary Prevention Project[23]; SAPAT, Double-Blind Trial of Aspirin in Primary Prevention of Myocardial Infarction in Patients with Stable Chronic Angina Pectoris[68]; TIPS-3, Polypill with or without Aspirin in Persons without Cardiovascular Disease[36]; TPT, Thrombosis Prevention Trial[22]; US PHS, US Physician Health Study[31]; WHS, Women's Health Study[19].

or stroke in the US, could also be recommended in Europe for evaluating the 10-year MACE risk because the alternative ESC European Systematic COronary Risk Evaluation (SCORE)[67] provided only the estimate of fatal cardiovascular events. Although it was possible to use approximative conversion factors to obtain the risk for total (fatal plus non-fatal) MACEs, the utilization of SCORE could lead to an inaccurate total MACE risk estimation. The 2021 ESC Guidelines for cardiovascular prevention[6] have, however, recently introduced the SCORE2, which now allows risk estimates for 10-year fatal and non-fatal cardio- and cerebrovascular events. SCORE2 also allows additional precision in risk stratification based on the European country of membership, and can therefore currently be proposed as the most updated way for risk estimate, useful to decide on the use of aspirin in primary prevention.

Conclusion

Aspirin is an effective drug in the context of secondary cardiovascular prevention; however, its use is not applicable *tout court* in primary prevention. Because of obvious benefits associated with relatively rare and mostly reversible side effects, a combination of healthy diet, physical exercise, and smoking cessation constitute the most relevant lifestyle changes to be recommended and adopted. Among medical treatments, administration of statins and antihypertensive drugs are probably the most effective way to curb cardiovascular risk in primary prevention. Once lipid levels and blood pressure have been addressed, it is currently recommended to perform a proper risk stratification to identify patients who might benefit from aspirin administration in primary prevention, and then to have a discussion of risks and benefits with individual patients who may differ in preferences. In line with data provided by the most recent clinical trials, this recommendation should be restricted to patients at the highest end of the spectrum of cardiovascular risk (>20% risk of MACE at 10 years), and—possibly—those at intermediate risk (10–20% risk of MACEs at 10 years), whenever a prohibitive bleeding risk can be excluded. The benefit of such antithrombotic therapy is amplified by the simultaneous treatment of other risk factors, including lipid-lowering and antihypertensive drugs. A practical flow chart for the use of aspirin in primary prevention is provided in ➔ Figure 14.2.

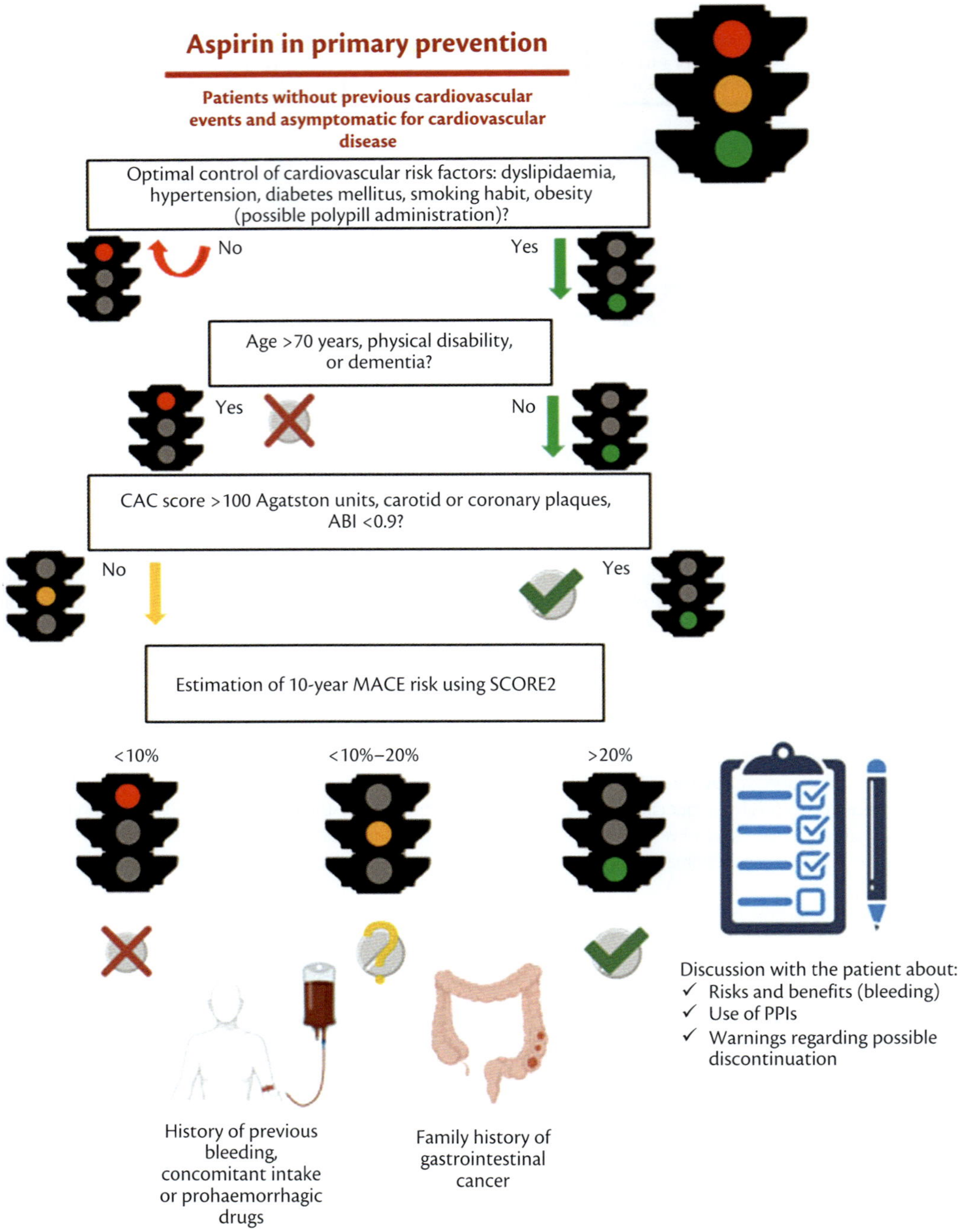

Figure 14.2 A decision-making algorithm for aspirin use in primary cardiovascular prevention (asymptomatic patients without known overt cardiovascular disease). Patients in primary prevention should first achieve optimal control of cardiovascular risk factors, if appropriate by administration of antihypertensive/cardioprotective and lipid-lowering drugs, even in a polypill combination. Subsequently, patients aged under 70 years without physical disability and/or dementia should be screened for subclinical atherosclerotic disease, by calculation of coronary artery calcium (CAC) score, possible documentation of coronary plaques at coronary angio-computed tomography (CT) or carotid plaques at echo-colour Doppler, and measurement of ankle–brachial index (ABI), to identify a population at increased risk that may benefit from aspirin administration in primary prevention. If negative at screening, patients should be stratified using Systematic COronary Risk Estimation 2 (SCORE2) into (a) those at low cardiovascular risk [10-year major adverse cardiovascular event (MACE) risk <10%]; (b) intermediate (between 10% and 20%); or (c) high (>20%). In the first group, aspirin administration is not recommended because of the proven little clinical benefit as opposed to increased bleeding risk. In intermediate-risk patients, aspirin therapy may be considered, particularly in patients with a family history of gastrointestinal cancer and in the absence of previous irreversible bleedings and/or concomitant therapy with pro-haemorrhagic medications. In subjects with 10-year MACE risk greater than 20%, aspirin therapy should be undertaken, after reasonable discussion with the patient regarding the potential risks and benefits (with particular attention to bleeding) and the importance of concomitant proton pump inhibitor (PPI) intake. The danger of the possible rebound effect associated with discontinuation of regular and prolonged aspirin therapy, not justified by surgery and/or bleeding, should, in addition, be considered.

What's new

- A recently published trial, TIPS-3, has provided new evidence regarding the potential efficacy of aspirin in primary prevention in selected populations at intermediate cardiovascular risk and low bleeding risk.
- TIPS-3 results underline the important role of concomitant risk factors control by co-administration of lipid-lowering and antihypertensive drugs.
- The 2021 ESC Guidelines for cardiovascular prevention have introduced an updated score, SCORE2, for estimating the 10-year risk of fatal and non-fatal major cardio- and cerebrovascular events.
- CAC score, detection of carotid artery plaques at carotid ultrasound, measurement of the ABI, and CT coronary angiography are non-invasive tests, which improve cardiovascular risk estimation in primary prevention.
- Proton pump inhibitors are an effective tool to reduce gastrointestinal bleeding in patient on aspirin therapy and high risk of haemorrhagic events.
- In patients with essential thrombocythaemia and obesity, twice-daily aspirin administration may be required.
- In patients in primary prevention, a Swedish study showed a 28% increase of cardiovascular events after aspirin withdrawal, possibly due to a prothrombotic rebound.
- The results of meta-regression showing the relationship of MACEs and major bleeding as a function of baseline cardiovascular risk, conducted on the basis of all clinical trials of aspirin in primary prevention so far available, show that the net clinical benefit increases as a function of cardiovascular risk.

Guideline recommendations

Aspirin is the cornerstone of antiplatelet therapy in the setting of secondary prevention. Both most recent US and European guidelines strongly recommend the use of aspirin in subjects with previous atherothrombotic events, established coronary artery disease, or symptomatic lower extremities arterial disease if no contraindications exist. For primary prevention, in US guidelines aspirin administration may be considered in selected younger patients at higher cardiovascular risk without high risk of bleeding and is not recommended in patients older than 70 years of age or with increased risk of bleeding. Conversely, in the context of primary prevention, European guidelines recommend the use of aspirin only in patients with diabetes at high or very high cardiovascular risk and contraindicate its use in adults with low/moderate risk because of the prevailing bleeding risk in this category.

What's next

There is limited evidence based on randomized control trials on the use of aspirin in patients at high or even intermediate cardiovascular risk. More trials in such patients would still be welcomed.

Drug dosing

Low-dose aspirin (75–100 mg once daily). In particular conditions (so far essential thrombocythaemia, perhaps in obese patients) featuring accelerated platelet turnover, a twice-daily aspirin recommendation (100 mg twice daily) can be recommended. In such conditions, probably even 50 mg twice daily is effective, and theoretically more effective than 100 mg once daily. Two of the four contemporary trials described in this chapter used enteric-coated aspirin formulations, but with no conclusive evidence of advantages or disadvantages.

References

1. Montinari MR, Minelli S, De Caterina R. The first 3500 years of aspirin history from its roots—a concise summary. Vascul Pharmacol. 2019;113:1–8.
2. Roth GJ, Stanford N, Majerus PW. Acetylation of prostaglandin synthase by aspirin. Proc Natl Acad Sci U S A. 1975;72(8): 3073–6.
3. Ibanez B, James S, Agewall S, et al. 2017 ESC Guidelines for the management of acute myocardial infarction in patients presenting with ST-segment elevation: the Task Force for the management of acute myocardial infarction in patients presenting with ST-segment elevation of the European Society of Cardiology (ESC). Eur Heart J. 2018;39(2):119–77.
4. Collet JP, Thiele H, Barbato E, et al. 2020 ESC Guidelines for the management of acute coronary syndromes in patients presenting without persistent ST-segment elevation. Eur Heart J. 2021;42(14):1289–367.
5. Cosentino F, Grant PJ, Aboyans V, et al. 2019 ESC Guidelines on diabetes, pre-diabetes, and cardiovascular diseases developed in collaboration with the EASD. Eur Heart J. 2020;41(2):255–323.
6. Visseren FLJ, Mach F, Smulders YM, et al. 2021 ESC Guidelines on cardiovascular disease prevention in clinical practice. Eur Heart J. 2021;42(34):3227–337.
7. Arnett DK, Blumenthal RS, Albert MA, et al. 2019 ACC/AHA guideline on the primary prevention of cardiovascular disease: executive summary: a report of the American College of Cardiology/American Heart Association Task Force on Clinical Practice Guidelines. J Am Coll Cardiol. 2019;74(10):1376–414.
8. Aimo A, De Caterina R. Aspirin for primary prevention of cardiovascular disease: advice for a decisional strategy based on risk stratification. Anatol J Cardiol. 2020;23(2):70–8.
9. Knuuti J, Wijns W, Saraste A, et al. 2019 ESC Guidelines for the diagnosis and management of chronic coronary syndromes. Eur Heart J. 2020;41(3):407–77.
10. Kleindorfer DO, Towfighi A, Chaturvedi S, et al. 2021 guideline for the prevention of stroke in patients with stroke and transient ischemic attack: a guideline from the American Heart Association/American Stroke Association. Stroke. 2021;52(7):e364–467.
11. Aboyans V, Ricco JB, Bartelink MEL, et al. 2017 ESC Guidelines on the diagnosis and treatment of peripheral arterial diseases, in collaboration with the European Society for Vascular Surgery (ESVS): document covering atherosclerotic disease of extracranial carotid and vertebral, mesenteric, renal, upper and lower extremity arteries. Endorsed by: the European Stroke Organization (ESO), The

Task Force for the Diagnosis and Treatment of Peripheral Arterial Diseases of the European Society of Cardiology (ESC) and of the European Society for Vascular Surgery (ESVS). Eur Heart J. 2018;39(9):763–816.

12. Collins R, Baigent C, Sandercock P, Peto R. Antiplatelet therapy for thromboprophylaxis: the need for careful consideration of the evidence from randomised trials. Antiplatelet Trialists' Collaboration. BMJ. 1994;309(6963):1215–17.
13. Antiplatelet Trialists' Collaboration. Secondary prevention of vascular disease by prolonged antiplatelet treatment. Br Med J (Clin Res Ed). 1988;296(6618):320–31.
14. Baigent C, Blackwell L, Collins R, et al. Aspirin in the primary and secondary prevention of vascular disease: collaborative meta-analysis of individual participant data from randomised trials. Lancet. 2009;373(9678):1849–60.
15. Patrono C. Low-dose aspirin in primary prevention: cardioprotection, chemoprevention, both, or neither? Eur Heart J. 2013;34(44):3403–11.
16. Cleland JG. Is aspirin useful in primary prevention? Eur Heart J. 2013;34(44):3412–18.
17. Bibbins-Domingo K. Aspirin use for the primary prevention of cardiovascular disease and colorectal cancer: U.S. Preventive Services Task Force Recommendation Statement. Ann Intern Med. 2016;164(12):836–45.
18. Guirguis-Blake JM, Evans CV, Senger CA, O'Connor EA, Whitlock EP. Aspirin for the primary prevention of cardiovascular events: a systematic evidence review for the U.S. Preventive Services Task Force. Ann Intern Med. 2016;164(12):804–13.
19. Ridker PM, Cook NR, Lee IM, et al. A randomized trial of low-dose aspirin in the primary prevention of cardiovascular disease in women. N Engl J Med. 2005;352(13):1293–304.
20. Gaziano JM, Brotons C, Coppolecchia R, et al. Use of aspirin to reduce risk of initial vascular events in patients at moderate risk of cardiovascular disease (ARRIVE): a randomised, double-blind, placebo-controlled trial. Lancet. 2018;392(10152):1036–46.
21. Ikeda Y, Shimada K, Teramoto T, et al. Low-dose aspirin for primary prevention of cardiovascular events in Japanese patients 60 years or older with atherosclerotic risk factors: a randomized clinical trial. JAMA. 2014;312(23):2510–20.
22. The Medical Research Council's General Practice Research Framework. Thrombosis prevention trial: randomised trial of low-intensity oral anticoagulation with warfarin and low-dose aspirin in the primary prevention of ischaemic heart disease in men at increased risk. Lancet. 1998;351(9098):233–41.
23. de Gaetano G. Low-dose aspirin and vitamin E in people at cardiovascular risk: a randomised trial in general practice. Collaborative Group of the Primary Prevention Project. Lancet. 2001;357(9250):89–95.
24. McNeil JJ, Wolfe R, Woods RL, et al. Effect of aspirin on cardiovascular events and bleeding in the healthy elderly. N Engl J Med. 2018;379(16):1509–18.
25. Fowkes FG, Price JF, Stewart MC, et al. Aspirin for prevention of cardiovascular events in a general population screened for a low ankle brachial index: a randomized controlled trial. JAMA. 2010;303(9):841–8.
26. Bowman L, Mafham M, Wallendszus K, et al. Effects of aspirin for primary prevention in persons with diabetes mellitus. N Engl J Med. 2018;379(16):1529–39.
27. Ogawa H, Nakayama M, Morimoto T, et al. Low-dose aspirin for primary prevention of atherosclerotic events in patients with type 2 diabetes: a randomized controlled trial. JAMA. 2008;300(18):2134–41.
28. Belch J, MacCuish A, Campbell I, et al. The prevention of progression of arterial disease and diabetes (POPADAD) trial: factorial randomised placebo controlled trial of aspirin and antioxidants in patients with diabetes and asymptomatic peripheral arterial disease. BMJ. 2008;337:a1840.
29. The Early Treatment Diabetic Retinopathy Study (ETDRS) Investigators. Aspirin effects on mortality and morbidity in patients with diabetes mellitus. Early Treatment Diabetic Retinopathy Study report 14. JAMA. 1992;268(10):1292–300.
30. Hansson L, Zanchetti A, Carruthers et al. Effects of intensive blood-pressure lowering and low-dose aspirin in patients with hypertension: principal results of the Hypertension Optimal Treatment (HOT) randomised trial. HOT Study Group. Lancet. 1998;351(9118):1755–62.
31. Steering Committee of the Physicians' Health Study. Final report on the aspirin component of the ongoing Physicians' Health Study. N Engl J Med. 1989;321(3):129–35.
32. Peto R, Gray R, Collins R, et al. Randomised trial of prophylactic daily aspirin in British male doctors. Br Med J (Clin Res Ed). 1988;296(6618):313–16.
33. Patrono C, Baigent C. Role of aspirin in primary prevention of cardiovascular disease. Nat Rev Cardiol. 2019;16(11):675–86.
34. Gaziano JM. Aspirin for primary prevention: clinical considerations in 2019. JAMA. 2019;321(3):253–5.
35. Patrignani P, Patrono C. Aspirin and cancer. J Am Coll Cardiol. 2016;68(9):967–76.
36. Yusuf S, Joseph P, Dans A, et al. Polypill with or without aspirin in persons without cardiovascular disease. N Engl J Med. 2021;384(3):216–28.
37. SCORE2 working group and ESC Cardiovascular risk collaboration. SCORE2 risk prediction algorithms: new models to estimate 10-year risk of cardiovascular disease in Europe. Eur Heart J. 2021;42(25):2439–54.
38. Greenland P, Blaha MJ, Budoff MJ, Erbel R, Watson KE. Coronary calcium score and cardiovascular risk. J Am Coll Cardiol. 2018;72(4):434–47.
39. Detrano R, Guerci AD, Carr JJ, et al. Coronary calcium as a predictor of coronary events in four racial or ethnic groups. N Engl J Med. 2008;358(13):1336–45.
40. Nielsen LH, Botker HE, Sorensen HT, et al. Prognostic assessment of stable coronary artery disease as determined by coronary computed tomography angiography: a Danish multicentre cohort study. Eur Heart J. 2017;38(6):413–21.
41. Stein JH, Korcarz CE, Hurst RT, et al. Use of carotid ultrasound to identify subclinical vascular disease and evaluate cardiovascular disease risk: a consensus statement from the American Society of Echocardiography Carotid Intima-Media Thickness Task Force. Endorsed by the Society for Vascular Medicine. J Am Soc Echocardiogr. 2008;21(2):93–111.
42. Peters SA, den Ruijter HM, Bots ML, Moons KG. Improvements in risk stratification for the occurrence of cardiovascular disease by imaging subclinical atherosclerosis: a systematic review. Heart. 2012;98(3):177–84.
43. Fowkes FG, Murray GD, Butcher I, et al. Ankle brachial index combined with Framingham Risk Score to predict cardiovascular events and mortality: a meta-analysis. JAMA. 2008;300(2):197–208.
44. Nakanishi R, Budoff MJ. A new approach in risk stratification by coronary CT angiography. Scientifica (Cairo). 2014;2014:278039.
45. Patrono C, Baigent C, Hirsh J, Roth G. Antiplatelet drugs: American College of Chest Physicians Evidence-Based Clinical Practice Guidelines (8th Edition). Chest. 2008;133(6 Suppl):199s–233s.
46. Pascale S, Petrucci G, Dragani A, et al. Aspirin-insensitive thromboxane biosynthesis in essential thrombocythemia is explained by accelerated renewal of the drug target. Blood. 2012;119(15):3595–603.
47. Rocca B, Santilli F, Pitocco D, et al. The recovery of platelet cyclooxygenase activity explains interindividual variability in

responsiveness to low-dose aspirin in patients with and without diabetes. J Thromb Haemost. 2012;10(7):1220–30.

48. De Stefano V, Rocca B, Tosetto A, et al. The Aspirin Regimens in Essential Thrombocythemia (ARES) phase II randomized trial design: implementation of the serum thromboxane B(2) assay as an evaluation tool of different aspirin dosing regimens in the clinical setting. Blood Cancer J. 2018;8(6):49.
49. García Rodríguez LA, Hernández-Díaz S, de Abajo FJ. Association between aspirin and upper gastrointestinal complications: systematic review of epidemiologic studies. Br J Clin Pharmacol. 2001;52(5):563–71.
50. Antithrombotic Trialists' Collaboration. Collaborative meta-analysis of randomised trials of antiplatelet therapy for prevention of death, myocardial infarction, and stroke in high risk patients. BMJ. 2002;324(7329):71–86.
51. Lanas A, Chan FKL. Peptic ulcer disease. Lancet. 2017;390(10094): 613–24.
52. Agewall S, Cattaneo M, Collet JP, et al. Expert position paper on the use of proton pump inhibitors in patients with cardiovascular disease and antithrombotic therapy. Eur Heart J. 2013;34(23):1708–13.
53. Eikelboom JW, Connolly SJ, Bosch J, et al. Rivaroxaban with or without aspirin in stable cardiovascular disease. N Engl J Med. 2017;377(14):1319–30.
54. Lanas A, Polo-Tomas M, Casado-Arroyo R. The aspirin cardiovascular/gastrointestinal risk calculator—a tool to aid clinicians in practice. Aliment Pharmacol Ther. 2013;37(7):738–48.
55. De Caterina R, Aimo A, Ridker PM. Aspirin therapy for primary prevention: the case for continuing prescribing to patients at high cardiovascular risk—a review. Thromb Haemost. 2020;120(2): 199–206.
56. Ridker PM. Should aspirin be used for primary prevention in the post-statin era? N Engl J Med. 2018;379(16):1572–4.
57. Ridker PM, Danielson E, Fonseca FA, et al. Rosuvastatin to prevent vascular events in men and women with elevated C-reactive protein. N Engl J Med. 2008;359(21):2195–207.
58. Yusuf S, Lonn E, Pais P, et al. Blood-pressure and cholesterol lowering in persons without cardiovascular disease. N Engl J Med. 2016;374(21):2032–43.
59. Sundström J, Hedberg J, Thuresson M, Aarskog P, Johannesen KM, Oldgren J. Low-dose aspirin discontinuation and risk of cardiovascular events: a Swedish nationwide, population-based cohort study. Circulation. 2017;136(13):1183–92.
60. Vial JH, McLeod LJ, Roberts MS. Rebound elevation in urinary thromboxane B2 and 6-keto-PGF1 alpha excretion after aspirin withdrawal. Adv Prostaglandin Thromboxane Leukot Res. 1991;21A:157–60.
61. McDonald JW, Ali M. Recovery of cyclooxygenase activity after aspirin in populations of platelets separated on stractan density gradients. Prostaglandins Leukot Med. 1983;12(3):245–52.
62. Doutremepuich C, Aguejouf O, Desplat V, Eizayaga FX. Paradoxical thrombotic effects of aspirin: experimental study on 1000 animals. Cardiovasc Hematol Disord Drug Targets. 2010;10(2):103–10.
63. Halvorsen S, Andreotti F, ten Berg JM, et al. Aspirin therapy in primary cardiovascular disease prevention: a position paper of the European Society of Cardiology working group on thrombosis. J Am Coll Cardiol. 2014;64(3):319–27.
64. Criqui MH, Langer RD, Fronek A, et al. Mortality over a period of 10 years in patients with peripheral arterial disease. N Engl J Med. 1992;326(6):381–6.
65. Halliday A, Harrison M, Hayter E, et al. 10-year stroke prevention after successful carotid endarterectomy for asymptomatic stenosis (ACST-1): a multicentre randomised trial. Lancet. 2010;376(9746):1074–84.
66. D'Agostino RB Sr, Vasan RS, Pencina MJ, et al. General cardiovascular risk profile for use in primary care: the Framingham Heart Study. Circulation. 2008;117(6):743–53.
67. Piepoli MF, Hoes AW, Agewall S, et al. 2016 European Guidelines on cardiovascular disease prevention in clinical practice: the Sixth Joint Task Force of the European Society of Cardiology and Other Societies on Cardiovascular Disease Prevention in Clinical Practice (constituted by representatives of 10 societies and by invited experts): developed with the special contribution of the European Association for Cardiovascular Prevention & Rehabilitation (EACPR). Eur J Prev Cardiol. 2016;23(11):NP1–96.
68. Juul-Möller S, Edvardsson N, Jahnmatz B, Rosén A, Sørensen S, Omblus R. Double-blind trial of aspirin in primary prevention of myocardial infarction in patients with stable chronic angina pectoris. The Swedish Angina Pectoris Aspirin Trial (SAPAT) Group. Lancet. 1992;340(8833):1421–5.

CHAPTER 15

Antithrombotic strategies in patients undergoing elective percutaneous coronary interventions and in chronic coronary syndromes without interventions

Antonio Greco and Davide Capodanno

Contents

Summary

Antithrombotic therapy plays a key role in the treatment and secondary prevention of coronary artery disease. After elective percutaneous coronary intervention or chronic coronary syndrome, dual antiplatelet therapy (DAPT) with aspirin and a $P2Y_{12}$ receptor inhibitor is usually indicated for 6 months. However, a risk stratification approach considering and weighing both the ischaemic and bleeding risks is of the utmost importance when it comes to tailoring antithrombotic therapy for the individual patient. A number of ischaemic, bleeding, and net benefit risk scores are available and should be used to inform the selection of the optimal antithrombotic regimen. Different approaches can be adopted according to the individual patient risk profile, including strategies aimed at minimizing the risk of bleeding (i.e. shortening DAPT duration by stopping either the $P2Y_{12}$ receptor inhibitor or aspirin) or at enhancing antithrombotic protection (i.e. prolonging DAPT duration with clopidogrel, prasugrel, or low-dose ticagrelor, switching from clopidogrel to prasugrel or ticagrelor, or adding a low-dose anticoagulant to aspirin in the context of a dual pathway inhibition). Also, long-term monotherapy should be carefully selected to improve the benefits of antithrombotic therapy for secondary prevention: although aspirin has long been the drug of choice, evidence on $P2Y_{12}$ inhibitor monotherapy (i.e. clopidogrel or ticagrelor) is accruing and it can represent a promising option. The choice of the antithrombotic regimen is even more challenging among patients who require, per se, long-term oral anticoagulation, such as those with atrial fibrillation, in whom a triple therapy is theoretically indicated but unfeasible over the long term due to the excess bleeding risk: current guidelines recommend a very short triple therapy (i.e. up to 1 week) followed by dual antithrombotic therapy with clopidogrel and a direct inhibitor of the activated factor II (i.e. dabigatran) or X (i.e. apixaban, edoxaban, or rivaroxaban) up to 6 months, and finally by lifelong oral anticoagulation alone. Gaps in knowledge still remain in the field of antithrombotic therapy for patients undergoing elective percutaneous coronary intervention or with chronic coronary syndrome, so further trials are warranted to inform clinical practice and future guidelines on the optimal regimen to be selected for each specific setting and condition.

Introduction

The practice of administering antithrombotic therapy in patients with coronary artery disease (CAD) dates back to 1980, when a small randomized trial demonstrated a survival benefit of vitamin K antagonists (VKAs) compared with placebo after a myocardial infarction (MI).[1] In the 1990s, aspirin was the first antiplatelet agent to be tested for the purpose of preventing MI in a randomized placebo-controlled trial of patients with stable angina.[2] Combining aspirin and VKA then became an option following the introduction of percutaneous coronary intervention (PCI) that, at the time, was performed mostly without implanting coronary stents.[3] The era of PCI procedures with stent implantation established the need for a better strategy to mitigate the risk of stent-related thrombotic complications. In another trial, dual antiplatelet therapy (DAPT)—consisting of aspirin in combination with the $P2Y_{12}$ receptor inhibitor ticlopidine—was better than aspirin, oral anticoagulation (OAC), or their combination, and thus became the standard of care for patients undergoing PCI.[4,5] However, a major and unavoidable drawback of DAPT is its increased risk of major bleeding, which is known to exert detrimental prognostic effects.[6]

The emerging paradigm of tailored therapy led to the conceptualization of a number of DAPT strategies aimed at achieving the sweet spot between protection at the level of stented and non-stented coronary segments and the risk of bleeding events.[7] While the introduction of clopidogrel addressed some of the side effects of ticlopidine (e.g. neutropenia, diarrhoea, and rash) and established the paradigm of a 12-month course of DAPT after stent implantation, the availability of newer iterations of coronary stents and several technical advances in PCI practice also enabled the administration of shorter and safer DAPT regimens in patients with and without high bleeding risk (HBR).[8]

To date, a number of antithrombotic strategies are available for the treatment and secondary prevention of patients undergoing elective PCI or presenting with chronic coronary syndrome (CCS).[8] These include several types and durations of DAPT, and the combination of aspirin with the low-dose anticoagulant rivaroxaban. This chapter aims at reviewing the body of knowledge supporting current guideline recommendations and future directions in the field of antithrombotic therapy for CCS patients with or without PCI.

Risk stratification

Choosing the optimal antithrombotic regimen is a major clinical challenge since one strategy does not fit all patients. Indeed, a large amount of clinical and procedural factors influence the propensity of a patient to experience thrombotic or bleeding complications.[7] A risk stratification approach that simultaneously estimates the individual risks of thrombotic and bleeding events is key; this approach must aim at identifying the most prevalent risk and inform treatment decisions (i.e. to select a strategy that confers higher ischaemic protection or reduces the risk of bleeding). Of note, these two opposed but intertwined risks are dynamic and strongly dependent on factors that are extremely variable; hence, risk assessment should be repeated over time.[9]

Several risk-based approaches are available to support decision-making after elective PCI or in patients with CCS. Complex PCI is frequently considered a surrogate of thrombotic risk, and broadly accepted as one of the following circumstances: three coronary vessels treated, at least three stents implanted, at least three lesions treated, bifurcation with two stents implanted, a total stent length greater than 60 mm, and the presence of a chronic total occlusion.[10,11] A number of additional conditions were associated with a higher risk of thrombotic complications, including diabetes, premature or accelerated CAD, history of recurrent MI, peripheral artery disease, concomitant systemic inflammatory diseases, and chronic kidney disease.[12]

Defining the risk of bleeding is also essential when antithrombotic therapy is decided. The most used bleeding scales are the Bleeding Academic Research Consortium (BARC), Global Strategies for Opening Occluded Coronary Arteries (GUSTO), International Society on Thrombosis and Haemostasis (ISTH), and Thrombolysis In Myocardial Infarction (TIMI) classifications, which use different parameters to grade bleeding based on severity.[13–16] Bleeding risk stratification tools also exist; the PRECISE-DAPT score, which is recommended by the guidelines from the European Society of Cardiology (ESC), was derived from a pooled analysis of eight trials encompassing almost 15,000 PCI patients and included five variables (i.e. age, creatinine clearance, haemoglobin, white blood cell count, and prior spontaneous bleeding) to predict the risk of TIMI major or minor bleeding at 1 year. The score was conceived as a tool to calculate out-of-hospital bleeding, with a cut-off value of 25 or greater indicating HBR on DAPT. More recently, the Academic Research Consortium (ARC) produced a consensus document, also recommended by the ESC Guidelines, that provides a dichotomic definition of HBR for patients undergoing PCI. Twenty risk factors were selected and classified as major or minor according to the associated risk of BARC major or fatal bleeding at 1 year (i.e. ≥4% or ≥1%, respectively); patients with at least one major or two minor criteria were categorized as HBR.[17] These criteria were also externally validated in different registries, showing good predictive performances among patients with either acute coronary syndrome or CCS.[18–21] Although the ARC-HBR approach is semiquantitative and dichotomic, it is not surprising that fulfilling more criteria is associated with a stepwise higher risk of bleeding events.[21]

An important goal of a good risk stratification approach is the ability to balance the risks of thrombosis and bleeding to identify subgroups of patients who are candidates for one or another strategy. The DAPT score uses nine clinical or procedural variables (i.e. age, smoking status, diabetes, presentation with MI, history of PCI or MI, heart failure or left ventricular ejection fraction <30%, and implantation of paclitaxel-eluting stent(s), stents with diameter <3 mm, or stents at the level of vein grafts) to predict the risk of both thrombosis and bleeding after 12 months of uneventful DAPT; a DAPT score greater than 2 means that the thrombotic risk prevails over the risk of bleeding, thereby implying a preference for prolonged DAPT.[22] Another trade-off approach was introduced by the ARC-HBR task force.[23]

Antithrombotic strategies for chronic coronary syndrome patients in sinus rhythm

The current ESC Guidelines on the management of CCS recommend secondary prevention with aspirin 75–100 mg in patients with a previous MI or revascularization [class of recommendation (COR) I, level of evidence (LOE) A] or in those with evidence of CAD on imaging (COR IIb, LOE C); clopidogrel 75 mg is an alternative in patients with aspirin intolerance (COR I, LOE B) or in patients with peripheral artery disease or a history of stroke or transient ischaemic attack (COR IIb, LOE B).[11] In patients undergoing PCI with stent implantation, DAPT with aspirin 75–100 mg and clopidogrel 75 mg is recommended for 6 months (COR I, LOE A).[11]

Based on risk assessment and its expected trade-off, antithrombotic therapy can be modulated to be either less or more intense (➔ Figure 15.1). However, the interplay of ischaemia and bleeding remains a matter of debate, especially because several patients present with high risk of both thrombosis and bleeding. In a pooled analysis of 14,963 patients from eight randomized trials, those undergoing complex PCI showed an increased risk of thrombosis and benefited from prolonged DAPT only in the absence of HBR features.[7] As such, HBR seems the first aspect to consider when deciding the antithrombotic regimen based on risk stratification, regardless of PCI complexity or thrombotic risk.

Shortening the duration of dual antiplatelet therapy by withdrawing the $P2Y_{12}$ inhibitor

While different options to modulate the intensity of DAPT have been proposed for patients with acute coronary syndrome (i.e. shortening DAPT duration or switching from prasugrel or ticagrelor to clopidogrel at some point in time),[24] the main strategy for CCS patients consists of stopping early one of the two components of DAPT and continuing with single antiplatelet therapy.

A large body of evidence supports the practice of shortening DAPT duration by early discontinuation of the $P2Y_{12}$ inhibitor at 3–6 months and continuation of aspirin monotherapy, which reduces the risk of bleeding compared with standard DAPT (i.e. 12 months).[25–34] Although these investigations were not individually powered for the evaluation of infrequent thrombotic endpoints, their collective evidence suggests that the decreased incidence of bleeding does not come at the price of higher rates of MI and stent thrombosis.[35]

Based on these trials, current ESC Guidelines on CCS recommend to shorten DAPT by withdrawing the $P2Y_{12}$ inhibitor at 3 months after PCI in patients at high risk of life-threatening bleeding (COR IIa, LOE A) or even after 1 month if this risk is very high (COR IIb, LOE C).[11]

Recently, in the One-Month DAPT trial (n = 3020), 1-month DAPT followed by aspirin monotherapy was non-inferior to 6–12-month DAPT with respect to net adverse cardiac events (NACE) at 1 year [5.9% vs 6.5%, absolute difference −0.7%, upper limit of one-sided 97.5% confidence interval (CI) 1.33%; P <0.00 for non-inferiority].[36] In addition, a significant interaction for the treatment effect by clinical presentation was noted, with a significant reduction with short DAPT observed in patients with CCS but not in those with acute coronary syndromes (P = 0.005 for interaction).[37]

Shortening the duration of dual antiplatelet therapy by stopping aspirin

Several criticisms have been raised on the role of aspirin as the cornerstone of antithrombotic therapy, and the advent of more potent drugs than clopidogrel (i.e. prasugrel and ticagrelor) has paved the way for the paradigm of aspirin-free strategies of $P2Y_{12}$ inhibitor monotherapy. No recommendations on short DAPT followed by $P2Y_{12}$ inhibitor monotherapy were included in the 2019 ESC Guidelines on CCS because of the scarce body of evidence available at the time. However, this option was included in subsequent guidelines for acute coronary syndromes,[12] and will probably be considered by future updates in CCS.

Paralleling similar studies in the acute setting, two trials investigated 3-month DAPT followed by $P2Y_{12}$ inhibitor monotherapy in elective PCI patients.[38] The SMART-CHOICE trial (n = 2993) compared 3-month DAPT followed by $P2Y_{12}$ inhibitor monotherapy to 12-month DAPT after PCI: short DAPT was non-inferior to standard DAPT in terms of ischaemic events (2.9% vs 2.5%, absolute difference 0.4%, upper limit of one-sided 95% CI 1.3%; P = 0.007 for non-inferiority) and was associated with lower rates of bleeding [2.0% vs 3.4%, hazard ratio (HR) 0.58, 95% CI 0.36–0.92; P = 0.02].[39] However, it should be noted that this trial enrolled only East-Asian patients,[40] clopidogrel was the most used $P2Y_{12}$ inhibitor (~77%), and approximately 20% of enrolled patients did not adhere to the investigational strategy. Importantly, the results of the trial were consistent also in the high-risk subgroups of patients with high platelet reactivity or undergoing complex PCI.[41,42] Similarly, in the TWILIGHT trial (n = 7119), PCI patients who were treated uneventfully with 3

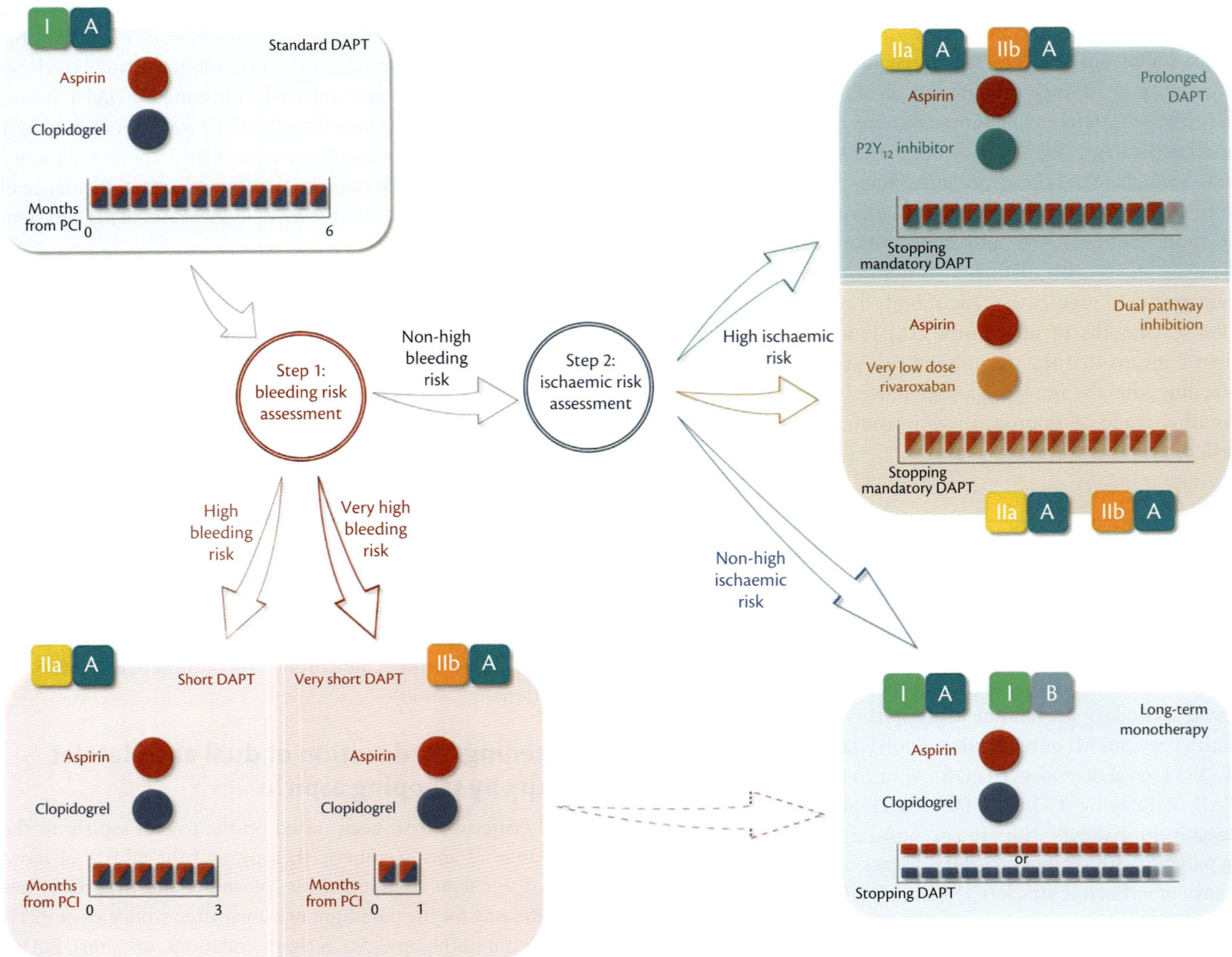

Figure 15.1 Antithrombotic strategies and guideline recommendations in patients with chronic coronary syndrome or undergoing elective percutaneous coronary intervention and in sinus rhythm. Patients in sinus rhythm with chronic coronary syndrome or undergoing percutaneous coronary intervention are usually administered a standard course of dual antiplatelet therapy (DAPT) as in the top left panel. However, if the risk of bleeding is high, short DAPT durations (bottom left panel) should be considered, followed by long-term antiplatelet monotherapy (bottom right panel). Patients who are not at high bleeding risk undergo the assessment of their ischaemic risk to select the antithrombotic regimen to be administered after completing the mandatory initial DAPT period: adding a second antithrombotic drug (either prolonged DAPT or dual pathway inhibition) is an option for patients at high ischaemic risk over the long term (top right panel); by contrast, patients without a substantial ischaemic risk are referred to long-term antiplatelet monotherapy (bottom right panel). Strategies of adding a second antithrombotic drug are supported by a class IIa or IIb recommendation in patients at high risk or moderately increased risk of ischaemic events, respectively. Long-term monotherapy is supported by a level of evidence A or B for aspirin and clopidogrel, respectively.

months of DAPT with aspirin and ticagrelor were randomized to ticagrelor monotherapy or standard ticagrelor-based DAPT for 12 additional months; at 1 year, ticagrelor monotherapy was associated with a reduced incidence of major bleeding (4.0% vs 7.1%, HR 0.56, 95% CI 0.45–0.68; P <0.001) and was non-inferior in terms of ischaemic events (3.9% vs 3.9%, absolute difference −0.06%, 95% CI −0.97 to 0.84; HR 0.99, 95% CI 0.78–1.25; P <0.001 for non-inferiority).[43] There was no statistical interaction by HBR status or PCI complexity,[44,45] but ticagrelor monotherapy was more effective in reducing bleeding in patients with acute coronary syndrome than in those with CCS (P = 0.03 for interaction).[46]

Another option consists of very short DAPT (i.e. 1 month) followed by $P2Y_{12}$ inhibitor monotherapy.[38] The GLOBAL LEADERS trial randomized 15,968 all-comer patients undergoing PCI to 1-month DAPT followed by ticagrelor monotherapy for 23 months or 12-month DAPT followed by aspirin monotherapy for additional 12 months; at 2 years, there were no between-group significant differences in terms of neither ischaemic events (3.81% vs 4.37%, rate ratio 0.87, 95% CI 0.75–1.01; P = 0.073) nor major bleeding (2.04% vs 2.12%, rate ratio 0.97, 95% CI 0.78–1.20; P = 0.77).[47] Interestingly, the treatment effect of ticagrelor monotherapy was again affected by clinical presentation, with signals of bleeding reduction observed in patients with acute coronary syndromes but not in those with CCS (P = 0.007 for interaction).[48] There were also signals of more pronounced benefit of ticagrelor monotherapy in other high-risk settings, including complex PCI, multivessel PCI, stenting of the left anterior descending artery, and long stenting.[49–52] To account for the lack of endpoint adjudication in GLOBAL LEADERS, the GLASSY adjudication substudy was performed, which showed the non-inferiority of ticagrelor monotherapy in terms of death or Q-wave MI (7.14% vs 8.41%, rate ratio 0.85, 95% CI 0.72–0.99; P <0.001 for non-inferiority), and no difference in bleeding (2.48% vs 2.48%, rate ratio 1.00, 95% CI 0.75–1.33; P = 0.986).[53] The STOPDAPT-2 trial (n = 3045) randomly compared 1-month DAPT with aspirin and clopidogrel or prasugrel followed by clopidogrel monotherapy to 12-month DAPT in East-Asian PCI patients. At 1 year, short DAPT was superior to standard DAPT with respect to NACE (2.36% vs 3.0%, HR 0.64, 95% CI 0.42–0.98; P = 0.04 for superiority) and bleeding (0.41% vs 1.54%, HR 0.26, 95% CI 0.11–0.64; P = 0.004) and non-inferior with respect to ischaemic outcomes (1.96% vs 2.51%, absolute difference −0.55%, 95% CI −1.62% to 0.52%; HR 0.79, 95% CI 0.49–1.29; P = 0.005 for non-inferiority; P = 0.34 for superiority).[54] These results were confirmed in subgroup analyses of patient at HBR or undergoing complex PCI.[55,56] Meta-analyses of the above-mentioned trials showed that shortening DAPT with transition to $P2Y_{12}$ inhibitor monotherapy (either at 1 or 3 months after PCI) is an effective strategy for PCI patients to reduce the incidence of bleeding that does not significantly increase the risk of thrombotic or ischaemic events.[57,58]

Shortening the duration of dual antiplatelet therapy by stopping either drug

The newest trial on short DAPT at the time of writing this chapter is the MASTER DAPT, which allowed for the shortening of DAPT at 1 month by either withdrawing the $P2Y_{12}$ inhibitor or aspirin. In this randomized trial enrolling 4434 HBR patients, an abbreviated DAPT regimen was non-inferior to prolonged DAPT (i.e. at least 3 months) in terms of NACE (7.5% vs 7.7%; absolute difference −0.23%, 95% CI −1.80 to 1.33; P <0.001 for non-inferiority) and ischaemic events (6.1% vs 5.9%, absolute difference 0.11%, 95% CI −1.29 to 1.51; P = 0.001 for non-inferiority), while significantly reduced the risk of bleeding (6.5% vs 9.4%, absolute difference −2.82%, 95% CI −4.40 to −1.24; P <0.001).[59] These results were also confirmed among patients undergoing complex PCI.[60]

Prolonging the duration of dual antiplatelet therapy

When the risk of stent thrombosis and ischaemic events is considered to be higher than the risk of bleeding complications, the intensity of antithrombotic therapy can be increased by prolonging DAPT duration. Despite some small trials of prolonged DAPT showing neutral findings, this strategy was tested in the large DAPT trial (n = 9961), which randomized PCI patients who completed an uneventful 12-month course of DAPT with aspirin and clopidogrel or prasugrel to either stop the $P2Y_{12}$ inhibitor immediately or continue DAPT for additional 18 months. Prolonged DAPT was associated with reduced rates of stent thrombosis (0.4% vs 1.4%, HR 0.29, 95% CI 0.17–0.48; P <0.001) and ischaemic events (4.3% vs 5.9%, HR 0.71, 95% CI 0.59–0.85; P <0.001) but increased bleeding (2.5% vs 1.6%; P <0.001).[22] The benefit of prolonged DAPT was consistent regardless of PCI complexity.[61]

Another strategy of prolonged DAPT was tested in the PEGASUS-TIMI 54 trial (n = 21,162) that randomized patients with a prior MI 1–3 years before to ticagrelor 90 mg twice daily, ticagrelor 60 mg twice daily, or placebo on top of aspirin. At 3 years, both ticagrelor regimens reduced the incidence of ischaemic events compared with placebo (7.85% for 90 mg vs 7.77% for 60 mg vs 9.04% for placebo; HR for 90 mg vs placebo 0.85, 95% CI 0.75–0.96; P = 0.008; HR for 60 mg vs placebo 0.84, 95% CI 0.74–0.95; P = 0.004), but increased major bleeding (2.60% for 90 mg vs 2.30% for 60 mg vs 1.06% for placebo; HR for 90 mg vs placebo 2.69, 95% CI 1.96–3.70; P <0.001; HR for 60 mg vs placebo 2.32, 95% CI 1.68–3.21; P <0.001).[62] Prolonged DAPT with ticagrelor 60 mg twice daily was then preferred by regulators over DAPT with the highest dose because of the better expected net benefit.

Current ESC Guidelines on CCS recommend to add a second antithrombotic drug to aspirin over the long term in patients without features of HBR and with a high (COR IIa, LOE A) or moderate risk (COR IIb, LOE A) of ischaemic events (i.e. multivessel or diffuse CAD, diabetes, recurrent MI, peripheral artery disease, heart failure, or moderate-to-severe chronic kidney disease).[11]

Adding a low-dose anticoagulant to aspirin

Guideline recommendations on adding a second antithrombotic drug to aspirin also refer to the so-called dual pathway inhibition, defined as the combination of aspirin and rivaroxaban 2.5 mg twice daily. This strategy was tested in the COMPASS trial (n = 27,395), which randomized patients with stable CAD or peripheral artery disease to rivaroxaban 5 mg twice daily, rivaroxaban 2.5 mg twice daily plus aspirin, or aspirin alone. At a mean follow-up of 23 months, while rivaroxaban 5 mg twice daily did not improve cardiovascular outcomes, dual pathway inhibition reduced the rates of NACE (4.7% vs 5.5%, HR 0.80, 95% CI 0.70–0.91; P <0.001) and ischaemic events (4.1% vs 5.4%, HR 0.76, 95% CI 0.66–0.86; P <0.001) with a parallel increase in major bleeding (3.1% vs 2.8%, HR 1.70, 95% CI 1.40–2.05; P <0.001) compared to aspirin alone.[63]

Intensifying the potency of $P2Y_{12}$ inhibition

A theoretical option to enhance anti-ischaemic protection in PCI patients is to adopt a potent $P2Y_{12}$ inhibitor (i.e. prasugrel or ticagrelor) instead of clopidogrel. However, the evidence supporting this strategy in elective PCI is lacking. In the SASSICAIA trial, 781 patients undergoing elective PCI were randomized to receive a loading dose of either prasugrel (60 mg) or clopidogrel (600 mg) followed by DAPT with aspirin and clopidogrel in both groups. The trial was prematurely stopped due to slow recruitment at a time when it did not show any difference between the two strategies in terms of 30-day NACE [17.3% vs 18.6%, odds ratio (OR) 0.92, 95% CI 0.63–1.32; P = 0.64] and bleeding (4.2% vs 4.8%, OR 0.87, 95% CI 0.44–1.73; P = 0.70).[64] In the ALPHEUS trial, 1910 high-risk patients undergoing elective PCI were randomized to receive ticagrelor (180 mg loading dose followed by aspirin and ticagrelor 90 mg twice daily for 30 days) or clopidogrel (300–600 mg loading dose followed by aspirin and clopidogrel 75 mg daily for 30 days); there was no difference in the incidence of periprocedural MI or injury (35% vs 36%, OR 0.97, 95% CI 0.80–1.17; P = 0.75) nor was there any difference in 30-day NACE (10.1% vs 9.0%, OR 1.19, 95% CI 0.77–1.84; P = 0.43).[65]

To tackle specifically high-risk patients, DAPT escalation strategies guided by platelet function testing or genotyping were also investigated. Three trials conducted in patients with high on-treatment platelet reactivity did not show benefits of escalating from clopidogrel to a more potent $P2Y_{12}$ inhibitors over standard DAPT.[66–68] Subsequent trials tested DAPT escalation as a strategy (i.e. testing vs no testing in all-comer PCI patients), with mixed results. The largest of these trials was the TAILOR-PCI (n = 5302) study, which randomized PCI patients to genotype-guided DAPT (i.e. ticagrelor or clopidogrel administered to patients with or without CYP2C19 loss-of-function variants, respectively) or clopidogrel-based DAPT. There was no difference in ischaemic events between the two strategies (4.4% vs 5.3%, HR 0.84, 95% CI 0.65–1.07; P = 0.16), which were also similar in the subgroup of patients with CYP2C19 loss-of-function variants.[69]

Current guidelines recommend that prasugrel and ticagrelor may be considered, particularly in the initial postprocedural period, only in specific high-risk settings (e.g. suboptimal stent deployment, procedural features determining a high risk of stent thrombosis, complex left main stem disease, or multivessel stenting) or if DAPT cannot be administered due to aspirin intolerance (COR IIb, LOE C).[11]

More recently, the THEMIS trial (n = 19,220) focused on patients with stable CAD and diabetes, who were randomized to DAPT with ticagrelor or aspirin alone; at a median follow-up of 39.9 months, ticagrelor reduced the incidence of ischaemic events (7.7% vs 8.5%, HR 0.90, 95% CI 0.81–0.99; P = 0.04) but increased major bleeding (2.2% vs 1.0%, HR 2.32, 95% CI 1.82–2.94; P <0.001).[70]

Long-term monotherapy

Regardless of the duration of DAPT (i.e. standard, short, or prolonged), the vast majority of patients become candidates to discontinue DAPT and transition to a single antiplatelet therapy at a certain point in time after PCI. Whether aspirin or a $P2Y_{12}$ inhibitor should be preferred as a long-term monotherapy for secondary prevention of CAD is still a matter of debate. Among 19,185 patients with atherosclerotic disease (i.e. recent MI, stroke, or symptomatic peripheral artery disease), clopidogrel 75 mg outperformed aspirin 325 mg in the reduction of the composite of vascular death, MI, or ischaemic stroke (5.32% vs 5.83%, relative risk reduction 8.7%, 95% CI 0.3–16.5; P = 0.043) at a median follow-up of 1.9 years; there was no difference in bleeding between the two treatments, but clopidogrel was associated with less gastrointestinal haemorrhages than aspirin (1.99% vs 2.66%, P <0.002).[71] A landmark analysis of the GLOBAL LEADERS trial reported results between 12 and 24 months (i.e. for the comparison between ticagrelor and aspirin monotherapies): ticagrelor was associated with a lower incidence of ischaemic events compared to aspirin (1.90% vs 2.60%, adjusted HR 0.74, 95% CI 0.58–0.96; P = 0.022) and a significant increase in major bleeding (0.5% vs 0.3%, adjusted HR 1.89, 95% CI 1.03–3.45; P = 0.005).[72] A true head-to-head comparison of aspirin and a $P2Y_{12}$ inhibitor was performed in the HOST-EXAM trial, which randomized 5530 East-Asian patients after 6–18 months from PCI to receive either aspirin or clopidogrel monotherapy. At 2 years, compared to aspirin, clopidogrel reduced the incidence of NACE (5.70% vs 7.70%, HR 0.73, 95% CI 0.59–0.90; P = 0.0035), ischaemic events (3.70% vs 5.50%, HR 0.68, 95% CI 0.52–0.87; P = 0.003) and bleeding (2.30% vs 3.30%, HR 0.70, 95% CI 0.51–0.98; P = 0.036).[73] These findings were confirmed at a median follow-up of 5.8 years in the HOST-EXAM Extended Study, where clopidogrel was associated with reduced rates of NACE (12.8% vs 16.9%, HR 0.74, 95% CI 0.63–0.86, P <0.001), ischaemic events (7.9% vs 11.9%, HR 0.66, 95% CI 0.55–0.79; P <0.001), and bleeding (4.5% vs 6.1%, HR 0.74, 95% CI 0.57–0.94; P = 0.016) compared to aspirin.[74]

A network meta-analysis of 19 studies including 73,126 patients showed the potential net benefit of $P2Y_{12}$ inhibition following DAPT discontinuation in PCI patients: compared to $P2Y_{12}$ inhibitor monotherapy, aspirin was associated with a higher risk of MI (risk ratio 1.32, 95% CI 1.08–1.62), without any difference in death (risk ratio 1.00, 95% CI 0.80–1.26) and major bleeding (risk ratio 1.12, 95% CI 0.82–1.53).[75] Finally, an individual patient data meta-analysis of seven randomized trials including 24,325 CAD patients showed that, compared to aspirin, $P2Y_{12}$ inhibitor monotherapy reduced the risk of NACE (6.4% vs 7.2%, HR 0.89, 95% CI 0.81–0.98; P = 0.020) and ischaemic events (5.5% vs 6.3%, HR 0.88, 95% CI 0.79–0.97; P = 0.014), mainly driven by a reduction in MI (2.3% vs 3.0%, HR 0.77, 95% CI 0.66–0.90; P <0.001), with no difference in major bleeding (1.2% vs 1.4%, HR 0.87, 95% CI 0.70–1.09; P = 0.23).[76]

Antithrombotic strategies for chronic coronary syndrome patients with atrial fibrillation

In patients with atrial fibrillation, the management of antithrombotic therapy is different because both DAPT and OAC are theoretically indicated for the first period after PCI (➔ Figure 15.2). Four randomized trials were performed to investigate dual antithrombotic therapy (DAT) with clopidogrel and a direct oral anticoagulant (DOAC) inhibiting thrombin (i.e. dabigatran) or the activated factor X (i.e. apixaban, edoxaban, rivaroxaban) after a short triple therapy.[77] In the PIONEER AF-PCI, DAT with rivaroxaban 15 mg once daily plus a $P2Y_{12}$ inhibitor was associated with less bleeding at 1 year compared to triple therapy with aspirin, clopidogrel and VKA, with no significant difference

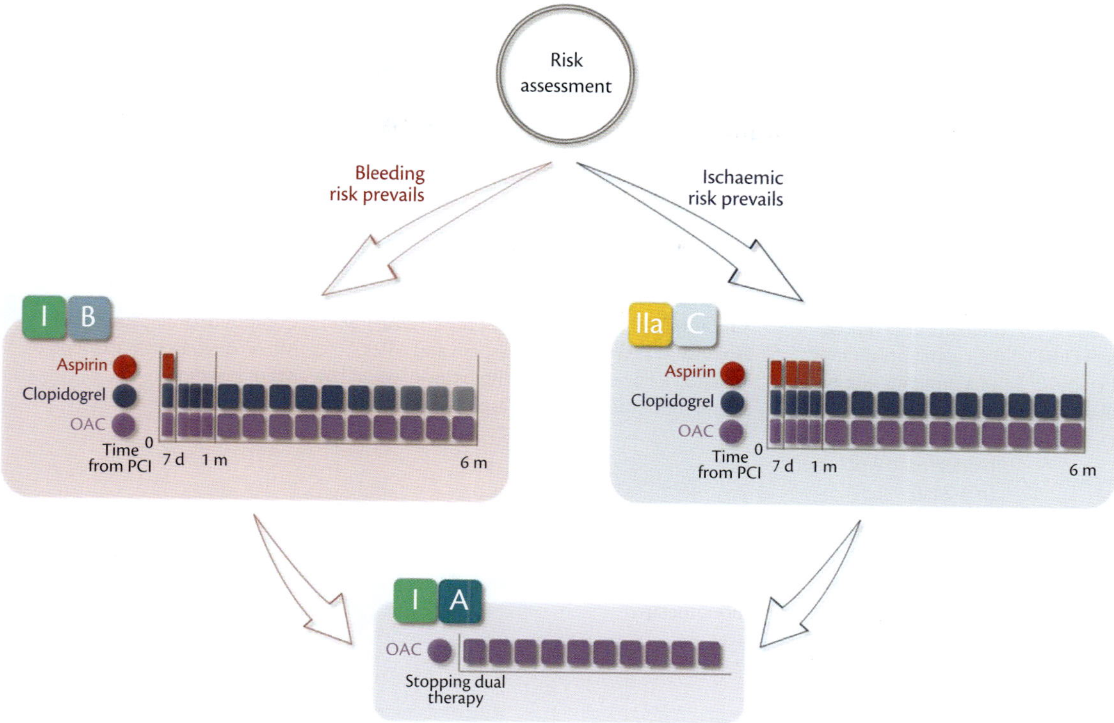

Figure 15.2 Antithrombotic strategies and guideline recommendations in patients with chronic coronary syndrome or undergoing elective percutaneous coronary intervention and with an indication for long-term oral anticoagulation (OAC). Patients with chronic coronary syndrome or undergoing percutaneous coronary intervention and with an indication for long-term OAC should undergo risk stratification to assess whether bleeding (left panel) or ischaemia (right panel) represents the prevailing risk. After an initial period of triple antithrombotic therapy followed by dual antithrombotic therapy, patients are referred to long-term OAC. d, days; m, months.

in ischaemic outcomes.[78] In the RE-DUAL PCI trial, DAT with dabigatran 110 mg twice daily and DAT with dabigatran 150 mg twice daily were respectively superior and non-inferior to triple therapy in reducing bleeding.[79] The AUGUSTUS trial implemented a 2 × 2 factorial design to explore the relative contributions of apixaban versus VKA and DAT versus triple therapy: compared to VKA, apixaban reduced the incidence of bleeding and the composite of death or hospitalization; in addition, dropping aspirin reduced the rates of bleeding and did not increase death or hospitalization nor the composite ischaemic endpoint.[80] Finally, in the ENTRUST-AF PCI trial, edoxaban-based DAT was non-inferior but not superior to VKA-based triple therapy in terms of bleeding, without any difference in the ischaemic endpoints.[81] In aggregate, these trials showed that DAT with a DOAC was associated with less bleeding without significant drawbacks in ischaemic protection as compared to long-term VKA-based triple therapy.[82]

Current ESC Guidelines for patients with CCS and atrial fibrillation recommend to use a DOAC in preference to a VKA in combination with antiplatelet therapy (COR I, LOE A).[11,83] In general, recommended doses of DOACs for the prevention of stroke should be used; however, if the risk of bleeding is higher than that of stent thrombosis or ischaemic stroke, rivaroxaban 15 mg once daily and dabigatran 110 mg twice daily should be preferred over their highest doses for the duration of concomitant antiplatelet therapy (COR IIa, LOE B).[83] In CCS patients undergoing PCI, when the risk of stent thrombosis is lower than the bleeding risk, it is recommended to discontinue triple therapy (i.e. aspirin, clopidogrel, and a DOAC) after 1 week in favour of DAT with OAC and clopidogrel; the latter will be continued up to 6 months (COR I, LOE B); otherwise, triple therapy should be maintained up to 1 month (COR IIa, LOE C).[83] Prasugrel and ticagrelor should not be part of a triple therapy (COR III, LOE C), but can be adopted with OAC as an alternative to triple therapy in patients with a moderate or high risk of stent thrombosis (COR IIb, LOE C).[11]

Future directions

Despite accruing evidence in the field, several areas of uncertainties remain when it comes to select the optimal antithrombotic regimen for patients with CCS or undergoing elective PCI. Randomized trials are ongoing (➔ Table 15.1) to address some of the remaining questions: among them, the OPTIMIZE-APT trial (ClinicalTrials.gov Identifier: NCT05418556) will compare 1-month DAPT followed by clopidogrel monotherapy to standard DAPT in CCS patients; the SMART-CHOICE 3 trial (ClinicalTrials.gov Identifier: NCT04418479) will randomize PCI patients at high thrombotic risk to receive either aspirin or clopidogrel after 1 year of DAPT. A similar information on the long-term antithrombotic regimen to be preferred after PCI will

Table 15.1 Ongoing randomized trials in patients with CCS or undergoing elective PCI

Trial (ClinicalTrials.gov Identifier)	Population	Interventional strategy	Control strategy	Primary outcome(s)	Follow-up
AQUATIC (NCT04217447)	Patients on OAC with stabilized CAD (n = 2000)	Full-dose OAC plus aspirin	Full-dose OAC plus placebo	*Ischaemic*: MACE *Bleeding*: major bleeding	4 years
ASA-IN (NCT05347069)	Patients with CCS not eligible for revascularization (n = 2890)	Aspirin	No aspirin	Composite of all-cause death, MI, stroke, coronary or peripheral revascularization, or critical limb ischaemia	5 years
Comparison Three vs Twelve Months of Dual Anti-Platelet Therapy After Stent Implantation (NCT03008083)	Patients undergoing PCI with implantation of a sirolimus-eluting stent with abluminal grooves containing a biodegradable polymer (n = 2446)	3-month DAPT with aspirin and a $P2Y_{12}$ inhibitor, followed by aspirin monotherapy	12-month DAPT with aspirin and a $P2Y_{12}$ inhibitor, followed by aspirin monotherapy	Composite of all-cause death, MI, cerebrovascular accident, or major bleeding	18 months
OPTIMIZE-APT (NCT05418556)[a]	Patients undergoing optimized DES implantation guided by intravascular imaging (n = 3944)	1-month DAPT with aspirin and clopidogrel, followed by clopidogrel monotherapy	12-month DAPT with aspirin and clopidogrel	*Ischaemic*: composite of all-cause death, MI, ischaemia-driven TVR, or stent thrombosis *Bleeding*: clinically relevant bleeding *Net*: NACE	12 months
PARTHENOPE (NCT04135989)[b]	Patients undergoing PCI (n = 2106)	DAPT for 3 months or 24 months in patients with low or high DAPT score, respectively	DAPT for 12 months	NACE	2 years
POPular CABG (NCT02352402)	Patients undergoing CABG with one or more saphenous vein grafts	DAPT with aspirin and ticagrelor for 1 year	Aspirin and placebo for 1 year	Saphenous vein graft occlusion	1 year
SMART-CHOICE 2 (NCT03119012)	Patients who underwent PCI with bioresorbable scaffold at least 12 months before (n = 1520)	$P2Y_{12}$ inhibitor monotherapy for 24 months	DAPT with aspirin and a $P2Y_{12}$ inhibitor for 24 months	Composite of death, MI, or cerebrovascular events	3 years
SMART-CHOICE 3 (NCT04418479)	Patients at high risk for recurrent ischaemic events who underwent PCI at least 12 months before (n = 5000)	Clopidogrel monotherapy	Aspirin monotherapy	Composite of all-cause death, MI, or stroke	1 year

[a] The OPTIMIZE-APT trial is investigating different antiplatelet strategies for patients with either acute or chronic coronary syndromes; only details on chronic coronary syndrome patients are reported in this table.

[b] PARTHENOPE is a factorial 2 × 2 trial investigating both stent type and antiplatelet regimens; only details on the comparison of antiplatelet strategies in patients with chronic coronary syndrome are reported in this table.

CABG, coronary artery bypass grafting; CAD, coronary artery disease; CCS, chronic coronary syndrome; DAPT, dual antiplatelet therapy; DES, drug-eluting stent; MACE, major adverse cardiovascular events; MI, myocardial infarction; n = number; OAC, oral anticoagulation; NACE, net adverse cardiovascular events; PCI, percutaneous coronary intervention; TVR, target vessel revascularization.

come from the 10-year median follow-up of the HOST-EXAM Extended study.

Conclusion

Patients undergoing elective PCI and also patients with CCS treated conservatively are at risk of disease progression and ischaemic events, and therefore require antithrombotic therapy for secondary prevention purposes. Risk stratification that takes individual ischaemic and bleeding risk profiles into account plays a key role for the selection of a tailored antithrombotic regimen. Different modulation strategies are available to shift the balance of antithrombotic therapy towards higher protection from ischaemic events or better avoidance of bleeding complications, including shortening or prolonging DAPT duration, intensifying the potency of the $P2Y_{12}$ inhibition, or adding a low-dose anticoagulant to aspirin over the long term. The management of antithrombotic drugs can be further complicated by concomitant indications to OAC, therefore requiring specific considerations on selecting drugs and adjusting therapy duration. Several gaps in knowledge still remain when it comes to selecting the optimal antithrombotic regimen, which warrant further high-quality evidence from randomized investigations.

What's new

- A risk stratification approach is of key importance to determine the individual trade-off between the risks of ischaemia and bleeding and should be always considered for selection of antithrombotic therapy.
- A strategy to be adopted in patients at high risk of bleeding is represented by shortening the duration of DAPT, which can be obtained by either withdrawing the $P2Y_{12}$ receptor inhibitor or stopping aspirin.
- Adding a second antithrombotic drug for long-term antithrombotic secondary prevention is an alternative to standard therapy to treat patient at high risk of thrombosis. Despite prolonged DAPT being an option, dual pathway inhibition with aspirin and a low dose of the direct activated factor X inhibitor rivaroxaban showed favourable results in patients with stable coronary artery disease.
- $P2Y_{12}$ receptor inhibitor monotherapy has also been investigated as an alternative to aspirin for the long-term antiplatelet monotherapy phase after the mandatory period of DAPT.
- In patients with an established indication for OAC undergoing PCI, a very short (i.e. up to 1 week) triple therapy with aspirin, clopidogrel, and a direct inhibitor of thrombin or activated factor X is indicated. After this period, a DAT with clopidogrel and an OAC should be maintained up to 6 months.

Guideline recommendations

- Aspirin 75–100 mg daily is recommended in patients with a previous MI or revascularization. (I, A)
- Clopidogrel 75 mg daily is recommended as an alternative to aspirin in patients with aspirin intolerance. (I, B)
- Clopidogrel 75 mg daily may be considered in preference to aspirin in symptomatic or asymptomatic patients, with either peripheral artery disease or a history of ischaemic stroke or transient ischaemic attack. (IIb, B)
- Aspirin 75–100 mg daily may be considered in patients without a history of MI or revascularization, but with definitive evidence of coronary artery disease on imaging. (IIb, C)
- Aspirin 75–100 mg daily is recommended following stenting. (I, A)
- Clopidogrel 75 mg daily following appropriate loading (e.g. 600 mg or >5 days of maintenance therapy) is recommended, in addition to aspirin, for 6 months following coronary stenting, irrespective of stent type, unless a shorter duration (1–3 months) is indicated due to risk or the occurrence of life-threatening bleeding. (I, A)
- Clopidogrel 75 mg daily following appropriate loading (e.g. 600 mg or >5 days of maintenance therapy) should be considered for 3 months in patients with a higher risk of life-threatening bleeding. (IIa, A)
- Clopidogrel 75 mg daily following appropriate loading (e.g. 600 mg or >5 days of maintenance therapy) may be considered for 1 month in patients with very high risk of life-threatening bleeding. (IIb, C)
- Adding a second antithrombotic drug to aspirin for long-term secondary prevention should be considered in patients with a high risk of ischaemic events and without HBR. (IIa, A)
- Adding a second antithrombotic drug to aspirin for long-term secondary prevention may be considered in patients with at least a moderately increased risk of ischaemic events and without HBR. (IIb, A)
- Prasugrel or ticagrelor may be considered, at least as initial therapy, in specific high-risk situations of elective stenting (e.g. suboptimal stent deployment or other procedural characteristics associated with high risk of stent thrombosis, complex left main stem, or multivessel stenting) or if DAPT cannot be used because of aspirin intolerance. (IIb, C)
- When OAC is initiated in a patient with atrial fibrillation who is eligible for a DOAC, a DOAC is recommended in preference to a vitamin K antagonist. (I, A)
- In patients at HBR, rivaroxaban 15 mg once daily should be considered in preference to rivaroxaban 20 mg once daily for the duration of concomitant single or DAPT, to mitigate bleeding risk. (IIa, B)
- In patients at HBR, dabigatran 110 mg twice daily should be considered in preference to dabigatran 150 mg twice daily for the duration of concomitant single or DAPT, to mitigate bleeding risk. (IIa, B)
- After uncomplicated PCI, early cessation (i.e. within 1 week) of aspirin and continuation of dual therapy with an OAC and clopidogrel for up to 6 months is recommended if the risk of stent thrombosis is low or if concerns about bleeding risk prevail over concerns about risk of stent thrombosis, irrespective of the type of stent used. (I, B)
- Triple therapy with aspirin, clopidogrel, and an OAC for longer than 1 week should be considered when risk of stent thrombosis outweighs the bleeding risk, with the total duration (within 1 month) decided according to assessment of these risks, and the treatment plan should be clearly specified at hospital discharge. (IIa, C)
- The use of ticagrelor or prasugrel is not recommended as part of triple antithrombotic therapy with aspirin and an OAC. (III, C)
- Dual therapy with an OAC and either ticagrelor or prasugrel may be considered as an alternative to triple therapy with an OAC, aspirin, and clopidogrel in patients with a moderate or high risk of stent thrombosis, irrespective of the type of stent used. (IIb, C)

What's next

- $P2Y_{12}$ receptor inhibitor monotherapy may be a promising alternative either after shortening DAPT duration to 3 or even 1 month(s) or for long-term secondary prevention. Further investigations and the extended follow-up of the

HOST-EXAM trial will shed additional light on the role of this attractive option.

- Fulfilling the concept of precision medicine, risk stratification tools (i.e. risk scores, platelet function testing, and genotyping) are expected to gain importance to guide the selection of the optimal antithrombotic therapy in the individual patient.
- New antithrombotic regimens consisting of combinations of currently available drugs (i.e. aspirin, $P2Y_{12}$ receptor inhibitors, and OACs) are expected to be explored to optimize the ischaemic protection while minimizing bleeding in patients with CCS or after elective PCI.

Drug dosing

- Apixaban: 5 mg twice daily.
- Aspirin: 75–100 mg once daily.
- Clopidogrel: 600 mg loading dose; 75 mg once daily.
- Dabigatran: 110 mg twice daily or 150 mg twice daily.
- Edoxaban: 60 mg once daily.
- Prasugrel: 60 mg loading dose; 10 mg once daily.
- Rivaroxaban: 20 mg once daily or 15 mg once daily or 2.5 mg twice daily.
- Ticagrelor: 180 mg loading dose; 90 mg twice daily or 60 mg twice daily.

References

1. Sixty Plus Reinfarction Study Research Group. A double-blind trial to assess long-term oral anticoagulant therapy in elderly patients after myocardial infarction. Lancet. 1980;316(8202):989–94.
2. Juul-Möller S, Edvardsson N, Jahnmatz B, Rosén A, Sørensen S, Omblus R. Double-blind trial of aspirin in primary prevention of myocardial infarction in patients with stable chronic angina pectoris. The Swedish Angina Pectoris Aspirin Trial (SAPAT) Group. Lancet. 1992;340(8833):1421–5.
3. ten Berg JM, Kelder JC, Suttorp MJ, et al. Effect of coumarins started before coronary angioplasty on acute complications and long-term follow-up: a randomized trial. Circulation. 2000;102(4):386–91.
4. Schömig A, Neumann F-J, Kastrati A, et al. A randomized comparison of antiplatelet and anticoagulant therapy after the placement of coronary-artery stents. N Engl J Med. 1996;334(17):1084–9.
5. Leon MB, Baim DS, Popma JJ, et al. A clinical trial comparing three antithrombotic-drug regimens after coronary-artery stenting. N Engl J Med. 1998;339(23):1665–71.
6. Kwok CS, Khan MA, Rao SV, et al. Access and non-access site bleeding after percutaneous coronary intervention and risk of subsequent mortality and major adverse cardiovascular events: systematic review and meta-analysis. Circ Cardiovasc Interv. 2015;8(4):e001645.
7. Costa F, Van Klaveren D, Feres F, et al. Dual antiplatelet therapy duration based on ischemic and bleeding risks after coronary stenting. J Am Coll Cardiol. 2019;73(7):741–54.
8. Angiolillo DA, Galli M, Collet J-P, Kastrati A, O'Donoghue MOD. Antiplatelet therapy after percutaneous coronary intervention. EuroIntervention. 2022;17(17):e1371–96.
9. Buccheri S, D'Arrigo P, Franchina G, Capodanno D. Risk stratification in patients with coronary artery disease: a practical walkthrough in the landscape of prognostic risk models. Interv Cardiol. 2018;13(3):112–20.
10. Giustino G, Chieffo A, Palmerini T, et al. Efficacy and safety of dual antiplatelet therapy after complex PCI. J Am Coll Cardiol. 2016;68(17):1851–64.
11. Knuuti J, Wijns W, Saraste A, et al. 2019 ESC Guidelines for the diagnosis and management of chronic coronary syndromes. Eur Heart J. 2020;41(3):407–77.
12. Collet J-P, Thiele H, Barbato E, et al. 2020 ESC Guidelines for the management of acute coronary syndromes in patients presenting without persistent ST-segment elevation. Eur Heart J. 2021;42(14):1289–367.
13. Mehran R, Rao SV, Bhatt DL, et al. Standardized bleeding definitions for cardiovascular clinical trials: a consensus report from the Bleeding Academic Research Consortium. Circulation. 2011;123(23):2736–47.
14. The GUSTO Investigators. An international randomized trial comparing four thrombolytic strategies for acute myocardial infarction. N Engl J Med. 1993;329(10):673–82.
15. Chesebro JH, Knatterud G, Roberts R, et al. Thrombolysis in Myocardial Infarction (TIMI) trial, phase I: a comparison between intravenous tissue plasminogen activator and intravenous streptokinase. Clinical findings through hospital discharge. Circulation. 1987;76(1):142–54.
16. Schulman S, Kearon C. Definition of major bleeding in clinical investigations of antihemostatic medicinal products in non-surgical patients. J Thromb Haemost. 2005;3(4):692–4.
17. Urban P, Mehran R, Colleran R, et al. Defining high bleeding risk in patients undergoing percutaneous coronary intervention. Circulation. 2019;140(3):240–61.
18. Ueki Y, Bär S, Losdat S, et al. Validation of the Academic Research Consortium for High Bleeding Risk (ARC-HBR) criteria in patients undergoing percutaneous coronary intervention and comparison with contemporary bleeding risk scores. EuroIntervention. 2020;16(5):371–9.
19. Natsuaki M, Morimoto T, Shiomi H, et al. Application of the Academic Research Consortium high bleeding risk criteria in an all-comers registry of percutaneous coronary intervention. Circ Cardiovasc Interv. 2019;12(11):e008307.
20. Cao D, Mehran R, Dangas G, et al. Validation of the Academic Research Consortium high bleeding risk definition in contemporary PCI patients. J Am Coll Cardiol. 2020;75(21):2711–22.
21. Corpataux N, Spirito A, Gragnano F, et al. Validation of high bleeding risk criteria and definition as proposed by the academic research consortium for high bleeding risk. Eur Heart J. 2020;41(38):3743–9.
22. Mauri L, Kereiakes DJ, Yeh RW, et al. Twelve or 30 months of dual antiplatelet therapy after drug-eluting stents. N Engl J Med. 2014;371(23):2155–66.
23. Urban P, Gregson J, Owen R, et al. Assessing the risks of bleeding vs thrombotic events in patients at high bleeding risk after coronary stent implantation. JAMA Cardiol. 2021;6(4):410–19.
24. Laudani C, Greco A, Occhipinti G, et al. Short duration of DAPT versus de-escalation after percutaneous coronary intervention for acute coronary syndromes. JACC Cardiovasc Interv. 2022;15(3):268–77.

25. Gwon H-C, Hahn J-Y, Park KW, et al. Six-month versus 12-month dual antiplatelet therapy after implantation of drug-eluting stents. Circulation. 2012;125(3):505–13.
26. Kim B-K, Hong M-K, Shin D-H, et al. A new strategy for discontinuation of dual antiplatelet therapy: the RESET Trial (REal Safety and Efficacy of 3-month dual antiplatelet Therapy following Endeavor zotarolimus-eluting stent implantation). J Am Coll Cardiol. 2012;60(15):1340–8.
27. Feres F, Costa RA, Abizaid A, et al. Three vs twelve months of dual antiplatelet therapy after zotarolimus-eluting stents. JAMA. 2013;310(23):2510–22.
28. Colombo A, Chieffo A, Frasheri A, et al. Second-generation drug-eluting stent implantation followed by 6- versus 12-month dual antiplatelet therapy. J Am Coll Cardiol. 2014;64(20):2086–97.
29. Schulz-Schupke S, Byrne RA, ten Berg JM, et al. ISAR-SAFE: a randomized, double-blind, placebo-controlled trial of 6 vs. 12 months of clopidogrel therapy after drug-eluting stenting. Eur Heart J. 2015;36(20):1252–63.
30. Gilard M, Barragan P, Noryani AAL, et al. 6- versus 24-month dual antiplatelet therapy after implantation of drug-eluting stents in patients nonresistant to aspirin. J Am Coll Cardiol. 2015;65(8):777–86.
31. Han Y, Xu B, Xu K, et al. Six versus 12 months of dual antiplatelet therapy after implantation of biodegradable polymer sirolimus-eluting stent. Circ Cardiovasc Interv. 2016;9(2):e003145.
32. Hong S-J, Shin D-H, Kim J-S, et al. 6-month versus 12-month dual-antiplatelet therapy following long everolimus-eluting stent implantation. JACC Cardiovasc Interv. 2016;9(14):1438–46.
33. Nakamura M, Iijima R, Ako J, et al. Dual antiplatelet therapy for 6 versus 18 months after biodegradable polymer drug-eluting stent implantation. JACC Cardiovasc Interv. 2017;10(12):1189–98.
34. Byoung-Kwon L, Jung-Sun K, Oh-Huyn L, et al. Safety of six-month dual antiplatelet therapy after second-generation drug-eluting stent implantation: OPTIMA-C randomised clinical trial and OCT substudy. EuroIntervention. 2018;13(16):1923–30.
35. Palmerini T, Benedetto U, Bacchi-Reggiani L, et al. Mortality in patients treated with extended duration dual antiplatelet therapy after drug-eluting stent implantation: a pairwise and Bayesian network meta-analysis of randomised trials. Lancet. 2015;385(9985):2371–82.
36. Hong S-J, Kim J-S, Hong SJ, et al. 1-month dual-antiplatelet therapy followed by aspirin monotherapy after polymer-free drug-coated stent implantation. JACC Cardiovasc Interv. 2021;14(16):1801–11.
37. Yong-Joon L, Jae Young C, Kyeong Ho Y, et al. Impact of one-month DAPT followed by aspirin monotherapy in patients undergoing percutaneous coronary intervention according to clinical presentation: a post hoc analysis of the randomised one-month DAPT trial. EuroIntervention. 2022;18(6):471–81.
38. Greco A, Mauro MS, Capodanno D, Angiolillo DJ. P2Y12 inhibitor monotherapy: considerations for acute and long-term secondary prevention post-PCI. Rev Cardiovasc Med. 2022;23(10):348.
39. Hahn J-Y, Song YB, Oh J-H, et al. Effect of P2Y12 inhibitor monotherapy vs dual antiplatelet therapy on cardiovascular events in patients undergoing percutaneous coronary intervention: the SMART-CHOICE randomized clinical trial. JAMA. 2019;321(24):2428–37.
40. Greco A, Capodanno D, Angiolillo D. The conundrum surrounding racial differences on ischaemic and bleeding risk with dual antiplatelet therapy. Thromb Haemost. 2019;119(1):9–13.
41. Lee SH, Lee SY, Chun WJ, et al. Clopidogrel monotherapy in patients with and without on-treatment high platelet reactivity: a SMART-CHOICE substudy. EuroIntervention. 2021;17(11):e888–97.
42. Roh JW, Hahn J-Y, Oh J-H, et al. P2Y12 inhibitor monotherapy in complex percutaneous coronary intervention: a post-hoc analysis of SMART-CHOICE randomized clinical trial. Cardiol J. 2021;28(6):855–63.
43. Mehran R, Baber U, Sharma SK, et al. Ticagrelor with or without aspirin in high-risk patients after PCI. N Engl J Med. 2019;381(21):2032–42.
44. Escaned J, Cao D, Baber U, et al. Ticagrelor monotherapy in patients at high bleeding risk undergoing percutaneous coronary intervention: TWILIGHT-HBR. Eur Heart J. 2021;42(45):4624–34.
45. Dangas G, Baber U, Sharma S, et al. Ticagrelor with or without aspirin after complex PCI. J Am Coll Cardiol. 2020;75(19):2414–24.
46. Baber U, Dangas G, Angiolillo DJ, et al. Ticagrelor alone vs. ticagrelor plus aspirin following percutaneous coronary intervention in patients with non-ST-segment elevation acute coronary syndromes: TWILIGHT-ACS. Eur Heart J. 2020;41(37):3533–45.
47. Vranckx P, Valgimigli M, Jüni P, et al. Ticagrelor plus aspirin for 1 month, followed by ticagrelor monotherapy for 23 months vs aspirin plus clopidogrel or ticagrelor for 12 months, followed by aspirin monotherapy for 12 months after implantation of a drug-eluting stent: a multicentre, open-label, randomised superiority trial. Lancet. 2018;392:940–9.
48. Vranckx P, Valgimigli M, Odutayo A, et al. Efficacy and safety of ticagrelor monotherapy by clinical presentation: pre-specified analysis of the GLOBAL LEADERS trial. J Am Heart Assoc. 2021;10(18):e015560.
49. Serruys PW, Takahashi K, Chichareon P, et al. Impact of long-term ticagrelor monotherapy following 1-month dual antiplatelet therapy in patients who underwent complex percutaneous coronary intervention: insights from the Global Leaders trial. Eur Heart J. 2019;40(31):2595–604.
50. Takahashi K, Serruys PW, Chichareon P, et al. Efficacy and safety of ticagrelor monotherapy in patients undergoing multivessel PCI. J Am Coll Cardiol. 2019;74(16):2015–27.
51. Takahashi K, Wang R, Kawashima H, et al. Efficacy and safety of one-month DAPT followed by 23-month ticagrelor monotherapy in patients undergoing proximal LAD stenting: insights from the GLOBAL LEADERS trial. Int J Cardiol. 2020;320:27–34.
52. Takahashi K, Chichareon P, Modolo R, et al. Impact of ticagrelor monotherapy on two-year clinical outcomes in patients with long stenting: a post hoc analysis of the GLOBAL LEADERS trial. EuroIntervention. 2020;16(8):634–44.
53. Franzone A, McFadden E, Leonardi S, et al. Ticagrelor alone versus dual antiplatelet therapy from 1 month after drug-eluting coronary stenting. J Am Coll Cardiol. 2019;74(18):2223–34.
54. Watanabe H, Domei T, Morimoto T, et al. Effect of 1-month dual antiplatelet therapy followed by clopidogrel vs 12-month dual antiplatelet therapy on cardiovascular and bleeding events in patients receiving PCI: the STOPDAPT-2 randomized clinical trial. JAMA. 2019;321(24):2414–27.
55. Yamamoto K, Watanabe H, Morimoto T, et al. Very short dual antiplatelet therapy after drug-eluting stent implantation in patients who underwent complex percutaneous coronary intervention: insight from the STOPDAPT-2 trial. Circ Cardiovasc Interv. 2021;14(5):e010384.
56. Watanabe H, Domei T, Morimoto T, et al. Very short dual antiplatelet therapy after drug-eluting stent implantation in patients with high bleeding risk. Circulation. 2019;140(23):1957–9.
57. O'Donoghue ML, Murphy SA, Sabatine MS. The safety and efficacy of aspirin discontinuation on a background of a P2Y12 inhibitor in patients after percutaneous coronary intervention: a systematic review and meta-analysis. Circulation. 2020;142(6):538–45.
58. Valgimigli M, Gragnano F, Branca M, et al. P2Y12 inhibitor monotherapy or dual antiplatelet therapy after coronary revascularisation:

individual patient level meta-analysis of randomised controlled trials. BMJ. 2021;373:n1332.

59. Valgimigli M, Frigoli E, Heg D, Tijssen J, Jüni P, Vranckx P, et al. Dual antiplatelet therapy after PCI in patients at high bleeding risk. N Engl J Med. 2021;385:1643–55.
60. Valgimigli M, Smits PC, Frigoli E, et al. Duration of antiplatelet therapy after complex percutaneous coronary intervention in patients at high bleeding risk: a MASTER DAPT trial sub-analysis. Eur Heart J. 2022;43(33):3100–14.
61. Yeh RW, Kereiakes DJ, Steg PG, et al. Lesion complexity and outcomes of extended dual antiplatelet therapy after percutaneous coronary intervention. J Am Coll Cardiol. 2017;70(18):2213–23.
62. Bonaca MP, Bhatt DL, Cohen M, et al. Long-term use of ticagrelor in patients with prior myocardial infarction. N Engl J Med. 2015;372(19):1791–800.
63. Eikelboom JW, Connolly SJ, Bosch J, et al. Rivaroxaban with or without aspirin in stable cardiovascular disease. N Engl J Med. 2017;377(14):1319–30.
64. Mehilli J, Baquet M, Hochholzer W, et al. Randomized comparison of intensified and standard P2Y12-receptor-inhibition before elective percutaneous coronary intervention. Circ Cardiovasc Interv. 2020;13(6):e008649.
65. Silvain J, Lattuca B, Beygui F, et al. Ticagrelor versus clopidogrel in elective percutaneous coronary intervention (ALPHEUS): a randomised, open-label, phase 3b trial. Lancet. 2020;396(10264):1737–44.
66. Price MJ, Berger PB, Teirstein PS, et al. Standard- vs high-dose clopidogrel based on platelet function testing after percutaneous coronary intervention: the GRAVITAS randomized trial. JAMA. 2011;305(11):1097–105.
67. Collet J-P, Cuisset T, Rangé G, et al. Bedside monitoring to adjust antiplatelet therapy for coronary stenting. N Engl J Med. 2012;367(22):2100–9.
68. Trenk D, Stone GW, Gawaz M, et al. A randomized trial of prasugrel versus clopidogrel in patients with high platelet reactivity on clopidogrel after elective percutaneous coronary intervention with implantation of drug-eluting stents: results of the TRIGGER-PCI (Testing Platelet Reactivity In Patients Undergoing Elective Stent Placement on Clopidogrel to Guide Alternative Therapy With Prasugrel) study. J Am Coll Cardiol. 2012;59(24):2159–64.
69. Pereira NL, Farkouh ME, So D, et al. Effect of genotype-guided oral P2Y12 inhibitor selection vs conventional clopidogrel therapy on ischemic outcomes after percutaneous coronary intervention: the TAILOR-PCI randomized clinical trial. JAMA. 2020;324(8):761–71.
70. Steg PG, Bhatt DL, Simon T, et al. Ticagrelor in patients with stable coronary disease and diabetes. N Engl J Med. 2019;381(14): 1309–20.
71. Committee CS. A randomised, blinded, trial of clopidogrel versus aspirin in patients at risk of ischaemic events (CAPRIE). CAPRIE Steering Committee. Lancet. 1996;348(9038):1329–39.
72. Ono M, Hara H, Kawashima H, et al. Ticagrelor monotherapy versus aspirin monotherapy at 12 months after percutaneous coronary intervention: a landmark analysis of the GLOBAL LEADERS trial. EuroIntervention. 2022;18(5):e377–88.
73. Koo B-K, Kang J, Park KW, et al. Aspirin versus clopidogrel for chronic maintenance monotherapy after percutaneous coronary intervention (HOST-EXAM): an investigator-initiated, prospective, randomised, open-label, multicentre trial. Lancet. 2021;397(10293):2487–96.
74. Kang J, Park KW, Lee H, et al. Aspirin vs. clopidogrel for chronic maintenance monotherapy after percutaneous coronary intervention: the HOST-EXAM extended study. Circulation. 2023;147(2):108–17.
75. Andò G, De Santis G, Greco A, et al. P2Y12 inhibitor or aspirin following dual antiplatelet therapy after percutaneous coronary intervention: a network meta-analysis. JACC Cardiovasc Interv. 2022;15(22):2239–49.
76. Valgimigli M. PANTHER: P2Y12 inhibitor versus aspirin monotherapy in patients with coronary artery disease. Presented at ESC Congress; August 26–29 2022; Barcelona, Spain. 2022.
77. Greco A, Laudani C, Rochira C, Capodanno D. Antithrombotic management in atrial fibrillation patients following percutaneous coronary intervention: a European perspective. Int Cardiol Rev. 2023;18:e05.
78. Gibson CM, Mehran R, Bode C, et al. Prevention of bleeding in patients with atrial fibrillation undergoing PCI. N Engl J Med. 2016;375(25):2423–34.
79. Cannon CP, Bhatt DL, Oldgren J, et al. Dual antithrombotic therapy with dabigatran after PCI in atrial fibrillation. N Engl J Med. 2017;377(16):1513–24.
80. Lopes RD, Heizer G, Aronson R, et al. Antithrombotic therapy after acute coronary syndrome or PCI in atrial fibrillation. N Engl J Med. 2019;380(16):1509–24.
81. Vranckx P, Valgimigli M, Eckardt L, et al. Edoxaban-based versus vitamin K antagonist-based antithrombotic regimen after successful coronary stenting in patients with atrial fibrillation (ENTRUST-AF PCI): a randomised, open-label, phase 3b trial. Lancet. 2019;394(10206):1335–43.
82. Capodanno D, Di Maio M, Greco A, et al. Safety and efficacy of double antithrombotic therapy with non-vitamin K antagonist oral anticoagulants in patients with atrial fibrillation undergoing percutaneous coronary intervention: a systematic review and meta-analysis. J Am Heart Assoc. 2020;9(16):e017212.
83. Hindricks G, Potpara T, Dagres N, et al. 2020 ESC Guidelines for the diagnosis and management of atrial fibrillation developed in collaboration with the European Association for Cardio-Thoracic Surgery (EACTS). Eur Heart J. 2021;42(5):373–498.

CHAPTER 16

Antithrombotic therapy in ST-elevation acute myocardial infarction and non-ST elevation acute coronary syndromes

William A.E. Parker, Raffaele De Caterina, David J. Moliterno, Steen Dalby Kristensen, and Robert F. Storey

Contents

Summary

Atherothrombosis is the central pathological process in acute coronary syndromes (ACS). Antithrombotic therapy is, therefore, a cornerstone of ACS treatment. As soon as ACS is suspected, aspirin should be commenced to reduce the risk of major adverse cardiovascular events. Addition of an oral $P2Y_{12}$ inhibitor further reduces risk. Parenteral anticoagulation is indicated for any patient undergoing percutaneous coronary intervention (PCI) or thrombolysis, and for patients with non-ST elevation ACS where an early invasive treatment strategy is not pursued. In some cases of PCI for ST-elevation myocardial infarction, a platelet glycoprotein inhibitor may be utilized. Where timely primary PCI cannot be performed for ST-elevation myocardial infarction, thrombolysis with a tissue plasminogen activator may be recommended. Where there is an additional requirement for oral anticoagulation, in general patients treated by PCI should receive a short period of aspirin plus P2Y12 inhibitor plus oral anticoagulation before stopping aspirin, and then receive oral anticoagulation alone from 1 year.

Introduction

Acute coronary syndromes (ACS) are both common and serious. For example, coronary artery disease causes over half a million deaths per year in the European Union, the majority as a direct or indirect result of ACS events.[1] ACS most commonly results from atherothrombosis within the epicardial coronary arteries, typically triggered by plaque rupture or erosion. Where associated with myocardial damage, this indicates type 1 myocardial infarction (MI).[2] If there is no myocardial injury but the clinical and electrocardiogram findings indicate an unpredictable pattern of chest pain, this is termed unstable angina.

ACS can be further defined by the presence or absence of ST-segment elevation on the electrocardiogram. In the appropriate clinical context, presence of significant, territorial ST elevation typically signifies ST-elevation myocardial infarction (STEMI) secondary to acute total occlusion of a major epicardial coronary artery, resulting, if left without treatment, in a transmural infarction. ACS without ST elevation [termed non-ST-elevation acute coronary syndrome (NSTE-ACS)] is usually associated with transient or partial coronary artery occlusion, and more often results in subendocardial MI or, in unstable angina, with no detectable myocardial damage (➔ Figure 16.1).[2]

Atherothrombosis is the central pathological process driving most ACS. It is therefore rational that antithrombotic therapy is at the forefront of its management. Since the last decades of the 20th century, significant stepwise advances have been made in the development of antithrombotic drugs, establishing a strong evidence base for their use in ACS. With new targets and new drugs becoming available, a multiplicity of available treatments, feasible combinations and durations, and differing clinical characteristics at presentation, choosing the right drug regimen can be complex. Striking the right balance between antithrombotic benefits and anti-haemostatic risks is at the centre of treatment decisions.

Rationale for antithrombotic therapy in acute coronary syndromes

The key aims of antithrombotic therapy in patients with ACS are summarized in ➔ Figure 16.2.

Antithrombotic therapy in acute coronary syndromes: evidence and current recommendations

There is evidence for a range of antithrombotic drugs in the treatment of ACS. Current European Society of Cardiology (ESC) recommendations for antithrombotic therapy in ACS are found in the 2017 STEMI and 2020 NSTE-ACS ESC Guidelines.[3,4] Key recommendations relating to the initial phase of ACS treatment are summarized in ➔ Figure 16.3.

Oral antithrombotic drugs in acute coronary syndromes

Aspirin

(See also ➔ Chapter 5.) Evidence for the efficacy of aspirin in ACS comes, for example, from the landmark International Study

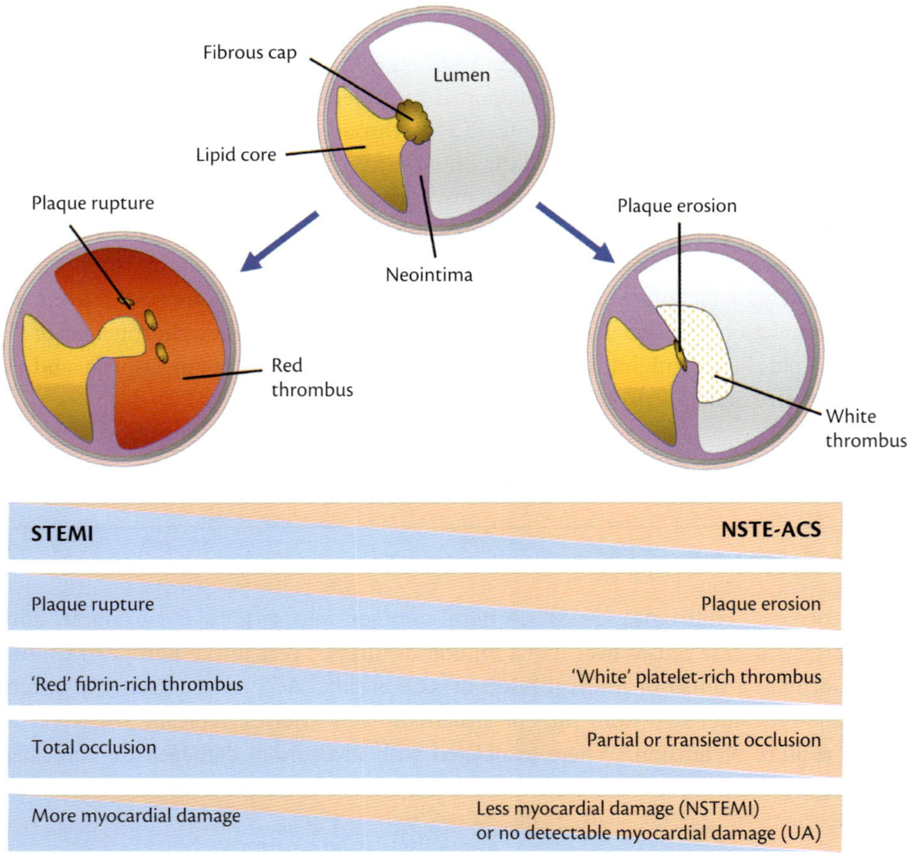

Figure 16.1 Pathophysiological features of atherothrombosis in the ACS spectrum. NSTE-ACS, non-ST-elevation acute coronary syndromes; NSTEMI, non-ST-elevation myocardial infarction; STEMI, ST-elevation myocardial infarction; UA, unstable angina.

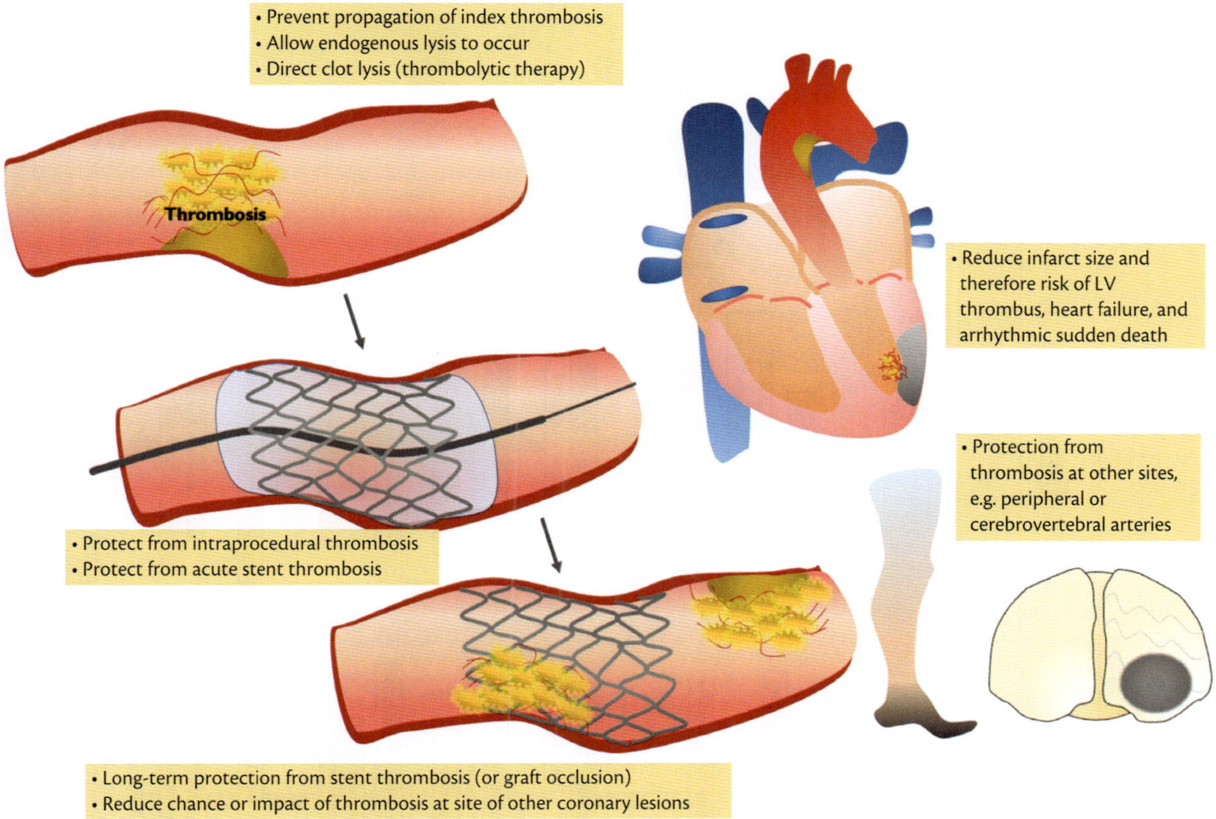

Figure 16.2 Summary of the rationale for antithrombotic therapy in patients with ACS. LV, left ventricular.

of Infarct Survival (ISIS)-2, which randomized 17,187 patients with suspected acute MI to receive aspirin versus placebo and streptokinase versus placebo in a 2 × 2 factorial design.[5] The trial showed that, at 5 weeks after MI, aspirin, given at a dose of 160 mg once daily, conferred a magnitude of benefit similar to thrombolysis with streptokinase (5-week vascular mortality odds reduction ± standard deviation: thrombolysis vs placebo 25% ± 4%, aspirin vs placebo 23% ± 4%); and when the two treatments were combined this led to a much lower risk of vascular death than either alone (odds reduction ± standard deviation for both treatments vs neither: 42 ± 5%).

There is also strong evidence for continuation of aspirin long term beyond the initial post-MI period. For example, the Antithrombotic Trialists' Collaboration performed a meta-analysis demonstrating that antiplatelet therapy, predominantly aspirin monotherapy, was associated with a significantly lower frequency of major adverse cardiovascular events (MACE; defined unless otherwise specified as cardiovascular death, MI, or stroke) compared with the control group using data from 12 trials including 20,006 patients with prior MI.[6,7] This analysis also suggested that daily aspirin doses of 75–150 mg were at least as effective as higher doses in the secondary prevention of cardiovascular events.

Current ESC Guidelines recommend an initial loading dose of aspirin of 150–300 mg orally or 75–250 mg intravenously for all patients with either STEMI (class of recommendation I, level of evidence B) or NSTE-ACS (I, A), followed by an oral maintenance dose of 75–100 mg once daily long term.[3,4]

$P2Y_{12}$ inhibition

(See also ➔ Chapter 6.) There is good evidence from randomized controlled trials (RCTs) that adding a $P2Y_{12}$ inhibitor to aspirin [dual antiplatelet therapy (DAPT)] improves clinical outcomes among patients with ACS (➔ Table 16.1). In trials including patients with NSTE-ACS [Clopidogrel in Unstable Angina to Prevent Recurrent Events Trial (CURE)] or STEMI [Clopidogrel as Adjunctive Reperfusion Therapy—Thrombolysis in Myocardial Infarction (CLARITY TIMI) 28; and ClOpidogrel and Metoprolol in Myocardial Infarction Trial (COMMIT)], addition of the oral thienopyridine clopidogrel to aspirin significantly and consistently reduced occurrence of the respective primary composite clinical outcome endpoints, with some evidence of increased risk of bleeding, but concluded that the balance of clinical benefit strongly favoured intensified treatment.[8–10]

Increasing the pharmacodynamic efficacy and reliability of $P2Y_{12}$ inhibition during DAPT leads to improved cardiovascular outcomes in patients with ACS (➔ Table 16.2). In the Trial to Assess Improvement in Therapeutic Outcomes by Optimizing Platelet Inhibition with Prasugrel (TRITON)—TIMI 38 trial, prasugrel-based DAPT was associated with a lower frequency of MACE in patients with ACS and planned invasive management compared with clopidogrel-based treatment. However, there was

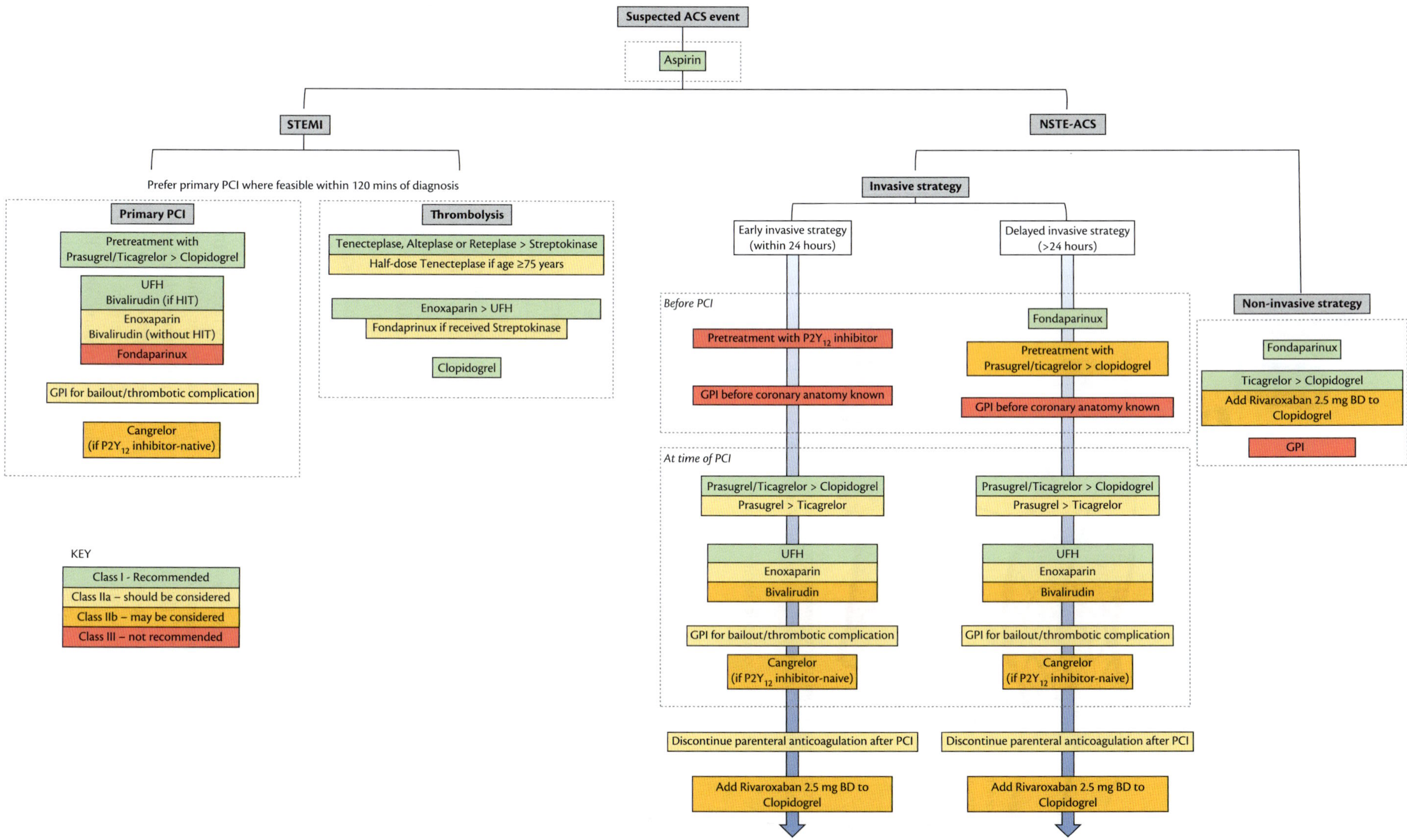

Figure 16.3 Summary of current ESC Guidelines for initial antithrombotic therapy in patients with ACS and without an existing indication for oral anticoagulation.[3,4] ACS, acute coronary syndrome; GPI, glycoprotein IIb/IIIa inhibitor; NSTE-ACS, non-ST-elevation acute coronary syndrome; PCI, percutaneous coronary intervention; STEMI, ST-elevation myocardial infarction; UFH, unfractionated heparin.

Collet J-P, Thiele H, Barbato E, Barthélémy O, Bauersachs J, Bhatt DL, et al. 2020 ESC Guidelines for the management of acute coronary syndromes in patients presenting without persistent ST-segment elevation: The Task Force for the management of acute coronary syndromes in patients presenting without persistent ST-segment elevation of the European Society of Cardiology (ESC). Eur Heart J. 2021;42(14):1289–367.

Table 16.1 Key randomized controlled trials of dual antiplatelet therapy in acute coronary syndromes

Trial, reference	N	ACS group included	Study medication group	Control group	Primary outcomes	Key safety endpoints
CURE[8]	12,562	NSTE-ACS	Aspirin + clopidogrel	Aspirin + placebo	CV death/MI/stroke: RR 0.80 (95% CI 0.72–0.90; P <0.001) CV death/MI/stroke/refractory ischaemia: RR 0.87 (95% CI 0.79–0.94; P <0.001)	Major bleeding: RR 1.38 (95% CI 1.13–1.67; P = 0.001) No significant difference in life-threatening bleeding, fatal bleeding, or haemorrhagic stroke
CLARITY[9]	3491	STEMI	Aspirin + clopidogrel	Aspirin + placebo	Occluded infarct-related artery on angiography/death (all cause) or recurrent MI before angiography/death or recurrent MI before discharge or day 8 in those not undergoing angiography: odds reduction 36% (95% CI 24–47%; P <0.001)	No significant difference in major bleeding at 24 hours post angiography, intracranial bleeding, or bleeding post CABG
COMMIT[68]	45,852	STEMI	Aspirin + clopidogrel	Aspirin + placebo	Death/reinfarction/stroke: OR 0.91 (95% CI 0.86–0.97; P = 0.002) Death (all cause): OR 0.93 (95% CI 0.87–0.99; P = 0.03)	No significant differences in fatal or non-fatal cerebral or non-cerebral bleeding

ACS, acute coronary syndrome; CABG, coronary artery bypass grafting; CV, cardiovascular; HR, hazard ratio; MI, myocardial NSTE-ACS, non-ST elevation ACS; OR, odds ratio; RR, relative risk; STEMI, ST elevation MI.

no significant difference in efficacy between the two regimens in patients with medically managed ACS in the Targeted Platelet Inhibition to Clarify the Optimal Strategy to Medically Manage Acute Coronary Syndromes (TRILOGY ACS) trial. In the Study of Platelet Inhibition and Patient Outcomes (PLATO), ticagrelor, when compared to clopidogrel in aspirin-treated ACS patients, significantly reduced MACE across the spectrum of ACS types and treatment strategies.[11]

A more recent open-label RCT, Intracoronary Stenting and Antithrombotic Regimen: Rapid Early Action for Coronary Treatment (ISAR-REACT) 5, demonstrated higher rates of death, MI, or stroke with a ticagrelor-based strategy versus a prasugrel-based

Table 16.2 Key trials of prasugrel or ticagrelor versus clopidogrel in patients receiving dual antiplatelet therapy for acute coronary syndromes

Trial, reference	N	ACS group included	Study medication group	Control group	Primary outcomes	Key safety endpoints
TRITON-TIMI 38[69]	13,608	All ACS with scheduled PCI	Aspirin + prasugrel	Aspirin + clopidogrel	CV death/MI/stroke in both NSTE-ACS (HR 0.82, 95% CI 0.73–0.93; P = 0.002) and STEMI (HR 0.79, 95% CI 0.65–0.97; P = 0.02) groups	Major bleeding (HR 1.32, 95% CI 1.03–1.68; P = 0.03) Life-threatening bleeding (HR 1.52, 95% CI 1.08–2.13; P = 0.01) CABG-related major bleeding (HR 4.73, 95% CI 1.90–11.82; P <0.001) No significant difference in cerebral haemorrhage or non-bleeding-related serious adverse events
TRILOGY ACS[70]	7243	NSTE-ACS with medical management	Aspirin + prasugrel	Aspirin + clopidogrel	No significant difference in CV death/MI/stroke, although trend towards benefit with prasugrel after 12 months (P = 0.07)	No significant differences in GUSTO or TIMI-defined severe/life-threatening/fatal bleeding TIMI major or minor bleeding (HR 1.54, 95% CI 1.06–2.23; P = 0.02) No significant difference in non-haemorrhagic serious adverse events
PLATO[11]	18,624	All ACS (STEMI patients included only if for primary PCI)	Aspirin + ticagrelor	Aspirin + clopidogrel	CV death/MI/stroke (HR 0.84, 95% CI 0.77–0.92; P <0.001)	No significant differences in major, fatal, life-threatening, or CABG-related bleeding Increased non-CABG-related major bleeding (P = 0.03) Intracranial bleeding (P = 0.06)/fatal intracranial bleeding (P = 0.02) Reduced non-intracranial fatal bleeding (P = 0.03) Increased dyspnoea (P <0.001) Increased ventricular pauses in 1st week (P = 0.01) but not at 30 days and no significant difference in syncope or PPM requirement

ACS, acute coronary syndrome; CABG, coronary artery bypass grafting; CV, cardiovascular; GUSTO, Global Use of Strategies for Opening Occluded Coronary Arteries; HR, hazard ratio; MI, myocardial NSTE-ACS, non-ST elevation ACS; PCI, percutaneous coronary intervention; PPM, permanent pacemaker; STEMI, ST elevation MI; TIMI, Thrombolysis in Myocardial Infarction.

strategy in invasively-managed ACS patients [hazard ratio (HR) 1.34, 95% confidence interval (CI) 1.09–1.70; P = 0.006],[12] although high rates of femoral access and unexpectedly high rates of stent thrombosis (these latter in the ticagrelor group) have raised questions about the wider applicability of these findings to contemporary practice.[13,14]

Current ESC Guidelines on STEMI recommend administration of a $P2Y_{12}$ inhibitor, preferably prasugrel or ticagrelor, before a primary percutaneous coronary intervention (PCI) and continued for a default duration of 12 months (I, A).[3] Similarly, in NSTE-ACS, 12 months of a $P2Y_{12}$ inhibitor is recommended (I, A), with ticagrelor or prasugrel as the recommended agents (I, B). It is advised that prasugrel be considered in preference to ticagrelor for patients with NSTE-ACS proceeding to PCI without pretreatment (IIa, B).[15]

Oral anticoagulants

(See also ➔ Chapter 9–11.) Atherothrombosis involves not only platelet activation, but also triggering of the coagulation cascade, leading to the generation of thrombin, which cleaves soluble fibrinogen to insoluble fibrin, forming networks of strands.[16] Thrombin also leads to platelet activation via protease activated receptors (PAR)-1 and -4, and, conversely, activated platelets contribute to thrombin generation via membrane scramblase activity. Drugs targeting platelets therefore can also influence coagulation, and anticoagulants may also reduce platelet activation.[17]

Patients with ACS and a separate indication for full-dose oral anticoagulation (OAC), such as atrial fibrillation (AF), present particular challenges and are considered later in this chapter and also in ➔ Chapters 20, 26 and 28.

The Anti-Xa Therapy to Lower Cardiovascular Events in Addition to Standard Therapy in Subjects with ACS 2 (ATLAS-ACS 2)-TIMI 51 trial demonstrated that the addition of a low dose of the non-vitamin K antagonist oral anticoagulant (NOAC) rivaroxaban 2.5 mg twice daily in ACS patients treated with aspirin and clopidogrel significantly reduced the occurrence of cardiovascular death, MI, or stroke when compared to placebo (HR 0.84, 95% CI 0.72–0.97; P = 0.02).[18] There was a converse increase in TIMI major non-coronary artery bypass graft (CABG)-related bleeding (HR 3.46, 95% CI 2.08–5.77; P <0.001). Addition of low-dose rivaroxaban to DAPT with the newer $P2Y_{12}$ inhibitors has not been robustly tested and, similarly, clinical outcomes when receiving the combination of aspirin, clopidogrel, and low-dose rivaroxaban have not been compared with prasugrel- or ticagrelor-based DAPT in ACS. Current ESC Guidelines for treatment of NSTE-ACS include a recommendation that adding a rivaroxaban 2.5 mg twice-daily regimen to aspirin and clopidogrel may be considered where there is no prior stroke/transient ischaemic attack, bleeding risk is low, and ischaemic risk high (IIb, B).[4]

Parenteral antithrombotic therapy in acute coronary syndromes

Heparins

(See also ➔ Chapter 8.) In 1996, a meta-analysis of six individually negative trials including 1353 aspirin-treated patients with unstable angina suggested that intravenous unfractionated heparin (UFH) given for 2–7 days reduced the risk of MI or death by one-third [relative risk (RR) 0.67, 95% CI 0.44–1.02; P = 0.06].[19] Though this narrowly missed the threshold for statistical significance, the authors and wider community recommended giving heparin alongside aspirin in the initial management of patients with NSTE-ACS. Despite the advantage of rapid onset and offset, administration of intravenous UFH can be challenging in practice, with the requirement for a continuous infusion, frequent monitoring, and often low time spent in the therapeutic range. There is also the possibility of developing heparin-induced thrombocytopenia that complicates antithrombotic and procedural management.[20] Low-molecular-weight heparins (LMWHs) have the advantage of more reliable pharmacokinetics when given as an intermittent subcutaneous dose, meaning that monitoring of drug activity levels is not commonly required, and they also have a lower risk of heparin-induced thrombocytopenia.[21] A meta-analysis of 12 trials involving a total of 17,157 patients with NSTE-ACS found that pooling trials testing UFH or LMWHs versus placebo demonstrated a significant benefit of heparins on rates of MI or death (OR 0.53, 95% CI 0.38–0.73; P = 0.0001).[22] Despite the potential pharmacological advantages, there was no evidence of a significant difference between outcomes with LMWH versus UFH (OR 0.88, 95% CI 0.69–1.12; P = 0.34) among the pooled data, though individual trials, such as Efficacy and Safety of Subcutaneous Enoxaparin in Unstable Angina and Non-Q-Wave MI (ESSENCE; n = 3171; death, MI, or recurrent angina at 14 days: 16.6% vs 19.8%; P = 0.019) and TIMI-IIB (n = 3910; death, MI, or urgent revascularization; OR 0.83, 95% CI 0.69–1.00; P = 0.048), have demonstrated marginal superiority of LMWH.[23] UFH remains the most commonly used agent to prevent intraprocedural thrombosis during PCI or CABG.

ESC Guidelines recommend anticoagulation for all patients in addition to antiplatelet therapy during primary PCI (I, C).[3] Routine use of UFH is recommended in this setting (I, C), but intravenous enoxaparin can also be considered (IIa, A). In those with NSTE-ACS, parenteral anticoagulation is recommended for all patients at the time of diagnosis and, especially, during revascularization procedures (I, A).[4] UFH to achieve an activated clotting time of 250–350 seconds, or 200–250 seconds if given with a glycoprotein IIb/IIIa inhibitor (GPI), is recommended during PCI (I, A), and intravenous enoxaparin can be considered where patients have been pre-treated with subcutaneous LMWH (IIa, B).

Fondaparinux

(See also ➔ Chapter 8.) The pentasaccharide heparin analogue fondaparinux selectively inhibits activated factor X.[24] Fondaparinux (2.5 mg once daily) was compared with LMWH (enoxaparin 1 mg/kg twice daily) in the Fifth Organization to Assess Strategies in Acute Ischemic Syndromes (OASIS-5) trial, which randomized 20,078 patients age 60 years or over with ACS within 24 hours of symptom onset.[25] Treatment was for a mean of 6 days. The primary endpoint of death, MI, or refractory ischaemia at 9 days occurred at similar rates in the two groups (HR 1.01, 95% CI 0.90–1.13) and met criteria for non-inferiority. Notably, however, major bleeding was significantly less frequent among those receiving fondaparinux (at day 9: HR 0.52, 95% CI 0.44–0.61; P <0.001), and combining the primary efficacy endpoint and major bleeding demonstrated a clear net clinical benefit of fondaparinux over LMWH (HR 0.81, 95% CI 0.73–0.89; P <0.001).

Though there is rationale for commencing fondaparinux 2.5 mg/day as soon as NSTE-ACS is suspected, potentially in the prehospital setting, and this includes the prevention of venous thromboembolism in patients bed-ridden while awaiting for PCI and for few days thereafter, treatment is only currently recommended in cases of NSTE-ACS where early invasive management (within 24 hours of diagnosis) is not planned and patients who undergo PCI when receiving fondaparinux should also receive UFH (I, B).[4] Fondaparinux is not a recommended anticoagulant before or during primary PCI for STEMI (III, B).[3]

Bivalirudin

(See also ➔ Chapter 8.) Bivalirudin, a synthetic version of the naturally occurring anticoagulant substance hirudin found in leeches, acts as a direct thrombin inhibitor. Bivalirudin was tested alone, and in combination with a GPI, against heparin plus GPI in the Acute Catheterization and Urgent Intervention Triage Strategy (ACUITY) trial.[26] Assessed at 30 ± 5 days after randomization, there were no significant differences in the rates of the primary ischaemic endpoint of death, MI, or unplanned revascularization when comparing bivalirudin plus GPI or bivalirudin alone with heparin plus GPI. However, rates of non-CABG-related major bleeding were significantly lower when receiving bivalirudin alone vs heparin plus GPI (RR 0.52, 95% CI 0.44–0.61; P < 0.001), as were combined efficacy and safety outcomes (RR 0.85, 95% CI 0.77–0.97; P = 0.015). Bivalirudin alone was further compared with UFH plus GPI in the setting of primary PCI for STEMI in another open-label trial, Harmonizing Outcomes with Revascularization and Stents in Acute MI (HORIZONS-AMI).[27] While bivalirudin led to a lower rate of 30-day net adverse clinical events (RR 0.76, 95% CI 0.63–0.92; P = 0.005), driven by reduced non-CABG major bleeding, there was a significant increase in the number of acute stent thrombosis episodes (1.3% vs 0.3%; P <0.001). Subsequently, bivalirudin was compared with heparin in two trials. In Unfractionated Heparin versus Bivalirudin in Primary Percutaneous Coronary Intervention (HEAT-PPCI), an open-label, single-centre RCT, UFH was associated with a significantly lower occurrence of the primary efficacy outcome of all-cause mortality, stroke, MI, or unplanned target lesion revascularization (8.7% vs 5.7%, RR 1.52, 95% CI 1.09–2.13; P = 0.01) without a significant difference in safety outcomes.[28] Similarly, in Bivalirudin versus Heparin in ST-Segment and Non–ST-Segment Elevation Myocardial Infarction in Patients on Modern Antiplatelet Therapy in the Swedish Web System for Enhancement and Development of Evidence-based Care in Heart Disease Evaluated according to Recommended Therapies Registry Trial (VALIDATE-SWEDEHEART), there was no evidence of benefit of bivalirudin over heparin (12.3% vs 12.8%, HR 0.96, 95% CI 0.83–1.10; P = 0.54) in the occurrence of the composite endpoint of all-cause mortality, MI, or major bleeding.[29] Most recently, the Bivalirudin With Prolonged Full-Dose Infusion During Primary PCI Versus Heparin Trial (BRIGHT)-4 compared a strategy of bivalirudin (given during PCI followed by a high-dose infusion for 2–4 hours after PCI) with UFH (given only during PCI) in 6016 patients with STEMI undergoing primary PCI using a randomized open-label design.[30] The primary composite endpoint of all-cause mortality or Bleeding Academic Research Consortium (BARC) type 3–5 bleeding at 30 days occurred significantly less frequently in the bivalirudin group (4.39% in the heparin group vs 3.06% in the bivalirudin group; HR 0.69, 95% CI 0.53–0.91; P = 0.007). Limitations of interpretation include that, as well as the drug, duration of therapy was different between the study arms, and that approximately one-third of patients did not receive a potent oral $P2Y_{12}$ inhibitor; yet these data may support ongoing infusion of parenteral anticoagulant therapy after primary PCI.

ESC Guidelines recommend that routine use of bivalirudin, as an alternative to UFH, may be considered during primary PCI for STEMI (IIa, A) or NSTE-ACS (IIb, A).[3,4] Bivalirudin is the recommended parenteral anticoagulant for patients with a history of heparin-induced thrombocytopenia undergoing PCI for ACS (I, C).

Cangrelor

(See also ➔ Chapter 6.) Cangrelor, an intravenously administered, reversibly binding $P2Y_{12}$ inhibitor, is a potent and rapidly acting antiplatelet drug. An analogue of adenosine triphosphate, it has an ultra-short half-life related to its rapid metabolism by dephosphorylation to a main metabolite that does not bind to $P2Y_{12}$.[31] Cangrelor was tested in the Cangrelor versus Standard Therapy to Achieve Optimal Management of Platelet Inhibition (CHAMPION) programme of trials. The first two (CHAMPION PCI and PLATFORM) failed to meet their primary endpoints.[32,33] Conversely, the CHAMPION PHOENIX study, a randomized double-blind, placebo-controlled trial carried out in 11,145 patients undergoing PCI for STEMI (18%), NSTE-ACS (25%), or stable angina (55%)[34] had favourable results. Participants were randomized as initial therapy to either parenteral cangrelor or oral clopidogrel. The primary efficacy endpoint, a composite of all-cause mortality, MI, ischaemia-driven revascularization, and stent thrombosis at 48 hours, occurred significantly less frequently in the group receiving cangrelor than that receiving clopidogrel (4.7% vs 5.9%, OR 0.78, 95% CI 0.66–0.93; P = 0.005). Diagnosis at presentation did not affect the benefit of cangrelor (interaction P = 0.98).

The clinical benefits of cangrelor have not been well compared with the newer more potent and reliable oral $P2Y_{12}$ inhibitors. However, limited studies using pharmacodynamic, physiological and imaging endpoints have suggested that cangrelor, for example, leads to a greater degree of $P2Y_{12}$ inhibition than ticagrelor during primary PCI for STEMI, but that variables such as coronary flow and infarct size are similar between the treatments.[35]

ESC Guidelines recommend that cangrelor may be considered during PCI for STEMI or NSTE-ACS in patients who have not received an oral $P2Y_{12}$ inhibitor (IIb, A).[3,4]

Glycoprotein (GP)-IIb/IIIa inhibitors

(See also ➔ Chapter 7.) Platelet–platelet binding, mediated by activated GPIIb/IIIa complexes on the cell membrane with fibrinogen or von Willebrand factor as bridging factors, is the final common pathway of platelet aggregation. Three platelet GPIs have been extensively studied. Abciximab is the fragment antigen-binding region of a monoclonal murine anti-human GPIIb/IIIa antibody, binding tightly to the receptor and providing a high level of receptor blockade during intravenous infusion. However, high cost and associated rare risk of severe thrombocytopenia have led to its withdrawal from the market. Eptifibatide and tirofiban are both small-molecule inhibitors of GPIIb/IIIa derived from snake venom. Both have short half-lives and are usually given as continuous infusions for this reason.

Studies such as the ReoPro and Primary PTCA Organization and Randomized Trial (RAPPORT)[36] and Abciximab before Direct Angioplasty and Stenting in Myocardial Infarction Regarding Acute and Long-Term Follow-up (ADMIRAL)[37] demonstrated the benefit of GPIs in the setting of primary PCI in reducing vascular events, but $P2Y_{12}$ inhibitors were either not given or were given after PCI. Subsequent studies in the era of pretreatment with an oral $P2Y_{12}$ inhibitor such as the Bavarian Reperfusion Alternatives Evaluation (BRAVE)-3[38] and Ongoing Tirofiban In Myocardial infarction Evaluation (On-TIME) 2 trials[39] failed to demonstrate significant effects of GPI administration on key outcomes such as MACE, though, in On-TIME 2, there was some evidence of improvements in other markers, such as time to resolution of ST-segment elevation.

Current ESC Guidelines recommend considering use of a GPI as a bailout strategy if there is no-reflow phenomenon or a thrombotic complication during PCI for STEMI or NSTE-ACS (IIa, C), but not where coronary anatomy is not known (III, A).[3,4] Some operators also advocate GPIs during primary PCI where there is concern regarding the oral absorption of $P2Y_{12}$ inhibitors, for example, where the patient has received opiates.[40]

Thrombolytic agents

(See also Chapter 13.) While antiplatelet and anticoagulant drugs can help to prevent the initiation or propagation of thrombosis and can tip the balance towards endogenous clot lysis, they cannot themselves lead to dissolution of fibrin clot. Tissue plasminogen activators, in contrast, act as fibrinolytics, and can therefore directly lead to clot lysis and vessel recanalization. These include streptokinase and the recombinant tissue plasminogen activators alteplase, reteplase, and tenecteplase. Landmark trials such as Gruppo Italiano per la Sperimentazione della Streptochinasi nell'Infarto Miocardico (GISSI) 1 demonstrated the benefit of thrombolysis on mortality in patients with MI and significant ST changes.[41] Later trials such as TIMI-IIIB clarified that thrombolysis was of no significant benefit in NSTE-ACS, and therefore it became recommended routinely only in the setting of STEMI.[42] Use of the recombinant drugs over streptokinase became recommended when these were shown to lead to better 30-day mortality, likely due to greater fibrin specificity, as well as the more practical advantage of allowing repeat administration due to lack of immunogenicity.[43]

In current practice, on the basis of evidence from numerous trials, primary PCI is the preferred reperfusion strategy for patients with acute STEMI where this is feasible within 2 hours of diagnosis (I, A).[3,44] However, where this cannot be performed, fibrinolysis is recommended if within 12 hours of symptom onset and no contraindications (I, A). A fibrin-specific agent (i.e. recombinant tissue plasminogen activator rather than streptokinase) is recommended (I, B) and, in the case of patients aged 75 years or older, half-dose tenecteplase should be considered (IIa, B). As with STEMI managed by primary PCI, aspirin (I, B) and a $P2Y_{12}$ inhibitor should be given, but, as there is very limited evidence for use of ticagrelor or prasugrel in patients undergoing thrombolysis, clopidogrel remains the recommended agent in current ESC Guidelines (I, A). Parenteral anticoagulation should also be given alongside the thrombolytic drug. Intravenous followed by subcutaneous enoxaparin is the preferred regimen (I, A), but alternatives are UFH (I, B), or fondaparinux if streptokinase is used (IIa, B).

Contemporary debates in antithrombotic therapy for acute coronary syndromes

Duration of dual antiplatelet therapy after acute coronary syndromes

The current 'default' duration of DAPT after ACS remains 12 months; however, several important trials have now examined whether alternative (primarily shortened) durations offer a better profile of efficacy and safety in certain patient groups.

The role of DAPT extended beyond 12 months after ACS in certain groups into the chronic coronary syndrome phase is covered in Chapter 15. Conversely, recent trials have also tested durations of DAPT less than 12 months, including in patients with ACS. The largest of these are summarized in Table 16.3.

ESC Guidelines for treatment of NSTE-ACS endorse considering de-escalating from DAPT to aspirin alone at 3 months in cases treated with PCI where there is high bleeding risk (e.g., PRECISE-DAPT score ≥25) (IIa, B) or to $P2Y_{12}$ inhibitor monotherapy at 3–6 months where the balance of ischaemic and bleeding risk is felt to favour this approach (IIa, A).[4] An alternative option in those treated with prasugrel- or ticagrelor-based DAPT is to de-escalate to clopidogrel, either unguided or guided by platelet function and/or genotyping to determine the presence of clopidogrel resistance (IIb, A) (Chapter 29).

Future research and guidelines will likely focus on better determining the circumstances in which to lengthen or shorten DAPT after ACS depending on individual ischaemic and bleeding profiles. The ongoing open-label Duration of Dual Anti-Platelet Therapy (DUAL ACS) trial (ClinicalTrials.gov Identifier: NCT03252249) may provide further insights; however, recruitment was terminated early due to resource limitation issues that may limit the study value.

Approach to the patient with an indication for full-dose anticoagulation

Patients with ACS who also have an indication for full-dose OAC, for example, in AF with a more-than-minimal stroke risk, present unique challenges, especially when treated by PCI.

Table 16.3 Randomized clinical trials of shortened dual antiplatelet therapy in acute coronary syndromes

Study short title, reference	Year published	N	Randomized population	Experimental regimen	Comparator	Primary endpoint	Primary safety endpoint[a]	ACS subgroup (primary endpoint)
GLOBAL LEADERS[71]	2018	15,968	Patients undergoing PCI for CCS (53%) or ACS (47%), between angiography and PCI	Aspirin 75–100 mg OD and ticagrelor 90 mg BD for 1 month, then ticagrelor 90 mg BD for 23 months	Aspirin 75–100 mg OD plus either clopidogrel 75 mg OD (CCS) or ticagrelor 90 mg BD (ACS) for 12 months, then aspirin 75–100 mg OD for 12 months	All-cause death or new Q-wave MI at 730 days: 3.81% vs 4.37% (RR 0.87, 95% CI 0.75–1.01; P = 0.073)	BARC grade 3–5 bleeding: 2.04% vs 2.12% (RR 0.97, 95% CI 0.78–1.20; P = 0.77)	Between 31 and 365 days, primary endpoint: 1.5% vs 2.0% (HR 0.73, 95% CI 0.51–1.03; P = 0.07) BARC type 3 or 5 bleeding: 0.8% vs 1.5%, (HR 0.52, 95% CI 0.33–0.81; P = 0.004)[72]
TWILIGHT[73]	2019	7119	'High-risk' patients undergoing PCI for CCS (35%) or non-ST elevation ACS (65%), after 3 event-free months of DAPT with aspirin 75 mg OD and ticagrelor 90 mg BD	Ticagrelor 90 mg BD plus placebo for 3 years	Aspirin 81–100 mg OD plus ticagrelor 90 mg BD for 3 years	BARC grade 2, 3, or 5 bleeding: 4.0% vs 7.1% (HR 0.56; 95% CI 0.45–0.68; P <0.001)	All-cause death, non-fatal MI, or non-fatal stroke: 3.9% vs 3.9% [HR 0.99; 95% CI 0.78–1.25; P (non-inferiority) <0.001]	3.6% vs 7.6% (HR 0.47, 95% CI 0.36–0.61; P <0.001)[74]
MASTER DAPT[75]	2021	4434	Patients at high bleeding risk undergoing PCI for stable angina (36%), ACS (54%), or silent ischaemia (10%) biodegradable-polymer sirolimus-eluting stent implantation, randomized at 1 month	Antiplatelet monotherapy [~70% $P2Y_{12}$ inhibitor (mostly clopidogrel), 30% aspirin]	Aspirin plus $P2Y_{12}$ inhibitor (mostly clopidogrel) continued for at least an additional 2 months	All-cause death, MI, stroke, or major bleeding at 1 year: 7.5% vs 7.7% (difference −0.23%, 95% CI −1.80% to 1.33%; P <0.001 for non-inferiority)	Major or clinically relevant non-major bleeding: 6.5% vs 9.4% (difference −2.82%, 95% CI −4.40% to −1.24%; P <0.001 for superiority)	Difference in primary endpoint (ITT) ACS: −0.75 (95% CI −3.13 to 1.63); stable coronary artery disease: −0.30 (95% CI −2.32 to 1.72)
STOP DAPT ACS2[76]	2022	4136	Patients undergoing PCI with cobalt chromium everolimus-eluting stents for ACS (56% STEMI, 20% NSTEMI)	1–2 months of DAPT followed by clopidogrel monotherapy	12 months of DAPT with aspirin and clopidogrel	CV death, MI, stroke, definite stent thrombosis, or TIMI major/minor bleeding, assessed at 12 months: 3.2% vs 2.8% (absolute difference 0.37%, 95% CI −0.68% to 1.42%; HR 1.14, 95% CI 0.80–1.62; P for non-inferiority = 0.06)	TIMI major/minor bleeding: 0.5% vs 1.2% (absolute difference −0.63%, 95% CI −1.20% to −0.06%; HR 0.46, 95% CI 0.23–0.94)	N/A
TICO[77]	2020	3056	Patients undergoing PCI for ACS with ultrathin bioresorbable polymer sirolimus-eluting stents	3 months of aspirin plus ticagrelor, then ticagrelor monotherapy	12 months of aspirin plus ticagrelor	All-cause death, MI, stent thrombosis, stroke, target-vessel revascularization, or TIMI major bleeding, at 12 months: 3.9% vs 5.9% (absolute difference −1.98%, 95% CI −3.50% to −0.45%, HR 0.66, 95% CI 0.48–0.92; P = 0.01)	TIMI major bleeding: 1.7% of patients with ticagrelor monotherapy after 3-month DAPT and in 3.0% of patients with ticagrelor-based 12-month DAPT (HR 0.56, 95% CI 0.34–0.91; P = 0.02)	N/A

[a] Or key secondary safety endpoint if no primary safety endpoint defined.

ACS, acute coronary syndrome; BARC, Bleeding Academic Research Consortium; BD, twice daily; CCS, chronic coronary syndromes; CI, confidence interval; DAPT, dual antiplatelet therapy; HR, hazard ratio; ITT, intention-to-treat; MI, myocardial infarction; NSTEMI, non-ST-elevation MI; OD, once daily; PCI, percutaneous coronary intervention; RR, relative risk; STEMI, ST-elevation MI; TIMI, Thrombolysis in Myocardial Infarction.

There is a need to treat the index coronary event and prevent stent thrombosis, mediated primarily by platelet activation, while also protecting from left atrial thrombosis and subsequent cardioembolism, mediated primarily by activation of the coagulation cascade. Yet, combining OAC with antiplatelet therapy leads to increased bleeding among patients who often have comorbidities and may have high baseline bleeding risk. Balancing these risks is key to optimal antithrombotic therapy in this setting.

There is now a reasonable body of evidence to support treatment recommendations. Data from the small-scale What is the Optimal antiplatElet & Anticoagulant Therapy in Patients With Oral Anticoagulation and Coronary StenTing? (WOEST) study suggested treatment with an OAC plus clopidogrel reduced bleeding following PCI compared to triple therapy with aspirin, clopidogrel, and an OAC.[45] While WOEST was underpowered to detect a meaningful difference in ischaemic events, there was no clear signal of harm when de-escalating antiplatelet therapy. Subsequently, larger RCTs have also supported this approach. An Open-label, 2 × 2 Factorial, Randomized Controlled, Clinical Trial to Evaluate the Safety of Apixaban vs Vitamin K Antagonist and Aspirin vs Aspirin Placebo in Patients With AF and ACS or PCI (AUGUSTUS) is the largest of these to date, randomizing 4614 patients with AF and ACS and/or recent PCI (61% for ACS), due to receive a $P2Y_{12}$ inhibitor for 6 months, to receive aspirin versus placebo, plus apixaban (5 mg twice daily, or 2.5 mg twice daily where indicated) versus warfarin.[46] The investigators concluded that (1) receiving aspirin increased the risk of the primary endpoint of International Society of Thrombosis and Haemostasis major or clinically-relevant non-major bleeding (HR 1.89, 95% CI 1.59–2.24; P <0.001) without significantly reducing the incidence of the secondary endpoint of death or ischaemic events (HR 0.89, 95% CI 0.71–1.11), and (2) receiving a NOAC led to significantly less bleeding than a vitamin K antagonist (VKA) (HR 0.69, 95% CI 0.58–0.81; P <0.001) without increasing the incidence of death or ischaemic events (HR 0.89, 95% CI 0.71–1.11).

There remains debate regarding the timing of de-escalation of DAPT to single antiplatelet therapy (SAPT) after PCI in ACS patients receiving concurrent OAC, and whether this should be, for example, immediately after PCI, at hospital discharge, 1 week after PCI, or later.[47] Though trials in this population have generally stopped aspirin rather than the $P2Y_{12}$ inhibitor when transitioning from triple to double therapy (OAC plus SAPT), there is little evidence to inform whether this is the best strategy or if it would be equivalent or better to discontinue the $P2Y_{12}$ inhibitor and continue aspirin instead.

While there is general consensus that ticagrelor or prasugrel should not be routinely used as part of triple therapy, it is feasible that in selected cases where coronary thrombotic risk is high but cardioembolic risk low (e.g., a relatively low CHA_2DS_2VASc score), temporary interruption of OAC to give DAPT with aspirin and a potent $P2Y_{12}$ inhibitor may be a valid strategy and is one currently being tested.[48]

The 2020 ESC NSTE-ACS Guidelines emphasize the importance of continuing OAC for AF where this is indicated using usual CHA_2DS_2VASc thresholds (I–IIa, A-B).[4] During PCI for ACS, parenteral anticoagulation should still be administered if the patient is receiving either a NOAC or a VKA if the international normalized ratio (INR) is less than 2.5 (I, C). After PCI, around a week or less of triple therapy with aspirin plus $P2Y_{12}$ inhibitor (preferably clopidogrel) plus OAC (preferably a NOAC) is recommended (I, A), at which point one antiplatelet drug can be discontinued, which, based on recent trial protocols, is typically aspirin. Discontinuation of the remaining antiplatelet drug can then usually occur at 12 months, leaving the patients on OAC alone long term. The potent $P2Y_{12}$ inhibitors ticagrelor and prasugrel are not recommended for use in triple therapy, but in combination with OAC alone can be considered (IIb, C). In medically managed patients, there is less robust evidence, but in general continuing one antiplatelet agent for 12 months alongside long-term OAC should be considered (IIa, C).

$P2Y_{12}$ inhibitor pretreatment versus no pretreatment

There is consensus that a loading dose of aspirin should be administered as soon as ACS is suspected, but it has been less clear when to initiate treatment with a $P2Y_{12}$ inhibitor. In cases of STEMI, the only large trial that has investigated the timing of $P2Y_{12}$ inhibition is the Administration of Ticagrelor in the Cath Lab or in the Ambulance for New STEMI to Open the Coronary Artery (ATLANTIC) study, which randomized 1862 patients to receive treatment with ticagrelor in the prehospital phase versus on arrival to the catheterization laboratory.[49] Between the strategies, there was no significant difference in the co-primary endpoints of at least 70% ST-segment elevation resolution before PCI (OR 0.93, 95% CI 0.69–1.25; P = 0.63) and TIMI grade 3 flow in the infarct-related artery angiography (OR 0.97, 95% CI 0.75–1.25; P = 0.82). Mitigating the lack of benefit may have been the fact that the average difference in administration time between the strategies was only 31 minutes, plus the previously underappreciated issue that concurrent treatment with opiates slows the absorption of oral $P2Y_{12}$ inhibitors,[50,51] limiting any benefit of earlier administration. There are no data supporting delaying $P2Y_{12}$ inhibitor administration until after angiography in STEMI. Current ESC Guidelines recommend administering a potent $P2Y_{12}$ inhibitor before primary PCI for STEMI (I, A).[3]

In NSTE-ACS, it is less clear whether initiation of a $P2Y_{12}$ inhibitor should occur before angiography ('pretreatment') or between angiography and PCI, particularly in cases where early (<24 hours after diagnosis) invasive management is planned. Arguments for pretreatment include the earlier termination of ongoing thromboinflammatory processes, a greater likelihood of adequate platelet inhibition in the peri-PCI period leading to reduced risk of stent thrombosis, and, in patients not undergoing immediate invasive treatment, an increased likelihood of detecting $P2Y_{12}$ inhibitor intolerance. Counter arguments are that pretreatment increases the risk of access site and other bleeding, that inappropriate therapy may be initiated in cases where it becomes apparent that the diagnosis is not ACS at angiography, or may delay or even be prohibitive for CABG or other surgery, such as for aortic dissection, where this is urgently indicated. The Comparison of Prasugrel at the Time of PCI or as Pretreatment at the Time of Diagnosis in Patients with NSTEMI (ACCOAST) trial randomized 4033 patients with NSTE-ACS scheduled to undergo angiography within 2–48 hours to receive one of two regimens of prasugrel: either 30 mg pre-angiography plus 30 mg at time of PCI, or 60 mg at time of PCI. At day 7, pretreatment was not associated with any difference in the composite of cardiovascular death, MI, stroke, urgent revascularization, or GPI rescue therapy (HR 1.02, 95% CI 0.84–1.25; P = 0.81). Conversely, however, pretreatment was associated with an increased risk of TIMI major bleeding (HR 1.90, 95% CI 1.19–3.02; P = 0.006). In ISAR-REACT 5, a strategy of ticagrelor pretreatment was tested against on-table administration of prasugrel in the subgroup with NSTE-ACS,[52] demonstrating superiority of prasugrel, consistent with the overall findings of the trial as discussed above. The contribution of the timing of $P2Y_{12}$ inhibitor initiation to these observations remains, however, unclear.

ESC Guidelines on treatment of NSTE-ACS advise to consider pretreatment where there is not high bleeding risk and where an early invasive strategy is not planned (IIb, C).[4] Conversely, pretreatment is not *routinely* recommended where coronary anatomy is unknown and early invasive management is envisaged (III, A). In the authors' opinion pretreatment is likely futile, and possibly dangerous, if PCI is planned very early (within 4–6 hours?) in such patients, but should be given if longer times before PCI are expected, provided a reasonable ruling-out of aortic dissection or the need of urgent surgery can be made.

Concerns around procedural bleeding are mitigated by utilizing radial rather than femoral access for angiography/PCI.[53] Similarly, new technologies for reversal of ticagrelor effects, such as the monoclonal antibody antidote bentracimab, currently in phase III development, or adsorbent devices for removing the drug during cardiopulmonary bypass, may hypothetically reduce the risks of pretreatment with this particular agent.[54–56]

Aspirin dosing in acute coronary syndromes

(See also ➔ Chapter 5.) Historically, a relatively wide range of daily aspirin doses have been utilized for maintenance treatment of ACS. When administered with ticagrelor, there is evidence that daily aspirin doses of 300 mg or greater are associated with worse outcomes than doses of less than 300 mg.[57]

Frequency of aspirin dosing in ACS may also be open to optimization. Because aspirin is only present in the circulation for a short time after each dose, new platelets released between doses remain uninhibited by aspirin until the next administration.[58] Twice-daily dosing of aspirin may reduce the proportion of uninhibited platelets present at any one time.[59] Particular groups of patients have higher-than-average platelet turnover, such as those with diabetes or obesity, those undergoing cardiac surgery, and current smokers. As yet, any clinical benefits of twice-daily over once-daily aspirin dosing in ACS remain uncertain, but the ongoing Aspirin Twice a Day in Patients With Diabetes and Acute Coronary Syndrome (ANDAMAN) trial (ClinicalTrials.gov Identifier: NCT02520921) is exploring this in patients with ACS and diabetes, obesity, or already receiving once-daily low-dose aspirin at the time of their ACS event. Synergism of aspirin and $P2Y_{12}$ inhibition may mean lower-than-standard doses of aspirin might hypothetically provide sufficient platelet inhibition while minimizing harmful effects, for example, on haemostasis, endothelial inhibition, and gastric erosion.[60] A novel regimen of very-low-dose (20 mg) twice-daily aspirin in ticagrelor-treated ACS patients leads to reduced peak-trough variation in effect, improving haemostasis, but maintains 24-hour antiplatelet effect.[61] Any influence on clinical outcomes remains to be determined.

Antiplatelet therapy for type 2 myocardial infarction

Type 2 MI, caused by a mismatch in myocardial oxygen supply and demand for a reason other than acute coronary thrombosis, cardiac surgery, or PCI and not associated with sudden death, can be challenging to diagnose and treat.[2] Representing a broad range of underlying aetiologies, different strategies may be valid depending on the individual circumstances of the case. For example, the patient with normal coronary arteries who suffers type 2 MI secondary to gastrointestinal blood loss will usually warrant different management to a patient with significant underlying coronary artery disease who suffers type 2 MI secondary to severe respiratory infection. Alongside treating the underlying cause for oxygen supply–demand mismatch (e.g., stopping bleeding or treating infection), it is reasonable in most patients without high bleeding risk to use at least SAPT, particularly where underlying coronary artery disease is demonstrated or suspected. Patients with type 2 MI due to cardioembolism may warrant OAC alone unless an indication for adjunctive SAPT exists. Patients with type 2 MI due to spontaneous coronary artery dissection may benefit from early cessation of DAPT, particularly once coronary blood flow normalizes. However, more evidence is required to guide management of different type 2 MI scenarios.[62]

The future of antithrombotic therapy in acute coronary syndromes

In addition to the ongoing trials discussed above, there are other areas in which progress is anticipated in the coming years. Some examples are as follows.

- New antithrombotic drugs are continually in development, and several in particular have clear potential in the treatment of ACS. Selatogrel is a subcutaneously administered reversible $P2Y_{12}$ inhibitor.[63] A single dose reliably and potently inhibits ADP-induced platelet aggregation within 15 minutes, the effect lasting for around 8 hours. Selatogrel is currently being tested in a phase III trial of prehospital administration for suspected MI (ClinicalTrials.gov Identifier: NCT04957719). In addition to providing a potential new option for platelet inhibition in ACS, it will also help clarify the issue of whether pretreatment is beneficial without the limitation of enteral drug absorption. Similarly, any clinical benefit of cangrelor during primary/early PCI in patients who have received potent oral $P2Y_{12}$ inhibitors remains to be determined.

- In the field of anticoagulants, factor (F)-XI or activated FXI inhibition (➔ Chapter 12) is a promising area. FXIa appears to play an important part in the pathological thrombotic response, but a relatively minor role in haemostasis. There is hope that FXIa inhibition translates into a benefit of reduced thrombotic risk with minimal effect on bleeding risk. For example, the oral FXIa inhibitor asundexian has recently been tested in acute MI as an adjunct to DAPT in the Study to Gather Information About the Proper Dosing and Safety of the Oral FXIa Inhibitor BAY 2433334 in Patients Following an Acute Heart Attack (PACIFIC-AMI) trial.[64] There was no evidence of efficacy or safety concerns and phase III trials are awaited. Milvexian, another oral FXIa inhibitor, has been studied in several clinical scenarios in phase II trials, and large phase III trials for secondary stroke prevention, MACE reduction after ACS, and versus a NOAC in AF are being planned.
- Manipulating previously under-recognized processes within the thrombotic response might also play a role in optimizing antithrombotic therapy for ACS. For example, hypofibrinolysis is now proven to be an independent risk factor for cardiovascular events after ACS and is not specifically targeted by current treatments.[65] Drugs that restore normal fibrinolysis have the potential to improve outcomes, perhaps without increasing bleeding risk.
- The thrombomodulatory role of specific microribonucleic acids (miRNAs), small non-coding genetic fragments, continues to be explored. Particular miRNAs have been determined to be platelet derived and have a role in platelet activation and atherothrombosis.[66] Furthermore, levels are altered by current antiplatelet drugs.[67] It is possible to target specific miRNAs using, for example, antagomirs. Whether specific targeting of platelet-related miRNAs in the clinical setting is feasible and moreover whether it has advantages over current antithrombotic approaches remains to be determined.

Conclusion

Most ACS are driven by atherothrombosis and, accordingly, can be treated with antithrombotic therapy. Various antiplatelet, anticoagulant, and fibrinolytic agents are available and recommended for treatments of ACS. There remain promising areas for future developments and a continually evolving evidence base on which to make recommendations.

What's new

- The 'default' recommended duration of DAPT with aspirin and a potent $P2Y_{12}$ inhibitor after ACS remains 12 months; however, prolonging DAPT in patients at high ischaemic risk but low bleeding risk, and shortening in patients at high bleeding risk, can optimize the net clinical outcome.
- There remain several options for parenteral anticoagulation. In patients with NSTE-ACS who are not progressing to immediate invasive management, subcutaneous fondaparinux remains a rational treatment. UFH, LMWH, or bivalirudin can be used in those undergoing PCI.
- Studies of patients with ACS plus an indication for OAC have led to the recommended strategy of a short period of triple therapy (preferably aspirin, clopidogrel, and a NOAC) followed by early discontinuation of aspirin.
- The ISAR REACT 5 trial suggested that prasugrel may be more efficacious than ticagrelor for patients with invasively managed ACS.

What's next

- Anticipated availability of a specific antidote to ticagrelor, bentracimab, might reduce concerns over intensifying antithrombotic therapy in some higher-risk groups of ACS patients.
- Novel antithrombotic drugs such as oral FXIa inhibitors may hypothetically lead to less bleeding than current OACs and might potentially find a role in the treatment of ACS.
- Aspirin dosing in ACS may be further optimized. For example, the ongoing ANDAMAN trial is testing twice-daily versus once-daily dosing in patients at high risk of poor aspirin response.
- Strategies may be developed to target as yet unaddressed abnormalities of the thrombotic response. For example, hypofibrinolysis has been linked with adverse outcomes after ACS and drugs that specifically target this may potentially be of benefit.
- The question of whether prasugrel or ticagrelor is the preferred $P2Y_{12}$ inhibitor after invasively managed ACS remains to be fully answered.
- New ESC Guidelines on the management of ACS will be published in 2023.

Guideline recommendations

Key recommendations on antithrombotic therapy from the ESC STEMI Guidelines 2017

Recommendation	Class of recommendation	Level of evidence
Reperfusion therapy		
Reperfusion therapy is indicated in all patients with symptoms of ischaemia of ≤12 h duration and persistent ST-segment elevation	I	A
A primary PCI strategy is recommended over fibrinolysis within indicated timeframes	I	A
If timely primary PCI cannot be performed after STEMI diagnosis, fibrinolytic therapy is recommended within 12 h of symptom onset in patients without contraindications	I	A
Antiplatelet therapy in primary PCI		
A potent $P2Y_{12}$ inhibitor (prasugrel or ticagrelor), or clopidogrel if these are not available or are contraindicated, is recommended before (or at latest at the time of) PCI and maintained over 12 months, unless there are contraindications such as excessive risk of bleeding	I	A
Aspirin (oral or IV if unable to swallow) is recommended as soon as possible for all patients without contraindications	I	B
GPIIb/IIIa inhibitors should be considered for bailout if there is evidence of no-reflow or a thrombotic complication	IIa	C
Cangrelor may be considered in patients who have not received $P2Y_{12}$ receptor inhibitors	IIb	A
Anticoagulant therapy in primary PCI		
Anticoagulation is recommended for all patients in addition to antiplatelet therapy during primary PCI	I	C
Routine use of UFH is recommended	I	C
In patients with heparin-induced thrombocytopenia, bivalirudin is recommended as the anticoagulant agent during primary PCI	I	C
Routine use of enoxaparin IV should be considered	IIa	A
Routine use of bivalirudin should be considered	IIa	A
Fondaparinux is not recommended for primary PCI	III	B
Fibrinolytic therapy		
When fibrinolysis is the reperfusion strategy, it is recommended to initiate this treatment as soon as possible after STEMI diagnosis, preferably in the prehospital setting	I	A
A fibrin-specific agent (i.e. tenecteplase, alteplase, or reteplase) is recommended	I	B
A half-dose of tenecteplase should be considered in patients >75 years of age	IIa	B
Antiplatelet co-therapy with fibrinolysis		
Oral or IV aspirin is indicated	I	B
Clopidogrel is indicated in addition to aspirin	I	A
DAPT (in the form of aspirin plus a $P2Y_{12}$ inhibitor) is indicated for up to 1 year in patients undergoing fibrinolysis and subsequent PCI	I	C
Anticoagulation co-therapy with fibrinolysis		
Anticoagulation is recommended in patients treated with lytics until revascularization (if performed) or for the duration of hospital stay up to 8 days. The anticoagulant can be:	I	A
◆ Enoxaparin IV followed by SC (preferred over UFH)	I	A
◆ UFH given as a weight-adjusted IV bolus followed by infusion	I	B
◆ In patients treated with streptokinase: fondaparinux IV bolus followed by an SC dose 24 h later	IIa	B

Key recommendations on antithrombotic therapy from the ESC NSTE-ACS Guidelines 2020

Recommendation	Class of recommendation	Level of evidence
Patients with NSTE-ACS without atrial fibrillation		
Antiplatelet treatment		
Aspirin is recommended for all patients without contraindications at an initial oral loading dose of 150–300 mg (or 75–250 mg IV), and at a maintenance dose of 75–100 mg once daily for long-term treatment	I	A

Recommendation	**Class of recommendation**	**Level of evidence**
A $P2Y_{12}$ receptor inhibitor is recommended in addition to aspirin, and maintained over 12 months unless there are contraindications or an excessive risk of bleeding Options are:	I	A
Prasugrel in $P2Y_{12}$ receptor inhibitor-naïve patients proceeding to PCI (60 mg loading dose, 10 mg/day as standard dose, 5 mg/day for patients aged ≥75 years or with a body weight <60 kg)	I	B
Ticagrelor irrespective of the planned treatment strategy (invasive or conservative) (180 mg loading dose, 90 mg twice daily)	I	B
Clopidogrel (300–600 mg loading dose, 75 mg daily dose), only when prasugrel or ticagrelor are not available, cannot be tolerated, or are contraindicated	I	C
Prasugrel should be considered in preference to ticagrelor for NSTE-ACS patients who proceed to PCI	IIa	B
GPIIb/IIIa antagonists should be considered for bail-out if there is evidence of no-reflow or a thrombotic complication	IIa	C
Cangrelor may be considered in $P2Y_{12}$ receptor inhibitor-naïve patients undergoing PCI	IIb	A
Pretreatment with a $P2Y_{12}$ receptor inhibitor may be considered in patients with NSTE-ACS who are not planned to undergo an early invasive strategy and do not have a high bleeding risk	IIb	C
Treatment with GPIIb/IIIa antagonists in patients in whom coronary anatomy is not known is not recommended	III	A
It is not recommended to administer routine pretreatment with a $P2Y_{12}$ receptor inhibitor in patients in whom coronary anatomy is not known and an early invasive management is planned	III	A
Peri-interventional anticoagulant treatment		
Parenteral anticoagulation is recommended for all patients, in addition to antiplatelet treatment, at the time of diagnosis and, especially, during revascularization procedures according to both ischaemic and bleeding risks	I	A
UFH (weight-adjusted IV bolus during PCI of 70–100 IU/kg, or 50–70 IU/kg in combination with a GPIIb/IIIa inhibitor; activated clotting time target range of 250–350 s, or 200–250 s if a GPIIb/IIIa inhibitor is given) is recommended in patients undergoing PCI	I	A
In cases of medical treatment or logistical constraints for transferring the patient to PCI within the required time frame, fondaparinux is recommended and, in such cases, a single bolus of UFH is recommended at the time of PCI	I	B
Enoxaparin (IV) should be considered in patients pre-treated with subcutaneous enoxaparin	IIa	B
Bivalirudin may be considered as an alternative to UFH	IIb	A
Patients with NSTE-ACS requiring chronic oral anticoagulation		
Stroke prevention is recommended to AF patients with ≥1 non-sex CHA_2DS_2-VASc stroke risk factors (score of ≥1 in males or ≥2 in females). For patients with ≥2 non-sex stroke risk factors, OAC is recommended	I	A
For patients with 1 non-sex stroke risk factor, OAC should be considered and treatment may be individualized based on net clinical benefit and consideration of patient values and preferences	IIa	B
Patients undergoing coronary stenting		
Anticoagulation		
During PCI, additional parenteral anticoagulation is recommended, irrespective of the timing of the last dose of all NOACs and if INR is <2.5 in VKA-treated patients	I	C
In patients with an indication for OAC with VKA in combination with aspirin and/or clopidogrel, the dose intensity of VKA should be carefully regulated with a target INR of 2.0–2.5 and a time in the therapeutic range >70%	IIa	B
Uninterrupted therapeutic anticoagulation with VKA or NOACs should be considered during the periprocedural phase	IIa	C
Antiplatelet treatment		
In patients with AF and CHA_2DS_2-VASc score ≥1 in men and ≥2 in women, after a short period of triple antithrombotic therapy (TAT) (up to 1 week from the acute event), dual antithrombotic therapy (DAT) is recommended as the default strategy using a NOAC at the recommended dose for stroke prevention and a single oral antiplatelet agent (preferably clopidogrel)	I	A
Periprocedural DAPT administration consisting of aspirin and clopidogrel up to 1 week is recommended	I	A
Discontinuation of antiplatelet treatment in patients treated with an OAC is recommended after 12 months	I	B

Recommendation	Class of recommendation	Level of evidence
DAT (with an OAC and either ticagrelor or prasugrel) may be considered as an alternative to TAT (with an OAC, aspirin, and clopidogrel) in patients with a moderate or high risk of stent thrombosis, irrespective of the type of stent used	IIb	C
The use of ticagrelor or prasugrel as part of TAT is not recommended	III	C
Medically managed patients		
One antiplatelet agent in addition to an OAC should be considered for up to 1 year	IIa	C
In patients with AF, apixaban 5 mg twice daily and single antiplatelet therapy (clopidogrel) for at least 6 months may be considered	IIb	B

IV, intravenous; SC, subcutaneous.

Source data from Ibanez B, James S, Agewall S, Antunes MJ, Bucciarelli-Ducci C, Bueno H, et al. 2017 ESC Guidelines for the management of acute myocardial infarction in patients presenting with ST-segment elevation: The Task Force for the management of acute myocardial infarction in patients presenting with ST-segment elevation of the European Society of Cardiology (ESC). Eur Heart J. 2017;39(2):119–77; and Collet J-P, Thiele H, Barbato E, Barthélémy O, Bauersachs J, Bhatt DL, et al. 2020 ESC Guidelines for the management of acute coronary syndromes in patients presenting without persistent ST-segment elevation: The Task Force for the management of acute coronary syndromes in patients presenting without persistent ST-segment elevation of the European Society of Cardiology (ESC). Eur Heart J. 2021;42(14):1289–367.

Drug dosing

Drug	Dosing recommendation
Abciximab	Bolus 0.25 mg/kg IV then 0.125 mcg/kg/min infusion (max. 10 mcg/min) for 12 hours
Alteplase	15 mg IV then 0.75 mg/kg IV (up to 50 mg) over 30 minutes then 0.5 mg/kg (up to 35 mg) over 60 minutes
Aspirin	Loading dose 150–300 mg PO or 75–250 mg IV, followed by maintenance dose 75–100 mg OD
Bivalirudin	Bolus of 0.75 mg/kg IV then 1.75 mg/kg/h for up to 4 hours after PCI
Cangrelor	30 mcg/kg bolus IV then 4 mcg/kg/min for at least 2 hours or duration of procedure (whichever is longer)
Clopidogrel	Loading dose 300–600 mg PO (or 75 mg ≥75 years and receiving thrombolysis), followed by maintenance dose 75 mg OD
Enoxaparin	PCI: 0.5 mg/kg IV bolus With thrombolysis: 30 mg IV bolus then 1 mg/kg SC BD starting 15 minutes later (first two doses not to exceed 100 mg each) If ≥75 years, omit IV bolus and use 0.75 mg/kg SC BD (max. 75 mg for each of the first two doses) If eGFR <30 mL/min/1.73 m^2 then give OD rather than BD regardless of age
Eptifibatide	Bolus of 180 mcg/kg IV then 180 mcg/kg after 10 minutes, then infusion 2.0 mcg/kg/min for up to 18 hours
Fondaparinux	Thrombolysis with streptokinase: 2.5 mg IV then 2.5 mg OD SC NSTE-ACS without early invasive strategy: 2.5 mg OD SC
Prasugrel	Loading dose 60 mg PO, followed by 10 mg OD (or 5 mg OD if weight ≤60 kg or age ≥75 years)
Reteplase	10 units IV then 10 units after 30 minutes
Rivaroxaban	ACS in combination with aspirin and clopidogrel: 2.5 mg BD PO
Streptokinase	1.5 megaunits over 30–60 minutes IV
Tenecteplase	Single IV bolus of 30–50 mg depending on weight. Half dose in patients ≥75 years
Ticagrelor	Loading dose 180 mg PO, followed by 90 mg BD
Tirofiban	25 mcg/kg over 3 minutes IV then 0.15 mcg/kg/min for up to 18 hours
Unfractionated heparin	Before/during PCI: 70–100 IU/kg IV bolus, or 50–70 IU/kg if given alongside GPI Thrombolysis: 60 IU/kg bolus IV (max. 4000 IU) then 12 IU/kg for 24–48 hours (max. 1000 IU/h), titrated to aPTT 50–70 seconds or 1.5–2.0 times control value

aPTT, activated partial thromboplastin time; BD, twice daily; GPI, glycoprotein IIb/IIIa inhibitor; IV, intravenous; OD, once daily; PCI, percutaneous coronary intervention; PO, oral; SC, subcutaneous.

References

1. Eurostat. Deaths due to coronary heart diseases in the EU. 2022. Available at: https://ec.europa.eu/eurostat/web/products-eurostat-news/-/edn-20200928-1
2. Thygesen K, Alpert JS, Jaffe AS, et al. Fourth universal definition of myocardial infarction (2018). Eur Heart J. 2018;40(3):237–69.
3. Ibanez B, James S, Agewall S, et al. 2017 ESC Guidelines for the management of acute myocardial infarction in patients presenting with ST-segment elevation: the Task Force for the management of acute myocardial infarction in patients presenting with ST-segment elevation of the European Society of Cardiology (ESC). Eur Heart J. 2017;39(2):119–77.
4. Collet J-P, Thiele H, Barbato E, et al. 2020 ESC Guidelines for the management of acute coronary syndromes in patients presenting without persistent ST-segment elevation: the Task Force for the management of acute coronary syndromes in patients presenting without persistent ST-segment elevation of the European Society of Cardiology (ESC). Eur Heart J. 2021;42(14):1289–367.
5. ISIS-2 (Second International Study of Infarct Survival) Collaborative Group. Randomised trial of intravenous streptokinase, oral aspirin, both, or neither among 17,187 cases of suspected acute myocardial infarction: ISIS-2. Lancet. 1988;2(8607):349–60.
6. Antithrombotic Trialists' (ATT) Collaboration, Baigent C, Blackwell L, et al. Aspirin in the primary and secondary prevention of vascular disease: collaborative meta-analysis of individual participant data from randomised trials. Lancet. 2009;373(9678):1849–60.
7. Antithrombotic Trialists' Collaboration. Collaborative meta-analysis of randomised trials of antiplatelet therapy for prevention of death, myocardial infarction, and stroke in high risk patients. BMJ. 2002;324(7329):71–86.
8. Yusuf S, Zhao F, Mehta S, Chrolavicius S, Tognoni G, Fox K. Effects of clopidogrel in addition to aspirin in patients with acute coronary syndromes without ST-segment elevation. N Eng J Med. 2001;345:494–502.
9. Sabatine MS, Cannon CP, Gibson CM, et al. Addition of clopidogrel to aspirin and fibrinolytic therapy for myocardial infarction with ST-segment elevation. N Engl J Med. 2005;352(12):1179–89.
10. Chen ZM, Jiang LX, Chen YP, et al. Addition of clopidogrel to aspirin in 45,852 patients with acute myocardial infarction: randomised placebo-controlled trial. Lancet. 2005;366(9497):1607–21.
11. Wallentin L, Becker RC, Budaj A, et al. Ticagrelor versus clopidogrel in patients with acute coronary syndromes. N Engl J Med. 2009;361(11):1045–57.
12. Schupke S, Neumann FJ, Menichelli M, et al. Ticagrelor or prasugrel in patients with acute coronary syndromes. N Engl J Med. 2019;381(16):1524–34.
13. Zwart B, Yazdani M, Ow KW, et al. Use of glycoprotein IIb/IIIa antagonists to prevent stent thrombosis in morphine-treated patients with ST-elevation myocardial infarction. Platelets. 2019;31(2):174–8.
14. Gosling R, Yazdani M, Parviz Y, et al. Comparison of P2Y 12 inhibitors for mortality and stent thrombosis in patients with acute coronary syndromes: single center study of 10 793 consecutive 'real-world' patients. Platelets. 2017;28(8):767–73.
15. Crea F, Thiele H, Sibbing D, et al. Debate: prasugrel rather than ticagrelor is the preferred treatment for NSTE-ACS patients who proceed to PCI and pretreatment should not be performed in patients planned for an early invasive strategy. Eur Heart J. 2021;42(31):2973–85.
16. Ajjan R, Grant PJ. Coagulation and atherothrombotic disease. Atherosclerosis. 2006;186(2):240–59.
17. Sumaya W, Parker WAE, Fretwell R, et al. Pharmacodynamic effects of a 6-hour regimen of enoxaparin in patients undergoing primary percutaneous coronary intervention (PENNY PCI study). Thromb Haemost. 2018;118(7):1250–6.
18. Mega JL, Braunwald E, Wiviott SD, et al. Rivaroxaban in patients with a recent acute coronary syndrome. N Engl J Med. 2012;366(1):9–19.
19. Oler A, Whooley MA, Oler J, Grady D. Adding heparin to aspirin reduces the incidence of myocardial infarction and death in patients with unstable angina. A meta-analysis. JAMA. 1996;276(10):811–5.
20. Warkentin TE. Heparin-induced thrombocytopenia: pathogenesis and management. Br J Haematol. 2003;121(4):535–55.
21. Klein W, Buchwald A, Hillis SE, et al. Comparison of low-molecular-weight heparin with unfractionated heparin acutely and with placebo for 6 weeks in the management of unstable coronary artery disease: Fragmin in Unstable Coronary Artery Disease Study (FRIC). Circulation. 1997;96:61–8.
22. Eikelboom JW, Anand SS, Malmberg K, Weitz JI, Ginsberg JS, Yusuf S. Unfractionated heparin and low-molecular-weight heparin in acute coronary syndrome without ST elevation: a meta-analysis. Lancet. 2000;355(9219):1936–42.
23. Cohen M, Demers C, Gurfinkel EP, et al. A comparison of low-molecular-weight heparin with unfractionated heparin for unstable coronary artery disease. N Engl J Med. 1997;337:447–52.
24. Cheng JW. Fondaparinux: a new antithrombotic agent. Clin Ther. 2002;24(11):1757–69.
25. Fifth Organization to Assess Strategies in Acute Ischemic Syndromes Investigators, Yusuf S, Mehta SR, et al. Comparison of fondaparinux and enoxaparin in acute coronary syndromes. N Engl J Med. 2006;354(14):1464–76.
26. Stone GW, McLaurin BT, Cox DA, et al. Bivalirudin for patients with acute coronary syndromes. N Engl J Med. 2006;355(21):2203–16.
27. Stone GW, Witzenbichler B, Guagliumi G, et al. Bivalirudin during primary PCI in acute myocardial infarction. N Engl J Med. 2008;358(21):2218–30.
28. Shahzad A, Kemp I, Mars C, et al. Unfractionated heparin versus bivalirudin in primary percutaneous coronary intervention (HEAT-PPCI): an open-label, single centre, randomised controlled trial. Lancet. 2014;384:1849–58.
29. Erlinge D, Omerovic E, Fröbert O, et al. Bivalirudin versus heparin monotherapy in myocardial infarction. N Engl J Med. 2017;377(12):1132–42.
30. Li Y, Liang Z, Qin L, et al. Bivalirudin plus a high-dose infusion versus heparin monotherapy in patients with ST-segment elevation myocardial infarction undergoing primary percutaneous coronary intervention: a randomised trial. Lancet. 2022;400(10366):1847–57.
31. Parker WA, Bhatt DL, Prats J, et al. Characteristics of dyspnoea and associated clinical outcomes in the CHAMPION PHOENIX study. Thromb Haemost. 2017;117(6):1093–100.
32. Bhatt DL, Lincoff AM, Gibson CM, et al. Intravenous platelet blockade with cangrelor during PCI. N Engl J Med. 2009;361(24):2330–41.
33. Harrington RA, Stone GW, McNulty S, et al. Platelet inhibition with cangrelor in patients undergoing PCI. N Engl J Med. 2009;361(24):2318–29.
34. Bhatt DL, Stone GW, Mahaffey KW, et al. Effect of platelet inhibition with cangrelor during PCI on ischemic events. N Engl J Med. 2013;368(14):1303–13.
35. Ubaid S, Ford TJ, Berry C, et al. Cangrelor versus ticagrelor in patients treated with primary percutaneous coronary intervention: impact on platelet activity, myocardial microvascular function

and infarct size: a randomized controlled trial. Thromb Haemost. 2019;119(7):1171–81.

36. Brener SJ, Barr LA, Burchenal JEB, et al. Randomized, placebo-controlled trial of platelet glycoprotein IIb/IIIa blockade with primary angioplasty for acute myocardial infarction. Circulation. 1998;98: 734–41.
37. Montalescot G, Barragan P, Wittenberg O, et al. Platelet glycoprotein IIb/IIIa inhibition with coronary stenting for acute myocardial infarction. N Engl J Med. 2001;344(25):1895–903.
38. Mehilli J, Kastrati A, Schulz S, et al. Abciximab in patients with acute ST-segment-elevation myocardial infarction undergoing primary percutaneous coronary intervention after clopidogrel loading: a randomized double-blind trial. Circulation. 2009;119(14):1933–40.
39. Van't Hof AW, Ten Berg J, Heestermans T, et al. Prehospital initiation of tirofiban in patients with ST-elevation myocardial infarction undergoing primary angioplasty (On-TIME 2): a multicentre, double-blind, randomised controlled trial. Lancet. 2008;372(9638):537–46.
40. Sumaya W, Parker WAE, Judge HM, et al. Prolonged enoxaparin therapy compared with standard-of-care antithrombotic therapy in opiate-treated patients undergoing primary percutaneous coronary intervention. Platelets. 2021;32(4):555–9.
41. Gruppo Italiano per lo Studio della Streptochinasi nell'Infarto Miocardico (GISSI). Effectiveness of intravenous thrombolytic treatment in acute myocardial infarction. Lancet. 1986;327(8478):397–402.
42. Effects of tissue plasminogen activator and a comparison of early invasive and conservative strategies in unstable angina and non-Q-wave myocardial infarction. Results of the TIMI IIIB Trial. Thrombolysis in Myocardial Ischemia. Circulation. 1994;89(4):1545–56.
43. GUSTO investigators. An international randomized trial comparing four thrombolytic strategies for acute myocardial infarction. N Engl J Med. 1993;329(10):673–82.
44. Keeley EC, Boura JA, Grines CL. Primary angioplasty versus intravenous thrombolytic therapy for acute myocardial infarction: a quantitative review of 23 randomised trials. The Lancet. 2003;361:13–20.
45. Dewilde WJ, Oirbans T, Verheugt FW, et al. Use of clopidogrel with or without aspirin in patients taking oral anticoagulant therapy and undergoing percutaneous coronary intervention: an open-label, randomised, controlled trial. Lancet. 2013;381(9872):1107–15.
46. Lopes RD, Heizer G, Aronson R, et al. Antithrombotic therapy after acute coronary syndrome or PCI in atrial fibrillation. N Engl J Med. 2019;380(16):1509–24.
47. De Caterina R, Agewall S, Andreotti F, et al. Great debate: triple antithrombotic therapy in patients with atrial fibrillation undergoing coronary stenting should be limited to 1 week. Eur Heart J. 2022;43(37):3512–27.
48. Limbruno U, De Sensi F, Cresti A, Picchi A, Lena F, De Caterina R. Optimal antithrombotic treatment of patients with atrial fibrillation early after an acute coronary syndrome—triple therapy, dual antithrombotic therapy with an anticoagulant… or, rather, temporary dual antiplatelet therapy? J Clin Med. 2020; 9(8):2673.
49. Montalescot G, van 't Hof AW, Lapostolle F, et al. Prehospital ticagrelor in ST-segment elevation myocardial infarction. N Engl J Med. 2014;371(11):1016–27.
50. Thomas MR, Morton AC, Hossain R, et al. Morphine delays the onset of action of prasugrel in patients with prior history of ST-elevation myocardial infarction. Thromb Haemost. 2016;116:96–102.
51. Silvain J, Storey RF, Cayla G, et al. P2Y12 receptor inhibition and effect of morphine in patients undergoing primary PCI for ST-segment elevation myocardial infarction. The PRIVATE-ATLANTIC study. Thromb Haemost. 2016;116(2):369–78.
52. Valina C, Neumann FJ, Menichelli M, et al. Ticagrelor or prasugrel in patients with non-ST-segment elevation acute coronary syndromes. J Am Coll Cardiol. 2020;76(21):2436–46.
53. Valgimigli M, Gagnor A, Calabró P, et al. Radial versus femoral access in patients with acute coronary syndromes undergoing invasive management: a randomised multicentre trial. Lancet. 2015;385(9986):2465–76.
54. Bhatt Deepak L, Pollack Charles V, Mazer CD, et al. Bentracimab for ticagrelor reversal in patients undergoing urgent surgery. NEJM Evid. 2022;1(3):EVIDoa2100047.
55. Hassan K, Kannmacher J, Wohlmuth P, Budde U, Schmoeckel M, Geidel S. Cytosorb adsorption during emergency cardiac operations in patients at high risk of bleeding. Ann Thorac Surg. 2019;108(1):45–51.
56. Tripathi R, Morales J, Lee V, et al. Antithrombotic drug removal from whole blood using haemoadsorption with a porous polymer bead sorbent. Eur Heart J Cardiovasc Pharmacother. 2022;8(8):847–56.
57. Mahaffey KW, Wojdyla DM, Carroll K, et al. Ticagrelor compared with clopidogrel by geographic region in the Platelet Inhibition and Patient Outcomes (PLATO) trial. Circulation. 2011;124(5):544–54.
58. Rocca B, Santilli F, Pitocco D, et al. The recovery of platelet cyclooxygenase activity explains interindividual variability in responsiveness to low-dose aspirin in patients with and without diabetes. J Thromb Haemost. 2012;10(7):1220–30.
59. Cavalca V, Rocca B, Veglia F, et al. On-pump cardiac surgery enhances platelet renewal and impairs aspirin pharmacodynamics: effects of improved dosing regimens. Clin Pharmacol Ther. 2017;102(5):849–58.
60. Parker WAE, Thorneycroft K, Judge HM, Storey RF. Additive effects of aspirin and potent P2Y12 inhibition on platelet macro- and microaggregation of relevance to acute thrombotic stroke. Presented at ESC Heart & Stroke; 24–25 January 2020. Barcelona, Spain.
61. Parker WAE, Orme RC, Hanson J, et al. Very-low-dose twice-daily aspirin maintains platelet inhibition and improves haemostasis during dual-antiplatelet therapy for acute coronary syndrome. Platelets. 2019;30(2):148–57.
62. DeFilippis AP, Chapman AR, Mills NL, et al. Assessment and treatment of patients with type 2 myocardial infarction and acute nonischemic myocardial injury. Circulation. 2019;140(20):1661–78.
63. Parker W, Storey R. Pharmacology and potential role of selatogrel, a subcutaneous platelet P2Y12 receptor antagonist. Expert Opin Emerg Drugs. 2020;25(1):1–6.
64. Rao SV, Kirsch B, Bhatt DL, et al. A multicenter, phase 2, randomized, placebo-controlled, double-blind, parallel-group, dose-finding trial of the oral factor XIa inhibitor asundexian to prevent adverse cardiovascular outcomes after acute myocardial infarction. Circulation. 2022;146(16):1196–206.
65. Sumaya W, Wallentin L, James SK, et al. Fibrin clot properties independently predict adverse clinical outcome following acute coronary syndrome: a PLATO substudy. Eur Heart J. 2018;39(13):1078–85.
66. Czajka P, Fitas A, Jakubik D, et al. Microrna as potential biomarkers of platelet function on antiplatelet therapy: a review. Front Physiol. 2021;12:652579.
67. Parker WAE, Schulte C, Barwari T, et al. Aspirin, clopidogrel and prasugrel monotherapy in patients with type 2 diabetes mellitus: a double-blind randomised controlled trial of the effects on thrombotic markers and microRNA levels. Cardiovasc Diabetol. 2020;19(1):3.

68. Chen ZM, Jiang LX, Chen YP, et al. Addition of clopidogrel to aspirin in 45 852 patients with acute myocardial infarction: randomised placebo-controlled trial. Lancet. 2005;366(9497):1607–21.
69. Wiviott S, Braunwald E, McCabe C, et al. Prasugrel versus clopidogrel in patients with acute coronary syndromes. New Eng J Med. 2007;357: 2001–15.
70. Roe MT, Armstrong PW, Fox KA, et al. Prasugrel versus clopidogrel for acute coronary syndromes without revascularization. N Engl J Med. 2012;367(14):1297–309.
71. Vranckx P, Valgimigli M, Juni P, et al. Ticagrelor plus aspirin for 1 month, followed by ticagrelor monotherapy for 23 months vs aspirin plus clopidogrel or ticagrelor for 12 months, followed by aspirin monotherapy for 12 months after implantation of a drug-eluting stent: a multicentre, open-label, randomised superiority trial. Lancet. 2018;392(10151):940–9.
72. Tomaniak M, Chichareon P, Onuma Y, et al. Benefit and risks of aspirin in addition to ticagrelor in acute coronary syndromes: a post hoc analysis of the randomized GLOBAL LEADERS trial. JAMA Cardiol. 2019;4(11):1092–101.
73. Mehran R, Baber U, Sharma SK, et al. Ticagrelor with or without aspirin in high-risk patients after PCI. N Engl J Med. 2019;381(21):2032–42.
74. Baber U, Dangas G, Angiolillo DJ, et al. Ticagrelor alone vs. ticagrelor plus aspirin following percutaneous coronary intervention in patients with non-ST-segment elevation acute coronary syndromes: TWILIGHT-ACS. Eur Heart J. 2020;41(37):3533–45.
75. Valgimigli M, Frigoli E, Heg D, et al. Dual antiplatelet therapy after PCI in patients at high bleeding risk. N Engl J Med. 2021;385(18):1643–55.
76. Watanabe H, Morimoto T, Natsuaki M, et al. Comparison of clopidogrel monotherapy after 1 to 2 months of dual antiplatelet therapy with 12 months of dual antiplatelet therapy in patients with acute coronary syndrome: the STOPDAPT-2 ACS randomized clinical trial. JAMA Cardiol. 2022;7(4):407–17.
77. Kim B-K, Hong S-J, Cho Y-H, et al. Effect of ticagrelor monotherapy vs ticagrelor with aspirin on major bleeding and cardiovascular events in patients with acute coronary syndrome: the TICO randomized clinical trial. JAMA. 2020;323(23):2407–16.

CHAPTER 17

Antithrombotic therapy for patients with prosthetic valves and during structural percutaneous interventions

Naoki Misumida, Mohamad Alkhouli, and David J. Moliterno

Contents

Summary

Prosthetic heart valves are effective in alleviating symptoms of dysfunctional native valves. However, prosthetic valves are inherently inferior to native valves regarding haemodynamics, durability, and thrombogenicity. Antithrombotic therapy reduces the long-term risk of prosthetic valve thrombosis after mechanical valve replacement and can potentially mitigate the risk of acute or subacute leaflet thrombosis after bioprosthetic valve replacement. With the increasing complexity of patient undergoing valve replacement and the advent and growing use of direct oral anticoagulants, antithrombotic management among patients with valvular heart disease and prosthetic valves has become more intricate. This chapter reviews the current prophylactic and therapeutic strategies for the prevention and treatment of valve thrombosis and discusses future directions in this field.

Introduction and pathogenesis of valve thrombosis

Prosthetic valve thrombosis is a complex multifactorial phenomenon. According to the principles of Virchow's triad, the mechanisms implicated in endovascular thrombus formation include surface-, haemodynamic-, and haemostasis-related factors.[1,2] Artificial surfaces promote clotting through a complex series of interconnected processes that include protein adsorption, adhesion of platelets and leucocytes, thrombin generation, and complement activation.[1,2] Haemodynamic factors include turbulent flow which alters local shear stress and produces focal stasis leading to increased blood coagulability and neointimal injury.[1,2] Haemostatic factors include primary or secondary hypercoagulability as well as local tissue injury during valve implantation that can expose tissue factor to the blood, thereby inducing local activation of the extrinsic coagulation pathway.[1,2]

The risk of thrombus formation differs by the type of valve prosthesis as well as its location.[1] Mechanical valves are highly thrombogenic due to the inherent thrombogenicity of the surface materials, the presence of turbulent flow and high shear stress around the hinges, and the presence of backflow jets which damage blood cells and activate clotting pathways.[3,4] Bioprosthetic valves are less thrombogenic than mechanical valves, but they still carry a risk of thromboembolic events particularly within the first few months after implantation prior to their endothelialization.[1,5] The risk of thrombus formation is higher in the mitral position compared to aortic position because the mitral valve has a larger surface area and more stagnant blood flow compared to aortic prosthesis.[6]

Contemporary trends in valve choice

Thrombus formation on artificial heart valves and subsequent systemic embolization is one of the most feared complications of prosthetic valve replacement. For mechanical valves, lifelong anticoagulation is required to avoid thrombus formation.[3,4] In contrast, bioprosthetic valves, generally made of either bovine pericardium or porcine aortic valves, are less thrombogenic and do not require lifelong anticoagulation.[3] However, the advantage of avoiding long-term anticoagulation with bioprosthetic valves is counterbalanced by the increased risk of structural valve degeneration (SVD), an extremely rare phenomenon with mechanical valves.

The choice between a mechanical and a bioprosthetic valve is hence determined by several factors including patient age, life expectancy, comorbidities, bleeding and ischaemic risks, lifestyle, and patient preference. With the advent of transcatheter valve replacement, the choice of valve and interventional route (open vs endovascular) is even more complex and requires a diligent shared decision-making process through which the indications, risks, benefits, and lifelong management are thoroughly considered.[7] Age is an important factor and is incorporated into the recommendations towards specific valve types in the current guidelines; however, life expectancy rather than actual age is a more meaningful parameter to guide the preferred valve selection.[7] For example, a bioprosthetic valve is a reasonable option for patients less than 60 years of age when multiple comorbidities exist and limit life expectancy to 10 years or less. Indeed, current guidelines assign a class I recommendation [level of evidence (LOE) C] for bioprosthetic valves in any patient whose life expectancy is shorter than the presumed durability of the bioprosthesis.[7]

Randomized comparisons between mechanical and bioprosthetic valves date back to the 1970s. In the first large pivotal trial of mechanical versus bioprosthetic valves, patients randomized to the Bjork–Shiley valve had better 15-year survival compared to those treated with bioprosthetic valves (34% vs 21%; $P = 0.02$).[8] Another trial published in 2009 randomized patients aged 55–70 years to a more contemporary mechanical valve (St. Jude Medical or CarboMedics) or a bioprosthetic valve. During 13-year follow-up, there was no difference in mortality or thromboembolism rates between the two groups; however, the rates of reoperation were higher with bioprosthetic valves.[9] Observational studies comparing long-term mortality after mechanical and bioprosthetic valve replacement yielded mixed results.[10,11] Thus, uncertainty remains on whether mechanical valve replacement is associated with a definite mortality benefit. However, the literature consistently shows lower risks of valve degeneration or reoperation and higher risks of bleeding with mechanical valves compared to bioprosthetic valves.[10,11] Regardless, the utilization of mechanical valves in the US has been steadily declining across all age groups.[3,10,12]

Valve durability remains a crucial factor when deciding on the optimal type of artificial valve. A major challenge in studying valve durability is the wide variability in its definition in the literature. A systematic review documented 11 different definitions for SVD in published studies. In this review, freedom from SVD with bioprosthesis valve replacement ranged from 78% to 98% at 10 years, 62% to 89% at 15 years, and 25% to 56% at 20 years.[13] The rate of SVD of bioprostheses is higher in younger patients.[8,10,13] Current guidelines recommend considering a mechanical valve first (class I indication; LOE C) for patients at high risk for accelerated SVD including patients aged less than 40 years.[7] Specific guideline recommendations for mechanical or bioprosthetic valve are summarized in ➔ Table 17.1. Mechanical valves are recommended for patients aged less than 65 years in the mitral position and aged less than 60 years in the aortic position (class IIa). For bioprosthetic aortic valve replacement, transcatheter aortic valve implantation (TAVI) has a class I recommendation (LOE A) for patients older than 75 years, and for patients who are high risk for surgery regardless of age if suitable for transfemoral TAVI.[7] Among various types of bioprosthesis, there seems to be no clear difference in long-term outcomes, but the available data are hindered by the lack of standardized definitions of SVD and inadequate long-term systematically collected data.[13]

The emergence, development, and ongoing refinements of valve-in-valve procedures over the last decade have expanded options for the lifetime management of valvular disease. Transcatheter implantation of bioprosthetic valves inside failed surgical valves (valve-in-valve implantation) has shown favourable outcomes in both aortic and mitral positions.[14,15] There is a newer-generation surgical valve with expandable valve frame that was specifically designed for future valve-in-valve procedure (INSPIRIS RESILIA aortic valve).[16] In addition, there are growing data documenting favourable outcomes of TAVI-in-TAVI procedures.[17] The feasibility of future valve-in-valve options needs to be assessed and incorporated in the decision-making at the time of index valve replacement procedure.[18] Implantation of an optimal size of surgical prosthesis (with or without root replacement) during the index surgery is essential to avoid patient–prosthesis mismatch with future valve-in-valve procedure. Similarity, valve type and implant depth during TAVI may impact future TAVI-in-TAVI procedures and needs to be considered at the outset.

For patients contemplating future pregnancy, detailed planning of the lifetime management of valvular disease is warranted. During pregnancy, there is an increase in the levels of prothrombotic factors resulting in a hypercoagulable state. Thus, women with mechanical valves are at high risk of both

Table 17.1 Guideline recommendations: valve selection

Recommendations	Class[a]	Level[b]
Mechanical prosthesis		
A mechanical prosthesis is recommended according to the desire of the informed patient and if there are no contraindications to long term anticoagulation	I	C
A mechanical prosthesis is recommended in patients at risk of accelerated structural valve deterioration including age less than 40, hyperthyroidism and haemodialysis	I	C
A mechanical prosthesis should be considered in patients already on anticoagulation because of a mechanical prosthesis in another valve position	IIa	C
A mechanical prosthesis should be considered in patients aged <60 years for prostheses in the aortic position and aged <65 years for prostheses in the mitral position	IIa	B
A mechanical prosthesis should be considered in patients with a reasonable life expectancy for whom future redo valve surgery or TAVI (if appropriate) would be at high risk	IIa	C
A mechanical prosthesis may be considered in patients already on long-term anticoagulation due to the high risk for thromboembolism	IIb	C
Bioprosthesis		
A bioprosthesis is recommended according to the desire of the informed patient	I	C
A bioprosthesis is recommended when good quality anticoagulation is unlikely, contraindicated because of high bleeding risk and in those patients whose life expectancy is lower than the presumed durability of the bioprosthesis	I	C
A bioprosthesis is recommended in case of reoperation for mechanical valve thrombosis despite good long-term anticoagulant control	I	C
A bioprosthesis should be considered in patients for whom there is a low likelihood and/or a low operative risk of future redo valve surgery	IIa	C
A bioprosthesis should be considered in young women contemplating pregnancy	IIa	C
A bioprosthesis should be considered in patients aged >65 years for a prosthesis in the aortic position or aged >70 years in a mitral position	IIa	C
A bioprosthesis may be considered in patients already on long-term NOACs due to the high risk for thromboembolism	IIb	B

TAVI, transcatheter aortic valve intervention; NOAC, novel oral anticoagulant.
[a] Class of recommendation. [b] Level of evidence.
Vahanian A, Beyersdorf F, Praz F, et al; ESC/EACTS Scientific Document Group. 2021 ESC/EACTS Guidelines for the management of valvular heart disease. Eur Heart J. 2022 Feb 12;43(7):561–632. doi: 10.1093/eurheartj/ehab395.

adverse fetal and maternal events during pre- and postpartum periods, primarily due to thromboembolic complications and the antithrombotic therapy administered to prevent thromboembolic complications.[19,20] Thus, a bioprosthesis should be considered in young women contemplating pregnancy (class IIa; LOE C).[7] When the bioprosthesis eventually fails, a re-do surgery with a mechanical valve may be a reasonable consideration.

Lifetime anticoagulation management of surgical valves

See ➲ Table 17.2.

Mechanical valves

Patients with mechanical valves require lifelong anticoagulation due to the increased risk of valve thrombosis and subsequent thromboembolic events (➲ Figure 17.1). The occurrence of major embolism in the absence of antithrombotic therapy is 4 per 100 patient-years, and it is reduced to 1 per 100 patient-years with appropriate anticoagulation therapy.[21] To date, vitamin K antagonists (VKAs; e.g. warfarin), remain the only approved antithrombotic agent for patients with mechanical valves.[7]

The risk for thromboembolism is highest in the first 30 days after implantation of mechanical valves.[22] Since achieving a therapeutic level of warfarin requires several days after therapy initiation, all patients require bridging anticoagulation with either unfractionated heparin (UFH) or low-molecular-weight heparin (LMWH) as soon as the bleeding risk falls into an acceptable range following surgery (usually within 12–24 hours).[7] Observational data have shown no difference in thromboembolic events or bleeding events between UFH and LMWH in patients with mechanical valves.[23] However, UFH is generally preferred in the acute phase because the risk of bleeding is also high and effective reversal of UFH can be achieved quickly with drug discontinuation and protamine administration. Once stable, and a therapeutic international normalized ratio (INR) is achieved for longer than 24 hours, heparin bridging can be discontinued.

The optimal intensity of chronic anticoagulation is the level at which valve thrombosis is effectively prevented without posing excessive bleeding risk. However, discerning and maintaining this level is quite challenging. In addition, a personalized INR target needs to consider the specific prosthesis thrombogenicity and position, as well as patient-specific risk factors.[7] Several randomized

Table 17.2 Guideline recommendation: medications

Recommendations	Class[a]	Level[b]
Surgical valve replacement		
OAC using a VKA is recommended lifelong for all patients with an MHV prosthesis	I	B
For patients with a VKA, INR self-management is recommended provided appropriate training and quality control are performed	I	B
OAC is recommended for patients undergoing implantation of a surgical BHV who have other indications for anticoagulation	I	C
NOACs should be considered over VKA after 3 months following surgical implantation of a BHV in patients with AF	IIa	B
In patients with no baseline indications for OAC, low-dose aspirin (75–100 mg/day) or OAC using a VKA should be considered for the first 3 months after surgical implantation of an aortic BHV	IIa	B
In patients with no baseline indications for OAC, OAC using a VKA should be considered for the first 3 months after surgical implantation of a bioprosthesis in the mitral or tricuspid position	IIa	B
The addition of low-dose aspirin (75–100 mg/ day) to VKA may be considered in selected patients with MHVs in case of concomitant atherosclerotic disease and low risk of bleeding	IIb	C
The addition of low-dose aspirin (75–100 mg/ day) to VKA should be considered after thromboembolism despite an adequate INR	IIa	C
NOACs may be considered over VKA within 3 months following surgical implantation of a BHV in mitral position in patients with AF	IIb	C
NOACs are not recommended in patients with a mechanical valve prosthesis	III	B
Transcatheter aortic valve implantation		
OAC is recommended lifelong for TAVI patients who have other indications for OAC	I	B
Lifelong SAPT is recommended after TAVI in patients with no baseline indication for OAC	I	A
Routine use OAC is not recommended after TAVI in patients with no baseline indication for OAC	III	B

AF, atrial fibrillation; BHV, biological heart valve; INR, protime international normalized ratio; MHV, mechanical heart valve; NOAC, novel oral anticoagulant; OAC, oral anticoagulant; SAPT, single antiplatelet therapy; TAVI, transcatheter aortic valve implantation; VKA, vitamin K antagonist.

[a] Class of recommendation. [b] Level of evidence.

trials investigated the optimal intensity of anticoagulation among patients with mechanical valves, and these serve as the foundation for the current guideline recommendations.[25] Valves with high prosthesis thrombogenicity are the historically older prostheses such as the ball-cage (Starr–Edwards) or single titling-disc (Björk–Shiley) valves.[7] Most contemporary mechanical aortic valves, including CarboMedics, Medtronic Hall, ATS, St. Jude Medical, Sorin Bicarbon™, and On-X®, carry low prosthesis thrombogenicity. A prosthesis in the mitral or tricuspid position poses a significantly higher risk of valve thrombosis compared to the aortic position.[6] Patient-specific prothrombotic risk factors include previous thromboembolism, atrial fibrillation (AF), mitral stenosis, and reduced left ventricular systolic function (ejection fraction <35%).

For patients with aortic mechanical valves without other thrombotic risk factors, a target INR of 2.5 is generally recommended. For patients with a low-risk prosthesis in the mitral position or those with one of the additional thrombotic risk factors, a target INR of 3.0 is preferred.[7] An INR greater than 3.5 significantly increased the risk of intracranial haemorrhage.[26] In the current guidelines, a target INR is provided instead of an INR range. This approach is deemed more effective in reducing the time the INRs are closer to either border of the limit of the range (conventionally, the acceptable range extends to 0.5 INR units on each side of the target).[7] Patient-specific risk factors for bleeding have not been incorporated in determining an optimal target INR value in the guidelines. The efficacy of lowering targets of anticoagulation beyond the aforementioned recommendations has been investigated in the PROACT trial.[27] Patients who underwent surgical aortic valve replacement (SAVR) with the On-X valve and had at least one risk factor for thromboembolism such as AF were randomized to high-intensity anticoagulation (warfarin with target INR of 2.0–3.0) versus low-intensity anticoagulation (target INR of 1.5–2.0 after 3 months of INR of 2.0–3.0). Both groups received concomitant low-dose aspirin. At 3.8-year follow-up, patients in the low-intensity anticoagulation group had less major bleeding events with comparable mortality and thrombotic event rates.[27] Thus, low-intensity anticoagulation (INR target of 1.5–2.0) beyond the first 3 months has become a commonly adopted strategy after SAVR with the On-X valve. Achieving and maintaining optimal levels of anticoagulation is often challenging and requires continuous effort from both the provider and the patient. Self-management of anticoagulation is a valuable option that can improve outcomes for suitably selected patients with willingness and adequate support. A patient-level meta-analysis of randomized trials showed that anticoagulation self-management led to lower thromboembolic events and comparable major bleeding events and mortality compared to the routine standard of care.[28] Current guidelines endorse self-management of anticoagulation (class I; LOE B) provided that appropriate training and quality control are performed.[7]

Driven by the unmet need for alternatives to warfarin in patients with mechanical valves, there has been a growing interest in the use of non-vitamin K oral anticoagulants (NOACs). However,

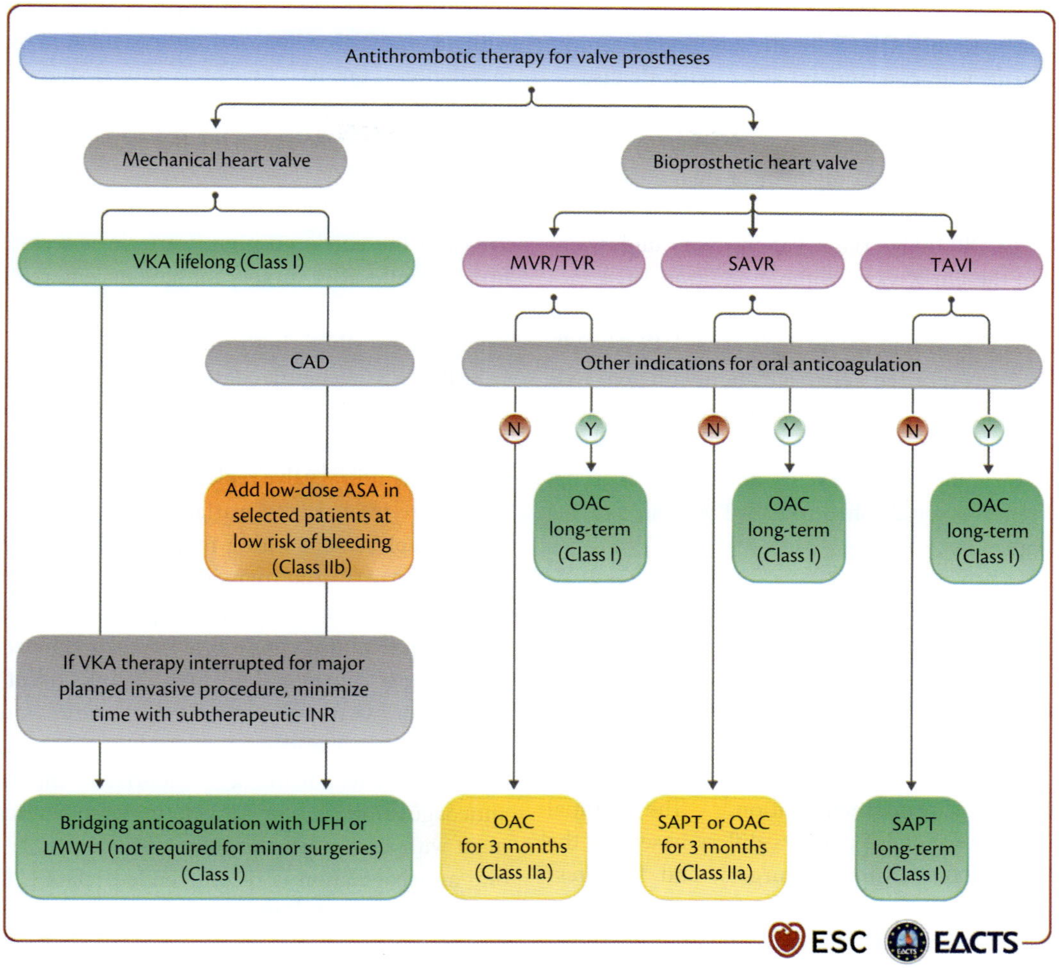

Figure 17.1 ESC/EACTS recommendation for antithrombotic therapy for valve prostheses (2021 ESC/EACTS Guidelines for the management of valvular heart disease). The figure summarizes the recommended antithrombotic therapy for patients with mechanical or bioprosthetic valves, according to the presence or absence of oral anticoagulation indications and to coronary artery disease. ASA, acetylsalicylic acid; CAD, coronary artery disease; INR, international normalized ratio; LMWH, low-molecular-weight heparin; MHV, mechanical heart valve; MVR, mitral valve replacement or repair; OAC, oral anticoagulation; SAPT, single antiplatelet therapy; SAVR, surgical aortic valve replacement; TAVI, transcatheter aortic valve implantation; TVR, tricuspid valve replacement or repair; UFH, unfractionated heparin; VKA, vitamin K antagonist.

the studies available to date have not yielded promising results. The use of the direct thrombin inhibitor, dabigatran, in patients with mechanical valves was investigated in the RE-ALIGN trial. Dabigatran use was associated with higher rates of thromboembolic and bleeding events compared with warfarin, and has since become contraindicated for patients with mechanical valves.[29] However, several issues in this trial warrant further consideration. One-third of the enrolled patients had mechanical valves in the mitral position, which poses a relatively higher risk of valve thrombosis compared to the aortic position. Also, most patients (79%) were enrolled in the acute phase following surgery, during which time the risk of thromboembolism as well as the risk of bleeding are heightened. Another small randomized trial (the RIWA study) randomized 44 patients to either rivaroxaban 15 mg twice daily versus warfarin. Although no significant difference was found in the primary outcome, this trial was underpowered and thus deemed inconclusive (no valve thrombosis event in either group).[30] To date, the use of anti-Xa direct oral anticoagulants has not been robustly assessed and is thus not recommended in the current guidelines (class III; LOE B).[7] The use of apixaban in patients with an aortic mechanical valve (On-X valve) is being studied in the PROACT Xa trial (ClinicalTrials.gov Identifier: NCT04142658) which plans to randomize 1000 patients to apixaban 2.5 mg or 5 mg twice daily versus warfarin with a target INR of 2.0–3.0.[31]

The benefits of aspirin in addition to oral anticoagulation among patients with mechanical valves remain uncertain. A randomized trial conducted in the 1980s reported lower mortality and thromboembolic events with the addition of aspirin to warfarin.[32] A similar reduction in thromboembolic events with the addition of aspirin was observed in a more contemporary trial.[33] However, a meta-analysis of 13 trials showed an increased frequency of bleeding events with the addition of aspirin,[34] although studies included in this meta-analysis had a low overall design quality and used various aspirin doses. Current guidelines assign a class IIb recommendation (LOE C) for the addition of aspirin to warfarin for patients with concomitant atherosclerotic disease and low risk of bleeding.[7] Tailoring target INR according to the use of concomitant antiplatelet therapy is not endorsed in the current guidelines. An investigational regimen of dual antiplatelet therapy (DAPT) in replacement for anticoagulation was tested in a separate arm of the PROACT trial.[35] Patients who underwent isolated SAVR with the On-X valve without additional risk factors for thromboembolism were randomized to DAPT (aspirin and clopidogrel) versus conventional warfarin (goal INR 2.0–3.0) plus aspirin. All patients received anticoagulation with goal INR 2.0–3.0 during the first 3 months and were randomized 3 months after the surgery. This arm of the study was terminated early due to excess cerebral thromboembolic events in the DAPT group. Thus, there is currently no established role for DAPT in patients with mechanical valves.

Bioprosthetic valves

After bioprosthetic surgical valve replacement, the risk of thromboembolism is highest in the acute phase, most prominently within the first 3 months, during which the valve leaflets undergo gradual endothelialization.[1,25] The optimal antithrombotic therapy for these patients differs based on the position of prosthesis, the timing of surgery, and the presence of other indications for oral anticoagulation (e.g. AF) or antiplatelets (e.g. atherosclerotic disease). In addition, new-onset postoperative AF complicates up to 40% of patients undergoing valve surgery, which warrants oral anticoagulation in many of the patients.[36] In the acute phase after surgery, bridging anticoagulation with either UFH or LMWH is considered for patients with a newly implanted bioprosthesis who are planned to be treated with long-term warfarin. For those who are planned to be treated with a NOAC, bridging anticoagulation is not required due to the rapid onset of action of these agents.

Optimal antithrombotic therapy after bioprosthetic SAVR in patients without a concurrent indication for oral anticoagulation is an area of ongoing debate. A randomized trial comparing warfarin (target INR 2.0–3.0) versus aspirin 150 mg daily for the first 3 months after surgery showed similar thromboembolic and bleeding event rates.[37] A meta-analysis including four randomized trials and 11 cohort studies showed comparable thromboembolic and mortality rates between warfarin versus aspirin.[38] Recently, an analysis of 943 patients who underwent SAVR with a bioprosthesis in a series of TAVI versus transcatheter aortic valve replacement (TAVR) trials provided new insight for a potential benefit of anticoagulation in this cohort.[39] Anticoagulation after SAVR was associated with lower rates of strokes [1% versus 4% (crude event rates); adjusted hazard ratio 0.17; 95% confidence interval 0.05–0.60]. No significant differences in mortality or major bleeding were observed. Current guidelines reflect this clinical equipoise and recommend either low-dose aspirin (75–100 mg) or oral anticoagulation with warfarin for the first 3 months after surgery for aortic bioprosthetic valves in patients with no indication for oral anticoagulation (class IIa recommendation; LOE B).[7] An observational study suggested potential benefits of long-term aspirin 3 months after surgical aortic bioprosthesis implantation but the evidence base for this practice remains limited.[40]

In contrast to the above recommendations for bioprosthetic valves in the aortic position, warfarin is recommended for the first 3 months after surgery for patients without a concurrent indication for oral anticoagulation who undergo valve replacement using a bioprosthesis in the mitral or tricuspid position (class IIa; LOE B).[7] This recommendation stems from observational rather than randomized clinical data.[41,42] In one observational studies that included 1344 patients, stroke rates within 30 days were higher after mitral valve replacement (MVR) with a bioprosthesis (44% were treated with warfarin) compared to mitral valve repair or replacement with a mechanical valve (95% were treated with warfarin).[41] The frequency of thromboembolism in a later phase following surgery was comparable between MVR using a bioprosthesis and after mitral valve repair.[41] The target INR for this indication is generally 2.5. Upon completion of anticoagulation therapy for a 3-month period, long-term low-dose (75–100 mg) aspirin is recommended.

For patients with a concurrent indication for oral anticoagulation such as AF who undergo surgical valve replacement with a bioprosthetic valve (either aortic or mitral), chronic oral anticoagulation is recommended (class I; LOE C).[7] An increasingly relevant clinical question in this cohort requiring long-term anticoagulation is whether NOAC can be safely used in lieu of the conventional warfarin therapy. The 2017 joint European consensus document makes an important distinction when considering anticoagulation for patients with AF who also have valvular heart disease. In this document, AF is classified as (1) type 1, which refers to patients with AF who have valvular heart disease that requires warfarin therapy, thus including severe mitral stenosis and mechanical heart valves; and (2) type 2, which refers to patients with AF who has valvular heart disease that require either warfarin or NOAC, thus including all other forms of valvular heart disease encompassing patients with bioprostheses.[43]

Despite the growing literature on the use of NOAC for patients with bioprosthetic valves, conclusive data are lacking, and clinical equipoise remains. In the RIVER trial, a total of 1005 patients with AF or atrial flutter who underwent MVR with a bioprosthetic valve were randomized to either rivaroxaban (20 mg once daily) or warfarin (goal INR 2.5).[44] Rivaroxaban was non-inferior to warfarin regarding the primary endpoint, defined as a composite of death, major cardiovascular events, or major bleeding at 12 months, and superior for stroke prevention (hazard ratio 0.25; 95% confidence interval 0.07–0.88). A recent meta-analysis showed that NOAC was associated with lower risk of bleeding without increasing the risk of thromboembolic events compared to conventional warfarin therapy in patients with AF who underwent SAVR or MVR using a bioprosthesis.[45] Current guidelines assign NOAC a class IIb recommendation (LOE C) for patients with AF who undergo MVR using a bioprosthesis within

3 months after surgery.[7] Beyond 3 months, the use of NOAC is elevated to a class IIa recommendation (LOE B).[7]

Lifetime anticoagulation management of transcatheter valves

Thromboembolic events can occur both in the acute phase and late phase following TAVI.[46] DAPT (aspirin and clopidogrel) for 3–6 months after TAVI has been recommended in society guidelines (Figure 17.2) and has been the standard of care, though the practice largely stemmed from the antithrombotic regimen utilized in the early series of trials that established the efficacy and safety of TAVI.[47–49] See Table 17.2.

Several large-scale randomized trials recently provided further insights and guidance on the optimal medical therapy for patients post TAVI. Conventional DAPT after TAVI was challenged by the POPULAR TAVI trial (cohort A). In this trial, patients undergoing TAVI who did not have an indication for oral anticoagulation were randomized to either aspirin monotherapy versus DAPT with aspirin and clopidogrel. Patients in the aspirin monotherapy group had significantly fewer bleeding events than those treated with aspirin plus clopidogrel (Figure 17.3a) with comparable rates of stroke or death.[50] A meta-analysis comparing single antiplatelet therapy with DAPT in patients without indications for chronic anticoagulation found lower major bleeding events with comparable all-cause mortality.[51] Based on these data, current guidelines recommend lifelong single antiplatelet therapy for patients who have no indication for oral anticoagulation after TAVI (class I).[7] Regarding the selection of single antiplatelet therapy, the ongoing randomized REAC-TAVI 2 trial (1206 patients) will provide further insights on the strategy of aspirin monotherapy versus ticagrelor monotherapy for 12 months following TAVI (ClinicalTrials.gov Identifier: NCT 05283356).

The optimal antithrombotic therapy for post-TAVI patients with an indication for oral anticoagulation has been investigated by multiple trials. In a predefined arm of the POPULAR TAVI trial (cohort B) which included patients with an indication for oral anticoagulation, adding clopidogrel to anticoagulation with a VKA or a NOAC was compared to anticoagulation therapy alone. Findings from this cohort showed a significantly higher risk of bleeding among patients treated with clopidogrel along with anticoagulation compared to anticoagulation alone (Figure 17.3b) with no difference in the rates of ischaemic events.[52] Based on these data, oral anticoagulation alone is recommended in the guideline after TAVI for patients with an indication for oral anticoagulation (class I; LOE B).[7] These lines of evidence regarding post TAVI medical therapy revealed a better safety profile of less potent regimens (favouring single antiplatelet compared to dual antiplatelet and favouring anticoagulation

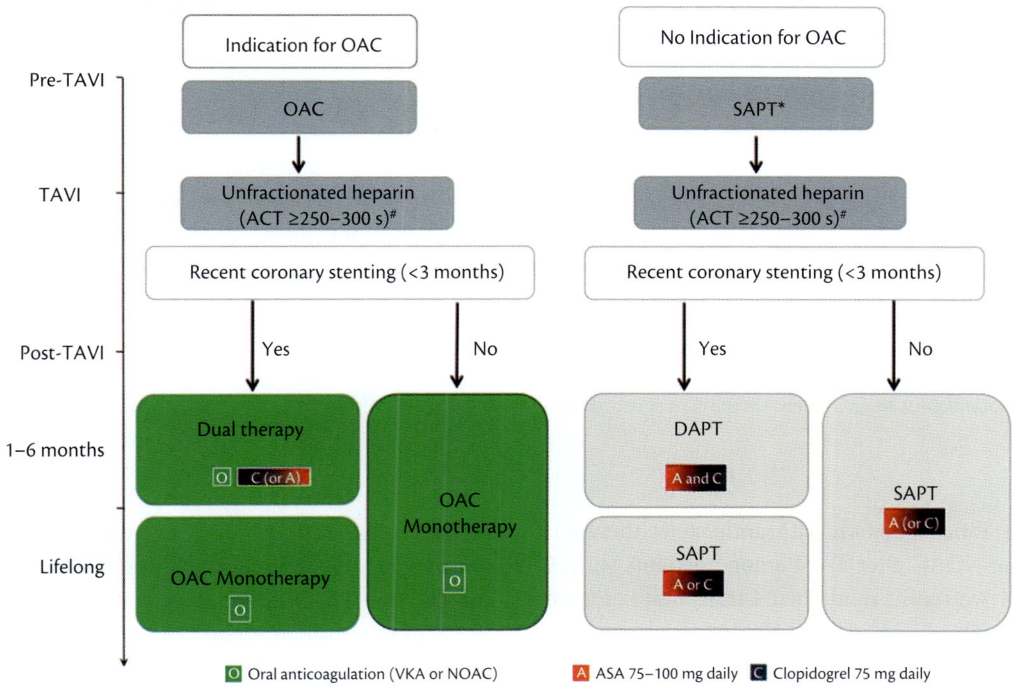

Figure 17.2 Antithrombotic treatment during and after transcatheter aortic valve implantation (2021 consensus document of the ESC working group on Thrombosis and the European Association of Percutaneous Cardiovascular Interventions). The figure summarizes the consensus for treating patients who are candidate for transcatheter aortic valve implantation, according to the presence or absence of oral anticoagulation indications and to recent coronary stenting. ACT, activated clotting time; ASA, aspirin; DAPT, dual antiplatelet therapy; NOAC, non-vitamin K antagonist oral anticoagulant; OAC, oral anticoagulation; SAPT, single antiplatelet therapy; VKA, vitamin K antagonist.

Ten Berg J, Sibbing D, Rocca B, et al. Management of antithrombotic therapy in patients undergoing transcatheter aortic valve implantation: a consensus document of the ESC Working Group on Thrombosis and the European Association of Percutaneous Cardiovascular Interventions (EAPCI), in collaboration with the ESC Council on Valvular Heart Disease. Eur Heart J. 2021 Jun 14;42(23):2265–2269. doi: 10.1093/eurheartj/ehab196. Copyright European Society of Cardiology. Reproduced with permission from Oxford University Press.

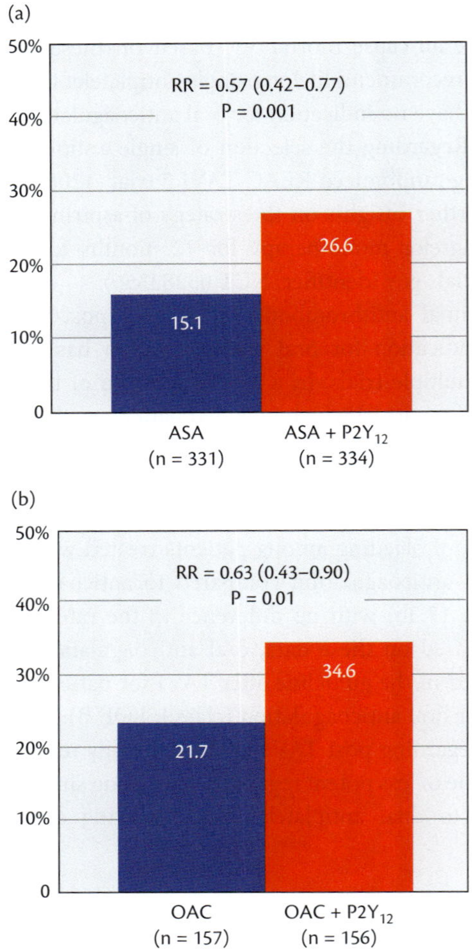

Figure 17.3 The primary outcomes (bleeding) of randomized clinical trials investigating optimal antithrombotic therapy among patients undergoing transcatheter aortic valve implantation (TAVI). (a) POPULAR TAVI trial (cohort A). Patients undergoing TAVI who did not have an indication for oral anticoagulation (OAC) were randomized to either aspirin monotherapy or DAPT with aspirin and clopidogrel. Patients in the aspirin monotherapy group had significantly fewer bleeding events than those treated with aspirin plus clopidogrel with comparable rates of stroke or death. (b) POPULAR TAVI trial (cohort B). Patients undergoing TAVI who had an indication for oral anticoagulation were randomized to either anticoagulation alone or anticoagulation with clopidogrel. Patients treated with clopidogrel along with anticoagulation had a significantly higher rate of bleeding compared to anticoagulation alone with no difference in the rates of ischaemic events. RR=risk ratio.

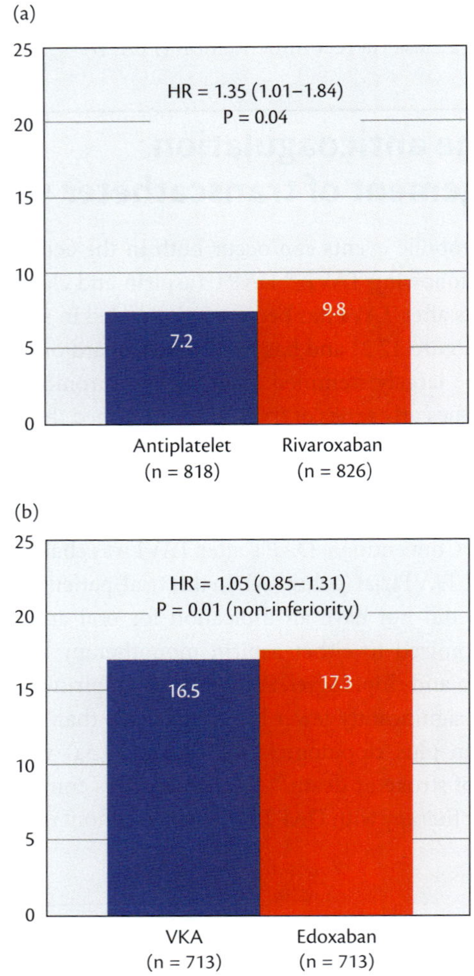

Figure 17.4 The primary outcomes (ischaemic) of clinical trials investigating optimal antithrombotic therapy among patients undergoing transcatheter aortic valve implantation (TAVI). (a) GALILEO trial. Patients undergoing TAVI who did not have an indication for oral anticoagulation were randomized to either 10 mg of rivaroxaban or dual antiplatelet therapy (DAPT). Patients treated with rivaroxaban had significantly higher rates of bleeding and death compared to DAPT.[58] (b) ENVISAGE-TAVI AF trial. Patients undergoing TAVI who had an indication for oral anticoagulation were randomized to edoxaban versus vitamin K antagonists (VKAs). This trial found that edoxaban was non-inferior to VKAs for the composite primary outcome of adverse clinical events. HR=hazard ratio.

alone compared to anticoagulation with antiplatelet therapy).[53] The potential role of NOAC after TAVI among patients with AF was investigated in two recent randomized trials that compared NOAC with VKAs. The ENVISAGE-TAVI AF trial compared edoxaban versus VKAs and found that edoxaban was non-inferior to VKAs for the composite primary outcome of adverse clinical events (➔ Figure 17.4a).[54] Another randomized study, the ATLANTIS trial (stratum 1), compared apixaban with a VKA (standard of care) and showed that apixaban was non-inferior to a VKA regarding the primary efficacy endpoint and primary safety endpoints.[55]

Reduced leaflet motion suggestive of subclinical leaflet thrombosis has been reported with both transcatheter and surgical bioprosthetic valves, but more commonly with transcatheter valves.[56] Observational data suggest that oral anticoagulation can prevent and reverse subclinical leaflet thrombosis.[57] In this context, the GALILEO trial randomized patients post TAVI to 10 mg of rivaroxaban versus DAPT. GALILEO documented a reduced rates of transcatheter aortic valve leaflet thrombosis with rivaroxaban; however, the trial was stopped early due to increased rates of bleeding and death in the NOAC group (➔ Figure 17.4b).[58] Later, two additional randomized trials investigated a NOAC in comparison with antiplatelet therapy in post TAVI patients who had no indication for chronic anticoagulation. The ADAPT TAVR trial compared edoxaban with DAPT and found a numerically lower, albeit statistically non-significant, reduction of leaflet thrombosis with edoxaban.[59] A separate arm of the ATLANTIS trial (stratum 2) compared apixaban with antiplatelet therapy and found a lower occurrence of valve thrombosis with a signal of higher non-cardiovascular mortality.[55] Current guidelines recommend against the routine use of oral anticoagulation in patients with no other indication for oral anticoagulation (class III; LOE B).[7]

Percutaneous MVR for patients with a failed surgical bioprosthesis is a less invasive alternative than re-do surgical replacement with preliminary data suggesting favourable outcomes.[15] A large majority of patients with failed mitral bioprostheses have a chronic indication for oral anticoagulation (e.g. AF) and are therefore commonly treated with oral anticoagulation after the procedure (>80% at discharge).[15] The reported occurrence of stroke was 1.1% at 30 days based on the largest registry data of this cohort.[15] No randomized data are available to guide antithrombotic management after the procedure in this cohort.

Intraprocedural anticoagulation management for patients with artificial valves

When patients with mechanical valves require a major surgery that warrants interruption of anticoagulation, bridging anticoagulation with UFH or LMWH is generally recommended (class I; LOE C).[7] However, bridging anticoagulation increases perioperative bleeding risk by twofold.[60] Thus, the risks and benefits of this approach need to be carefully considered for individual patients. Forgoing bridging anticoagulation may be considered in patients with current generation bileaflet mechanical aortic valves who have no or limited other thrombotic risks (AF, previous thromboembolism, or reduced left ventricular function). For patients who have aortic mechanical valves with additional thrombotic risks factors and for patients with mechanical mitral valves, bridging anticoagulation is preferred. The VKA should be held 3–5 days prior to the planned surgery, aiming for an INR less than 1.5 at the time of surgery (class I; LOE C).[7] Bridging anticoagulation with either UFH or LMWH should be initiated once the INR falls below the therapeutic range (class I; LOE C). Bridging intravenous anticoagulation will be resumed, once the postoperative bleeding risk is acceptable, and continued until the INR returns to a therapeutic level.

When patients with bioprosthetic valves on chronic anticoagulation require a major surgery that warrants interruption of anticoagulation, bridging anticoagulation is generally not required. The indication for bridging in this setting is mainly due to other high-risk indications for thromboembolism such as AF with history of embolic stroke or thromboembolism within the last 3 months. In a randomized study that evaluated perioperative bridging with a LMWH, dalteparin, among patients with AF, the presence of a mechanical valve was a trial exclusion, but patients with valvular AF were included. Perioperative bridging anticoagulation did not reduce the risk of thromboembolism but increased the rates of major bleeding.[60] Bridging anticoagulation is generally not indicated for patients chronically taking NOACs given the short half-life and relatively quick onset of these agents.

Treatment of valve thrombosis

Prosthetic valve thrombosis is a pathological entity characterized by thrombus formation on the various prosthetic structures.[1] Valve thrombosis may cause valve stenosis, regurgitation, and systemic thromboembolism. Valve thrombosis should be suspected when patients with either mechanical or bioprosthetic valves develop embolic events, worsening heart failure symptoms, or an unexpected rise in transvalvular gradient. The diagnosis of prosthetic valve thrombosis can be made by echocardiography, high-resolution computed tomography, or cinefluoroscopic evaluation (for mechanical valves).

Treatment options for prosthetic valve thrombosis include anticoagulation, fibrinolysis, or surgery, and should be guided by the type of prosthesis, severity of valve dysfunction, size of thrombus, as well as patients' clinical status (e.g. recurrent embolism) and risk factors. For critical obstructive thrombosis of a mechanical valve, emergent or urgent valve replacement is recommended for operative candidates.[7] If surgery is deemed a prohibitive risk, systemic fibrinolysis can be considered (class IIa; LOE B), but it carries significant risks of serious bleeding complications. For non-obstructive thrombosis of a mechanical valve, anticoagulation with UFH with bridging to warfarin is recommended. For non-obstructive valve thrombosis with large (>10 mm) thrombus and systemic embolism, surgery should be considered (class IIa; LOE C). For obstructive thrombosis of a bioprosthetic valve, anticoagulation with UFH with bridging to warfarin is recommended prior to considering re-intervention, since anticoagulation alone may resolve thrombus and restore normal valve haemodynamics.[7] Reduced leaflet motion suggestive of subclinical leaflet thrombosis has been reported with both transcatheter and surgical bioprosthetic valves.[56] Observational data suggested that oral anticoagulation can prevent and reverse subclinical leaflet thrombosis.[57] Anticoagulation is recommended in patients with leaflet thickening and reduced leaflet motion leading to a meaningfully elevated valvular gradient (class IIa; LOE B).[7]

After valve thrombotic events, anticoagulation management needs to be carefully reconsidered and optimized. If valve thrombosis is deemed to be primarily due to inadequate anticoagulation either by underdosing or inadequate compliance, care should be optimized by adjusting dosage, providing further patient education, as well as more frequent monitoring of the INR. If valve thrombus occurs despite maintaining a targeted INR, targeting a higher level of INR is a reasonable consideration.[7] If a patient not previously taking an antiplatelet agent develops valve thrombosis, antiplatelet therapy such as low-dose aspirin should be initiated (class IIa; LOE C).[7] For recurrent valve thrombosis despite adequate INR, haematological investigation and consultation are prudent.

Future directions

Several important ongoing randomized trials will further guide the optimal anticoagulation management of prosthetic heart valves. The RENOVATE (ClinicalTrials.gov Identifier: NCT 04258488) and PROACT Xa (ClinicalTrials.gov Identifier: NCT 04142658) trials will evaluate the efficacy and safety of anti-Xa direct oral anticoagulation inhibitors among patients with mechanical aortic valves. Also, optimal antiplatelet and anticoagulation management for patients post TAVI continues to be the subject of several ongoing studies. Advancements in transcatheter valves and interventions, including valve-in-valve procedures, will also impact the lifetime management of valvular disease. Until mechanical valves are created with a lower thrombogenicity or bioprosthetic valves become more durable, the clinical challenge of balancing the risk of valve degeneration of tissue valves against the risks of thrombosis and bleeding with mechanical valves will be ongoing.

Conclusion

With the increasing complexity of patients with valvular heart disease, the expansion of transcatheter valve interventions, and the growing use of NOACs, antithrombotic management among patients with valvular heart disease and prosthetic valve has become more intricate. To date, VKAs remain the only approved agents for patients with mechanical valves. For patients with bioprostheses who have indications for chronic anticoagulation, emerging data suggest non-inferiority of NOACs compared to VKAs. Regarding post-TAVI medical therapy, recent randomized trials have shown a better safety profile with less potent antithrombotic regimens (favouring single antiplatelet therapy compared to DAPT, and favouring anticoagulation alone compared to anticoagulation with antiplatelet therapy). For post-TAVI patients who have an indication for chronic anticoagulation, emerging data suggest non-inferiority of NOACs compared to VKAs. Several important randomized trials of antithrombotic therapy are ongoing and will further guide the optimal management of prosthetic heart valves.

What's new

- The RE-ALIGN trial showed that dabigatran increases thromboembolic and bleeding events compared to warfarin among patients with mechanical heart valves.
- The RIVER trial showed that rivaroxaban is non-inferior to conventional warfarin in major cardiovascular events among patients with AF and a bioprosthetic mitral valve.
- The POPULAR TAVI trial (cohort A) showed that aspirin monotherapy decreases bleeding events compared to DAPT with comparable rates of stroke or death after TAVI.
- The POPULAR TAVI trial (cohort B) showed that oral anticoagulation alone decreases bleeding events compared to oral anticoagulation and clopidogrel in post-TAVI patients with an indication for anticoagulation.
- The GALILEO trial showed that rivaroxaban increases risk of bleeding and death compared to DAPT in patients post TAVI without an indication for anticoagulation.
- The ENVISAGE-TAVI AF trial showed that edoxaban is non-inferior to a VKA in post-TAVI patients with an indication for anticoagulation.
- The ATLANTIS trial (stratum 1) showed that apixaban is non-inferior to a VKA (standard of care) in post-TAVI patients with an indication for anticoagulation.

What's next

- An ongoing randomized trial will evaluate the efficacy and safety of an anti-Xa direct oral anticoagulation inhibitor in patients with a mechanical aortic valve (PROACT Xa trial).
- Optimal antiplatelet and anticoagulation management for patients post TAVI will further investigated by ongoing randomized trials.
- Further advancements of transcatheter interventions will refine the lifetime management of valvular disease.

References

1. Dangas GD, Weitz JI, Giustino G, Makkar R, Mehran R. Prosthetic heart valve thrombosis prosthetic heart valve thrombosis. J Am Coll Cardiol. 2016;68:2670–89.
2. Puri R, Auffret V, Rodés-Cabau J. Bioprosthetic valve thrombosis. J Am Coll Cardiol. 2017;69:2193–211.
3. Head SJ, Çelik M, Kappetein AP. Mechanical versus bioprosthetic aortic valve replacement. Eur Heart J. 2017;38:2183–91.
4. Dasi LP, Simon HA, Sucosky P, Yoganathan AP. Fluid mechanics of artificial heart valves. Clin Exp Pharmacol Physiol. 2009;36:225–37.
5. Heras M, Chesebro JH, Fuster V, et al. High risk of thromboemboli early after bioprosthetic cardiac valve replacement. J Am Coll Cardiol. 1995;25:1111–19.
6. Cannegieter SC, Rosendaal FR, Briet E. Thromboembolic and bleeding complications in patients with mechanical heart valve prostheses. Circulation. 1994;89:635–41.
7. Vahanian A, Beyersdorf F, Praz F, et al. 2021 ESC/EACTS Guidelines for the management of valvular heart disease. Eur Heart J. 2022;43(7):561–632.
8. Hammermeister K, Sethi GK, Henderson WG, Grover FL, Oprian C, Rahimtoola SH. Outcomes 15 years after valve replacement with a mechanical versus a bioprosthetic valve: final report of the Veterans Affairs randomized trial. J Am Coll Cardiol. 2000;36:1152–8.
9. Stassano P, Tommaso L Di, Monaco M, et al. Aortic valve replacement. a prospective randomized evaluation of mechanical versus

biological valves in patients ages 55 to 70 years. J Am Coll Cardiol. 2009;54:1862–8.
10. Goldstone AB, Chiu P, Baiocchi M, et al. Mechanical or biologic prostheses for aortic-valve and mitral-valve replacement. N Engl J Med. 2017;377:1847–57.
11. Chikwe J, Chiang YP, Egorova NN, Itagaki S, Adams DH. Survival and outcomes following bioprosthetic vs mechanical mitral valve replacement in patients aged 50 to 69 years. JAMA. 2015;313:1435–42.
12. Alkhouli M, Alqahtani F, Kawsara A, Pislaru S, Schaff HV, Nishimura RA. National trends in mechanical valve replacement in patients aged 50 to 70 years. J Am Coll Cardiol. 2020;76:2687–8.
13. Fatima B, Mohananey D, Khan FW, et al. Durability data for bioprosthetic surgical aortic valve: a systematic review. JAMA Cardiol. 2019;4:71–80.
14. Webb JG, Murdoch DJ, Alu MC, et al. 3-year outcomes after valve-in-valve transcatheter aortic valve replacement for degenerated bioprostheses: the PARTNER 2 Registry. J Am Coll Cardiol. 2019;73:2647–55.
15. Whisenant B, Kapadia SR, Eleid MF, et al. One-year outcomes of mitral valve-in-valve using the SAPIEN 3 transcatheter heart valve. JAMA Cardiol. 2020;5:1245–52.
16. Bavaria JE, Griffith B, Heimansohn DA, et al. Five-year outcomes of the COMMENCE trial investigating aortic valve replacement with RESILIA tissue [published online ahead of print, 2022 Jan 20]. Ann Thorac Surg. 2022;S0003-4975(22)00063-7.
17. Landes U, Sathananthan J, Witberg G, et al. Transcatheter replacement of transcatheter versus surgically implanted aortic valve bioprostheses. J Am Coll Cardiol. 2021;77:1–14.
18. Medranda GA, Jimenez CES, Torguson R, et al. Lifetime management of patients with symptomatic severe aortic stenosis: a computed tomography simulation study. Eurointervention. 2022;18(5):e407–16.
19. Verhamme P, Herregods MC, Van Dewerf F. Anticoagulation of pregnant women with mechanical heart valves: protecting mother or child? Eur Heart J. 2017;38:1517–19.
20. Van Hagen IM, Roos-Hesselink JW, Ruys TPE, et al. Pregnancy in women with a mechanical heart valve. Circulation. 2015;132:132–42.
21. Cannegieter SC, Rosendaal FR, Briët E. Thromboembolic and bleeding complications in patients with mechanical heart valve prostheses. Circulation. 1994;89:635–41.
22. Allou N, Piednoir P, Berroëta C, et al. Incidence and risk factors of early thromboembolic events after mechanical heart valve replacement in patients treated with intravenous unfractionated heparin. Heart. 2009;95:1694–700.
23. Caldeira D, David C, Santos AT, Costa J, Pinto FJ, Ferreira JJ. Efficacy and safety of low molecular weight heparin in patients with mechanical heart valves: systematic review and meta-analysis. J Thromb Haemost. 2014;12:650–9.
24. Acar J, Iung B, Boissel JP, et al. AREVA: multicenter randomized comparison of low-dose versus standard- dose anticoagulation in patients with mechanical prosthetic heart valves. Circulation. 1996;94:2107–12.
25. Meschengieser SS, Fondevila CG, Frontroth J, Santarelli MT, Lazzari MA. Low-intensity oral anticoagulation plus low-dose aspirin versus high-intensity oral anticoagulation alone: a randomized trial in patients with mechanical prosthetic heart valves. J Thorac Cardiovasc Surg. 1997;113:910–16.
26. Singer DE, Chang Y, Fang MC, et al. Should patient characteristics influence target anticoagulation intensity for stroke prevention in nonvalvular atrial fibrillation? The ATRIA study. Circ Cardiovasc Qual Outcomes. 2009;2:297–304.
27. Puskas J, Gerdisch M, Nichols D, et al. Reduced anticoagulation after mechanical aortic valve replacement: interim results from the Prospective Randomized On-X Valve Anticoagulation Clinical Trial randomized Food and Drug Administration investigational device exemption trial. J Thorac Cardiovasc Surg. 2014;147:1202–11.e2.
28. Heneghan C, Ward A, Perera R, et al. Self-monitoring of oral anticoagulation: systematic review and meta-analysis of individual patient data. Lancet. 2012;379:322–34.
29. Eikelboom JW, Connolly SJ, Brueckmann M, et al. Dabigatran versus warfarin in patients with mechanical heart valves. N Engl J Med. 2013;369:1206–14.
30. Duraes AR, de Souza Lima Bitar Y, Schonhofen IS, et al. Rivaroxaban versus warfarin in patients with mechanical heart valves: open-label, proof-of-concept trial—the RIWA study. Am J Cardiovasc Drugs 2021;21:363–71.
31. Jawitz OK, Wang TY, Lopes RD, et al. Rationale and design of PROACT Xa: a randomized, multicenter, open-label, clinical trial to evaluate the efficacy and safety of apixaban versus warfarin in patients with a mechanical On-X Aortic Heart Valve. Am Heart J. 2020;227:91–9.
32. Turpie A, Gent M, Laupacis A, et al. A comparison of aspirin with placebo in patients treated with warfarin after heart-valve replacement. N Engl J Med.2010;329:524–9.
33. Dong MF, Ma ZS, Ma SJ, et al. Anticoagulation therapy with combined low dose aspirin and warfarin following mechanical heart valve replacement. Thromb Res.2011;128:e91–4.
34. Massel DR, Little SH. Antiplatelet and anticoagulation for patients with prosthetic heart valves. Cochrane Database Syst Rev. 2013;2013:CD003464.
35. Puskas JD, Gerdisch M, Nichols D, et al. Anticoagulation and antiplatelet strategies after On-X mechanical aortic valve replacement. J Am Coll Cardiol. 2018;71:2717–26.
36. Asher CR, Miller DP, Grimm RA, Cosgrove DM, Chung MK. Analysis of risk factors for development of atrial fibrillation early after cardiac valvular surgery. Am J Cardiol. 1998;82:892–5.
37. Rafiq S, Steinbrüchel DA, Lilleør NB, et al. Antithrombotic therapy after bioprosthetic aortic valve implantation: warfarin versus aspirin, a randomized controlled trial. Thromb Res. 2017;150:104–10.
38. Papak JN, Chiovaro JC, Noelck N, et al. Antithrombotic strategies after bioprosthetic aortic valve replacement: a systematic review. Ann Thorac Surg. 2019;107:1571–81.
39. Chakravarty T, Patel A, Kapadia S, et al. Anticoagulation after surgical or transcatheter bioprosthetic aortic valve replacement. J Am Coll Cardiol. 2019;74:1190–200.
40. Blair KL, Hatton AC, White WD, et al. Comparison of anticoagulation regimens after Carpentier-Edwards aortic or mitral valve replacement. Circulation. 1994;90:II214–19.
41. Russo A, Grigioni F, Avierinos JF, et al. Thromboembolic complications after surgical correction of mitral regurgitation: incidence, predictors, and clinical implications. J Am Coll Cardiol. 2008;51:1203–11.
42. Butnaru A, Shaheen J, Tzivoni D, Tauber R, Bitran D, Silberman S. Diagnosis and treatment of early bioprosthetic malfunction in the mitral valve position due to thrombus formation. Am J Cardiol. 2013;112:1439–44.
43. Lip GYH, Collet JP, De Caterina R, et al. Antithrombotic therapy in atrial fibrillation associated with valvular heart disease: a joint consensus document from the European Heart Rhythm Association (EHRA) and European Society of Cardiology Working Group on Thrombosis, endorsed by the ESC Working Group on Valvular Heart Disease, Cardiac Arrhythmia Society of Southern Africa (CASSA), Heart Rhythm Society (HRS), Asia Pacific Heart Rhythm Society (APHRS), South African Heart (SA Heart) Association and Sociedad Latinoamericana de Estimulación Cardíaca y Electrofisiología (SOLEACE). Europace. 2017;19:1757–8.

44. Guimarães HP, Lopes RD, de Barros e Silva PGM, et al. Rivaroxaban in patients with atrial fibrillation and a bioprosthetic mitral valve. N Engl J Med. 2020;383:2117–26.
45. Yokoyama Y, Briasoulis A, Ueyama H, et al. Direct oral anticoagulants versus vitamin K antagonists in patients with atrial fibrillation and bioprosthetic valves: a meta-analysis [published online ahead of print, 2021 Jul 29]. J Thorac Cardiovasc Surg. 2021;S0022-5223(21)01133-8.
46. Backer O De, Butt JH, Wong YH, et al. Early and late risk of ischemic stroke after TAVR as compared to a nationwide background population. Clin Res Cardiol. 2020;109:791–801.
47. Baumgartner H, Falk V, Bax JJ, et al. 2017 ESC/EACTS Guidelines for the management of valvular heart disease. Eur Heart J. 2017;38:2739–91.
48. Leon MB, Smith CR, Mack M, et al. Transcatheter aortic-valve implantation for aortic stenosis in patients who cannot undergo surgery. N Engl J Med. 2010;363:1597–607.
49. Adams DH, Popma JJ, Reardon MJ, et al. Transcatheter aortic-valve replacement with a self-expanding prosthesis. N Engl J Med. 2014;370:1790–8.
50. Brouwer J, Nijenhuis VJ, Delewi R, et al. Aspirin with or without clopidogrel after transcatheter aortic-valve implantation. N Engl J Med. 2020;383:1447–57.
51. Guedeney P, Sorrentino S, Mesnier J, et al. Single versus dual antiplatelet therapy following TAVR: a systematic review and meta-analysis of randomized controlled trials. JACC Cardiovasc Interv. 2021;14:234–6.
52. Nijenhuis VJ, Brouwer J, Delewi R, et al. Anticoagulation with or without clopidogrel after transcatheter aortic-valve implantation. N Engl J Med. 2020;382:1696–707.
53. Capodanno D, Collet JP, Dangas G, et al. Antithrombotic therapy after transcatheter aortic valve replacement. JACC Cardiovasc Interv. 2021;14:1688–703.
54. Van Mieghem NM, Unverdorben M, Hengstenberg C Edoxaban versus vitamin K antagonist for atrial fibrillation after TAVR. N Engl J Med. 2021;385:2150–60.
55. Collet J-P, Van Belle E, Thiele H, et al. Apixaban vs. standard of care after transcatheter aortic valve implantation: the ATLANTIS trial. Eur Heart J. 2022;43:2783–97.
56. Chakravarty T, Søndergaard L, Friedman J, et al. Subclinical leaflet thrombosis in surgical and transcatheter bioprosthetic aortic valves: an observational study. Lancet. 2017;389:2383–92.
57. Makkar RR, Fontana G, Jilaihawi H, et al. Possible subclinical leaflet thrombosis in bioprosthetic aortic valves. N Engl J Med. 2015;373:2015–24.
58. Dangas GD, Tijssen JGP, Wöhrle J, et al. A controlled trial of rivaroxaban after transcatheter aortic-valve replacement. N Engl J Med. 2020;382:120–9.
59. Park D-W, Ahn J-M, Kang D-Y, et al. Edoxaban versus dual antiplatelet therapy for leaflet thrombosis and cerebral thromboembolism after TAVR: the ADAPT-TAVR randomized clinical trial. Circulation. 2022;146:466–79.
60. Douketis JD, Spyropoulos AC, Kaatz S, et al. Perioperative bridging anticoagulation in patients with atrial fibrillation. N Engl J Med. 2015;373:823–33.

CHAPTER 18

Antithrombotic therapies in ischaemic stroke

Hans Christoph Diener, Graeme J. Hankey, and John W. Eikelboom

Contents

Summary

Most cases of ischaemic stroke are caused by cerebrovascular thrombosis or thromboembolism as a complication of underlying cardiovascular diseases. The acute treatment of ischaemic stroke in stroke centres includes chemical lysis and/or mechanical aspiration of occlusive thrombi to restore perfusion of any salvageable ischaemic penumbra. Early initiation and long-term maintenance of antithrombotic therapies with antiplatelet or anticoagulant drugs are effective adjuncts to vascular risk factor control and revascularization procedures, where appropriate, for preventing early and long-term recurrent thromboembolic ischaemic stroke and other major adverse cardiovascular events.

Introduction

Stroke is the second-leading cause of death (accounting for 12% of all deaths) and the third-leading cause of death and disability combined (6% of total daily-adjusted life years) globally.[1] Each year, about 12 million new/incident cases of stroke are added to a pool of 100 million prevalent survivors of stroke. Ischaemic stroke constitutes 7.6 million (62%) of all incident strokes.[1] Thrombosis and thromboembolism are the most common pathophysiological mechanisms of ischaemic stroke. The main aetiological subtypes of ischaemic stroke include cardioembolic, large artery, small artery, and embolic stroke of undetermined cause (➔ Figure 18.1). Strategies to reduce the global burden of stroke include (primary) prevention of first stroke, acute treatment, and (secondary) prevention of recurrent stroke. In this chapter we discuss the rationale, effectiveness, and safety of treatments and prevention of cerebrovascular thrombosis and thromboembolism.

Acute ischaemic stroke

Reperfusion

The basic therapeutic principle of acute ischaemic stroke is recanalization of the thrombosed artery, as early as possible. This can be achieved by systemic thrombolysis with recombinant tissue-type plasminogen activator (alteplase, tenecteplase) or by mechanical thrombectomy (➔ Figure 18.2).

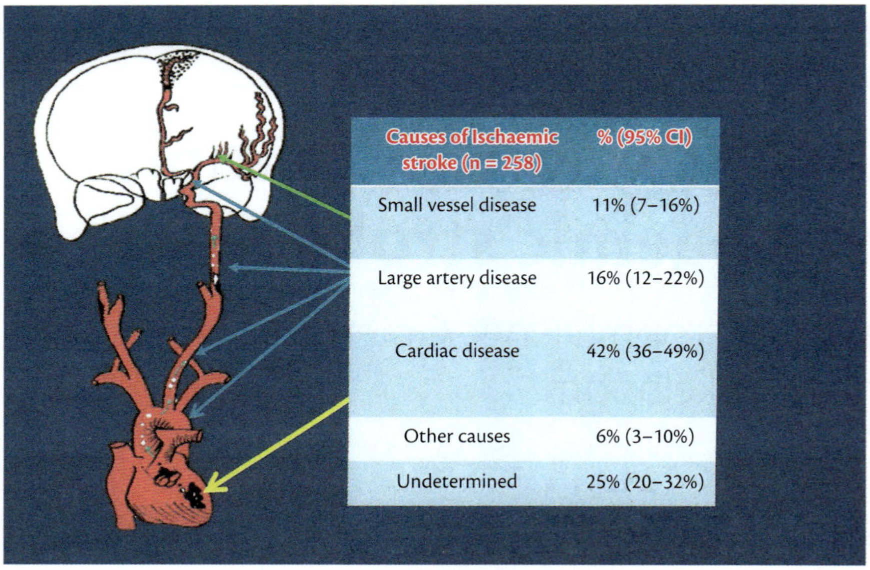

Figure 18.1 Causes of ischaemic stroke.

Thrombolysis

The benefit of systemic thrombolysis in the time window between 0 and 4.5 hours has been proven by a meta-analysis of eight randomized placebo-controlled trials in 6756 patients. A good functional outcome, as measured by the modified Rankin scale of 0–1, was observed in 34% of patients who received thrombolysis and in 29% of those receiving placebo.[2–4] The net absolute benefit from alteplase (treated within 4.5 hours of onset), that is, the difference between those who would do better if given alteplase and those who would do worse, was 55 patients per 1000 treated (95% confidence interval 13–91; P = 0.004).[3] Treatment within 3 hours resulted in a good outcome for 259 (32.9%) of 787 patients who received alteplase versus 176 (23.1%) of 762 who received a control [odds ratio (OR) 1.75, 95% confidence interval (CI) 1.35–2.27].[4]

For patients with an acute stroke who wake up with unknown time from symptom onset or who have an elapsed symptom onset time longer than 4.5–9 hours, and who have a salvageable ischaemic penumbra on advanced neuroimaging, thrombolysis also results in a higher likelihood of functional improvement at 3 months despite the increased risk of symptomatic intracerebral haemorrhage.[5]

For patients with acute ischaemic stroke who are receiving dual antiplatelet agents before being treated with intravenous (IV) thrombolysis, antiplatelet therapy was not associated with a higher risk of adverse outcomes after adjustment for potential confounders in nine observational studies.[6]

Thrombolysis is contraindicated in patients who are therapeutically anticoagulated. In patients treated with vitamin K antagonists, thrombolysis can be performed in patients with an international normalized ratio of less than 1.7.[7] The biological activity of dabigatran can be reversed by idarucizumab and allow IV thrombolysis.[8]

Tenecteplase, which is approved for treatment of acute coronary syndromes, has a longer half-life compared to alteplase, is more fibrin specific, and can be given as a single bolus injection. Five trials compared tenecteplase with alteplase in acute ischaemic stroke and found that tenecteplase is at least as efficacious as alteplase in terms of functional outcomes.[9,10] These studies also reported a trend towards improved safety profiles with the use of tenecteplase. A recent study in Canada in 1600 patients with acute ischaemic stroke found no difference in outcome and bleeding risk between intravenous tenecteplase (0.25 mg/kg to a maximum of 25 mg) vs alteplase (0.9 mg/kg to a maximum of 90mg; 0.09 mg/kg as a bolus and then a 60-min infusion of the remaining 0.81 mg/kg).[11] The NOR-TEST 2 study in patients with moderate-to-severe strokes observed an increased bleeding risk with a higher dose of intravenous tenecteplase (0.4 mg/kg) compared to standard dose alteplase (0.9 mg/kg).[10] A study in China observed no difference in functional outcomes comparing tenecteplase 0.25 mg/kg with standard dose alteplase in 1430 stroke patients.[11a]

Thrombectomy

Mechanical thrombectomy is the most effective therapy for acute ischaemic strokes caused by occlusion of the large arteries of the anterior and posterior cerebral circulation.[12]

An analysis of individual data for 1287 patients with ischaemic stroke caused by anterior circulation large artery occlusion who were enrolled in five randomized trials, among whom 634 were randomly assigned to endovascular thrombectomy (plus medical care) and 653 assigned to control (medical care), showed that endovascular thrombectomy in a 12-hour time window led to significantly reduced disability at 90 days compared with control (adjusted OR 2.49, 95% CI 1.76–3.53; P <0.0001).[13] In these initial randomized controlled trials, mechanical thrombectomy followed systemic thrombolysis in most patients.[13,14]

More recent studies have shown comparable recanalization rates and clinical outcomes when thrombectomy is performed directly, without prior systemic thrombolysis.[15] A study-level meta-analysis of six randomized controlled trials involving 1153 patients allocated to endovascular treatment and 1160 to intravenous thrombolysis plus endovascular treatment reported functional independence at 90 days in 49.1% of patients

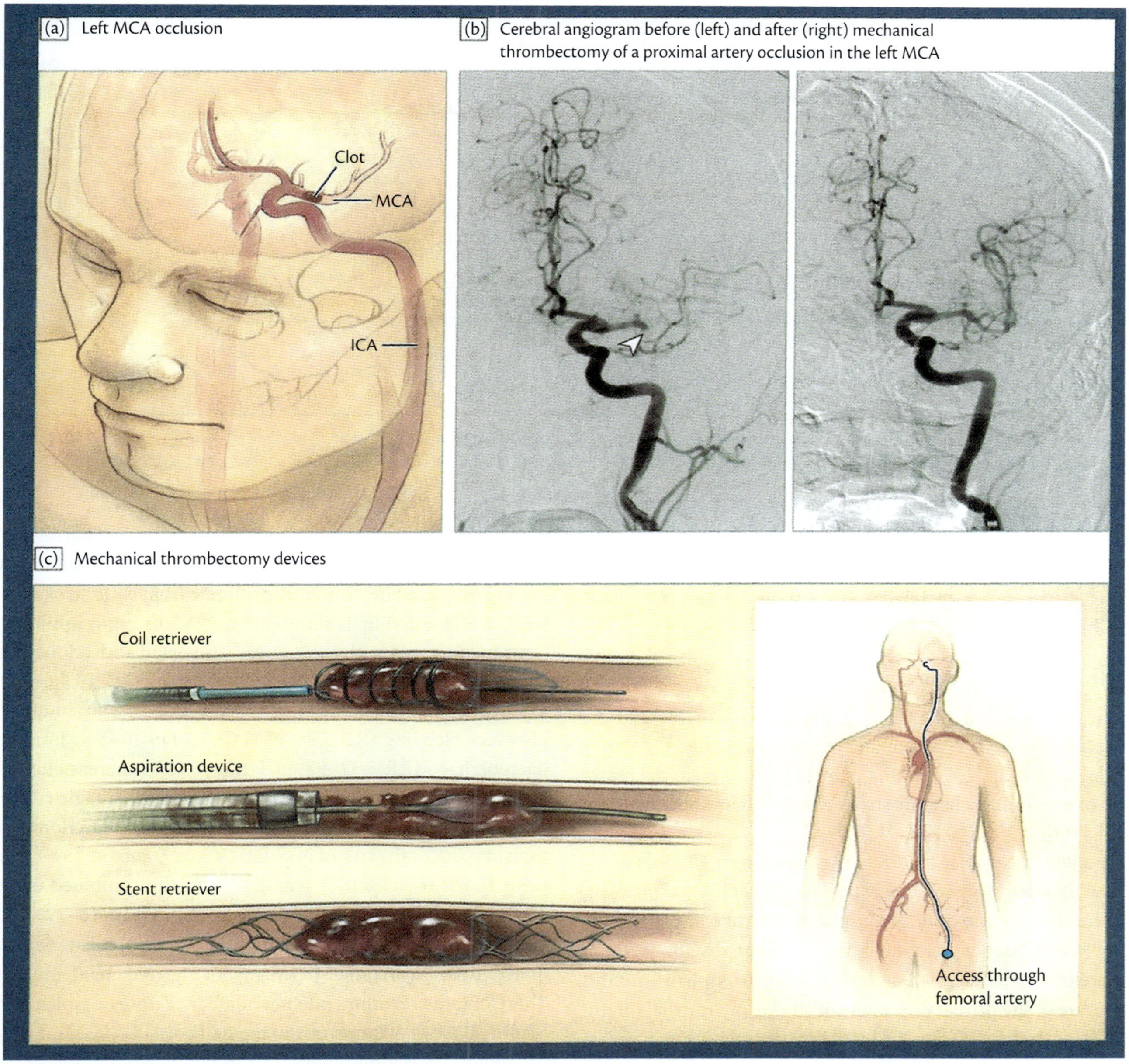

Figure 18.2 (a) Occlusion of the left middle cerebral artery (MCA). (b) Angiography prior to and after mechanical thrombectomy. (c) Thrombectomy devices. Modified from Prabhakaran S, Ruff I, Bernstein RA. Acute stroke intervention: a systematic review. JAMA. 2015 Apr 14;313(14):1451–62.

allocated thrombectomy and 50.9% of patients allocated thrombectomy plus thrombolysis (pooled unadjusted OR 0.93, 95% CI 0.79–1.10; risk difference: -1.9%, -5.9% to 2.1%).[15a] Three randomized controlled trials with 1092 individuals enrolled were included in a meta-analysis, including 543 (49.7%) who received endovascular thrombectomy alone and 549 (50.3%) who received IV thrombolysis plus endovascular thrombectomy. The primary outcome of 90-day functional independence, defined as modified Rankin scale score of 2 or less, was 44.6% (242/543) in the endovascular thrombectomy alone group versus 42.8% (235/549) in the alteplase with endovascular thrombectomy group (OR 1.08, 95% CI 0.85–1.38; P = 0.0539).[15] Another recent study showed that functional outcome can be improved when intra-arterial alteplase 0.225 mg/kg, (maximum dose 225 mg) is given after successful thrombectomy.[16] Periprocedural antithrombotic therapy with heparin, low-molecular-weight heparin, or platelet function inhibitors in ischaemic stroke patients undergoing thrombectomy should be avoided, as this does not improve the functional outcome and leads to an increased rate of major bleeding complications.[17]

Patients in whom neither thrombolysis nor thrombectomy can be performed should start immediate secondary prevention with single antiplatelet therapy or dual antiplatelet therapy (DAPT).

Secondary prevention of recurrent atherosclerotic ischaemic events

In patients with transient ischaemic attack (TIA) or ischaemic stroke, the risk of recurrent stroke is highest in the acute phase.[18,19] Predictors of early recurrent stroke are large artery atherosclerosis

Table 18.1 Secondary stroke prevention

Intervention	Risk of recurrent stroke (%)		Relative risk reduction (%)	Absolute risk reduction (%)
	Control	Intervention		
ASA vs placebo	2.5	2.1	19	0.4
Clopidogrel vs ASA	5.3	5.8	9	0.5
ASA plus clopidogrel vs ASA (90 days)	6.4	4.8	28	1.6
ASA plus ticagrelor vs ASA (30 days)	6.3	5.1	19	1.2
Anticoagulation in AF	12.0	4.7	66	7.3
VKA vs NOACs in AF	5.7	4.9	14	0.8
PFO-closure vs antithrombotic therapy	2.0	0.3	87	1.7
Revascularization in symptomatic carotid stenosis >70%	6.0	3.0	48	3.0

AF, atrial fibrillation; ASA, acetylsalicylic acid; NOAC, non-vitamin K oral anticoagulant; PFO, patent foramen ovale; VKA, vitamin K antagonist.
Source data from Diener HC, Hankey GJ. Primary and secondary prevention of ischemic stroke and cerebral hemorrhage: JACC focus seminar. J Am Coll Cardiol. 2020;75(15):1804–18.

as the underlying cause, shorter time since stroke onset, and multiple areas of infarction on brain imaging.

➔ Table 18.1 shows the relative and absolute risk reduction for different strategies of secondary stroke prevention.

Antiplatelet therapy

A Cochrane review of 11 trials comparing aspirin 160–300 mg with placebo in 42,226 participants with acute ischaemic stroke and followed for up to 6 months reported that aspirin decreases the risk of recurrent ischaemic stroke and death or dependency at 6 months (OR 0.95, 95% CI 0.91–0.99).[11]

In a pooled analysis of 15,778 participants from 12 trials of aspirin versus control in secondary stroke prevention, aspirin reduced the risk of early recurrent ischaemic stroke at 6 weeks by about 60% and disabling or fatal ischaemic stroke by about 70%.[20]

Ticagrelor monotherapy was not superior to aspirin in reducing the rate of the primary outcome of stroke, myocardial infarction (MI), or death at 90 days in 13,199 patients with a non-severe ischaemic stroke or high-risk TIA.[21]

A meta-analysis of 10,447 patients with acute non-cardioembolic TIA or minor ischaemic stroke[22] who were enrolled in three randomized trials found that adding clopidogrel to aspirin (DAPT) within 24 hours of symptom onset reduced the risk of non-fatal recurrent stroke at 90 days by 30% compared with aspirin [relative risk (RR) 0.70, 95% CI 0.61–0.80; absolute risk reduction 1.9%]. DAPT, however, increased the rate of moderate or severe extracranial bleeding (RR 1.71, 95% CI 0.92–3.20; absolute risk increase 0.2%).[23–26]

Among patients with a mild-to-moderate acute non-cardioembolic ischaemic stroke or TIA, the risk of the composite of stroke or death within 30 days was lower with a combination of ticagrelor and aspirin than with aspirin alone [hazard ratio (HR) 0.83, 95% CI 0.71–0.96; P = 0.02].[27] The incidence of disability did not differ significantly between the two groups. Severe bleeding was more frequent with ticagrelor. Most of the benefit of DAPT occurred within 10–21 days of randomization; thereafter the cumulative risk of bleeding with DAPT offsets any small benefit.

A pooled analysis of five randomized trials comparing a $P2Y_{12}$ receptor inhibitor plus aspirin with aspirin, started within 24 hours after an acute non-cardioembolic ischaemic stroke or TIA, with 21,808 individuals showed that $P2Y_{12}$ receptor inhibitor plus aspirin compared with aspirin was associated with a lower risk of recurrent stroke (RR 0.75, 95% CI 0.68–0.83).[28] Ticagrelor plus aspirin compared with aspirin was associated with a higher risk of severe bleeding (RR 3.98, 95% CI 1.74–9.10) and intracranial haemorrhage (RR 3.32, 95% CI 1.33–8.25), whereas clopidogrel plus aspirin versus aspirin had a similar haemorrhagic risk.

In the longer term, antiplatelet therapy with (predominantly) aspirin reduces the risk of non-fatal stroke by about 23% (reduced from 10.8% to 8.3% in 3 years),[29,30] and the combined endpoint of stroke, MI, and vascular death by about 13% (6–19%).[31] The efficacy of aspirin in secondary stroke prevention is independent of the dose in a range between 30 mg and 1600 mg/day.[31,32] Therefore, the recommended maintenance dose of aspirin (after a loading dose of 300 mg) is 100 mg daily.

Clopidogrel monotherapy (75 mg/day) was compared to aspirin (325 mg/day) in 19,185 patients with stroke, MI, or peripheral arterial disease and reduced the combined primary endpoint of stroke, MI, and vascular death in the CAPRIE trial by a relative risk reduction of 8.7% (0.3–16.3%).[33] In the subgroup of patient with previous TIA or ischaemic stroke, the relative risk reduction of clopidogrel versus aspirin was 7.3% (−5.7% to 18.7%). The combination of clopidogrel 75 mg and aspirin 75 mg was no more effective than clopidogrel monotherapy in preventing stroke or other major vascular events among high-risk patients with TIA or ischaemic stroke, whereas it did significantly increase bleeding complications.[34] The combination of clopidogrel and aspirin was also not more effective that aspirin monotherapy in preventing stroke and other major vascular events among 15,603 high vascular risk patients[35] or 3020 patients with a recent lacunar stroke[36] whereas it also increased bleeding rates in both populations compared with aspirin alone.

A direct, head-to-head, comparison of clopidogrel versus aspirin plus extended-release dipyridamole in 20,332 patients with ischaemic stroke followed for a mean period of 2.4 years found there was no difference in efficacy across all endpoints and no subgroup of patients.[37,38] Aspirin plus dipyridamole resulted in more intracranial bleeds and a higher drop-out rate due to headache compared with clopidogrel (5.9% vs 0.9%).

In Japanese patients, cilostazol (a phosphodiesterase III inhibitor) 100 mg twice daily reduced recurrent stroke by one-third compared with aspirin, from 8.3% (aspirin) to 5.5% (cilostazol) at 3 years (RR 0.67, 95% CI 0.52–0.86; absolute risk reduction 0.9% per year). The combination of cilostazol (100 mg twice daily) with aspirin or clopidogrel was associated with a reduced incidence of recurrent ischaemic stroke (2.2% per year dual therapy vs 4.5% per year monotherapy; HR 0.49, 95% CI 0.31–0.76), and a similar risk of severe or life-threatening bleeding (0.6% per year dual therapy vs 0.9% monotherapy; HR 0.66, 95% CI 0.27–1.60) compared with treatment with aspirin or clopidogrel alone in 1879 patients with high-risk non-cardioembolic ischaemic stroke followed for a median of 1.4 years.[39]

In conclusion, patients with a TIA or ischaemic stroke should be treated with aspirin, clopidogrel, or aspirin plus extended-release dipyridamole. Short-term use of DAPT for up to 21 days should be considered in patients with acute minor stroke or high-risk TIA and high risk of recurrence.

Clopidogrel is a prodrug that requires transformation to active metabolites by hepatic cytochrome P450 (CYP) enzymes. Reduced function of the *CYP2C19* gene, encoding the CYP2C19 enzyme, is associated with increased vascular risk in patients with stroke treated with clopidogrel.[40] In the CHANCE trial, in patients from China with minor ischaemic stroke or TIA, the use of clopidogrel plus aspirin compared with aspirin alone reduced the risk of a new stroke only in the subgroup of patients who were not carriers of the *CYP2C19* loss-of-function alleles.[41] The CHANCE 2 trial showed that, among 11,255 Chinese patients with minor ischaemic stroke or TIA who were screened, 6412 patients were carriers of *CYP2C19* loss-of-function alleles, and were randomized to ticagrelor (180 mg on day 1 followed by 90 mg twice daily on days 2 through 90; n = 3205) or clopidogrel (300 mg on day 1 followed by 75 mg once daily on days 2 through 90; n = 3207). Both groups received aspirin for 21 days. The risk of stroke at 90 days was modestly lower with ticagrelor than with clopidogrel (6.0% ticagrelor vs 7.6% clopidogrel; HR 0.77, 95% CI 0.64–0.94; P = 0.008). The risk of severe or moderate bleeding did not differ between the two treatment groups, but ticagrelor was associated with more total bleeding events than clopidogrel.[41] Among patients with minor stroke or TIA who carried *CYP2C19* loss-of-function alleles, benefit with ticagrelor and aspirin was present predominantly in the first week, with additional small benefit accruing in the next 2 weeks.[42]

Anticoagulation for secondary stroke prevention in the acute phase of ischaemic stroke

Routine anticoagulation with heparin in the early phase of ischaemic stroke does not reduce the risk of recurrent stroke and increases the risk of haemorrhage.[43–46] Low-dose low-molecular-weight heparin, however, reduced deep vein thrombosis and pulmonary embolism in patients with ischaemic stroke.[47]

At present, a new class of anticoagulants, the factor XI inhibitors, are being investigated for the prevention of early recurrent stroke in patients with TIA or ischaemic stroke. The hypothesis is that this class of drugs is as effective as traditional anticoagulants but has a lower bleeding rate. Milvexian, a small molecule oral factor XIa inhibitor, has been investigated in the AXIOMATIC-SSP trial. This was a phase II, double-blinded, placebo-controlled trial in 2366 patients with ischaemic stroke or high-risk TIA (ABCD^2 score ≥6, A = age ≥60 years, B = blood pressure ≥140/90 mmHg, C = clinical features of TIA, D = duration of symptoms, D = diabetes mellitus). Milvexian was given in five different doses and compared with placebo. Participants also received clopidogrel 75 mg daily for the first 21 days and aspirin 100 mg for 90 days. The primary endpoint was the composite of ischaemic stroke or incident infarct on magnetic resonance imaging (MRI). The results were presented at the Congress of the European Society of Cardiology (ESC) in August 2022. There was no dose response for the primary composite endpoint (symptomatic ischaemic stroke plus covert brain infarction). Milvexian was associated with fewer symptomatic ischaemic strokes at all doses except 200 mg twice daily. Doses from 25 mg to 100 mg twice daily showed similar relative risk reduction for symptomatic ischaemic stroke at approximately 30% versus placebo. The incidence of major bleeding was low (0.6–1.6%). There was a numerical increase in major bleeding at milvexian doses of 50 mg twice daily and above and the majority were gastrointestinal bleeds. No increase in symptomatic intracranial haemorrhage (ICH) bleeding versus placebo was observed.

Asundexian, another small molecule oral factor XIa inhibitor, has been investigated in the PACIFIC stroke trial. This was a phase II, double-blind, placebo-controlled trial in 1800 patients following an acute non-cardioembolic ischaemic stroke. Asundexian was given in three doses and compared with matching placebo. All participants received routine antiplatelet therapy. The primary endpoint was the composite of symptomatic ischaemic stroke or covert brain infarct detected by MRI. Asundexian did not reduce the composite of covert brain infarction or ischaemic stroke and did not increase the composite of major or clinically relevant non-major bleeding compared with placebo in patients with acute, non-cardioembolic ischaemic stroke.[48] The results of the two trials showed a small or no additional benefit of XIa inhibitors beyond antiplatelet therapy in patients with acute ischaemic stroke. For a final evaluation we need to wait for the results of the phase III trials with the use of the 50 mg daily dose of asundexian.

The COMPASS trial compared long-term oral anticoagulation with the combination of rivaroxaban 2.5 mg twice daily and aspirin 100 mg once daily with aspirin 100 mg once daily in patients with coronary and/or peripheral arterial disease.[49] Among the subgroup of 1032 participants in COMPASS with prior (>1 month) non-lacunar stroke, the rate of ischaemic/unknown stroke averaged 3.4% among aspirin-assigned patients, and was reduced by 67% with rivaroxaban plus aspirin (HR 0.33, 95% CI 0.14–0.77; P = 0.01; interaction P = 0.28).[50] The absolute reduction in recurrent stroke was 2.3% with rivaroxaban plus aspirin (number needed to treat for 1 year = 43).[50]

Anticoagulation in patients with atrial fibrillation and ischaemic stroke or transient ischaemic attack

Oral anticoagulation in patients with minor ischaemic stroke or TIA reduces the risk of recurrent stroke by about 66% in patients with atrial fibrillation (AF) compared with placebo (4% per year oral anticoagulation vs 12% per year placebo; HR 0.34, 95% CI 0.20–0.57).[51] The incidence of major bleeding events with anticoagulation was 2.8% per year.[51] Oral anticoagulation with warfarin is also more effective than aspirin in preventing vascular events (OR 0.67, 95% CI 0.50–0.91) and recurrent stroke (OR 0.49, 95% CI 0.33–0.72),[52] and the combination of aspirin and clopidogrel in patients with AF.[53]

Meta-analyses of all 71,683 participants enrolled in the non-vitamin K oral anticoagulant (NOAC) trials RE-LY, ROCKET AF, ARISTOTLE, and ENGAGE AF-TIMI 48 included 17,299 (24%) patients with AF and a history of prior stroke or TIA.[54] Among the 17,299 patients with AF and prior TIA or ischaemic stroke, the rate of stroke or systemic embolism over a median period of 1.8–2.8 years was 4.9% with a NOAC versus 5.7% with warfarin (RR 0.86, 95% CI 0.76–0.98). Stroke incidence was also lower with the NOACs as a group versus warfarin (RR 0.87, 95% CI 0.76–0.99). There were no significant differences for NOACs versus warfarin with respect to ischaemic stroke (RR 0.98, 95% CI 0.85–1.13). The incidence of intracerebral haemorrhage was halved (RR 0.50, 95% CI 0.36–1.00). The difference in terms of preventing cerebral haemorrhage for NOACs compared to warfarin was significant for apixaban, dabigatran, and edoxaban, but not for rivaroxaban.[54]

The optimal timing for starting oral anticoagulation after acute TIA or ischaemic stroke is currently based on registry data.[55,56] Randomized trials are ongoing. The empirical recommendation is to start anticoagulation on day 1 in patients with TIA, day 3–4 in patients with mild/moderate strokes, day 6 in patients with moderate strokes, and after 6–7 days in patients with severe stroke. Patients with AF who survive an ICH are at increased risk of subsequent ischaemic stroke. Determining the best approach for reducing further risk of stroke in patients with AF and previous ICH, or other clinically relevant bleeds, requires careful consideration of the associated risks. Several randomized controlled trials are investigating the risks and benefits of start of NOAC after ICH: ENRICH-AF (ClinicalTrials.gov Identifier: NCT03950076), SoSTART2 (ClinicalTrials.gov Identifier: NCT03153150), NASPAF-ICH (ClinicalTrials.gov Identifier: NCT02998905), and Prestige AF (ClinicalTrials.gov Identifier: NCT03996772). Until the results of these trials become available, we recommend to follow the ESC guidelines that after ICH, oral anticoagulation in AF patients may be reinitiated with a NOAC after 4–8 weeks provided the cause of bleeding or the relevant risk factor has been treated or controlled.[57]

In summary, patients with cardiac embolism, especially AF, should be treated with oral anticoagulation. Treatment options include vitamin K antagonists (international normalized ratio 2.0–3.0) or the NOACs apixaban, dabigatran, edoxaban, or rivaroxaban. Patients who have contraindications to oral anticoagulation or who do not wish to use it should receive interventional left atrial appendage closure (➔ Chapter 20) or be treated with aspirin or the combination of aspirin plus clopidogrel. NOACs are contraindicated in patients with moderate or severe mitral stenosis, rheumatic heart disease, or mechanical heart valves. In patients with TIA or minor stroke, oral anticoagulation may be initiated immediately after exclusion of cerebral haemorrhage.[57]

In a multicentre, double-blind study in 775 patients with AF, of whom 65 (9%) had a history of prior stroke or TIA, the new oral factor XIa inhibitor asundexian was compared with the factor Xa inhibitor apixaban. For the primary endpoint of International Society of Thrombosis and Haemostasis serious bleeding complications or clinically relevant non-serious bleeding, there was a 70% reduction in favour of the two doses of asundexian 20 mg and 50 mg compared to apixaban.[58]

Secondary stroke prevention in patients with embolic stroke of undetermined cause

Strokes were previously divided into large vessel disease, small vessel disease with lacunar infarcts, cardiac sources of embolism such as AF, rare causes such as vasculitis or drug abuse, and so-called cryptogenic strokes, in which the cause of stroke could not be classified.[59] More recently, the term cryptogenic stroke has been replaced by the term embolic stroke of undetermined source (ESUS). ESUS provides an operational definition and defines a diagnostic algorithm[60] (➔ Figure 18.3). Assuming that patients with ESUS may have undetected causes of emboli or silent paroxysmal AF, two large randomized trials comparing treatment with dabigatran or rivaroxaban with aspirin were conducted. In the RE-SPECT ESUS trial,[61] dabigatran, and in the NAVIGATE ESUS trial,[62] rivaroxaban, were not superior to aspirin therapy in secondary prevention. The ARCARDIA trial compares apixaban and aspirin in patients with ESUS and atrial cardiopathy.[63] The results were presented at ESOC 2023. There was no benefit of apixaban over aspirin. Strokes in patients with patent foramen ovale are no longer considered as ESUS.[64]

Carotid surgery or stenting in patients with asymptomatic and symptomatic high-grade stenosis of the internal carotid artery

According to the guidelines of the European Stroke Organisation (ESO) and based on moderate-quality evidence, carotid

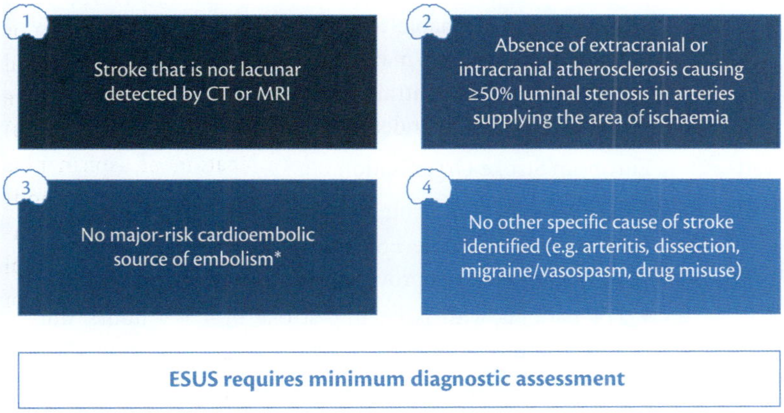

Figure 18.3 Diagnostic criteria for embolic stroke of unknown source (ESUS). * For example, permanent, persistent, or paroxysmal AF. CT, computed tomography; MRI, magnetic resonance imaging.

endarterectomy is recommended in patients with 60–99% asymptomatic carotid stenosis considered to be at increased risk of stroke on best medical treatment alone.[65] Medical care, however has dramatically improved since the randomized trials comparing endarterectomy with control were performed 20 years ago. At present, the stroke risk in patients with asymptomatic carotid stenosis is very low.[66] Therefore, it might be justified to keep these patients on best medical therapy alone.

Carotid surgery or stenting are highly effective in the secondary prevention of stroke in patients with stroke or TIA and high-degree symptomatic stenosis of the internal carotid artery.[67] Carotid endarterectomy was highly beneficial in participants with 70–99% stenosis of the internal carotid stenosis without near-occlusion (RR 0.53, 95% CI 0.42–0.67) in three studies with 1095 participants.[67] The reported perioperative risk of stroke or death associated with carotid endarterectomy for symptomatic high-grade carotid stenosis is approximately 7% (95% CI 6.2–8.0). In the longer term, the risk of stroke or death at 5 years was reduced by a quarter in patients with 50–69% stenosis (19% carotid endarterectomy vs 27% control, RR 0.72, 95% CI 0.58–0.86; absolute risk reduction 8%).[68] The benefit of surgery was greatest in men, elderly patients, patients with recent (rather than later) cerebral ischaemic events versus amaurosis fugax, patients with progressive carotid stenosis, and patients with ulcerated versus smooth carotid plaque.[69] Patients with less than 50% carotid stenosis did not benefit from carotid endarterectomy.

Internal carotid artery stenting has a lower risk of periprocedural MI, caudal cranial nerve lesion, and haematoma at the access site compared with carotid endarterectomy, but a higher risk of periprocedural stroke or death at 30 days (OR 1.71, 95% CI 1.38–2.11; ten randomized controlled trials, 5797 symptomatic patients), especially in patients aged 70 years or older. The long-term rate of stroke or death is higher with stenting than with carotid endarterectomy because of periprocedural risk differences.[70] Excluding procedural risks, long-term rates after carotid endarterectomy and carotid artery stenting are similar for ipsilateral stroke (4% at 9 years for stenting and carotid endarterectomy), fatal or disabling stroke, and functional outcome.[71–73] Restenosis is more common after stenting (10%), but is not associated with an increase in late ipsilateral stroke.

As a recommendation for clinical practice, symptomatic patients with greater than 60% stenosis of the internal carotid artery should undergo surgery. Stenting of the internal carotid artery is an alternative to endarterectomy in patients considered unfit or at high risk for endarterectomy. The preventive benefit of carotid surgery is highest in the first 2–4 weeks after a TIA or minor stroke. The benefit of carotid surgery is lower in patients with stenosis between 50% and 70%, in women, and when surgery is performed more than 12 weeks after the initial event. Patients do not benefit from surgery if the complication rate of the procedure exceeds 6%. Prophylaxis with aspirin before, during, and after endarterectomy is recommended. Carotid stenting has a slightly higher short-term complication rate compared with carotid surgery. Dual therapy with clopidogrel (75 mg) plus aspirin (75–100 mg) is recommended for 1–3 months in patients after carotid stenting, based on extrapolation from studies of coronary stenting. However, no data are available from carotid stenting studies.

Patients with symptomatic stenosis of the intracranial arteries have a very high risk of recurrence. Stenting of recently symptomatic atherosclerotic intracranial stenosis is associated with unacceptable periprocedural risks of stroke or death, compared with intensive medical therapy (14.7% stenting vs 5.8% medical) and higher stroke rates after 1 year (20.0% stenting vs 12.2% medical).[74,75]

Symptomatic vertebral artery stenosis is also associated with a high risk of recurrent stroke, and the risks are higher with intracranial than extracranial stenosis. However, the risks of periprocedural stroke or death with vertebral artery stenting are also higher for intracranial stenosis than for extracranial stenosis (16% vs 1%; $P < 0.0001$).[76] Compared with best medical therapy, there is no significant reduction in rates of any stroke with vertebral artery stenting (HR for stenting vs medical therapy only: 0.81%, 95% CI 0.45–1.44; $P = 0.47$). For extracranial stenosis alone, the HR was 0.63 (95% CI 0.27–1.46) and for intracranial stenosis alone it was 1.06 (95% CI 0.46–2.42; $P = 0.395$).

What's new

- Tenecteplase, at doses of 0.25–0.4 mg/kg in patients with ischaemic strokes has no additional benefit compared to alteplase 0.9 mg/kg and has at higher doses an increased bleeding risk. Alteplase is currently the only approved thrombolytic drug for ischaemic stroke. Tenecteplase is not available in many countries.
- Alteplase prior to thrombectomy has a small benefit in terms of recanalization rate.[77]
- Aspirin or unfractionated heparin, or both, during endovascular stroke treatment increase the risk of bleeding and have no additional benefit.[17]
- Intra-arterial alteplase following successful thrombectomy improves functional outcome in one trial.[16]
- In patients with AF treated with dabigatran who experience an acute ischaemic stroke, thrombolysis can be performed after normalizing coagulation with idarucizumab.[78]
- Two studies presented showed a clear benefit of thrombectomy over medical treatment in patients with basilar artery thrombosis.[78a,78b]

Guideline recommendations

Thrombolysis

American Heart Association/American Stroke Association

- In patients eligible for IV alteplase, benefit of therapy is time dependent, and treatment should be initiated as quickly as possible and not delayed for additional multimodal neuroimaging, such as computed tomography and MRI perfusion imaging.[79]
- IV alteplase (0.9 mg/kg, maximum dose 90 mg over 60 minutes with initial 10% of dose given as bolus over 1 minute) is recommended for selected patients who can be treated within 4.5 hours of ischaemic stroke symptom onset or patient last known well, or at baseline state.[79]
- IV alteplase (0.9 mg/kg, maximum dose 90 mg over 60 minutes with initial 10% of dose given as bolus over 1 minute) administered within 4.5 hours of stroke symptom recognition can be beneficial in patients with acute ischaemic stroke who awake with stroke symptoms or have unclear time of onset longer than 4.5 hours from last known well or at baseline state and who have a diffusion-weighted MRI lesion smaller than one-third of the middle cerebral artery territory and no visible signal change on fluid-attenuated inversion recovery (FLAIR).[79]
- Patients eligible for IV alteplase should receive IV alteplase even if mechanical thrombectomy is being considered.[79]
- Given the extremely low risk of unsuspected abnormal platelet counts or coagulation studies in a population, it is reasonable that urgent IV alteplase treatment not be delayed while waiting for haematological or coagulation testing if there is no reason to suspect an abnormal test.[79]
- IV aspirin should not be administered within 90 minutes after the start of IV alteplase.[79]
- It may be reasonable to choose tenecteplase (single IV bolus of 0.25 mg/kg, maximum 25 mg) over IV alteplase in patients without contraindications for IV fibrinolysis who are also eligible to undergo mechanical thrombectomy.[79]

European Stroke Organisation

- For patients with acute ischaemic stroke of less than 4.5 hours' duration, the ESO recommends IV thrombolysis with alteplase to improve functional outcome.[80]
- For patients with ischaemic stroke of 4.5–9 hours' duration (known onset time), or on awakening from sleep, and with computed tomography or MRI core/perfusion mismatch or MRI diffusion-weighted imaging/FLAIR mismatch, within 9 hours from the stoke onset or the midpoint of sleep, and for whom mechanical thrombectomy is either not indicated or not planned, the ESO recommends IV thrombolysis with alteplase.[80]
  - This new recommendation extends the time window recommended for thrombolysis treatment up to 9 hours after time of stroke where imaging findings suggest benefit.

Acute antithrombotic therapy

American Heart Association/American Stroke Association

- Administration of aspirin is recommended in patients with AIS within 24–48 hours after onset. For those treated with IV alteplase, aspirin administration is generally delayed until 24 hours later but might be considered in the presence of concomitant conditions for which such treatment given in the absence of IV alteplase is known to provide substantial benefit or withholding such treatment is known to cause substantial risk.[79]
- Urgent anticoagulation, with the goal of preventing early recurrent stroke, halting neurological worsening, or improving outcomes after AIS, is not recommended for treatment of patients with acute ischaemic stroke.[79]
- In patients presenting with minor non-cardioembolic ischaemic stroke (National Institutes of Health Stroke Scale (NIHSS) score ≤3) who did not receive IV alteplase, treatment with DAPT (aspirin and clopidogrel) started within 24 hours after symptom onset and continued for 21 days is effective in reducing recurrent ischaemic stroke for a period of up to 90 days from symptom onset.[79]

American Heart Association/American Stroke Association

- For patients with recent minor (NIHSS score ≤3) non-cardioembolic ischaemic stroke or high-risk TIA ($ABCD^2$ score ≥4), DAPT (aspirin plus clopidogrel) should be initiated early (ideally within 12–24 hours of symptom onset and at least within 7 days of onset) and continued for 21–90 days, followed by single antiplatelet therapy, to reduce the risk of recurrent ischaemic stroke.[81]
- For patients with recent (<24 hours) minor-to-moderate stroke (NIHSS score ≤5), high-risk TIA ($ABCD^2$ score

≥6), or symptomatic intracranial or extracranial 30% or greater stenosis of an artery that could account for the event, DAPT with ticagrelor plus aspirin for 30 days may be considered to reduce the risk of 30-day recurrent stroke but may also increase the risk of serious bleeding events, including ICH.[81]

- In patients with ischaemic stroke at low risk for haemorrhagic conversion in the setting of AF, it may be reasonable to initiate anticoagulation 2–14 days after the index event to reduce the risk of recurrent stroke.[81]

European Stroke Organisation

- In patients with acute non-cardioembolic high-risk TIA ($ABCD^2$ score of ≥4), the ESO recommends short-term DAPT with aspirin and clopidogrel over monotherapy, subsequently followed by monotherapy.[82]

Long-term antithrombotic therapy

American Heart Association/American Stroke Association

- For patients with non-cardioembolic ischaemic stroke or TIA, aspirin 50–325 mg daily, clopidogrel 75 mg, or the combination of aspirin 25 mg and extended-release dipyridamole 200 mg twice daily is indicated for secondary prevention of ischaemic stroke.[81]
- For patients with non-cardioembolic ischaemic stroke or TIA, the continuous use of DAPT (aspirin plus clopidogrel) for longer than 90 days or the use of triple antiplatelet therapy is associated with excess risk of haemorrhage.[81]
- In patients with non-valvular AF and stroke or TIA, the American Heart Association/American Stroke Association (AHA/ASA) recommends oral anticoagulation (e.g. apixaban, dabigatran, edoxaban, rivaroxaban, or warfarin) to reduce the risk of recurrent stroke.[81]
- In patients with ischaemic stroke or TIA and valvular AF (moderate-to-severe mitral stenosis or any mechanical heart valve), the AHA/ASA recommends warfarin to reduce the risk of recurrent stroke or TIA.[81]
- In patients with stroke or TIA and left ventricular thrombus, the AHA/ASA recommends anticoagulation with therapeutic warfarin for at least 3 months to reduce the risk of recurrent stroke.[81]
- In patients with ESUS, treatment with direct oral anticoagulants is not recommended to reduce risk of secondary stroke.[81]
- In patients 18–60 years of age with a non-lacunar ischaemic stroke of undetermined cause despite a thorough evaluation and a patent foramen ovale with high-risk anatomical features, the AHA/ASA considers it is reasonable to choose closure with a transcatheter device and long-term antiplatelet therapy over antiplatelet therapy alone for preventing recurrent stroke.[81]

European Stroke Organisation

- In patients with non-valvular AF and previous ischaemic stroke or TIA, the ESO recommends NOACs over vitamin K antagonists for secondary prevention of all events because they have a lower risk of major bleeding and death.[83]

What's next

- Despite major advances in therapeutics, ischaemic stroke remains a major cause of global disability and death.
- Delayed presentation of acute stroke limits the application of effective reperfusion strategies, and antithrombotic interventions for early and long-term treatment are incompletely effective and associated with risk of bleeding.
- Current efforts to improve stroke outcomes focus on community and physician education, implementation of expedited stroke protocols, refinement of available therapeutics, and their evaluation in special populations.
- Approaches currently under evaluation include new anticoagulant drugs that target the contact pathway (e.g. coagulation factor XI) and new approaches to individualized dosing of antiplatelet therapy based on pharmacodynamic or genetic testing, both of which are expected to be associated with more favourable benefit/risk profiles, and targeting of upstream drivers of haemostatic activation (e.g. inflammation, neutrophil extracellular traps, and polyphosphates).
- The most effective approach to reducing the burden of ischaemic stroke remains risk factor modification to prevent the proximal causes of vessel wall injury that lead to haemostatic activation and occlusive thrombus formation that characterizes acute stroke.

Disclosures

In the last 3 years, HCD received honoraria for participation in clinical trials, contribution to advisory boards or oral presentations from Abbott, BMS, Boehringer Ingelheim, Daiichi-Sankyo, Novo-Nordisk, Pfizer, Portola and WebMD Global. Boehringer Ingelheim provided financial support for research projects. HCD received research grants from the German Research Council (DFG) and German Ministry of Education and Research (BMBF). HCD serves as editor of *Neurologie up2date*, *Info Neurologie & Psychiatrie*, *Arzneimitteltherapie*, as co-editor of Cephalalgia, and on the editorial board of *Lancet Neurology and Drugs*.

GJH reports personal fees from the American Heart Association for serving as an Associate Editor of *Circulation*, from Bayer for consulting about stroke prevention in AF, from Bristol Myers Squibb for serving as a member of the Steering Committee of the AXIOMATIC-SSP trial of milvexian, a factor XIa inhibitor, added to DAPT after atherosclerotic TIA and mild ischaemic stroke, and from Janssen Research and Development for consultation.

JWE reports honoraria and/or research support Anthos, AZ, Bayer, BI, BMS, DSI, Janssen, Pfizer, Servier, and WebMD.

References

1. Global Burden of Disease 2019 Stroke Collaborators. Global, regional, and national burden of stroke and its risk factors, 1990–2019: a systematic analysis for the Global Burden of Disease Study 2019. Lancet Neurol. 2021;20(10):795–820.
2. Wardlaw JM, Murray V, Berge E, del Zoppo GJ. Thrombolysis for acute ischaemic stroke. Cochrane Database Syst Rev. 2014;2014(7):CD000213.
3. Lees KR, Emberson J, Blackwell L, et al. Effects of alteplase for acute stroke on the distribution of functional outcomes: a pooled analysis of 9 trials. Stroke. 2016;47(9):2373–9.
4. Emberson J, Lees KR, Lyden P, et al. Effect of treatment delay, age, and stroke severity on the effects of intravenous thrombolysis with alteplase for acute ischaemic stroke: a meta-analysis of individual patient data from randomised trials. Lancet. 2014;384(9958):1929–35.
5. Tsivgoulis G, Katsanos AH, Malhotra K, et al. Thrombolysis for acute ischemic stroke in the unwitnessed or extended therapeutic time window. Neurology. 2020;94(12):e1241–8.
6. Malhotra K, Katsanos AH, Goyal N, et al. Safety and efficacy of dual antiplatelet pretreatment in patients with ischemic stroke treated with IV thrombolysis: a systematic review and meta-analysis. Neurology. 2020;94(7):e657–66.
7. Xian Y, Liang L, Smith EE, et al. Risks of intracranial hemorrhage among patients with acute ischemic stroke receiving warfarin and treated with intravenous tissue plasminogen activator. JAMA. 2012;307(24):2600–8.
8. Kermer P, Eschenfelder CC, Diener HC, Grond M, Abdalla Y, Abraham A, et al. Antagonizing dabigatran by idarucizumab in cases of ischemic stroke or intracranial hemorrhage in Germany-—updated series of 120 cases. Int J Stroke. 2020;15(6):609–18.
9. Hailu K, Cannon C, Hayes S. Tenecteplase use in the management of acute ischemic stroke: literature review and clinical considerations. Am J Health Syst Pharm. 2022;79(12):944–9.
10. Kvistad CE, Næss H, Helleberg BH, et al. Tenecteplase versus alteplase for the management of acute ischaemic stroke in Norway (NOR-TEST 2, part A): a phase 3, randomised, open-label, blinded endpoint, non-inferiority trial. Lancet Neurol. 2022;21(6):511–19.
11. Menon BK, Buck BH, Singh N, et al. Intravenous tenecteplase compared with alteplase for acute ischaemic stroke in Canada (AcT): a pragmatic, multicentre, open-label, registry-linked, randomised, controlled, non-inferiority trial. Lancet. 2022;400(10347):161–9.

11a. Wang Y, Li S, Pan Y, et al. Tenecteplase versus alteplase in acute ischaemic cerebrovascular events (TRACE-2): a phase 3, multicentre, open-label, randomised controlled, non-inferiority trial. Lancet. 2023;401(10377):645–54.

12. Zhao Y, Zhao W, Guo Y, Li Y. Endovascular thrombectomy versus standard medical treatment for stroke patients with acute basilar artery occlusion: a systematic review and meta-analysis. J Neurointerv Surg. 2022;14(12):1173–9.
13. Goyal M, Menon BK, van Zwam WH, et al. Endovascular thrombectomy after large-vessel ischaemic stroke: a meta-analysis of individual patient data from five randomised trials. Lancet. 2016;387(10029):1723–31.
14. Roaldsen MB, Jusufovic M, Berge E, Lindekleiv H. Endovascular thrombectomy and intra-arterial interventions for acute ischaemic stroke. Cochrane Database Syst Rev. 2021;6(6):CD007574.
15. Chen J, Wan TF, Xu TC, Chang GC, Chen HS, Liu L. Direct endovascular thrombectomy or with prior intravenous thrombolysis for acute ischemic stroke: a meta-analysis. Front Neurol. 2021;12:752698.

15a. Turc G, Tsivgoulis G, Audebert HJ, et al. European Stroke Organisation-European Society for Minimally Invasive Neurological Therapy expedited recommendation on indication for intravenous thrombolysis before mechanical thrombectomy in patients with acute ischaemic stroke and anterior circulation large vessel occlusion. Eur Stroke J. 2022; 7: I–XXVI.

16. Renú A, Millán M, San Román L, et al. Effect of intra-arterial alteplase vs placebo following successful thrombectomy on functional outcomes in patients with large vessel occlusion acute ischemic stroke: the CHOICE randomized clinical trial. JAMA. 2022;327(9):826–35.
17. van der Steen W, van de Graaf RA, Chalos V, et al. Safety and efficacy of aspirin, unfractionated heparin, both, or neither during endovascular stroke treatment (MR CLEAN-MED): an open-label, multicentre, randomised controlled trial. Lancet. 2022;399(10329):1059–69.
18. Amarenco P, Lavallee PC, Labreuche J, et al. One-year risk of stroke after transient ischemic attack or minor stroke. N Engl J Med. 2016;374(16):1533–42.
19. Amarenco P, Lavallee PC, Monteiro Tavares L, et al. Five-year risk of stroke after TIA or minor ischemic stroke. N Engl J Med. 2018;378(23):2182–90.
20. Rothwell PM, Algra A, Chen Z, Diener HC, Norrving B, Mehta Z. Effects of aspirin on risk and severity of early recurrent stroke after transient ischaemic attack and ischaemic stroke: time-course analysis of randomised trials. Lancet. 2016;388(10042):365–75.
21. Johnston SC, Amarenco P. Ticagrelor versus aspirin in acute stroke or transient ischemic attack. N Engl J Med. 2016;375(14):1395.
22. Prasad K, Siemieniuk R, Hao Q, et al. Dual antiplatelet therapy with aspirin and clopidogrel for acute high risk transient ischaemic attack and minor ischaemic stroke: a clinical practice guideline. BMJ. 2018;363:k5130.
23. Kennedy J, Hill MD, Ryckborst KJ, Eliasziw M, Demchuk AM, Buchan AM. Fast assessment of stroke and transient ischaemic attack to prevent early recurrence (FASTER): a randomised controlled pilot trial. Lancet Neurol. 2007;6(11):961–9.
24. Johnston SC, Easton JD, Farrant M, et al. Clopidogrel and aspirin in acute ischemic stroke and high-risk TIA. N Engl J Med. 2018;379(3):215–25.
25. Wang Y, Wang Y, Zhao X, et al. Clopidogrel with aspirin in acute minor stroke or transient ischemic attack. N Engl J Med. 2013;369(1):11–19.
26. Hao Q, Tampi M, O'Donnell M, Foroutan F, Siemieniuk RA, Guyatt G. Clopidogrel plus aspirin versus aspirin alone for acute minor ischaemic stroke or high risk transient ischaemic attack: systematic review and meta-analysis. BMJ. 2018;363:k5108.
27. Johnston SC, Amarenco P, Denison H, et al. Ticagrelor and aspirin or aspirin alone in acute ischemic stroke or TIA. N Engl J Med. 2020;383(3):207–17.
28. Huang WY, Ovbiagele B, Lee M. P2Y12 receptor inhibitor plus aspirin versus aspirin treated within 24 hours of acute noncardioembolic ischemic stroke or TIA: Meta-analysis. J Formos Med Assoc. 2022;121(6):1053–61.
29. Antithrombotic Trialists' Collaboration. Collaborative meta-analysis of randomised trials of antiplatelet therapy for prevention of death, myocardial infarction, and stroke in high risk patients. BMJ. 2002;524:71–86.
30. Baigent C, Blackwell L, Collins R, et al. Aspirin in the primary and secondary prevention of vascular disease: collaborative

meta-analysis of individual participant data from randomised trials. Lancet. 2009;373(9678):1849–60.

31. Algra A, van Gijn J. Cumulative meta-analysis of aspirin efficacy after cerebral ischaemia of arterial origin. J Neurol Neurosurg Psychiatry. 1999;65:255.
32. Patrono C, Garcia Rodriguez LA, Landolfi R, Baigent C. Low-dose aspirin for the prevention of atherothrombosis. N Engl J Med. 2005;353(22):2373–83.
33. CAPRIE Steering Committee. A randomised, blinded, trial of clopidogrel versus aspirin in patients at risk of ischaemic events (CAPRIE). Lancet. 1996;348:1329–39.
34. Diener HC, Bogousslavsky J, Brass LM, et al. Aspirin and clopidogrel compared with clopidogrel alone after recent ischaemic stroke or transient ischaemic attack in high-risk patients (MATCH): randomised, double-blind, placebo-controlled trial. Lancet. 2004;364(9431):331–7.
35. Bhatt DL, Fox KA, Hacke W, et al. Clopidogrel and aspirin versus aspirin alone for the prevention of atherothrombotic events. N Engl J Med. 2006;354(16):1706–17.
36. SPS3 Investigators, Benavente OR, Hart RG, et al. Effects of clopidogrel added to aspirin in patients with recent lacunar stroke. N Engl J Med. 2012;367(9):817–25.
37. Sacco RL, Diener HC, Yusuf S, et al. Aspirin and extended-release dipyridamole versus clopidogrel for recurrent stroke. N Engl J Med. 2008;359(12):1238–51.
38. Diener HC, Sacco RL, Yusuf S, et al. Effects of aspirin plus extended-release dipyridamole versus clopidogrel and telmisartan on disability and cognitive function after recurrent stroke in patients with ischaemic stroke in the Prevention Regimen for Effectively Avoiding Second Strokes (PRoFESS) trial: a double-blind, active and placebo-controlled study. Lancet Neurol. 2008;7(10):875–84.
39. Toyoda K, Uchiyama S, Yamaguchi T, et al. Dual antiplatelet therapy using cilostazol for secondary prevention in patients with high-risk ischaemic stroke in Japan: a multicentre, open-label, randomised controlled trial. Lancet Neurol. 2019;18(6):539–48.
40. Lin J, Mo Y, Cai D, Mao D, Fu H, Wei D. CYP2C19 polymorphisms and clopidogrel efficacy in the secondary prevention of ischemic stroke: a retrospective observational study. Ann Palliat Med. 2021;10(12):12171–80.
41. Wang Y, Meng X, Wang A, et al. Ticagrelor versus clopidogrel in CYP2C19 loss-of-function carriers with stroke or TIA. N Engl J Med. 2021;385(27):2520–30.
42. Pan Y, Meng X, Jin A, et al. Time course for benefit and risk with ticagrelor and aspirin in individuals with acute ischemic stroke or transient ischemic attack who carry CYP2C19 loss-of-function alleles: a secondary analysis of the CHANCE-2 randomized clinical trial. JAMA Neurol. 2022;79(8):739–45.
43. Berge E, Abdelnoor M, Nakstad PH, Sandset PM. Low molecular-weight heparin versus aspirin in patients with acute ischaemic stroke and atrial fibrillation: a double-blind randomised study. HAEST Study Group. Heparin in Acute Embolic Stroke Trial. Lancet. 2000;355(9211):1205–10.
44. Chimowitz MI, Lynn MJ, Howlett-Smith H, et al. Comparison of warfarin and aspirin for symptomatic intracranial arterial stenosis. N Engl J Med. 2005;352(13):1305–16.
45. International Stroke Trial Collaborative Group. The International Stroke Trial (IST): a randomised trial of aspirin, subcutaneous heparin, both, or neither among 19435 patients with acute ischaemic stroke. Lancet. 1997;349(9065):1569–81.
46. Mohr JP, Thompson JL, Lazar RM, et al. A comparison of warfarin and aspirin for the prevention of recurrent ischemic stroke. N Engl J Med. 2001;345(20):1444–51.
47. Bath PM, Lindenstrom E, Boysen G, et al. Tinzaparin in acute ischaemic stroke (TAIST): a randomised aspirin-controlled trial. Lancet. 2001;358(9283):702–10.
48. Shoamanesh A, Mundl H, Smith EE, et al. Factor XIa inhibition with asundexian after acute non-cardioembolic ischaemic stroke (PACIFIC-Stroke): an international, randomised, double-blind, placebo-controlled, phase 2b trial. Lancet. 2022;400(10357):997–1007.
49. Eikelboom JW, Connolly SJ, Bosch J, et al. Rivaroxaban with or without aspirin in stable cardiovascular disease. N Engl J Med. 2017;377(14):1319–30.
50. Sharma M, Hart RG, Connolly SJ, et al. Stroke outcomes in the COMPASS trial. Circulation. 2019;139(9):1134–45.
51. European Atrial Fibrillation Trial (EAFT) Study Group. Secondary prevention in non-rheumatic atrial fibrillation after transient ischaemic attack or minor stroke. Lancet. 1993;342(8882):1255–62.
52. Saxena R, Koudstaal PJ. Anticoagulants for preventing stroke in patients with nonrheumatic atrial fibrillation and a history of stroke or transient ischemic attack. Stroke. 2004;35:1782–3.
53. Connolly S, Pogue J, Hart R, et al. Clopidogrel plus aspirin versus oral anticoagulation for atrial fibrillation in the Atrial fibrillation Clopidogrel Trial with Irbesartan for prevention of Vascular Events (ACTIVE W): a randomised controlled trial. Lancet. 2006;367(9526):1903–12.
54. Ntaios G, Papavasileiou V, Diener HC, Makaritsis K, Michel P. Nonvitamin-K-antagonist oral anticoagulants versus warfarin in patients with atrial fibrillation and previous stroke or transient ischemic attack: an updated systematic review and meta-analysis of randomized controlled trials. Int J Stroke. 2017;12(6):589–96.
55. Paciaroni M, Agnelli G, Ageno W, Caso V. Timing of anticoagulation therapy in patients with acute ischaemic stroke and atrial fibrillation. Thromb Haemost. 2016;116(3):410–6.
56. Mizoguchi T, Tanaka K, Toyoda K, et al. Early initiation of direct oral anticoagulants after onset of stroke and short- and long-term outcomes of patients with nonvalvular atrial fibrillation. Stroke. 2020;51(3):883–91.
57. Hindricks G, Potpara T, Dagres N, et al. 2020 ESC Guidelines for the diagnosis and management of atrial fibrillation developed in collaboration with the European Association for Cardio-Thoracic Surgery (EACTS): the Task Force for the diagnosis and management of atrial fibrillation of the European Society of Cardiology (ESC). Developed with the special contribution of the European Heart Rhythm Association (EHRA) of the ESC. Eur Heart J. 2021;42(5):373–498.
58. Piccini JP, Caso V, Connolly SJ, et al. Safety of the oral factor XIa inhibitor asundexian compared with apixaban in patients with atrial fibrillation (PACIFIC-AF): a multicentre, randomised, double-blind, double-dummy, dose-finding phase 2 study. Lancet. 2022;399(10333):1383–90.
59. Adams HP Jr, Bendixen BH, Kappelle LJ, et al. Classification of subtype of acute ischemic stroke. Definitions for use in a multicenter clinical trial. TOAST. Trial of Org 10172 in Acute Stroke Treatment. Stroke. 1993;24(1):35–41.
60. Hart RG, Diener HC, Coutts SB, et al. Embolic strokes of undetermined source: the case for a new clinical construct. Lancet Neurol. 2014;13(4):429–38.
61. Diener HC, Sacco RL, Easton JD, et al. Dabigatran for prevention of stroke after embolic stroke of undetermined source. N Engl J Med. 2019;380(20):1906–17.
62. Hart RG, Sharma M, Mundl H, et al. Rivaroxaban for stroke prevention after embolic stroke of undetermined source. N Engl J Med. 2018;378(23):2191–201.
63. Kamel H, Longstreth WT Jr, Tirschwell DL, et al. The AtRial cardiopathy and antithrombotic drugs in prevention after

cryptogenic stroke randomized trial: rationale and methods. Int J Stroke. 2019;14(2):207–14.

64. Diener HC, Easton JD, Hart RG, Kasner S, Kamel H, Ntaios G. Review and update of the concept of embolic stroke of undetermined source. Nat Rev Neurol. 2022;18(8):455–65.
65. Bonati LH, Kakkos S, Berkefeld J, et al. European Stroke Organisation guideline on endarterectomy and stenting for carotid artery stenosis. Eur Stroke J. 2021;6(2):I–XLVII.
66. Chang RW, Tucker L-Y, Rothenberg KA, et al. Incidence of ischemic stroke in patients with asymptomatic severe carotid stenosis without surgical intervention. JAMA. 2022;327(20):1974–82.
67. Rerkasem A, Orrapin S, Howard DP, Rerkasem K. Carotid endarterectomy for symptomatic carotid stenosis. Cochrane Database Syst Rev. 2020;9(9):CD001081.
68. Orrapin S, Rerkasem K. Carotid endarterectomy for symptomatic carotid stenosis. Cochrane Database Syst Rev. 2017;6:CD001081.
69. Rothwell PM, Warlow CP. Prediction on benefit from carotid endarterectomy in individual patients: a risk-modelling study. European Carotid Surgery Trialists' Collaborative Group. Lancet. 1999;353(9170):2105–10.
70. Muller MD, Lyrer P, Brown MM, Bonati LH. Carotid artery stenting versus endarterectomy for treatment of carotid artery stenosis. Cochrane Database Syst Rev. 2020;2:CD000515.
71. Bonati LH, Lyrer P, Ederle J, Featherstone R, Brown MM. Percutaneous transluminal balloon angioplasty and stenting for carotid artery stenosis. Cochrane Database Syst Rev. 2012;9:CD000515.
72. Bonati LH, Dobson J, Featherstone RL, et al. Long-term outcomes after stenting versus endarterectomy for treatment of symptomatic carotid stenosis: the International Carotid Stenting Study (ICSS) randomised trial. Lancet. 2015;385(9967):529–38.
73. Brott TG, Howard G, Roubin GS, et al. Long-term results of stenting versus endarterectomy for carotid-artery stenosis. N Engl J Med. 2016;374(11):1021–31.
74. Derdeyn CP, Chimowitz MI, Lynn MJ, et al. Aggressive medical treatment with or without stenting in high-risk patients with intracranial artery stenosis (SAMMPRIS): the final results of a randomised trial. Lancet. 2014;383(9914):333–41.
75. Chimowitz MI, Lynn MJ, Derdeyn CP, et al. Stenting versus aggressive medical therapy for intracranial arterial stenosis. N Engl J Med. 2011;365(11):993–1003.
76. Markus HS, Harshfield EL, Compter A, et al. Stenting for symptomatic vertebral artery stenosis: a preplanned pooled individual patient data analysis. Lancet Neurol. 2019;18(7):666–73.
77. LeCouffe NE, Kappelhof M, Treurniet KM, et al. A randomized trial of intravenous alteplase before endovascular treatment for stroke. N Engl J Med. 2021;385(20):1833–44.
78. Barber PA, Wu TY, Ranta A. Stroke reperfusion therapy following dabigatran reversal with idarucizumab in a national cohort. Neurology. 2020;94(19):e1968–72.
78a. Tao C, Nogueira RG, Zhu Y, et al. ATTENTION Investigators. Trial of endovascular treatment of acute basilar-artery occlusion. N Engl J Med. 2022;387(15):1361–72.
78b. Jovin TG, Li C, Wu L, et al. BAOCHE Investigators. Trial of thrombectomy 6 to 24 hours after stroke due to basilar-artery occlusion. N Engl J Med. 2022;387(15):1373–84.
79. Powers WJ, Rabinstein AA, Ackerson T, et al. Guidelines for the early management of patients with acute ischemic stroke: 2019 update to the 2018 guidelines for the early management of acute ischemic stroke: a guideline for healthcare professionals from the American Heart Association/American Stroke Association. Stroke. 2019;50(12):e344–418.
80. Berge E, Whiteley W, Audebert H, et al. European Stroke Organisation (ESO) guidelines on intravenous thrombolysis for acute ischaemic stroke. Eur Stroke J. 2021;6(1):I–LXII.
81. Kleindorfer DO, Towfighi A, Chaturvedi S, et al. 2021 guideline for the prevention of stroke in patients with stroke and transient ischemic attack: a guideline from the American Heart Association/American Stroke Association. Stroke. 2021;52(7):e364–467.
82. Fonseca AC, Merwick Á, Dennis M, et al. European Stroke Organisation (ESO) guidelines on management of transient ischaemic attack. Eur Stroke J. 2021;6(2):CLXIII–CLXXXVI.
83. Klijn CJ, Paciaroni M, Berge E, et al. Antithrombotic treatment for secondary prevention of stroke and other thromboembolic events in patients with stroke or transient ischemic attack and non-valvular atrial fibrillation: a European Stroke Organisation guideline. Eur Stroke J. 2019;4(3):198–223.

CHAPTER 19

Antithrombotic therapy in patients with patent foramen ovale (PFO), PFO closure, left ventricular mural thrombus, atrial thrombus, and catheter-related thrombosis

Jens Erik Nielsen-Kudsk, Asger Andersen, Kasper Korsholm, and Erik L. Grove

Contents

Summary

A patent foramen ovale (PFO) can give rise to paradoxical embolism and ischaemic stroke. In patients younger than 60–65 years with PFO-related ischaemic stroke, the risk of recurrent stroke can be reduced by about 60% by transcatheter PFO closure, while continuing antiplatelet therapy. Clinical history, age, presence of risk factors for stroke, ischaemic brain infarct location, and PFO anatomy are key factors when determining the probability of an ischaemic stroke being causally linked to a PFO. Heart–brain team assessment should be integral in the decision-making process for PFO closure. Technical success of transcatheter PFO closure is very high, and the complication rate is low. Dual antiplatelet therapy (aspirin and clopidogrel) should be given for 1–6 months after PFO closure followed by single antiplatelet therapy for up to 5 years. Oral anticoagulation is recommended over antiplatelets in patients with a PFO-related ischaemic stroke not eligible for transcatheter PFO closure. Thrombus formation on the PFO-closure device is a rare complication after PFO closure. Management of device-related thrombosis is outlined. Left ventricular mural thrombus is a serious complication occurring in the setting of regional or global left ventricular dysfunction. It is most often seen in association with acute myocardial infarction. Addition of oral anticoagulation with vitamin K antagonists to aspirin is the historical treatment; however, newer observational studies suggest direct oral anticoagulants to be a safe and equally effective alternative. Thrombus formation in the right and left atria can occur in association with atrial fibrillation, mitral and tricuspid valve stenosis, inflammatory disorders, coagulopathy, cancer, or congenital heart disease and in the setting of thrombosis on intracardiac catheters or pacing leads. Diagnosis and management of atrial thrombi and catheter-related thrombosis are discussed.

Introduction

Ischaemic stroke can be due to paradoxical embolism through a patent foramen ovale (PFO). When there is a high probability that a stroke is mediated through a PFO, it should be classified as a PFO-related stroke. Based on recent randomized clinical trials, transcatheter PFO closure has become a recommended therapy for patients younger than 60–65 years with PFO-related stroke. This chapter reviews the diagnosis, patient selection, treatment strategies including transcatheter PFO closure, medical therapy for patients with PFO-related stroke, and management of PFO device-related thrombosis (DRT).

The diagnosis and management of left ventricular (LV) mural thrombus, atrial thrombus, and catheter-related thrombosis (CRT) is also outlined in this chapter.

Patent foramen ovale

Foramen ovale is an opening in the anterior–superior part of the interatrial septum used in fetal life to shunt oxygenated blood from the placenta and inferior vena cava to the systemic circulation thereby bypassing the pulmonary circulation. It is a tunnel-like communication covered by a thin flap valve. With birth, there is a drop in right atrial pressure causing the flap valve to close and, over time, the foramen ovale will seal completely. A PFO will be formed if there is lack of fusion between the thin flap valve (primum septum) and the cranial rim of the interatrial septum (secundum septum). A PFO can be identified in approximately 25% of the general population from autopsies, and in approximately 12% it can be visualized with echocardiography in the healthy adult population.[1] A PFO is often asymptomatic, but with venous thromboembolism a blood clot can shunt through the PFO to the systemic circulation as a paradoxical embolus.

Patent foramen ovale-related ischaemic stroke

An embolus derived from thrombi in the veins, often in the lower extremities or lower part of the body, can be shunted through the PFO and embolize to the cerebral circulation causing a PFO-related ischaemic stroke. This causal mechanism was initially described by Dr Cohnheim in 1877 based on an autopsy of a young woman who died from an ischaemic stroke.[2] About 15–20% of embolic ischaemic strokes are of undetermined source (ESUS)[3] and approximately 40% of ESUS patients have a PFO suggesting a causal relationship.[4] The causal relationship of a PFO and ischaemic stroke was strengthened based on randomized studies of percutaneous PFO closure as add-on to medical therapy versus medical therapy alone in selected patients with ESUS (➔ Table 19.1).[5–11] A meta-analysis based on pooled individual participant data from the randomized trials showed an annualized hazard ratio (HR) of 0.41 [95% confidence interval (CI) 0.28–0.60] in favour of PFO closure as add-on to medical therapy to prevent recurrent ischaemic stroke.[12]

When to suspect a patent foramen ovale-related stroke

There is no clear-cut way to identify if an ischaemic stroke is PFO related or not, but brain imaging and clinical clues may increase the suspicion that an ischaemic stroke is caused by paradoxical embolism through a PFO.

Magnetic resonance imaging is the recommended imaging modality in ischaemic stroke as it can visualize the infarct in the first few hours after onset of symptoms.[13] Magnetic resonance imaging findings that increase suspicion of PFO-related ischaemic stroke are larger (>1.5 cm) solitary cortical strokes without signs of prior lesions, but smaller thalamic and cerebellar lacunar infarcts, and smaller infarcts in several vascular territories may also be embolic in origin.[13] Therefore, brain imaging can raise suspicion of, but cannot rule out, a PFO-related stroke mechanism.[1] Other important information provided by imaging is evaluation of a possible vascular source of thrombus by visualizing the carotid and cerebral arteries.[13]

Clinical clues that increase the suspicion of a PFO-related ischaemic stroke are presence of simultaneous venous thromboembolism, immobilization (surgery, travel, sedentary lifestyle), younger patients (<55 years), absence of other risk factors [atrial fibrillation (AF), diabetes, hypertension, smoking], Valsalva manoeuvre leading up to onset of symptoms (heavy lifting, coughing, defecating), and stroke on awakening in patients with obstructive sleep apnoea.

Another common source of embolic strokes is embolism from the left atrial appendage in patients with AF. To rule out AF in a patient with suspected embolic ischaemic stroke, an electrocardiogram (ECG), in-hospital telemetry, and 24-hour Holter ECG monitoring are recommended in younger patients (<55 years). In older patients, especially if they have risk factors for AF, longer ECG monitoring or insertable cardiac monitors are recommended to rule out AF. If a patient is diagnosed with AF, the patient should be treated with oral anticoagulation or left atrial appendage closure (in patients with high bleeding risk). Patients with AF and embolic ischaemic stroke should not routinely be evaluated for a PFO.[1]

Patients with a suspected PFO-related ischaemic stroke but no AF should be referred for imaging to diagnose if the patients have a PFO.

Diagnosis of patent foramen ovale

The diagnosis of a PFO aims to visualize venoarterial shunting across the interatrial septum and the PFO anatomy to identify high-risk PFO features. Key in the evaluation is contrast-enhanced imaging with agitated saline combined with an adequate Valsalva

Table 19.1 Randomized clinical trials and meta-analysis of closure of patent foramen ovale versus medical therapy in patients with patent foramen ovale-related ischaemic stroke

Study, reference	N	Main inclusion criteria	Endpoints	Results
Closure[10]	909	18–60 years and TIA, ischaemic stroke <6 months	Composite: death 0–30 days, neurological death >30 days, ischaemic stroke, TIA	2-year FU: HR 0.78, 95% CI 0.45–1.35
PC-Trial[7]	414	18–60 years and ischaemic stroke, TIA, or systemic embolism	Composite: death, ischaemic stroke, TIA, or systemic embolism	4.5-year FU: HR 0.63, 95% CI 0.24–1.62
RESPECT[5,6]	980	18–60 years and ischaemic stroke, TIA (confirmed on imaging)	Composite: early death (30–45 days), ischaemic stroke, or TIA	2.1-year FU: HR 0.49, 95% CI 0.22–1.11 5.9-year FU: HR 0.55, 95% CI 0.31–0.99
REDUCE[8]	664	18–59 years and ischaemic stroke, TIA (confirmed on imaging) <180 days	Co-primary: ischaemic stroke and new brain infarctions (on imaging)	3.2-year FU: Ischaemic stroke: HR 0.23, 95% CI 0.09–0.62 New brain infarctions: RR 0.51, 95% CI 0.29–0.91
CLOSE[9]	663	16–60 years and ischaemic stroke or TIA (both confirmed on imaging) and PFO with ASA and/or large shunt	Ischaemic stroke	5.3-year FU: HR 0.03, 95% CI 0.00–0.26
DEFENSE PFO[11]	120	Ischaemic stroke, TIA (confirmed on imaging) <180 days and high-risk PFO (ASA and/or >1 mm diastase).	Ischaemic stroke, death, or major bleeding	2-year FU: 0 events in the PFO group and 12.9% in the medical group (P = 0.013)
Kent et al. meta-analysis[12]	3740	Individual participant data pooled analysis from the studies above	Ischaemic stroke	Annualized: HR 0.41, 95% CI 0.28–0.60

ASA, atrial septum aneurysm; CI, confidence interval; FU, follow-up; HR, hazard ratio; PFO, patent foramen ovale; RR, relative risk; TIA, transient ischaemic attack.

manoeuvre to visualize bubbles shunted from the venous to the arterial circulation. To visualize shunting, contrast-enhanced transthoracic echocardiography (c-TTE, sensitivity of 88% and specificity of 82%) should be performed.[1] Contrast-enhanced transcranial Doppler (c-TCD, sensitivity of 94% and specificity of 92%) is an alternative. Limitations to c-TTE and c-TCD are inadequate Valsalva manoeuvre and the wash-away of bubbles injected through an arm vein from the region of the PFO in patients with a prominent inferior vena cava valve that directs the bloodstream directly towards the PFO (➔ Figure 19.1d). To increase the sensitivity of c-TTE and c-TCD, injection of agitated saline can be done through a femoral vein which directs the flow of bubbles directly to the interatrial septum.[14]

If a shunt is found, contrast-enhanced transoesophageal echocardiography (c-TOE) should be performed to visualize the anatomy of the PFO and to confirm that the bubbles are shunted through the PFO. On c-TOE it is important to visualize and report PFO-related anatomy and potential high-risk PFO features: the PFO channel length and diastasis (➔ Figure 19.1a); shunting of bubbles through the PFO and the PFO shunt with colour Doppler (➔ Figure 19.1b); interatrial septum mobility and if it is aneurysmatic (➔ Figure 19.1c); the presence of an inferior vena cava valve and Chiari network (➔ Figure 19.1c); and the size of the aortic root and thickness of the septum secundum and primum (➔ Figure 19.1c,d).

If a PFO is diagnosed in a patient with an embolic ischaemic stroke suspected to be PFO related and other causes of ischaemic stroke have been excluded (AF and vascular source of thrombus), the patient should have a diagnosis of PFO-related ischaemic stroke and an individualized treatment strategy should be chosen.

Patient selection and treatment strategy in patent foramen ovale-related ischaemic stroke

Selection of treatment strategy for a patient with a PFO-related ischaemic stroke should be done by an interdisciplinary 'heart–brain' team including neurologists and cardiologists (➔ Figure 19.2c) and the patient should be actively involved and informed in the decision process. Initial assessment should identify the risk of recurrence and the causal link between the PFO and ischaemic stroke based on brain imaging, clinical clues, and PFO anatomy. To aid in this decision, the Risk of Paradoxical Embolism (RoPE) score combined with the presence or absence of high-risk PFO features on c-TOE gives the PFO-Associated Stroke Causal Likelihood (PASCAL) of a PFO being causally related to the index stroke (➔ Figure 19.2a,b).[12] This score was developed based on analysis of the randomized PFO closure trials and limitations of the score are that it has not been prospectively tested and it does not account for all aspects of brain imaging, clinical clues, and PFO anatomy. Although the PASCAL score can be helpful, it should not replace the individual assessment of patients by the heart–brain team.

Younger patients (<65 years) with a high probability that the stroke was causally linked to the PFO and a high risk of recurrent stroke should be referred for transcatheter PFO closure. Oral anticoagulation can be used in patients with a low or unknown probability of a causal link and a low risk of recurrent stroke, but PFO closure can still be considered on an individual basis. Antiplatelets are rarely recommended if a PFO-related stroke is suspected.[1]

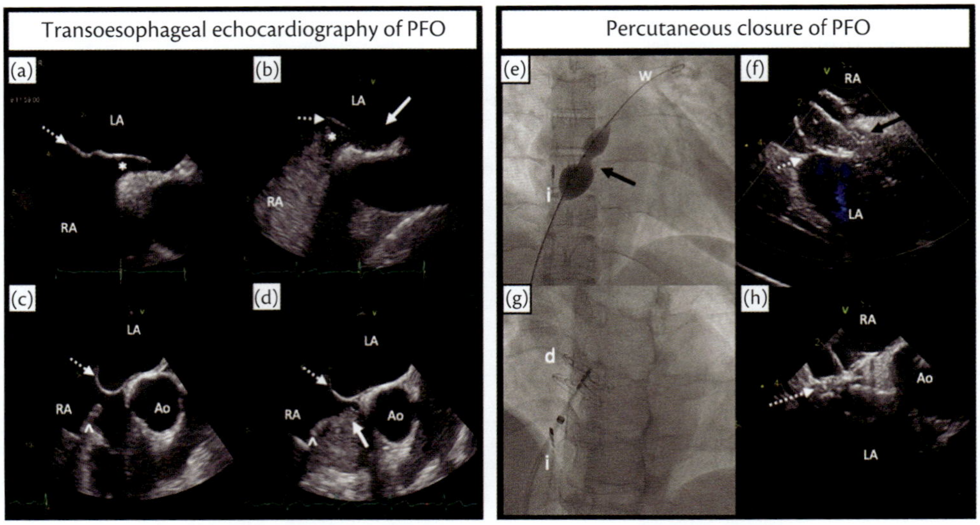

Figure 19.1 TOE and percutaneous closure of PFO. TOE of (a) measuring diastasis during Valsalva manoeuvre of the PFO (*). (b) Shunting of bubbles (white arrow) from agitated saline through the PFO during Valsalva manoeuvre. (c) Atrial septum aneurysm (dotted white arrow) and inferior venae cava valve (^). (d) Agitated saline flushed away from the atrial septum due to the inferior vena cava valve. (e) Fluoroscopy showing balloon sizing (black arrow) guided by intracardiac echocardiography (i) with guidewire (w) through the PFO channel and inserted into the left upper pulmonary vein. (f) Intracardiac echocardiography showing 'stop flow' during balloon sizing. (g) Fluoroscopy showing a PFO closure device with a disc on each site of the PFO (d). (h) Intracardiac echocardiography showing a PFO device straddling over the secundum septum and aorta (Ao). LA, left atrium; RA, right atrium.

Transcatheter closure of a patent foramen ovale

Closure of a PFO is done percutaneously with local analgesia through a femoral venous access guided by fluoroscopy and intracardiac echocardiography or TOE. A guidewire is advanced across the PFO channel to the left upper pulmonary vein, and a semi-compliant balloon inflated with contrast media may be used for sizing the PFO channel (➔ Figure 19.2e,f). Based on balloon sizing and echocardiographic evaluation of the PFO channel anatomy, an appropriate device is selected for closure. The device is advanced in a delivery sheath to the left atrium. The left atrial disc is formed in the left atrium and pulled gently towards the interatrial septum, and then the right atrial disc is deployed, allowing the device to straddle each side of the PFO (➔ Figure 19.2g,h). After the device is inserted, the correct position and sealing of the device is confirmed with echocardiography, fluoroscopy, and contrast-enhanced echocardiography.

Transcatheter PFO closure is a procedure with a high success rate and few complications. Technical success of transcatheter PFO closure is close to 100% and at 1 year, complete closure is seen in 93–96%.[1] Complications in the randomized trials are 2.6% with device thrombosis (1–2%) and device embolization (~1%) being the most common and minor complications occurring in 1–1.7%. Device erosion is a rare complication (<1:1000) that requires cardiac surgery.[1] The incidence of post-procedure AF in the randomized trials is 4.6% over 3.8 years of follow-up. Most AF cases occur within 45 days after closure and most of the AF episodes are of short duration.[15] The long-term effect of PFO closure on the incidence on AF is unclear and needs to be investigated.

Antithrombotic therapy after patent foramen ovale closure

It is recommended to continue antiplatelet therapy after PFO closure. The duration of antiplatelet therapy after PFO closure should be based on an individual evaluation, balancing risk of bleeding, device thrombosis, risk of non-PFO-related stroke recurrence, and comorbidities. At least 1–6 months of dual antiplatelet treatment is recommended after PFO closure to prevent DRT and, in most patients, it is recommended to continue single antiplatelet therapy for 5 years after PFO closure and possibly lifelong if a favourable risk/benefit ratio is expected.[1] In younger patients with a low cardiovascular risk and without coagulation disorders, retrospective observational reports have found it safe to discontinue antiplatelet therapy.[16] It is, however, important to note that the current recommendation is based on expert opinion, short follow-up in the randomized trials, and few observational reports, so it is a field that needs to be investigated further.

Medical therapy after patent foramen ovale-related ischaemic stroke

Oral anticoagulation is recommended over antiplatelets in patients with a PFO-related ischaemic stroke not eligible for

(a) **RoPE score calculator**

Characteristics	Points
No history of	
Hypertension	1
Diabetes	1
Stroke or TIA	1
Nonsmoker	1
Cortical infarct on imaging	1
Age, y	
18–29	5
30–39	4
40–49	3
50–59	2
60–69	1
Total RoPE score =	

(b) **PASCAL classification system**

High RoPE score (≥7)	High risk PFO features ASA and/or LS	PFO related Stroke
Absent	Absent	Unlikely
Absent	Present	Possible
Present	Absent	
Present	Present	Probable

(c)

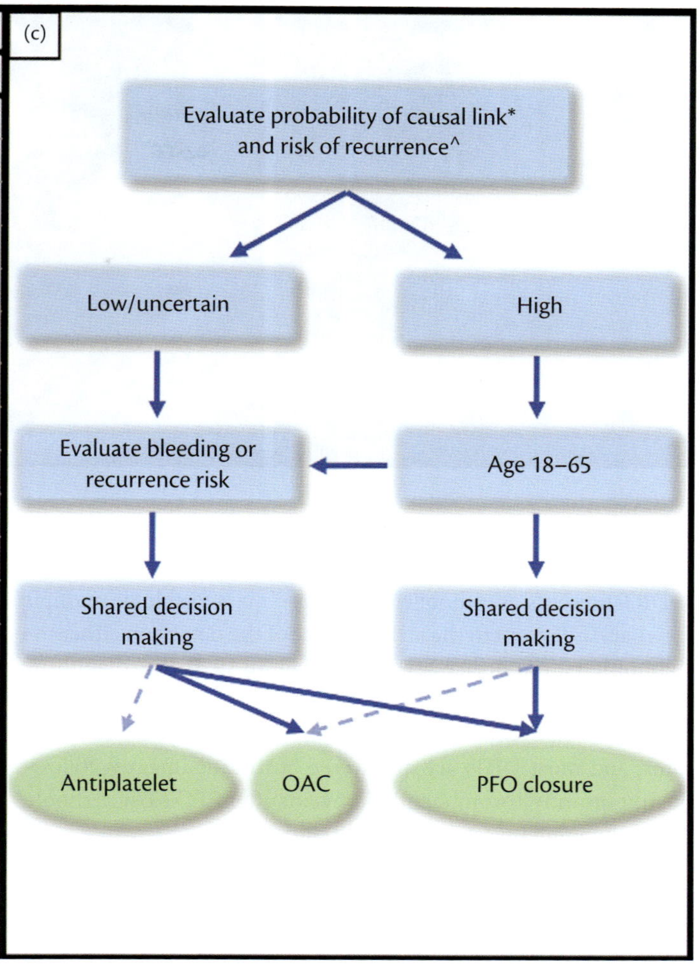

Figure 19.2 Secondary prevention of PFO-related ischaemic stroke, RoPE score, and PASCAL classification system. (a) The RoPE score assesses the probability that a PFO is pathogenically related to the cryptogenic stroke and not an incidental finding. Transient ischaemic attack (TIA), years (y). (b) The PASCAL score combines the RoPE score with the presence or absence of high-risk PFO features to assess the likelihood of a PFO being causally related to the index stroke. Large shunt (LS) size is greater than 20 left atrial bubbles on TOE; atrial septum aneurysm (ASA) is 10 mm or greater of excursion of the interatrial septum from midline. (c) Secondary prevention of PFO-related stroke. Oral anticoagulation (OAC). *High likelihood of causal link: ASA, atrial septal hypermobility, LS, simultaneous pulmonary embolism or deep venous thrombosis. Other features that should be considered when assessing likelihood: imaging supporting embolic stroke, PFO anatomy (size, tunnel length), Chiari network, prominent inferior vena cava valve, age less than 55 years, risk factors for stroke, PASCAL classification system, clinical evaluation (immobilization, recent surgery, previous pulmonary embolism/deep venous thrombosis, travel). ^High risk of recurrence: ASA, coagulation disorders. Other features that should be considered when assessing risk of recurrence: older age, PFO anatomy, other indication for antiplatelets/OAC, transient ischaemic attack or stroke as index event, stroke on antiplatelets/OAC.

transcatheter PFO closure and in patients eligible for PFO closure in the waiting time until the procedure can be performed.[1]

There are no adequately powered or well-designed randomized studies comparing anticoagulation to antiplatelets or to PFO closure in patients with a PFO-related ischaemic stroke. The recommendation is based on a meta-analysis using data from the CLOSE trial (➔ Table 19.1),[9] the small PICCS trial (n = 98)[17] that randomized patients with cryptogenic stroke and a PFO to warfarin or aspirin, and a subgroup of patients with a PFO included in the NAVIGATE ESUS trial (n = 534)[18] that randomized ESUS patients to rivaroxaban or aspirin. The meta-analysis found an odds ratio of 0.48 (95% CI 0.24–0.96)[18] in favour of anticoagulation over antiplatelets.

Device-related thrombosis in patent foramen ovale closure

Thrombus formation on the atrial surface of PFO-closure devices is rare but may cause pulmonary or systemic embolic complications. The incidence is less than 1% in the randomized trials[8,9,11] and reported at around 1–2% in observational reports including various non-contemporary device types.[19] The risk of DRT is highest in the early period after implantation until device endothelialization has occurred. Occurrence after 8-12 months is rare, but DRT has been observed up to 5 years after implantation.[20]

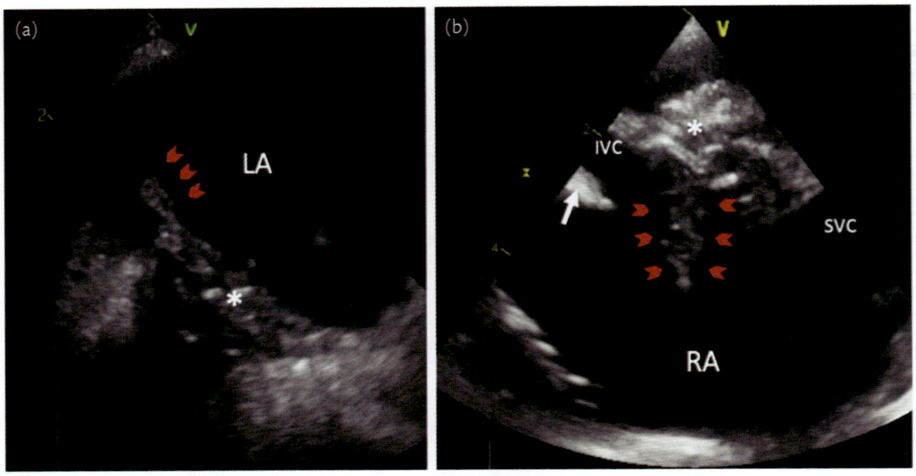

Figure 19.3 DRT on PFO closure device. DRT (red arrows) visualized (a) on the left atrial (LA) surface and (b) on the right atrial (RA) surface by TOE. The PFO device is marked by an asterisk. The white arrow marks an inferior vena cava (IVC) valve. SVC, superior vena cava.

DRT presents as a mobile echo-dense mass visible in multiple views and adherent to the atrial surface of the device on either the right or left atrial device surface (➔ Figure 19.3). The diagnostic ability of TTE is limited, and the diagnosis of DRT should rely on TOE or cardiac computed tomography. DRT rarely causes symptoms, and most DRTs are discovered at routine imaging follow-up. Importantly, thromboembolic events after PFO closure should lead to imaging investigations to exclude DRT.

Management of DRT includes intensified anticoagulation therapy. The majority resolve within 1–3 months with either low-molecular-weight heparin alone or in combination with warfarin.[19] Currently, only limited experience with direct oral anticoagulants exists, suggesting that they should be used with caution.[21] Surgical removal may be considered in selected patients with treatment failure such as thrombus progression or embolic complications despite anticoagulation.[20] Repeated imaging follow-up should be performed after 1–3 months to confirm DRT resolution or regression.

Left ventricular mural thrombus

LV mural thrombus is a serious complication occurring in the setting of regional or global LV dysfunction.[22,23] It is mainly described in association with acute myocardial infarction,[22,23] but may occur in most heart failure conditions with reduced LV systolic function regardless of aetiology.[23,24] The incidence has generally been declining after the introduction of primary percutaneous coronary intervention, yet LV thrombi may be found in up to 10% of patients with acute myocardial infarction.[24] Independent risk factors for LV thrombus include anterior myocardial infarction, reduced LV ejection fraction (<40%), larger LV end-diastolic and end-systolic volume, and presence of LV aneurysm.[25,26]

Patients with LV thrombi may face detrimental thromboembolic complications calling for careful imaging evaluation and initiation of anticoagulation therapy.[27] TTE is a cornerstone in the screening for LV thrombus due to the immediate availability but

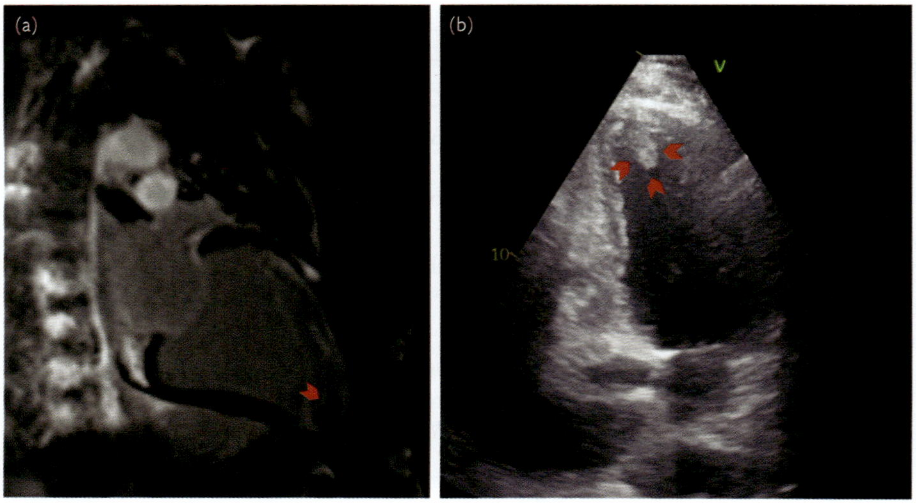

Figure 19.4 LV thrombus visualized by CMR and TTE. (a) Apical mural thrombus visualized on CMR in a patient with an anterior myocardial infarction (red arrow). (b) An apical mural thrombus (red arrows) on TTE in a patient with severe global LV systolic dysfunction secondary to tachycardia-induced cardiomyopathy.

may be limited by soft tissue delineation and impaired acoustic windows. The sensitivity of non-contrast TTE is around 30%,[28] which improves to around 60% with the use of echo contrast.[29] LV thrombus on TTE may appear as an echo-dense structure with a distinct border from the endocardium and different echogenicity and should be visible in multiple views with a typical location near an area of impaired contractility (➔ Figure 19.4). Cardiac magnetic resonance imaging (CMR) is considered the gold standard, with a sensitivity around 90% and a specificity of 99% compared to surgical findings.[29] Data indicate late gadolinium enhancement CMR to be superior to cine-CMR. Cardiac computed tomography has been described as an alternative diagnostic modality, but data on the diagnostic accuracy are lacking.[30] Application of contrast TTE and/or CMR should be considered at a low threshold in patients with risk factors for LV thrombus.

The incidence of LV thrombus secondary to ST-segment elevation myocardial infarction is 3% by TTE assessment, increasing to 9% in anterior myocardial infarcts.[31] The apparent underdiagnosis with TTE is evident from meta-analyses of CMR studies indicating an overall incidence of 6% in patients with ST-segment elevation myocardial infarction, increasing to 19% in patients with anterior myocardial infarction.[28]

Prophylactic oral anticoagulation in patients without imaging evidence of LV thrombus is debatable and not generally recommended as the efficacy is offset by increased risk of major bleeding events.[23,32] In the presence of LV thrombus, oral anticoagulation therapy is imperative in order to prevent thromboembolic complications.[27,33,34] Both the US and European guidelines include a class IIb, level of evidence C recommendation, reflecting that treatment evidence is based on observational data. Nevertheless, the risk of adverse events and mortality is significantly increased with the presence of LV thrombus,[34] with meta-analyses indicating a significant reduction of embolic complications with the addition of warfarin to aspirin.[35,36] Historically, treatment has consisted of heparin followed by dose-adjusted warfarin therapy (international normalized ratio 2–3). Efficacy and safety data associated with vitamin K antagonists and direct-acting oral anticoagulants (DOACs) are mainly derived from observational studies with conflicting results,[23] and randomized studies are ongoing. An open-label randomized trial ($n = 35$) reported non-inferiority of apixaban 5 mg twice daily compared to warfarin (international normalized ratio 2–3) for thrombus resolution, with numerically less bleeding in the apixaban group.[37] Similarly, rivaroxaban 20 mg was non-inferior to warfarin in the randomized NO-LVT trial including 79 patients. The real-life use of DOAC therapy in the setting of LV thrombus (and acute myocardial infarction) is likely higher than anticipated due to convenience and the safety profile demonstrated in other areas of cardiovascular medicine (AF, pulmonary embolism, etc.); however, further data are warranted to confirm the efficacy.

The duration of anticoagulation therapy in the presence of LV thrombus has not been clearly defined, but guidelines recommend at least 3–6 months with repeated imaging evaluation by either TTE or CMR.[27,33] Improved LV function reduces the risk of recurrence, whereas significant LV dysfunction and, for example, LV aneurysm indicates that anticoagulant therapy should be continued. Studies exploring recurrence rate and risk/benefit ratio of long-term anticoagulation therapy for prevention of LV thrombus recurrence are warranted.

Atrial thrombus

An intracardiac thrombus is typically formed either in the setting of low blood flow, or in the setting of a mechanical prosthetic heart valve and subtherapeutic anticoagulation. Atrial thrombosis is most often seen in the left atrial appendage in patients with AF or atrial flutter (➔ Chapters 3 and 21) and in patients with mitral valve stenosis; however, atrial thrombosis is not an infrequent finding in other settings. Although the risk of stroke and systemic embolism is obviously much higher in left atrial thrombosis, right atrial thrombosis is also an important marker of poor prognosis. Thrombus in the right atrial appendage is an underestimated cause of pulmonary embolism, especially in patients with AF.[38]

Key risk factors for atrial thrombosis include AF, mitral valve stenosis, tricuspid valve stenosis, inflammatory disorders, coagulopathy, cancer, and abnormal anatomy as seen, for example, in patients with congenital heart disease.[39] Moreover, any foreign body (pacing leads, indwelling central venous lines, occluder devices, etc.) also increases the risk of thrombosis.

Several scanning modalities (computed tomography, magnetic resonance imaging, etc.) of the chest or heart may raise the suspicion of an intracardiac thrombosis, but atrial thrombosis is most frequently diagnosed with echocardiography. Using multiple cross sections, the exact localization and size of the thrombus can be visualized. Importantly, the use of additional imaging should be considered to rule out differential diagnosis of atrial masses, including benign or malignant primary or metastatic tumours as well as valve vegetations. Contrast-enhanced computed tomography is more sensitive for detecting intraventricular thrombosis than TTE, whereas TOE is superior for detection of atrial thrombi.[40] Sometimes, differentiating a thrombus from a tumour (most frequently a myxoma) may be challenging[41] because of similar echo densities of myxoma and thrombi and, in such cases, the use of echo contrast should be considered, since contrast echocardiography helps distinguish thrombi without perfusion from tumours with varying degrees of perfusion.[42] Also, CMR provides superior specificity for evaluation of tissue characteristics and may help in differentiating thrombi from other masses.

The treatment of atrial thrombosis may include anticoagulant treatment, surgery, or catheter-based therapy[43] with the strategy depending on (1) symptoms, (2) thrombus site, (3) thrombus size, and (4) whether there is a free-floating thrombus with expected high risk of embolization.

Catheter-related thrombosis

The risk of thrombosis increases with the presence of all types of foreign body, including any type of central venous lines, haemodialysis catheters, and so on, since intravenous catheters cause endothelial trauma and inflammation and because the catheter surface may be procoagulant. Superficial vein thrombosis related to peripheral intravenous catheters are generally self-limiting once the catheter has been removed; however, some patients develop deep vein thrombosis with its inherent risk of embolism, and intracardiac CRT should not be managed conservatively.

An *intrinsic* CRT presents as an intraluminal thrombosis or a fibrin sheath thrombus surrounding the catheter, whereas an *extrinsic* thrombus forms outside the catheter and presents as atrial mural thrombosis or as central vein thrombosis, which may result in complete thrombosis of the vessel (i.e. deep vein thrombosis). Central venous thrombosis can occur in any vein through which the catheter traverses, such as the jugular, subclavian, or brachiocephalic vein, or the vena cava, and several vein segments may be involved.

Oedema, tenderness, and other classical symptoms of deep vein thrombosis are seen in CRT in the veins, whereas intracardiac thrombosis is often asymptomatic, although there may be dysfunction of the catheter. Rarely, signs and symptoms of embolization, either to the pulmonary circulation or paradoxically to the systemic arterial bed, may be the first sign of CRT.

In the presence of a venous catheter, signs and symptoms of thrombophlebitis are diagnostic for CRT, but in some cases (e.g. in the presence of catheter dysfunction but no other symptoms) imaging may be needed.[44] Diagnosing CRT with ultrasound is preferred, because it is inexpensive, non-invasive, and readily available; however, venography is more sensitive and in case of mechanical catheter problems, instillation of intravenous contrast into the catheter lumen under fluoroscopy may demonstrate a thrombus.

Risk factors for CRT include infection, a history of venous thrombosis, cancer, prothrombotic conditions, catheter malposition, chemical irritation, and multi-lumen catheters.[45] Systemic anticoagulation is the treatment of choice in most cases of CRT with the aim of relieving symptoms and preventing embolization. Low-molecular-weight heparin is most often used, but observational and smaller controlled studies have shown promising results with direct oral anticoagulants.[46] The catheter should be removed if it is no longer needed or in case of infection or catheter dysfunction. In contrast, a catheter that is functioning and for which there is an ongoing need, does not need to be removed. Systemic anticoagulation should be used if the catheter is used and for an additional 3 months after catheter removal to prevent thrombus progression. In selected cases, alternatives to systemic anticoagulation may be considered: (1) surgical thrombectomy; (2) intraluminal thrombolytic therapy (e.g. in an occluded dialysis catheter); or (3) catheter-directed therapy, such as catheter-directed or ultrasound-directed thrombolysis, or percutaneous catheter-directed suction thrombectomy. Systemic thrombolysis is not recommended.

What's new

- Recent randomized clinical trials have shown that transcatheter PFO closure reduces the risk of recurrent ischaemic stroke by about 60% in patients younger than 60–65 years with a PFO-related stroke.
- Clinical history, age, presence of risk factors for stroke, ischaemic brain infarct location, and PFO anatomy are key factors to determine the probability that an ischaemic stroke is causally linked to a PFO.
- Patients with an assumed PFO-related stroke should be individually assessed by a heart–brain team and actively involved in the decision on PFO closure.
- Oral anticoagulation is recommended over antiplatelets in patients with a PFO-related ischaemic stroke who are not eligible for transcatheter PFO closure.
- LV mural thrombus is a serious complication most often seen in association with acute myocardial infarction. Recent observational studies suggest that DOACs can be an alternative to vitamin K antagonist-based anticoagulation.
- Treatment strategies for atrial thrombi and CRT is outlined.

Guideline recommendations

- A position paper on the management of patients with PFO was published in 2019 from eight European academic societies including the European Society of Cardiology Working Group on Thrombosis.[1]

What's next

- Studies that clarify the role of transcatheter PFO closure in patients older than 60–65 years.
- Studies that clarify the role of transcatheter PFO closure in patients with an indication for anticoagulation (e.g. high-risk venous thromboembolism and thrombophilia).
- Studies that clarify the role of transcatheter PFO closure for primary prevention of stroke.
- Studies that address the potential role of PFO closure in migraine with aura.
- Studies on the long-term effects of PFO closure including the long-term risk of AF.
- Studies that clarify the role of DOACS in the treatment of LV mural thrombus.

References

1. Pristipino C, Sievert H, D'Ascenzo F, et al. European position paper on the management of patients with patent foramen ovale. General approach and left circulation thromboembolism. Eur Heart J. 2019;40(38):3182–95.
2. Andersen A, Nielsen JM, Peters CD, Schou UK, Sloth E, Nielsen-Kudsk JE. Effects of phosphodiesterase-5 inhibition by sildenafil in the pressure overloaded right heart. Eur J Heart Fail. 2008;10(12):1158–65.
3. Hart RG, Catanese L, Perera KS, Ntaios G, Connolly SJ. Embolic stroke of undetermined source: a systematic review and clinical update. Stroke. 2017;48(4):867–72.
4. Strambo D, Sirimarco G, Nannoni S, et al. Embolic stroke of undetermined source and patent foramen ovale: risk of paradoxical embolism score validation and atrial fibrillation prediction. Stroke. 2021;52(5):1643–52.
5. Carroll JD, Saver JL, Thaler DE, et al. Closure of patent foramen ovale versus medical therapy after cryptogenic stroke. N Engl J Med. 2013;368(12):1092–100.
6. Saver JL, Carroll JD, Thaler DE, et al. Long-term outcomes of patent foramen ovale closure or medical therapy after stroke. N Engl J Med. 2017;377(11):1022–32.
7. Meier B, Kalesan B, Mattle HP, et al. Percutaneous closure of patent foramen ovale in cryptogenic embolism. N Engl J Med. 2013;368(12):1083–91.
8. Sondergaard L, Kasner SE, Rhodes JF, et al. Patent foramen ovale closure or antiplatelet therapy for cryptogenic stroke. N Engl J Med. 2017;377(11):1033–42.
9. Mas JL, Derumeaux G, Guillon B, et al. Patent foramen ovale closure or anticoagulation vs. antiplatelets after stroke. N Engl J Med. 2017;377(11):1011–21.
10. Furlan AJ, Reisman M, Massaro J, et al. Closure or medical therapy for cryptogenic stroke with patent foramen ovale. N Engl J Med. 2012;366(11):991–9.
11. Lee PH, Song JK, Kim JS, et al. Cryptogenic stroke and high-risk patent foramen ovale: the DEFENSE-PFO trial. J Am Coll Cardiol. 2018;71(20):2335–42.
12. Kent DM, Saver JL, Kasner SE, et al. Heterogeneity of treatment effects in an analysis of pooled individual patient data from randomized trials of device closure of patent foramen ovale after stroke. JAMA. 2021;326(22):2277–86.
13. Aplin M, Andersen A, Brandes A, et al. Assessment of patients with a suspected cardioembolic ischemic stroke. A national consensus statement. Scand Cardiovasc J. 2021;55(5):315–25.
14. Hamann GF, Schatzer-Klotz D, Frohlig G, et al. Femoral injection of echo contrast medium may increase the sensitivity of testing for a patent foramen ovale. Neurology. 1998;50(5):1423–8.
15. Andersen A, Matzen KL, Andersen G, et al. Atrial fibrillation after closure of patent foramen ovale in the REDUCE clinical study. Catheter Cardiovasc Interv. 2022;99(5):1551–7.
16. Wintzer-Wehekind J, Alperi A, Houde C, et al. Impact of discontinuation of antithrombotic therapy following closure of patent foramen ovale in patients with cryptogenic embolism. Am J Cardiol. 2019;123(9):1538–45.
17. Homma S, Sacco RL, Di Tullio MR, Sciacca RR, Mohr JP, PFO in in Cryptogenic Stroke Study (PICSS) Investigators. Effect of medical treatment in stroke patients with patent foramen ovale: patent foramen ovale in Cryptogenic Stroke Study. Circulation. 2002;105(22): 2625–31.
18. Kasner SE, Swaminathan B, Lavados P, et al. Rivaroxaban or aspirin for patent foramen ovale and embolic stroke of undetermined source: a prespecified subgroup analysis from the NAVIGATE ESUS trial. Lancet Neurol. 2018;17(12):1053–60.
19. Krumsdorf U, Ostermayer S, Billinger K, et al. Incidence and clinical course of thrombus formation on atrial septal defect and patient foramen ovale closure devices in 1,000 consecutive patients. J Am Coll Cardiol. 2004;43(2):302–9.
20. Olasinska-Wisniewska A, Grygier M. Antithrombotic/antiplatelet treatment in transcatheter structural cardiac interventions—PFO/ASD/LAA occluder and interatrial shunt devices. Front Cardiovasc Med. 2019;6:75.
21. Bovin A, Vase H, Nielsen-Kudsk JE, Grove EL. Direct oral anticoagulants after percutaneous patent foramen ovale (PFO) closure: a call for caution. Am J Case Rep. 2020;21:e922467.
22. McCarthy CP, Murphy S, Venkateswaran RV, et al. Left ventricular thrombus: contemporary etiologies, treatment strategies, and outcomes. J Am Coll Cardiol. 2019;73(15):2007–9.
23. Camaj A, Fuster V, Giustino G, et al. Left ventricular thrombus following acute myocardial infarction: JACC state-of-the-art review. J Am Coll Cardiol. 2022;79(10):1010–22.
24. Allard L, Bernhard B, Windecker S, Valgimigli M, Grani C. Left ventricular thrombus in ischaemic heart disease: diagnosis, treatment and gaps of knowledge. Eur Heart J Qual Care Clin Outcomes. 2022;8(5):496–509.
25. Zhang Q, Zhang Z, Jin L, et al. Prognosis and new predictors of early left-ventricular thrombus following ST-elevation myocardial infarction. Int J Gen Med. 2021;14:8991–9000.
26. Driesman A, Hyder O, Lang C, Stockwell P, Poppas A, Abbott JD. Incidence and predictors of left ventricular thrombus after primary percutaneous coronary intervention for anterior ST-segment elevation myocardial infarction. Clin Cardiol. 2015;38(10):590–7.
27. Ibanez B, James S, Agewall S, et al. 2017 ESC Guidelines for the management of acute myocardial infarction in patients presenting with ST-segment elevation: the Task Force for the management of acute myocardial infarction in patients presenting with ST-segment elevation of the European Society of Cardiology (ESC). Eur Heart J. 2018;39(2):119–77.
28. Bulluck H, Chan MHH, Paradies V, et al. Incidence and predictors of left ventricular thrombus by cardiovascular magnetic resonance in acute ST-segment elevation myocardial infarction treated by primary percutaneous coronary intervention: a meta-analysis. J Cardiovasc Magn Reson. 2018;20(1):72.
29. Roifman I, Connelly KA, Wright GA, Wijeysundera HC. Echocardiography vs. cardiac magnetic resonance imaging for the diagnosis of left ventricular thrombus: a systematic review. Can J Cardiol. 2015;31(6):785–91.
30. Singh M, Aldiwani H, Abidov A. Utilization of coronary computed tomography angiogram in evaluation of left ventricular thrombus. J Cardiovasc Comput Tomogr. 2020;14(5):e82–4.
31. Robinson AA, Jain A, Gentry M, McNamara RL. Left ventricular thrombi after STEMI in the primary PCI era: a systematic review and meta-analysis. Int J Cardiol. 2016;221:554–9.
32. Homma S, Thompson JL, Pullicino PM, et al. Warfarin and aspirin in patients with heart failure and sinus rhythm. N Engl J Med. 2012;366(20):1859–69.
33. O'Gara PT, Kushner FG, Ascheim DD, et al. 2013 ACCF/AHA guideline for the management of ST-elevation myocardial infarction: a report of the American College of Cardiology Foundation/American Heart Association Task Force on Practice Guidelines. J Am Coll Cardiol. 2013;61(4):e78–140.
34. Lattuca B, Bouziri N, Kerneis M, et al. Antithrombotic therapy for patients with left ventricular mural thrombus. J Am Coll Cardiol. 2020;75(14):1676–85.

35. Andreotti F, Testa L, Biondi-Zoccai GG, Crea F. Aspirin plus warfarin compared to aspirin alone after acute coronary syndromes: an updated and comprehensive meta-analysis of 25,307 patients. Eur Heart J. 2006;27(5):519–26.
36. Vaitkus PT, Barnathan ES. Embolic potential, prevention and management of mural thrombus complicating anterior myocardial infarction: a meta-analysis. J Am Coll Cardiol. 1993;22(4):1004–9.
37. Alcalai R, Butnaru A, Moravsky G, et al. Apixaban versus warfarin in patients with left ventricular thrombus, a prospective multicenter randomized clinical trial. Eur Heart J Cardiovasc Pharmacother. 2022;8(7):660–7.
38. Anfinogenova ND, Vasiltseva OY, Vrublevsky AV, et al. Right atrial thrombosis and pulmonary embolism: a narrative review. Semin Thromb Hemost. 2020;46(8):895–907.
39. Silvey M, Brandão LR. Risk factors, prophylaxis, and treatment of venous thromboembolism in congenital heart disease patients. Front Pediatr. 2017;5:146.
40. de Bruijn SF, Agema WR, Lammers GJ, et al. Transesophageal echocardiography is superior to transthoracic echocardiography in management of patients of any age with transient ischemic attack or stroke. Stroke. 2006;37(10):2531–4.
41. Grove EL. Large atrial mass in a patient with Crohn's disease: organised thrombus mimicking a myxoma. BMJ Case Rep. 2017;2017:bcr2017222044.
42. Kirkpatrick JN, Wong T, Bednarz JE, et al. Differential diagnosis of cardiac masses using contrast echocardiographic perfusion imaging. J Am Coll Cardiol. 2004;43(8):1412–19.
43. Schultz J, Andersen A, Grove EL, Ilkjær LB, Nielsen-Kudsk JE. Large solid right atrial thrombus treated by angiovac catheter-based suction thrombectomy. Case Rep Cardiol. 2018;2018:7904064.
44. Gunawansa N, Sudusinghe DH, Wijayaratne DR. Hemodialysis catheter-related central venous thrombosis: clinical approach to evaluation and management. Ann Vasc Surg. 2018;51:298–305.
45. Liu GD, Ma WJ, Liu HX, Tang L, Tan YH. Risk factors associated with catheter-related venous thrombosis: a meta-analysis. Public Health. 2022;205:45–54.
46. Marin A, Bull L, Kinzie M, Andresen M. Central catheter-associated deep vein thrombosis in cancer: clinical course, prophylaxis, treatment. BMJ Support Palliat Care. 2021;11(4):371–80.

CHAPTER 20

Atrial fibrillation: current and forthcoming antithrombotic therapies

Raffaele De Caterina and Rossella Marcucci

Contents

Summary

Atrial fibrillation is the most common sustained arrhythmia, involving up to 1 out of 10 patients beyond 80 years of age. Its prevalence is increasing, only partly explained by the ageing of the population. Atrial fibrillation is a thrombogenic condition, with blood stasis in the left atrium/left atrial appendage and local structural abnormalities in the atrial walls favouring thrombus formation and distal embolization in the arterial circulation, causing 20–25% of ischaemic strokes. The risk of stroke in patients with atrial fibrillation is widely variable, from less than 1/100 patient-years (indistinguishable from the risk of the average population without the arrhythmia) to greater than 10/100 patient-years, depending on well-characterized risk factors, some of which are modifiable. Risk scores, such as the CHA_2DS_2-VASc, help in stratifying ischaemic risk, but are even more useful to identify patients who do not derive benefit—and possibly derive harm—from antithrombotic treatments. Anticoagulants are here the antithrombotic treatment of choice, and are clearly superior to aspirin for stroke prevention. In recent years, with few exceptions, the non-vitamin K antagonist oral anticoagulants have largely replaced vitamin K antagonists such as warfarin for stroke prevention, being at least equally effective and safer. An emerging role for stroke prevention is that of left atrial appendage occlusion, either percutaneous or surgical.

Introduction

Atrial fibrillation—definitions

Atrial fibrillation (AF) is a supraventricular tachyarrhythmia characterized by uncoordinated atrial activation with consequent deterioration of atrial mechanical function. AF features atrial wavelets propagating in different directions, causing disorganized atrial depolarization without effective atrial contraction.[1] On the electrocardiogram, AF is described by the replacement of consistent P waves by rapid oscillations (fibrillatory ('*f*') waves) that vary in size, shape, and timing, at a rate of 350–600 beats/min, associated with an irregular, frequently rapid ventricular response when atrioventricular conduction is intact.[2] The ventricular response to AF depends on the electrophysiological properties of the atrioventricular node, the level of vagal and sympathetic tone, and the action of drugs.[1]

By convention, an episode lasting at least 30 seconds or for an entire 12-lead electrocardiogram is considered diagnostic for clinical AF.[3] An emerging clinical condition is that of atrial high-rate episodes, which refers to the detection of high-rate episodes by various implanted devices or wearable monitors.[4] When occurring in the absence of symptoms, these configure the entity of 'subclinical AF', which is attracting a great deal of attention as a possible hidden cause of stroke.[3]

Pathophysiological mechanisms

Important progress in understanding AF mechanisms and thrombogenicity today considers the role of atrial cardiomyopathy, that is, atrial structural changes preceding and accompanying AF, with potentially relevant clinical manifestations[5] (these concepts are covered in detail in ➔ Chapter 3). Indeed, the atria of patients with AF display structural abnormalities beyond changes caused by the underlying heart disease.[5] Histological examinations have shown patchy fibrosis with juxtaposition of normal and diseased atrial fibres, which may account for the non-homogeneity of atrial refractoriness.[6] Fibrosis or fatty infiltration may also affect the sinus node, and may be a reaction to inflammatory or degenerative processes that are difficult to detect. The role of inflammation in the pathogenesis of AF has not yet been evaluated, but histological changes consistent with myocarditis were reported in 66% of atrial biopsy specimens from patients with lone AF,[6] and is supported by epidemiological data linking the use of steroidal and non-steroidal anti-inflammatory drugs with AF.[7] Atrial fibre hypertrophy has been described as a major feature in AF patients.[6] Atrial hypertrophy and dilatation may be either a cause or a consequence of persistent AF, because progressive atrial enlargement and changes in atrial contractility have been demonstrated echocardiographically.[8,9] Experimental studies have shown that heart failure facilitates the induction of sustained AF, mediated by extensive interstitial fibrosis.[10] In most patients, however, it is not possible to identify the underlying anatomical process responsible for the arrhythmia.

Importantly, AF is not only a risk factor for but also a marker of atrial cardiomyopathy, which could explain the lack of temporal relationship between detected AF and stroke.[11] More data are needed to define prognostic and treatment implications of the different atrial cardiomyopathy morphofunctional forms. It is clear, however, that there is a continuum from the initial alterations, possibly triggered by external factors (i.e. concomitant infective or inflammatory processes) to a stable condition sustained by permanent risk factors (i.e. hypertension), to the finally completed altered atrial structure that maintains a chronic alteration of the rhythm no longer modifiable by drugs or ablation procedures.

Classification

The pattern of AF may be defined in terms of the number of episodes, duration, frequency, mode of onset and possible triggers, and response to therapy, although these features are difficult to discern when AF is first encountered in an individual patient.

The most recent classification proposed by the European Society of Cardiology (ESC)[3] is the following:

- First diagnosed AF: when a patient presents AF for the first time, irrespective of the duration of the arrhythmia or the presence and severity of AF-related symptoms.
- Paroxysmal AF: when AF is self-terminating, usually within 48 hours. Although AF paroxysms may continue for up to 7 days, the 48-hour time point is clinically important because after this the likelihood of spontaneous conversion is low and anticoagulation must be considered.
- Persistent AF: when AF episodes either last longer than 7 days or require termination by either pharmacological or electrical cardioversion.
- Long-standing persistent AF: when AF has lasted for at least 1 year when adopting a rhythm control strategy is decided.
- Permanent AF: when the presence of AF is accepted by the patient (and the physician). Hence, rhythm control interventions are, by definition, not pursued in patients with permanent AF. Should a rhythm control strategy be adopted, the arrhythmia is redesignated as 'long-standing persistent AF'.

Terminology that should be abandoned includes lone AF, valvular/non-valvular AF, and chronic AF.

Epidemiology

AF is the most sustained arrhythmia encountered in clinical practice, accounting for approximately one-third of hospitalizations for cardiac rhythm disturbances.

AF affects 1–2% of the population[12] and its incidence appears to be increasing. The prevalence of AF increases with age, from <0.5% at 40–50 years to 5–15% at 80 years.[12,13] The age-adjusted prevalence is higher in men.[14] AF is most common in patients with congestive heart failure or valvular heart disease (VHD), and increases in prevalence with the severity of these conditions. The frequency of AF in patients with no history of cardiopulmonary disease ('lone' AF) varies from less than 12% of all cases of AF[15] to over 30% in some series.[16,17]

Secular trends of AF prevalence are informative of the epidemiology of this arrhythmia. In a study evaluating the prevalence rates of AF in patients with incident stroke and in age- and sex-matched controls over a 30-year period in a population of Rochester, Minnesota, USA,[18] consistent with other studies,[15,19–21] the authors observed that age is a potent risk factor for the development of AF: each decade of age was associated with a doubling of the odds for AF. However, even after adjustment for age, the prevalence of AF increased significantly during a 22-year period among men in the Framingham study[22] and during a 30-year period among men and women in the Rochester study.[18] The authors suggest that changes over time in the prevalence of comorbid conditions, such as hypertension, coronary heart disease, diabetes mellitus, and heart failure, may play an important role in the origin and propagation of this epidemic. Therefore, on the one hand an increasing number of persons now reach the age at which the risk of AF becomes common; on the other hand, a significantly higher proportion of the elderly population have comorbidities, which in themselves are risk factors for the development of AF. A possible pathophysiological link between these conditions and the development of AF is diastolic dysfunction, identified as a predictor of non-valvular AF.[23] Another explanation of the increasing prevalence of AF may be the increasing prevalence of VHD over time. Such an increasing prevalence is not only due to increased diagnosis, due to a more widespread use of echocardiography, but also to an actual increase in the number of older individuals developing degenerative valve disease.[24] Finally, other factors, such as alcohol consumption, sleep apnoea, thyroid disorders, infection, or pulmonary disease, which undoubtedly have themselves multiple causes, can also affect secular trends in the prevalence of AF.

A previous lifetime AF risk estimate of one in four individuals,[14,25] was recently revised to one in three individuals of European ancestry at index age of 55 years.[26,27] The observed impact of clinical risk factor burden/multiple comorbidities on AF risk suggests that an early intervention and modifiable risk factor control could reduce incident AF.

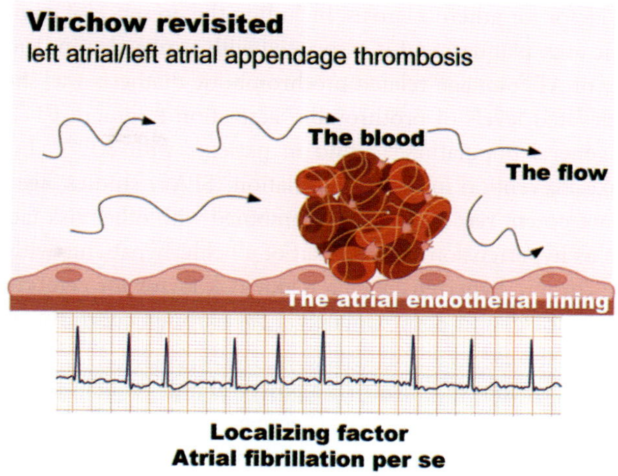

Figure 20.1 The pathophysiology of stroke in AF implicating stasis and thrombus formation in a structurally abnormal and dilated atrium, and possibly favoured by thrombophilia (this last factor is still of uncertain value), reproducing Virchow's triad.

Patient management

The simple Atrial fibrillation Better Care (ABC) holistic pathway ('A', Anticoagulation/Avoid stroke; 'B', Better symptom management; 'C', Cardiovascular and Comorbidity optimization)[3,28] streamlines integrated care of AF patients across all healthcare levels and among different specialties. In the prospective, randomized mobile AF Application (mAFA)-II trial, the composite outcome was significantly lowered with ABC pathway management intervention compared with usual care.[29]

The thromboembolic risk in atrial fibrillation

AF is an independent risk factor for stroke: overall, it confers a fivefold higher risk to affected patients compared with the unaffected population. One in five of all strokes is attributed to this arrhythmia.[30,31] Ischaemic strokes in association with AF are often fatal, and the survivors are more disabled and more likely suffer a recurrence than patients with other causes of stroke. The annualized stroke rate is about 3.2–3.3%, and has been considered similar in patients with paroxysmal AF and in patients with permanent AF.[32] Although an association of AF burden with AF-related outcomes has been more recently proposed,[33] it is insufficient to guide treatment and should not be factored in treatment decisions.[3]

The pathophysiology of stroke in AF traditionally implicates stasis and thrombus formation in a structurally abnormal and dilated atrium because of the contribution of the three factors of Virchow's triad: blood stasis, parietal abnormalities (endothelial dysfunction), and blood hypercoagulability[34] (➔ Figure 20.1). The occlusion of a cerebral artery would be thus due to an embolus dislodged from the left atrium. Thrombi arise most frequently in the left atrial appendage (LAA), the morphology and function of which can be assessed by transoesophageal echocardiography (TOE), computed cardiac tomography, or magnetic resonance imaging.[35] TOE demonstrates reduced flow velocities (stasis) in the LAA related to the loss of organized mechanical contractions and associated with the presence of spontaneous echo-contrast.[36,37] Endothelial dysfunction has been difficult to demonstrate as a distinct mechanism contributing to thrombus formation in patients with AF: increased levels of von Willebrand factor in the systemic circulation and in the atrial tissue in some patients may prove the existence of this mechanism.[38] Biochemical markers of coagulation and platelet activation may reflect a systemic hypercoagulable state associated with AF. Systemic fibrinogen degradation products and fibrin D-dimer levels, indicating active intravascular thrombogenesis, are increased in both permanent and paroxysmal AF; elevated beta-thromboglobulin and platelet factor 4 (PF4) in selected patients indicate platelet activation, but these data are relatively weak.[38] Such biochemical markers of coagulation and platelet activation do not distinguish between a reactive process secondary to intravascular coagulation and a primary hypercoagulable state. Some investigations suggest that AF may itself cause a hypercoagulable state[39,40] and that hypercoagulable state may be a 'marker' for other conditions predisposing to stroke (➔ Figure 20.1).

The rate of stroke is higher in patients with prior stroke or transient ischaemic attack[30,41] and in patients with mitral stenosis.[42] In subjects with AF in the absence of structural heart disease, the risk of stroke is largely governed by the presence and extent of additional risk factors. Cohort data, as well as the non-warfarin arms of clinical trials, have identified clinical and echocardiographic risk factors that can be related to an increased risk of stroke in AF. The frequency of stroke related to AF increases with age.[31] The effect of ageing in increasing the risk of stroke in AF is multifactorial: in such patients, ageing is associated with left atrial enlargement, reduced flow velocity in the LAA, and the presence of spontaneous echo-contrast.[8,43,44] Moreover, age is a risk factor for atherosclerosis, including the presence of complex aortic arch plaques, and is associated with stroke also independently of AF[45]; an age-related prothrombotic diathesis was shown by elevated levels of prothrombin activation fragment F1+2, in the general population[46–48] and in patients with AF.[49,50] In the Stroke Prevention in Atrial Fibrillation (SPAF) studies, age was a more potent risk factor when combined with other risk factors such as hypertension[50]: about half of all elderly patients with AF have chronic hypertension,[51] a major risk factor for cerebrovascular disease, and approximately 12% harbour cervical carotid artery stenoses.[52]

Hypertension, specifically, is a powerful independent predictor of stroke in patients with non-rheumatic AF,[51,53] and a history of hypertension was strongly associated with findings of left atrial stasis and the presence of thrombi at TOE and of complex aortic plaques, which all determine a high risk of thromboembolism.[54] Diabetes has also emerged as a risk factor for stroke,[55] although diabetes appears to be an extremely inhomogeneous condition, with insulin-treated diabetes mostly driving thromboembolic risk.[56,57]

Two systematic reviews[58,59] confirmed that prior stroke/transient ischaemic attack/thromboembolism, age, hypertension, diabetes, and structural heart disease are important risk factors. The presence of moderate-to-severe left ventricular systolic dysfunction on two-dimensional transthoracic echocardiography is considered the only independent echocardiographic risk factor for stroke on multivariable analysis, while on TOE the presence of left atrial thrombus, complex aortic plaques, spontaneous echocontrast, and low LAA velocities are independent predictors of stroke and thromboembolism.

Patients aged less than 60 years, with 'lone AF', that is, no clinical history or echocardiographic evidence of cardiovascular disease and no other risk factors, carry a very low cumulative stroke risk, estimated to be 1.3% over 15 years, similar to that of the overall population. However, it was recently emphasized that age as a risk factor is not a 'yes/no' phenomenon and the probability of stroke starts to rise from age over 65 years, and becomes very evident in patients aged 75 years and older (even with no other associated risk factors).[58,59] Also, the development of hypertension can modify the risk together with the advancing age. Some other risk factors were more recently highlighted[60]: moderate-to-severe left ventricular systolic dysfunction can be considered a risk factor for thromboembolism, while the presence of clinical sign and symptoms of heart failure with preserved ejection fraction cannot be strongly related to the risk; the presence of atherosclerotic vascular disease [myocardial infarction (but not angina per se), peripheral artery disease, complex aortic plaques in the descending aorta seen at TOE] may contribute to stroke risk; female sex also confers a higher risk of thromboembolism in patients with AF, although only in the presence of other risk factors.[3]

Atrial fibrillation and valvular heart disease

VHD is independently associated with AF, and more than one-third of patients with AF have some form of VHD.[61] Compared to AF patients without VHD, the risk of thromboembolism and stroke is higher among AF patients with VHD other than mitral stenosis and mechanical heart prostheses, mostly attributed to older age and more frequent comorbidities. The presence of some forms of VHD has implications for the use of non-vitamin K antagonist oral anticoagulants (NOACs). While patients with moderate-to-severe mitral stenosis (even without AF)[62] and patients with a mechanical prosthetic heart valve (➔ Chapter 17) require anticoagulation with vitamin K antagonists (VKAs), there is no evidence that the presence of other VHDs including aortic stenosis/regurgitation, mitral regurgitation, bioprostheses, or valve repair should modify the choice of oral anticoagulant (OAC).[63,64] In a meta-analysis of the four pivotal randomized controlled trials (RCTs) comparing NOACs with VKAs, the effects of NOACs versus VKAs in terms of stroke/systemic embolism and bleeding risk in patients with VHD other than mitral stenosis and mechanical prosthetic heart valves were consistent with those in the main RCTs.[65] In an observational study, NOACs were associated with better outcomes, with reduced rates of ischaemic stroke and major bleeding compared to warfarin in AF patients with mitral stenosis.[66] Such results are confirmed in the RIvaroxaban in mitral stenosis (RISE MS), a small randomized controlled trial with rivaroxaban versus warfarin.[67] Because of these considerations, the previously used terminology of 'valvular' versus 'non-valvular' AF should be abandoned, and recommendations restricted to specific subsets of VHD (➔ Table 20.1).

Atrial fibrillation without valvular heart disease

Assessing risk factors for stroke over time is crucial to optimize antithrombotic therapy in patients with AF. Prior stroke, transient ischaemic attack, or thromboembolism and age 75 years or older should be considered as 'major risk factors', together with the presence of some types of VHD (mitral stenosis or prosthetic mechanical heart valves). Heart failure [moderate-to-severe left ventricular systolic dysfunction, this latter arbitrarily defined as left ventricular ejection fraction ≤40%], hypertension, diabetes, age 65–74 years, vascular disease (myocardial infarction, peripheral artery disease, and the presence of complex aortic plaques), and female sex were once defined

Table 20.1 Specific settings of valvular heart disease with implications for the use of the non-vitamin K antagonist oral anticoagulants in patients with atrial fibrillation

Setting	Recommendation
Atrial fibrillation in the presence of a mechanical heart valve	Non-vitamin K oral anticoagulants are *contraindicated* in patients with a prosthetic *mechanical* valve
Atrial fibrillation in the presence of mitral stenosis	Use of non-vitamin K oral anticoagulants is *not* recommended in patients with atrial fibrillation and *moderate to severe mitral stenosis*

as 'clinically relevant non-major risk factors'.[60] Risk factors are cumulative, and this risk factor-based approach for patients with non-valvular AF can be summarized in risk assessment schemes, the simplest of which, and currently the one most in use, is the CHA_2DS_2-VASc score (➔ Table 20.2), an evolution of the former $CHADS_2$ score, and based on a point system in which 2 points are assigned to 'major risk factors' and 1 point each is assigned to 'clinically relevant non-major risk factors'. Proper antithrombotic therapy can be decided according to the patient's risk score.

As any clinical risk-factor-based score, CHA_2DS_2-VASc performs only modestly in predicting high-risk patients who will sustain thromboembolic events, but clearly identifies those at low risk. Indeed CHA_2DS_2-VASc scores = 0 (males), or = 1 (females) consistently have shown a very low risk of ischaemic stroke or mortality. Female sex is an age-dependent 'stroke risk modifier' rather than a risk factor per se. Observational studies have indeed shown that women with no other risk factors (CHA_2DS_2-VASc score = 1) have a low stroke risk, similar to men with a CHA_2DS_2-VASc score = 0.[68] The simplified CHA_2DS_2-VA score could guide the initial decision about OAC in AF patients, but not considering the sex component would underestimate stroke risk in women with AF.[69,70] This would be, however, only a minor limitation considering that the main purposes of these scores is to decide on the few patients with AF who should *not* be anticoagulated. In the presence of more than one non-sex stroke risk factor, women with AF consistently have significantly higher stroke risk than men.

Other scores, such as the ATRIA,[71] the R2CHADS,[72] the ABC[73] and ABC-AF,[74] the CHADS65,[75] a combination of CHA_2DS_2-VASc and HAS-BLED,[76] and others have been found in some reports of comparable or even better predictive power compared with the CHA_2DS_2-VASc. Because of the above considerations and the limited need for additional precision, their use is currently very low.

Table 20.2 The $CHADS_2$ and the CHA_2DS_2-VASc scores

$CHADS_2$		CHA_2DS_2-VASc	
Risk factor	**Score**	**Risk factor**	**Score**
Congestive heart failure/LV dysfunction	1	Congestive heart failure/LV dysfunction	1
Hypertension	1	Hypertension	1
Age ≥75 years	1	Age ≥75 years	2
Diabetes mellitus	1	Diabetes mellitus	1
Stroke/TIA/ thromboembolism	2	Stroke/TIA/ thromboembolism	2
		Vascular disease	1
		Age 65–74	1
		Sex category (female sex)	1

LV, left ventricular, TIA, transient ischaemic attack.

Risk of bleeding

Antithrombotic therapies—of any kind—confer an increased risk of bleeding. The most dreadful one is that of intracerebral haemorrhage, the rates of which are now considerably lower than in the past, ranging between 0.1 and 0.6 per 100 patient-years in contemporary reports,[60] probably reflecting lower anticoagulation intensity, more careful dose regulation, or better control of hypertension. Intracranial bleeding, including epidural haematoma, subdural haematoma, subarachnoid haemorrhage, and intracerebral haemorrhage, increases with international normalized ratio (INR) values greater than 3.5–4.0, while there is apparently no increase in bleeding risk with INR values between 2.0 and 3.0 compared with lower INR levels. The assessment of patient's basal bleeding risk is very important to minimize bleeding events. Various bleeding risk scores have been validated for bleeding risk in anticoagulated patients, with different components and leading to different stratifications. A simple bleeding risk score, HAS-BLED (➔ Table 20.3), was proposed in 2010,[77] and is now very popular, although not as accurate as one would wish.

A HAS-BLED score of 3 or greater indicates 'high risk' and would imply caution and regular review of the patient following the initiation of any antithrombotic therapy. A formal assessment of bleeding risk informs management of patients taking OAC, focusing attention on modifiable bleeding risk factors that should be managed and assessed at every patient contact, and identifying high-risk patients with non-modifiable bleeding risk factors who should be reviewed earlier (e.g. in 4 weeks rather than at 4–6 months) and more frequently.[78] A high bleeding risk score should not exempt AF patients from anticoagulation.[3]

Table 20.3 The HAS-BLED bleeding risk score

Letter	Definitions		Points
H	Hypertension	Systolic blood pressure >160 mmHg	1
A	Abnormal renal and liver function (1 point each)	Renal, defined as the presence of chronic dialysis or renal transplantation or serum creatinine ≥200 mmol/L; liver, defined as chronic hepatic disease or biochemical evidence of significant hepatic derangement (e.g. bilirubin >2 × upper normal limit, in association with aspartate aminotransferase/alanine aminotransferase/alkaline phosphatase >3 × upper normal limit, etc.)	1 or 2
S	Stroke	Stroke	1
B	Bleeding		1
L	Labile INRs	Unstable/high INRs or poor time in therapeutic range (e.g. <60%)	1
E	Elderly	E.g. age >65 years	1
D	Drugs or alcohol (1 point each)	Antiplatelet agents, non-steroidal anti-inflammatory drugs, or alcohol abuse, etc.	1 or 2

INR, international normalized ratio.

Table 20.4 Risk factors for bleeding

Non-modifiable	Potentially modifiable	Modifiable
Age >65 years	Extreme frailty	Hypertension/elevated systolic blood pressure
Previous major bleeding	Anaemia	concomitant antiplatelet agent/ NSAIDs
Dialysis or renal transplant	Reduced platelet count or function	Excessive alcohol intake
Cirrhosis	Creatinine clearance <60 mL/min	Non-adherence to oral anticoagulation
Malignancy		Hazardous hobbies/ occupations
Previous stroke		Bridging therapy with heparins
Cognitive impairment/ dementia		TTR on VKA
		Choice and dosage of the OAC

NSAIDs, non-steroidal anti-inflammatory agents; OAC, oral anticoagulant; TTR, time in therapeutic range; VKA, vitamin K antagonist.

Non-modifiable and partially modifiable bleeding risk factors (➔ Table 20.4) are important drivers of bleeding events in synergy with modifiable factors. Notably, and at variance from previous statements, a history of falls is not an independent predictor of bleeding on OAC: a study estimated that a patient would need to fall 295 times per year to allow the benefits of ischaemic stroke reduction with OAC to be outweighed by the potential for serious bleeding.[79]

The few absolute contraindications to OAC include active serious bleeding (where the source should then be identified and treated), associated comorbidities (e.g. severe thrombocytopenia at <50,000 platelets/μL, severe anaemia under investigation, and coagulopathies), or a recent high-risk bleeding event such as an intracranial haemorrhage.

Several other risk scores for bleeding have been proposed (comprehensively reviewed[80]), including ATRIA, ORBIT, and the ABC-bleeding risk scores, some of which, such as the ABC-bleeding risk score,[81] use circulating biomarkers to refine risk prediction. It has been pointed out that a high bleeding risk score should not lead to withholding OAC, 'as the net clinical benefit of OAC is even greater among such patients. However, the formal assessment of bleeding risk informs management of patients taking OAC, focusing attention on modifiable bleeding risk factors that should be managed and (re)assessed at every patient contact, and identifying high-risk patients with non-modifiable bleeding risk factors who should be reviewed earlier (for instance in 4 weeks rather than 4–6 months) and more frequently'.[3]

Antithrombotic therapies

These comprise pharmacological and non-pharmacological options. Among the former are OACs (including the VKAs and the NOACs), parenteral anticoagulants (heparins), and antiplatelet agents.

Vitamin K antagonists

Several clinical trials have provided an extensive evidence base for the use of antithrombotic therapy in AF. VKAs (including warfarin, acenocoumarol, phenprocoumon, and phenindione[82]) showed a 64% relative risk reduction of stroke compared with placebo,[83] despite being associated with a substantial higher risk for major bleeding (~1.2% per year), and have many pharmacokinetic limitations affecting their practical use.[82] VKAs are currently, however, the only treatment with established safety in AF patients with rheumatic mitral valve disease and/or mechanical heart valves.

VKA use entails a substantial risk of major bleeding, including intracranial haemorrhage, and they have a narrow therapeutic window, necessitating frequent coagulation monitoring to ensure appropriate dosing.[84] The marked variability in the dose–response relationship of OACs makes it unusually difficult to remain within the ideal INR range, which is 2–3 in the vast majority of AF patients. Absorption from the gastrointestinal tract of the various coumarin derivatives is generally quite good, but their dose response is influenced by many other factors, including (1) numerous drug interactions, (2) the dietary intake of vitamin K, (3) hepatic dysfunction, (4) changes in the gut flora, (5) patient compliance, and (6) alcohol intake. These factors are common, so that even within the controlled setting of older clinical trials it was not possible to stay within the therapeutic window [time in therapeutic range (TTR)] more than 50% of the time.[85] In more modern times, the highest TTR achieved for warfarin in a large RCT has been 68.4% of the treatment period (interquartile range, 56.5%–77.4%), as reported for the ENGAGE AF-TIMI 48 study.[86] Thus, even in the setting of a carefully conducted RCT, patients stay out of the therapeutic range more than 30% of the time.

This creates the necessity of unpleasant, frequent, and assiduous monitoring of the prothrombin time in every patient treated with OACs in order to reduce the risk of serious bleeding on the one hand, and of undertreatment on the other. Even with careful monitoring, patient selection is required to screen out patients who might be at increased risk of haemorrhage.[22,50,87,88] Several trials used some criteria to exclude patients from enrolment: dementia, elevated creatinine, anaemia with haemoglobin less than 100 g/L, blood pressure greater than 180/100 mmHg despite treatment, severe chronic alcoholism, previous intracranial haemorrhage, severe bleeding with a therapeutic INR while receiving a VKA, predisposition to head trauma, and requirement for non-steroidal anti-inflammatory drugs.[89–92] Patients with such risk features are common, limiting the viability of VKAs in the presence of reasonable alternatives.

The narrow therapeutic window of warfarin and other VKAs may be influenced by genetic variation. Single-nucleotide polymorphisms in the vitamin K epoxide reductase complex subunit 1 (VKORC1), one target enzyme of warfarin, were shown to be associated with the dose of warfarin required to achieve a target INR value.[93] Also genetic variants of cytochrome

P450 (CYP) were shown to affect warfarin dose requirements: patients requiring a low dose of warfarin on the basis of INR values and having an increased risk for haemorrhage during warfarin therapy, presumably because they metabolized the drug more slowly, often carry variant alleles of CYP2C9[94]; conversely, persons carrying a genetic variant in CYP4F2 might require an increase in the warfarin dose.[95] It has been suggested that testing patients for variations in VKORC1, CYP2C9, and CYP4F2 might provide information that might enhance clinical algorithms currently used to guide warfarin administration,[96] but such a pharmacogenetic approach is cumbersome and never proved really practical and effective.

Other reasons why VKAs for AF are so poorly tolerated and actually impractical for many patients include the clear disadvantage of having to be tied to the medical system for lifelong anticoagulation monitoring, with restriction of travelling, anxiety, cost, and loss of freedom, the need to avoid most non-steroidal anti-inflammatory drugs, to carefully control alcohol consumption, and of exerting caution in the use of other drugs and in changing dietary patterns because of potential drug interactions.

In summary, therapy with VKAs is complex, potentially dangerous, and unpleasant, and this has resulted in considerable difficulty in convincing physicians and patients to adhere to current practice guidelines, with a resulting undertreatment in a considerable proportion of patients at risk.[97]

Non-vitamin K antagonist oral anticoagulants

In four pivotal RCTs, dabigatran,[98] rivaroxaban,[99] apixaban,[100] and edoxaban[86] have all shown non-inferiority compared with warfarin in the prevention of stroke/systemic embolism. In a meta-analysis of these RCTs, NOACs were associated with a 19% significant stroke/systemic embolism risk reduction, a 51% reduction in haemorrhagic stroke, and similar ischaemic stroke risk reduction compared with VKAs, but NOACs were also associated with a significant 10% reduction in all-cause mortality.[101] There was a non-significant 14% reduction in major bleeding risk, a significant 52% reduction in intracranial haemorrhage, and a 25% increase in gastrointestinal bleeding with NOACs versus warfarin[101] (➔ Figure 20.2). All the four NOACs currently marketed have an absolute contraindication in patients with a mechanical heart valve (with or without AF), and are not advised (because of insufficient data) in patients with AF accompanying mitral stenosis (➔ Table 20.1).

Dabigatran etexilate (see also ➔ Chapter 10) is an oral prodrug that is rapidly converted by a serum esterase to dabigatran, a potent, direct, competitive inhibitor of thrombin. Dabigatran

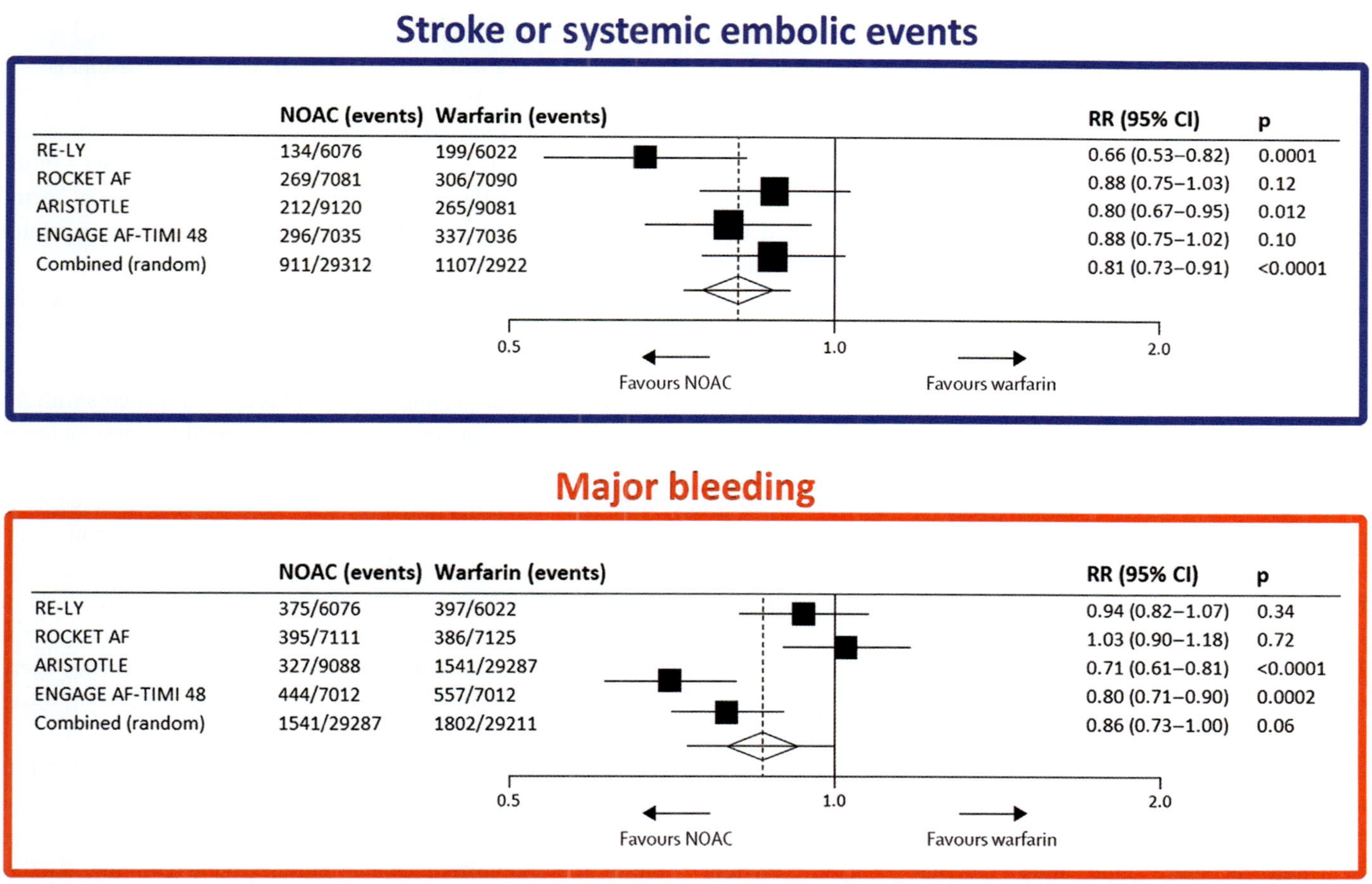

Figure 20.2 Efficacy and safety endpoints of the phase III trials comparing NOACs and warfarin in patients with atrial fibrillation. CI, confidence interval.
Reproduced from Ruff CT, Giugliano RP, Braunwald E, et al. Comparison of the efficacy and safety of new oral anticoagulants with warfarin in patients with atrial fibrillation: a meta-analysis of randomised trials. Lancet. 2014 Mar 15;383(9921):955–62. doi: 10.1016/S0140-6736(13)62343-0 with permission from Elsevier.

etexilate has an absolute bioavailability of 6.5%. Eighty per cent of the given dose is excreted by the kidneys, its serum half-life is 12–17 hours; the therapeutic window is fairly wide and it has therefore been tested in fixed doses (110 and 150 mg twice daily), not requiring regular monitoring.[102]

For patients with AF, dabigatran etexilate was evaluated in the Randomized Evaluation of Long-term anticoagulant therapY (RE-LY) trial,[98] a prospective, multicentre, parallel-group, non-inferiority trial comparing the efficacy and safety of two blinded doses of dabigatran etexilate with open-label warfarin for the prevention of stroke and systemic embolism in patients with non-valvular AF. At a dose of 150 mg twice daily, dabigatran etexilate was associated with lower rates of stroke and systemic embolism, with similar rates of major haemorrhage compared with VKA; at a dose of 110 mg twice daily the drug was non-inferior to VKA for the prevention of stroke and systemic embolism, with lower rates of major bleeding. Particularly, the rate of intracranial haemorrhage, the most devastating complication of warfarin therapy, with both doses of dabigatran etexilate, was less than one-third the rate with warfarin, without a reduction in the efficacy against ischaemic stroke, suggesting for the first time an important advantage of a NOAC as to this ominous side effect of anticoagulation. Gastrointestinal bleeding, however, was slightly increased with dabigatran 150 mg twice daily. There was a trend to higher rates of myocardial infarction with both dabigatran doses. Total mortality was similar for dabigatran and warfarin. Dabigatran has also been tested in a phase II trial against warfarin in patients with mechanical heart valves, with or without AF.[103] In that study, doses of 150, 210, and 300 mg twice daily were used, both in patients who had undergone aortic or mitral valve replacement within the past 7 days and in those who had undergone such replacement at least 3 months earlier. Warfarin in the control arm was titrated according to standard recommendations. Dabigatran was associated with increased rates of thromboembolic and bleeding complications, as compared with warfarin, thus showing no benefit and an excess risk,[103] warranting a class III recommendation at this time for all the NOACs[3] (➔ Table 20.1 and see also ➔ Chapter 17), despite that factor (F)-Xa inhibitors, potentially more similar to warfarin in interfering upstream with the coagulation cascade, might still warrant experiments in this setting.[104]

Apixaban, rivaroxaban, and edoxaban (see also ➔ Chapter 11) are direct inhibitors of FXa, as they do not require a plasma cofactor for their action, and are selective for FXa, as their Ki is at least 5000 times lower than that for any other serine protease. They inhibit the catalytic site of FXa. It has been shown that the direct inhibitors of FXa can inhibit FXa both in the fluid phase and in the context of the prothrombinase complex.

Rivaroxaban is a direct competitive, reversible, FXa inhibitor with higher than 10,000-fold greater selectivity for FXa than other serine proteases.[105] High bioavailability (≥ 80%) of 15 mg and 20 mg rivaroxaban is achieved when taken with food. Rivaroxaban has a high oral bioavailability and a rapid onset of action, reaching maximum plasma concentrations 2.5–4 hours after the administration. It has a half-life of up to 9 hours in healthy young subjects and 12–13 hours in healthy elderly subjects. It is eliminated via two routes: one-third is eliminated unchanged in the urine, and two-thirds after metabolic degradation (half of which is excreted via the kidney, half via the faecal route).[106]

Rivaroxaban 20 mg once daily (or 15 mg in patients with moderate renal impairment at screening) was compared with dose-adjusted warfarin for the prevention of stroke and systemic embolism in patients with AF at high risk of stroke, as evidenced by a $CHADS_2$-score of 2 or greater, in the Prospective, Randomized, Double-Blind, Parallel-Group, Multicenter, Non-inferiority Study Comparing the Efficacy and Safety of Rivaroxaban With Warfarin for the Prevention of Stroke and Non-Central Nervous System Systemic Embolism in Subjects With Non-Valvular AF (ROCKET-AF) trial.[99] Overall, rivaroxaban was non-inferior to warfarin in terms of the primary endpoint, a composite of stroke and non-central nervous system embolism, with similar rates of bleeding and adverse events. Such a treatment was superior to warfarin when investigators analysed the risk of stroke and non-central nervous system embolism in patients who remained on treatment over the course of the 40-month trial, although it was not superior to warfarin in the stricter intention-to-treat analysis.

Apixaban is a potent, selective, reversible inhibitor of FXa with a high oral bioavailability, rapid onset of action, and a half-life of about 12 hours. Food does not affect apixaban absorption, and changes in pH are unlikely to exert an effect. Apixaban has multiple elimination pathways of which about 25% are renal and 75% are non-renal.[107]

The Apixaban Versus Acetylsalicylic Acid (ASA) to Prevent Stroke in AF Patients Who Have Failed or Are Unsuitable for VKA Treatment (AVERROES) trial,[108] indicated that apixaban 5.0 mg twice daily reduced the risk of stroke or systemic embolism compared with aspirin (81–324 mg once daily) without significantly increasing the risk of major bleeding or intracranial haemorrhage in patients with AF and a $CHADS_2$-score of 1 or greater for whom VKA therapy was considered unsuitable.

That study started in parallel with the Apixaban for the Prevention of Stroke in Subjects with AF (ARISTOTLE trial),[100] which was—conversely—a comparison of apixaban 5.0 mg twice daily versus warfarin adjusted to an INR of 2.5 in patients with AF and a $CHADS_2$-score of 1 or greater. The results showed a lower incidence of the primary outcome of stroke or systemic embolism in the apixaban group compared with warfarin group. The rate of major bleeding was also lower for patients in the apixaban group compared with those in the warfarin group. Rates of haemorrhagic stroke and intracranial bleeding were significantly lower in patients treated with apixaban than with warfarin, while gastrointestinal bleeding was similar between the treatment arms. There was no difference in ischaemic stroke. Total mortality was lower for apixaban as compared with warfarin.

Edoxaban is an oral, direct, and competitive FXa inhibitor. It is rapidly absorbed, with a plasma half-life of 9–11 hours and a bioavailability of about 45%, not influenced by food intake.[109] The Phase 3, Randomized, Double-Blind, Double-Dummy, Parallel Group, Multi-Center, Multi-National Study for Evaluation of Efficacy and Safety of DU-176b Versus Warfarin In Subjects With AF—Effective Anticoagulation With Factor Xa Next Generation in

AF (ENGAGE AF-TIMI 48 trial)[86,110] compared edoxaban 30 mg or 60 mg once daily (dynamically adjusted during the trial in cases of changes in creatinine clearance, body mass index, or concomitant therapy with strong permeability glycoprotein inhibitors) with warfarin for the prevention of stroke and systemic embolism in 21,105 patients with AF and a $CHADS_2$ score of 2 or greater. Both once-daily regimens of edoxaban were non-inferior to warfarin with respect to the prevention of stroke or systemic embolism and were associated with significantly lower rates of bleeding and death from cardiovascular causes. The lower dose regimen, however, featured a trend to more ischaemic stroke/systemic embolism than warfarin,[86] and a choice was made not to recommend it clinically.

Post-marketing prospective registries on the effectiveness and safety of dabigatran,[111] rivaroxaban,[112,113] apixaban,[114] and edoxaban[115,116] have so far overall shown general consistency with the respective RCT.

Whereas patients with end-stage renal dysfunction were excluded from the pivotal RCTs, reduced dose regimens of rivaroxaban, apixaban, and edoxaban are feasible options for severe chronic kidney disease (creatinine clearance 15–30 mL/min using the Cockcroft–Gault equation).[117,118] Criteria for dose reduction of the currently used NOACs, because of renal function or other clinical features, are summarized in ➔ Table 20.5. Considering that inappropriate dose reductions are frequent in clinical practice,[119] thus increasing the risks of stroke/systemic embolism, hospitalization, and death, but without decreasing bleeding risk,[120] NOAC therapy should be optimized based on the efficacy and safety profile of each NOAC in different patient subgroups (➔ Table 20.5).

Heparins

Heparins (➔ Chapter 8) are a family of mucopolysaccharide chains of varying length and composition, with a mean molecular weight of 15,000 Da (range 3000–30,000 Da). Heparins contain a unique pentasaccharide unit with a high-affinity binding sequence for antithrombin (AT)-III, which is an inhibitor of coagulation serine proteases, including thrombin and activated FX, FIX, FXI, and FXII. Heparins form a complex with this AT-III, accelerating its inhibitory action. Unfractionated heparin (UFH) binds to endothelial cells, macrophages, numerous plasma proteins, and PF4: this explains the highly variable individual dose requirements to obtain the same antithrombotic effect, the need for therapeutic monitoring, and some side effects.[121] The most commonly used test for therapeutic monitoring of UFH is the activated partial thromboplastin time (aPTT). The range of aPTT relating to clinical efficacy of heparin is 1.5–2 times the basal value.[121] The most common and major side effect of heparin is bleeding. Another, less common, but severe, side effect is thrombocytopenia [heparin-induced thrombocytopenia (HIT)], two types of which are known[122]: early HIT, occurring during the first 5 days of treatment, with unknown aetiology, not severe and reversible; and late HIT, occurring between the fifth and the fifteenth day of treatment, due to antibodies against the heparin–PF4 complex, interacting with the CD32 receptor and causing abnormal platelet activation and the formation of prothrombotic platelet particles.[122] This latest type of HIT is often associated with venous and arterial thrombotic complications.

Low-molecular-weight heparins (LMWHs) are fractions of the heparin molecule, obtained by chemical or enzymatic depolymerization, with lesser dimensions (mean molecular weight 5000 Da, range 1000–10,000 Da), lesser capacity to inactivate thrombin compared to FXa (anti-FXa/AT-III ratio between 4:1 and 2:1; this ratio is 1:1 for UFH), and lesser capacity to bind plasma proteins, PF4, and endothelial cells. These characteristics result in a higher bioavailability (after subcutaneous injection: >90% vs 30% for UFH), reduced plasma clearance, longer half-life (anti-Xa activity 3–4 hours vs 30–150 minutes for UFH), less inter-individual variability of the anticoagulant response, and reduced risk of thrombocytopenia.[123] Therefore, LMWHs are more practical, cause less complications compared with UFH, and—to a large extent—they do not need monitoring.[123]

The use of heparins in AF is limited to few situations. In patients undergoing cardioversion for AF of short duration (i.e. <48 hours), heparins serve as anticoagulant coverage in the period around cardioversion; in patients with AF of duration longer than 48 hours with haemodynamic instability (angina, myocardial infarction, shock, or pulmonary oedema), in whom immediate cardioversion should be performed, UFH or LMWH should be administered before cardioversion (see below). In patients with high risk of thromboembolism, such as patients with AF, mechanical prosthetic heart valves, biological prosthetic heart valves or

Table 20.5 Criteria for dose selection of the non-vitamin K antagonist oral anticoagulants

	Dabigatran	Rivaroxaban	Apixaban	Edoxaban
Higher dose	150 mg BD	20 mg OD	5 mg BD	60 mg OD
Lower dose	110 mg BD			
Reduced dose		15 mg OD	2.5 mg BD	30 mg OD/15 mg OD
Dose-reduction criteria	110 mg BD if: (1) age ≥80 years; (2) concomitant use of verapamil; (3) increased bleeding risk	CrCl ≤15–49 mL/min	At least 2: (1) age ≥80 years; (2) body weight ≤60 kg; (3) serum creatinine ≥1.5 mg/dL Or single criterion: if creatinine clearance 15–29 mL/min	If any of the following: (1) CrCl 15–49 mL/min; (2) body weight ≤60 kg; (3) concomitant therapy with strong P-gp inhibitor

BD, twice daily; CrCl, creatinine clearance; OD, once daily; P-gp, permeability glycoprotein.

mitral valvular repair within the last 3 months, or recent venous thromboembolism (<3 months) plus thrombophilia, in whom it is necessary to interrupt oral anticoagulant therapy in preparation for elective surgical procedures, heparins provide an anticoagulant bridging therapy (see below).[124] VKAs should be stopped 5 days prior to surgery; a LMWH or UFH should be started 1 day after acenocoumarol interruption, and 2 days after warfarin interruption. The last dose of LMWH should be administered at least 12 hours before the procedure. LMWH are also an alternative to VKAs or NOACs in pregnancy, where the use of these drugs is partially (for VKAs) or totally (for NOACs) contraindicated.[125]

The use of LMWHs instead of UFH in patients with AF is based largely on extrapolations from data in trials of prevention of venous thromboembolism, in which LMWHs have proven as effective and safe as UFH.

Antiplatelet agents

The role of antiplatelet therapy, particularly monotherapy with aspirin, in the prevention of thromboembolism in patients with AF has always been thought as of lesser efficacy due to the modest protection that aspirin confers against stroke and systemic embolism in these patients. In the ACTIVE-A trial, patients unsuitable for anticoagulation had a lower rate of thromboembolic complications when clopidogrel was added to aspirin compared with aspirin alone, but with a significant increase in major bleeding.[126] Aspirin monotherapy was ineffective for stroke prevention compared with no antithrombotic treatment, and was associated with a higher risk of ischaemic stroke in elderly patients.[127] In the Atrial Fibrillation Clopidogrel Trial with Irbesartan for Prevention of Vascular Events (ACTIVE-W) trial, dual antiplatelet therapy (DAPT) with aspirin and clopidogrel was less effective than warfarin for prevention of stroke, systemic embolism, myocardial infarction, and vascular death (the annual risk of events being 5.6% vs 3.9%; $P = 0.0003$), with a similar rate of major bleeding.[128] Overall, antiplatelet monotherapy is ineffective for stroke prevention and is potentially harmful, especially among elderly AF patients,[129] whereas DAPT with aspirin and clopidogrel is associated with a bleeding risk similar to OAC therapy. Hence, antiplatelet therapy should not be used for stroke prevention in AF patients. No data are available with DAPT including aspirin in association with other, newer and more pharmacodynamically effective $P2Y_{12}$ inhibitors, such as ticagrelor or prasugrel.

The use of antiplatelet therapy remains, however, common in clinical practice, even in patients without an otherwise indication (e.g. for peripheral, coronary, or cerebrovascular disease) beyond AF.[130] There is limited evidence, and actually data against, to support the combination therapy solely for stroke prevention in AF, with no effect on reductions in stroke, myocardial infarction, or death, but with a substantial increase in the risk of major bleeding and intracranial haemorrhage.[131]

Non-pharmacological antithrombotic therapies: left atrial appendage exclusion

In patients with AF, studies have demonstrated that up to 90% of left atrial thrombi are localized to the LAA.[132,133] Increased thrombogenicity in the LAA is due to its narrow entrance orifice, coupled with its structure of trabeculated muscle of varying geometric shapes, which predisposes to blood stasis and thrombus formation.[35,134] Given the limitations of OACs, and specifically the increased risk of major bleeding—prohibitive in some occasions—non-pharmacological alternatives such as percutaneous LAA exclusion, performed with surgical approaches or through catheter-based occlusion [left atrial appendage occlusion (LAAO)], have emerged as a therapy that can reduce the risk of stroke among individuals with AF.[135] The two terms—exclusion and occlusion—are mostly today used interchangeably, although LAA *exclusion* is mostly referring to surgical approaches (by excision, ligation, suturing, or stapling).

Current catheter-based LAAOs are based on three different principles[136]:

1. Endovascular delivery of a device lobe or umbrella obstructing the neck of the LAA to prevent blood flow into the body of the LAA [WATCHMAN™ (Boston Scientific), WaveCrest® (Biosense Webster)].
2. Endovascular delivery of a device with a lobe or umbrella and an additional disc to seal the ostium of the LAA from the left atrial side [AMPLATZER™ Cardiac Plug (ACP)[137] and Amulet™ (both from Abbott Vascular);[137] Ultraseal™ LAA Occluder (Cardia),[138] LAmbre™ (Lifetech)].[139]
3. Ligation: LARIAT® (SentreHEART)[140] aims to snare and ligate the body of the LAA using both endocardial and epicardial approaches.

LAAO can be taken into consideration in the following clinical situations: patients with an absolute contraindication to OAC therapy; patients in whom OACs have failed; patients with kidney failure or under dialysis with a previous major bleeding on therapy; frail patients; and patients with coagulopathies associated with a significant higher bleeding risk.[141] LAA surgical exclusion is currently considered routinely in AF patients receiving other types of cardiac surgery.

Anatomical assessment of the LAA with TOE, computed tomography, or cardiac magnetic resonance imaging is critical to determine the technical feasibility of catheter-based LAAO, including optimal implant positioning and safety of device implantation. The selection of the type and size of the LAAO device used during implantation must account for anatomical characteristics of the LAA.[35]

The 4-year outcomes from the randomized, controlled PRAGUE-17 trial ($n = 402$) comparing LAAO (Watchman or Amulet) with NOACs (95% apixaban) in AF patients with a history of cardioembolism, showed that LAAO was non-inferior to NOACs for preventing major cardiovascular, neurological, or bleeding events.[142] A meta-analysis of 16 studies comprising 1428 patients suggested that LAAO combined with AF ablation is an effective and safe strategy. The rate of ischaemic stroke/transient ischaemic attack/systemic embolism during follow-up was 1%. The periprocedural adverse event rate (phrenic nerve palsy, intracoronary air embolus, device embolization, and periprocedural death) was 0%, procedure-related bleeding 3%, and pericardial effusion 0%.[143] Another meta-analysis of 42 studies showed that intracardiac echocardiography-guided implantation is feasible and safe, while reducing exposure to general anaesthesia and associated potential risks.[144] The next-generation Watchman FLX device approved by the US Food and Drug Administration in August 2020, is fully recapturable and repositionable, with shorter device length and an atraumatic closed distal end. The PINNACLE FLX study (n = 400) achieved the primary effectiveness endpoint in 100%. Device-related thrombus was reported in seven patients, no patients experienced pericardial effusion requiring open cardiac surgery, and there were no device embolizations.[145] A real-life analysis of the National Cardiovascular Data Registry (NCDR®) LAAO Registry (n = 49,357) suggested that women have a significantly higher risk of any in-hospital adverse events after LAAO (6.3% vs 3.9%; P <0.001), major adverse event (4.1% vs 2.0%; P <0.001) due to pericardial effusion requiring drainage (1.2% vs 0.5%) or major bleeding (1.7% vs 0.8%). Women were also more likely than men to experience a hospital stay longer than 1 day (16.0% vs 11.6%; P <0.001) or death (0.3% vs 0.1%; P <0.001).[146] In the Amulet IDE RCT trial (n = 1878) Amulet was non-inferior to Watchman for the primary safety endpoint (14.5% vs 14.7%; P <0.001 for non-inferiority). Major bleeding and all-cause death were similar between groups (10.6% vs 10.0% and 3.9% vs 5.1%, respectively). Procedure-related complications were higher for the Amulet occluder (4.5% vs 2.5%), largely related to more frequent pericardial effusion and device embolization. LAA occlusion was higher for the Amulet occluder than for the Watchman device (98.9% vs 96.8%; P <0.001 for non-inferiority; P = 0.003 for superiority).[137] Two retrospective studies suggested that LAAO can be safely performed with moderate conscious sedation and with same-day discharge.[147,148]

The surgical approach to LAA exclusion performed at the time of other cardiac surgery, despite being older, has been overall less frequently rigorously investigated. The procedure likely adds minimal risk in this clinical setting, contrasting with the risk in patients not undergoing surgery. Because of the paucity of randomized data, guidelines have so far been cautious in recommending LAA surgical exclusion at the time of cardiac surgery in patients with AF. The recent publication of the Left Atrial Appendage Occlusion Study III (LAAOS III) has now, however, provided robust data on this issue.[149] In this multicentre trial, 4811 AF patients with a CHA_2DS_2-VASc score of at least 2 were randomly assigned to LAAO during cardiac surgery or to standard care. OACs were recommended to be continued in all the patients. The trial found that the risk of ischaemic stroke or systemic thromboembolism (primary endpoint) was 33% lower with surgical LAAO than with standard care after 3.8 years (hazard ratio, 0.67). The surgical occlusion caused only minimal prolongation of bypass and cross-clamp times.[149] Because of the demonstrated benefits without appreciable risk, surgical LAAO is likely to be upgraded in future recommendations, to be performed at the time of other cardiac surgery in patients similar to those enrolled in the trial, with a continuation of anticoagulants. Although the trial has not involved patients without AF, and has enforced the continuation of OAC, its results should not be transferred to patients in sinus rhythm even considered at 'high risk' for AF, nor to patients who may have strong or absolute contraindication to OA, but will certainly foster new research in these important areas.[150]

Post-left atrial appendage occlusion antithrombotic management

The implantation of LAAO devices does not eliminate the short-term need for antithrombotic drugs in the postprocedural period due to the increased risk of device-related thrombosis before device endothelialization.[151,152] Thus, the postprocedural management period after LAAO implantation remains especially challenging, and the optimal postprocedural antithrombotic strategy is uncertain. The original protocols for antithrombotic therapy after the Watchman device implantation consisted of warfarin and aspirin at discharge, with scheduled follow-up and TOE at 45 ± 14 days to assess for peri-device leaks and device-related thrombosis. If a peri-device leak was detected, but estimated to be 5 mm or less, without evidence of device or atrial thrombosis, warfarin was discontinued and the patient started on DAPT until 6 months post implantation. After treatment with DAPT, ASA was to be continued indefinitely. Given the lack of RCTs for the ACP or Amulet devices, there are no published protocols or guidelines for the use of specific antithrombotic strategies after their implantation. DAPT is here commonly used for 1–3 months.[153,154]

For patients at very high bleeding risk due to a history of intracranial haemorrhage or major gastrointestinal bleeding, single antiplatelet therapy has been used post LAAO. In an analysis of the safety and effectiveness of LAAO with ACP and Amulet devices using aspirin alone as a post-implant antithrombotic treatment, Korsholm et al. reported on a single-centre experience of 110 patients with a median follow-up of 2.3 years. The rate of device-related thrombosis was 1.9% (2/107). Stroke occurred in 6/107 patients, with an annualized rate of 2.3%. The annualized risk of major bleeding was reduced by 57% compared with the predicted rate.[155] In the REgistry on Real-Life EXperience with Left Atrial Appendage Occlusion (RELAXIO), 469 consecutive patients with AF who had undergone LAAO with the Watchman or Amplatzer devices were retrospectively analysed to determine the incidence, predictors, and prognosis of device-related thrombosis. In this analysis, 36.2% of patients (170/469) received single antiplatelet therapy and 7.5% (n = 35/469) received no antithrombotic therapy after implantation of Watchman, ACP, or Amulet devices. Mean follow-up was 13 months, during which time 339 patients underwent imaging of the LAA. The incidence of device-related thrombosis was 7.2% per year.[156]

Overall, postprocedural antithrombotic regimens are highly variable, but real-world experience has demonstrated comparable effectiveness of single antiplatelet therapy, or DAPT, or NOACs with warfarin in the prevention of device-related thrombosis, thromboembolic events, and bleeding. While the majority of data around anticoagulant therapy are non-randomized and subject to numerous limitations, ongoing and future randomized studies aim to more effectively determine whether different antiplatelet and antithrombotic regimens are safe and effective after percutaneous LAAO, specifically for those patients who have contraindications to long-term OAC therapy.

Perspectives

Prevention of stroke in AF has made very important steps forward in the last 20 years. The most significant ones have been the introduction of the NOACs as alternatives to VKAs and catheter- or surgery-based LAA exclusion techniques. Issues of efficacy and safety are still challenging. Despite being quite effective, all currently used anticoagulants are incompletely effective, as recently shown by the added benefit of surgical LAA exclusion.[149] There are also residual important issues of safety with the new anticoagulants, including a non-negligible rate of gastrointestinal bleeding, and the still concerning risk of intracranial haemorrhages especially when the NOACs are combined with antiplatelet agents. Other limitations include areas where unfavourable results were reported (e.g. in patients with mechanical heart valves, and the antiphospholipid syndrome), settings in which the NOACs have not been adequately tested (e.g. extremes of renal function, impaired hepatic function, and extremes of body weight), still non-negligible interactions with other drugs, and indications not yet fully tested in clinical trials (e.g. mitral stenosis, with or without AF). The development of new drugs, such as the FXI inhibitors (reviewed in ➲ Chapter 12), and progresses in LAA exclusion will certainly further improve the fate of patients with this common disease in the years to come.

What's new

- To evaluate the thrombotic risk of patients with AF, the CHA_2DS_2-VASc score, an evolution of the former $CHADS_2$ score, includes congestive heart failure, hypertension, diabetes, and stroke (factors included in the $CHADS_2$ score), but also female sex, history of vascular disease, and age 65–75 years as additional risk factors. The main purpose of this score is to decide on the few patients with AF who should definitely *not* be anticoagulated.
- A CHA_2DS_2-VASc score = 0 (males), or = 1 (females), consistently has shown a very low risk of ischaemic stroke or death, so that such patients do *not* require an antithrombotic treatment. Female sex is an age-dependent 'stroke risk modifier' rather than a risk factor per se. For patients with a CHA_2DS_2-VASc score = 2 (males), or = 3 (females), OAC therapy is definitely recommended. In the presence of CHA_2DS_2-VASc = 1 (males), or = 2 (females), OAC therapy *should be considered.*
- NOACs are now recommended as first-line therapy in the vast majority of patients with AF requiring antithrombotic treatment.
- Patients with moderate-to-severe mitral stenosis (probably even without AF) and patients with a mechanical prosthetic heart valves require anticoagulation with VKAs. AF with other VHDs including aortic stenosis/regurgitation, mitral regurgitation, bioprostheses, or valve repair can now be treated with a NOAC. Valvular/non-valvular AF is a terminology that should be abandoned.
- A HAS-BLED score of 3 or greater indicates 'high bleeding risk' and would imply caution and regular review of the patient following the initiation of any antithrombotic therapy. A formal assessment of bleeding risk informs management of patients taking OAC. A high bleeding risk score should *not*, however, exempt AF patients from anticoagulation.
- Aspirin monotherapy is largely ineffective for stroke prevention in AF compared with no antithrombotic treatment, and is associated with a higher risk of ischaemic stroke compared with OAC, especially in elderly patients.
- Non-pharmacological alternatives such as percutaneous LAA exclusion, performed with surgical approaches or through catheter-based occlusion (LAAO), have emerged as a therapy that can reduce the risk of stroke among individuals with AF. LAAO can be taken into consideration in the following clinical situations: patients with an absolute contraindication to OAC therapy; patients in whom OACs have failed; patients with kidney failure or under dialysis with a previous major bleeding on therapy; frail patients; and patients with coagulopathies associated with a significant higher bleeding risk. LAA surgical exclusion is currently to be considered routinely in AF patients receiving other types of cardiac surgery. A recent study in surgical patients has demonstrated the added efficacy of surgical LAA exclusion on top of optimal OAC therapy.
- The implantation of LAAO devices does not, however, eliminate the short-term need for antithrombotic drugs in the postprocedural period due to the increased risk of device-related thrombosis. Post-LAAO antithrombotic regimens are highly variable, but real-world experience has demonstrated comparable effectiveness of single antiplatelet therapy, or DAPT, or NOACs with warfarin in the prevention of device-related thrombosis, thromboembolic events, and bleeding.

Guideline recommendations

Recommendations	Class[a]	Level[b]
For stroke prevention in AF patients who are eligible for OAC, NOACs are recommended in preference to VKAs (excluding patients with mechanical heart valves or moderate-to-severe mitral stenosis)	I	A
For stroke risk assessment, a risk-factor-based approach is recommended, using the CHA_2DS_2-VAS_c clinical stroke risk score to initially identify patients at 'low stroke risk' (CHA_2DS_2-VASc score = 0 in men, or 1 in women) who should not be offered antithrombotic therapy	I	A
OAC is recommended for stroke prevention in AF patients with CHA_2DS_2-VASc score ≥2 in men or ≥3 in women	I	A

Recommendations	Class[a]	Level[b]
OAC should be considered for stroke prevention in AF patients with a CHA_2DS_2-VASc score of 1 in men or 2 in women Treatment should be individualized based on net clinical benefit and consideration of patient values and preferences	IIa	B
For bleeding risk assessment, a formal structured risk-score-based bleeding risk assessment is recommended to help identify non-modifiable and address modifiable bleeding risk factors in all AF patients, and to identify patients potentially at high risk of bleeding who should be scheduled for early and more frequent clinical review and follow-up	I	B
For a formal risk-score-based assessment of bleeding risk, the HAS-BLED score should be considered to help address modifiable bleeding risk factors, and to identify patients at high risk of bleeding (HAS-BLED score ≥3) for early and more frequent clinical review and follow-up	IIa	B
Stroke and bleeding risk reassessment at periodic intervals is recommended to inform treatment decisions (e.g. initiation of OAC in patients no longer at low risk of stroke) and address potentially modifiable bleeding risk factors	I	B
In patients with AF initially at low risk of stroke, first reassessment of stroke risk should be made at 4–6 months after the index evaluation	IIA	B
If a VKA is used, a target INR of 2.0–3.0 is recommended, with individual TTR ≥70%	I	B
In patients on VKAs with low time in INR therapeutic range (e.g. TTR <70%), recommended options are:	I	B
• Switching to a NOAC but ensuring good adherence and persistence with therapy; or		
• Efforts to improve TTR (e.g. education/counselling and more frequent INR checks)	IIa	B
Antiplatelet therapy alone (monotherapy or aspirin in combination with clopidogrel) is not recommended for stroke prevention in AF	III	A
Estimated bleeding risk, in the absence of absolute contraindications to OAC, should not in itself guide treatment decisions to use OAC for stroke prevention	III	A
Clinical pattern of AF (i.e. first detected, paroxysmal, persistent, long-standing persistent, permanent) should not condition the indication to thromboprophylaxis	III	B
Recommendations for occlusion or exclusion of the LAA		
LAA occlusion may be considered for stroke prevention in patients with AF and contraindications for long-term anticoagulant treatment (e.g. intracranial bleeding without a reversible cause)	IIb	B
Surgical occlusion or exclusion of the LAA may be considered for stroke prevention in patients with AF undergoing cardiac surgery	IIb	C

[a] Class of recommendation. [b] Level of evidence.

What's next

The most significant progress made in this area comprises the introduction of the NOACs as alternatives to VKAs and catheter- or surgery-based LAA exclusion techniques. Issues of efficacy and safety are still challenging. Despite being quite effective, there are also residual important issues of safety with the new anticoagulants, including a non-negligible rate of gastrointestinal bleeding, and the still concerning risk of intracranial haemorrhage, especially when the NOACs are combined with antiplatelet agents. Other limitations include areas where unfavourable results were reported (e.g. in patients with mechanical heart valves, and the antiphospholipid syndrome), settings in which the NOACs have not been adequately tested (e.g. extremes of renal function, impaired hepatic function, and extremes of body weight), still non-negligible interactions with other drugs, and indications not yet fully tested in clinical trials (e.g. mitral stenosis, with or without AF). The development of new drugs, such as the FXI inhibitors, and progress in LAA exclusion will certainly further improve the fate of patients with this common disease in the years to come.

Drug dosing

	Dabigatran	Rivaroxaban	Apixaban	Edoxaban
Standard dose	150 mg BD	20 mg OD	5 mg BD	60 mg OD
Lower dose	110 mg BD			
Reduced dose		15 mg OD	2.5 mg BD	30 mg OD
Dose-reduction criteria	110 mg BD if: Age ≥80 years Use of verapamil Increased bleeding risk	CrCl 15–49 mL/min	At least 2 of 3 criteria: Age ≥80 years Body weight ≤60 kg Serum creatinine ≥1.5 mg/dL (133 micromol/L)	If any of the following: estimated CrCl 30–50 mL/min Body weight ≤60 kg Use of verapamil, quinidine, or dronedarone

BD, twice daily; CrCl, creatinine clearance; OD, once daily.

References

1. Nattel S, Dobrev D. Electrophysiological and molecular mechanisms of paroxysmal atrial fibrillation. Nat Rev Cardiol. 2016;13(10):575–90.
2. Bellet S. Clinical disorders of the heart beat. Clinics. 1946;5(1):190–234.
3. Hindricks G, Potpara T, Dagres N, et al. Corrigendum to: 2020 ESC Guidelines for the diagnosis and management of atrial fibrillation developed in collaboration with the European Association for Cardio-Thoracic Surgery (EACTS): The Task Force for the diagnosis and management of atrial fibrillation of the European Society of Cardiology (ESC) Developed with the special contribution of the European Heart Rhythm Association (EHRA) of the ESC. Eur Heart J. 2021;42(40):4194.
4. Gorenek B, Boriani G, Dan GA, et al. European Heart Rhythm Association (EHRA) position paper on arrhythmia management and device therapies in endocrine disorders, endorsed by Asia Pacific Heart Rhythm Society (APHRS) and Latin American Heart Rhythm Society (LAHRS). Europace. 2018;20(6):895–6.
5. Goette A, Lendeckel U. Atrial cardiomyopathy: pathophysiology and clinical consequences. Cells. 2021;10(10):2605.
6. Frustaci A, Chimenti C, Bellocci F, Morgante E, Russo MA, Maseri A. Histological substrate of atrial biopsies in patients with lone atrial fibrillation. Circulation. 1997;96(4):1180–4.
7. De Caterina R, Ruigomez A, Rodriguez LA. Long-term use of anti-inflammatory drugs and risk of atrial fibrillation. Arch Intern Med. 2010;170(16):1450–5.
8. Dittrich HC, Pearce LA, Asinger RW, et al. Left atrial diameter in nonvalvular atrial fibrillation: an echocardiographic study. Stroke Prevention in Atrial Fibrillation Investigators. Am Heart J. 1999;137(3):494–9.
9. Bianco F, De Caterina R, Chandra A, et al. Left atrial remodeling and stroke in patients with sinus rhythm and normal ejection fraction: ARIC-NCS. J Am Heart Assoc. 2022;11(9):e024292.
10. Li D, Fareh S, Leung TK, Nattel S. Promotion of atrial fibrillation by heart failure in dogs: atrial remodeling of a different sort. Circulation. 1999;100(1):87–95.
11. Brambatti M, Connolly SJ, Gold MR, et al. Temporal relationship between subclinical atrial fibrillation and embolic events. Circulation. 2014;129(21):2094–9.
12. Go AS, Hylek EM, Phillips KA, et al. Prevalence of diagnosed atrial fibrillation in adults: national implications for rhythm management and stroke prevention: the AnTicoagulation and Risk Factors in Atrial Fibrillation (ATRIA) Study. JAMA. 2001;285(18):2370–5.
13. Naccarelli GV, Varker H, Lin J, Schulman KL. Increasing prevalence of atrial fibrillation and flutter in the United States. Am J Cardiol. 2009;104(11):1534–9.
14. Lloyd-Jones DM, Wang TJ, Leip EP, et al. Lifetime risk for development of atrial fibrillation: the Framingham Heart Study. Circulation. 2004;110(9):1042–6.
15. Furberg CD, Psaty BM, Manolio TA, Gardin JM, Smith VE, Rautaharju PM. Prevalence of atrial fibrillation in elderly subjects (the Cardiovascular Health Study). Am J Cardiol. 1994;74(3):236–41.
16. Levy S, Maarek M, Coumel P, et al. Characterization of different subsets of atrial fibrillation in general practice in France: the ALFA study. The College of French Cardiologists. Circulation. 1999;99(23):3028–35.
17. Murgatroyd FD, Gibson SM, Baiyan X, et al. Double-blind placebo-controlled trial of digoxin in symptomatic paroxysmal atrial fibrillation. Circulation. 1999;99(21):2765–70.
18. Tsang TS, Petty GW, Barnes ME, et al. The prevalence of atrial fibrillation in incident stroke cases and matched population controls in Rochester, Minnesota: changes over three decades. J Am Coll Cardiol. 2003;42(1):93–100.
19. Benjamin EJ, Levy D, Vaziri SM, D'Agostino RB, Belanger AJ, Wolf PA. Independent risk factors for atrial fibrillation in a population-based cohort. The Framingham Heart Study. JAMA. 1994;271(11):840–4.
20. Feinberg WM, Blackshear JL, Laupacis A, Kronmal R, Hart RG. Prevalence, age distribution, and gender of patients with atrial fibrillation. Analysis and implications. Arch Intern Med. 1995;155(5):469–73.
21. Sudlow M, Thomson R, Thwaites B, Rodgers H, Kenny RA. Prevalence of atrial fibrillation and eligibility for anticoagulants in the community. Lancet. 1998;352(9135):1167–71.
22. Wolf PA, Benjamin EJ, Belanger AJ, Kannel WB, Levy D, D'Agostino RB. Secular trends in the prevalence of atrial fibrillation: the Framingham Study. Am Heart J. 1996;131(4):790–5.
23. Tsang TS, Gersh BJ, Appleton CP, et al. Left ventricular diastolic dysfunction as a predictor of the first diagnosed nonvalvular atrial fibrillation in 840 elderly men and women. J Am Coll Cardiol. 2002;40(9):1636–44.
24. Lindroos M, Kupari M, Heikkila J, Tilvis R. Prevalence of aortic valve abnormalities in the elderly: an echocardiographic study of a random population sample. J Am Coll Cardiol. 1993;21(5):1220–5.
25. Heeringa J, van der Kuip DA, Hofman A, et al. Prevalence, incidence and lifetime risk of atrial fibrillation: the Rotterdam study. Eur Heart J. 2006;27(8):949–53.
26. Magnussen C, Niiranen TJ, Ojeda FM, et al. Sex differences and similarities in atrial fibrillation epidemiology, risk factors, and mortality in community cohorts: results From the BiomarCaRE Consortium (Biomarker for Cardiovascular Risk Assessment in Europe). Circulation. 2017;136(17):1588–97.
27. Staerk L, Wang B, Preis SR, et al. Lifetime risk of atrial fibrillation according to optimal, borderline, or elevated levels of risk factors: cohort study based on longitudinal data from the Framingham Heart Study. BMJ. 2018;361:k1453.
28. Lip GYH. The ABC pathway: an integrated approach to improve AF management. Nat Rev Cardiol. 2017;14(11):627–8.
29. Guo Y, Lane DA, Wang L, et al. Mobile health technology to improve care for patients with atrial fibrillation. J Am Coll Cardiol. 2020;75(13):1523–34.
30. Wolf PA, Abbott RD, Kannel WB. Atrial fibrillation: a major contributor to stroke in the elderly. The Framingham Study. Arch Intern Med. 1987;147(9):1561–4.
31. Wolf PA, D'Agostino RB, Belanger AJ, Kannel WB. Probability of stroke: a risk profile from the Framingham Study. Stroke. 1991;22(3):312–8.
32. Friberg L, Hammar N, Rosenqvist M. Stroke in paroxysmal atrial fibrillation: report from the Stockholm Cohort of Atrial Fibrillation. Eur Heart J. 2010;31(8):967–75.
33. Chen LY, Chung MK, Allen LA, et al. Atrial fibrillation burden: moving beyond atrial fibrillation as a binary entity: a scientific statement from the American Heart Association. Circulation. 2018;137(20):e623–e44.
34. Bogousslavsky J, Cachin C, Regli F, Despland PA, Van Melle G, Kappenberger L. Cardiac sources of embolism and cerebral infarction—clinical consequences and vascular concomitants: the Lausanne Stroke Registry. Neurology. 1991;41(6):855–9.
35. Patti G, Pengo V, Marcucci R, et al. The left atrial appendage: from embryology to prevention of thromboembolism. Eur Heart J. 2017;38(12):877–87.

36. Daniel WG, Nellessen U, Schroder E, et al. Left atrial spontaneous echo contrast in mitral valve disease: an indicator for an increased thromboembolic risk. J Am Coll Cardiol. 1988;11(6):1204–11.
37. Li YH, Lai LP, Shyu KG, Hwang JJ, Kuan P, Lien WP. Clinical implications of left atrial appendage flow patterns in nonrheumatic atrial fibrillation. Chest. 1994;105(3):748–52.
38. De Caterina R, Renda G. Atrial fibrillation: antithrombotic therapy. In: Kristensen S, De Caterina R, Moliterno D, editors. Therapeutic Strategies in Thrombosis. Oxford: Clinical Publishing; 2006: 275–300.
39. Sohara H, Amitani S, Kurose M, Miyahara K. Atrial fibrillation activates platelets and coagulation in a time-dependent manner: a study in patients with paroxysmal atrial fibrillation. J Am Coll Cardiol. 1997;29(1):106–12.
40. Tsai LM, Chen JH, Tsao CJ. Relation of left atrial spontaneous echo contrast with prethrombotic state in atrial fibrillation associated with systemic hypertension, idiopathic dilated cardiomyopathy, or no identifiable cause (lone). Am J Cardiol. 1998;81(10):1249–52.
41. EAFT (European Atrial Fibrillation Trial) Study Group. Secondary prevention in non-rheumatic atrial fibrillation after transient ischaemic attack or minor stroke. Lancet. 1993;342(8882):1255–62.
42. Chimowitz MI, DeGeorgia MA, Poole RM, Hepner A, Armstrong WM. Left atrial spontaneous echo contrast is highly associated with previous stroke in patients with atrial fibrillation or mitral stenosis. Stroke. 1993;24(7):1015–9.
43. Goldman ME, Pearce LA, Hart RG, et al. Pathophysiologic correlates of thromboembolism in nonvalvular atrial fibrillation: I. Reduced flow velocity in the left atrial appendage (The Stroke Prevention in Atrial Fibrillation [SPAF-III] study). J Am Soc Echocardiogr. 1999;12(12):1080–7.
44. Asinger RW, Koehler J, Pearce LA, et al. Pathophysiologic correlates of thromboembolism in nonvalvular atrial fibrillation: II. Dense spontaneous echocardiographic contrast (The Stroke Prevention in Atrial Fibrillation [SPAF-III] study). J Am Soc Echocardiogr. 1999;12(12):1088–96.
45. Blackshear JL, Pearce LA, Hart RG, et al. Aortic plaque in atrial fibrillation: prevalence, predictors, and thromboembolic implications. Stroke. 1999;30(4):834–40.
46. Hursting MJ, Stead AG, Crout FV, Horvath BZ, Moore BM. Effects of age, race, sex, and smoking on prothrombin fragment 1.2 in a healthy population. Clin Chem. 1993;39(4):683–6.
47. Cushman M, Psaty BM, Macy E, et al. Correlates of thrombin markers in an elderly cohort free of clinical cardiovascular disease. Arterioscler Thromb Vasc Biol. 1996;16(9):1163–9.
48. Lowe GD, Rumley A, Woodward M, et al. Epidemiology of coagulation factors, inhibitors and activation markers: the Third Glasgow MONICA Survey. I. Illustrative reference ranges by age, sex and hormone use. Br J Haematol. 1997;97(4):775–84.
49. Feinberg WM, Cornell ES, Nightingale SD, et al. Relationship between prothrombin activation fragment F1.2 and international normalized ratio in patients with atrial fibrillation. Stroke Prevention in Atrial Fibrillation Investigators. Stroke. 1997;28(6):1101–6.
50. Hart RG, Pearce LA, McBride R, Rothbart RM, Asinger RW. Factors associated with ischemic stroke during aspirin therapy in atrial fibrillation: analysis of 2012 participants in the SPAF I-III clinical trials. The Stroke Prevention in Atrial Fibrillation (SPAF) Investigators. Stroke. 1999;30(6):1223–9.
51. Risk factors for stroke and efficacy of antithrombotic therapy in atrial fibrillation. Analysis of pooled data from five randomized controlled trials. Arch Intern Med. 1994;154(13):1449–57.
52. Kanter MC, Tegeler CH, Pearce LA, et al. Carotid stenosis in patients with atrial fibrillation. Prevalence, risk factors, and relationship to stroke in the Stroke Prevention in Atrial Fibrillation Study. Arch Intern Med. 1994;154(12):1372–7.
53. The SPAF III Writing Committee for the Stroke Prevention in Atrial Fibrillation Investigators. Patients with nonvalvular atrial fibrillation at low risk of stroke during treatment with aspirin: Stroke Prevention in Atrial Fibrillation III Study. JAMA. 1998;279(16):1273–7.
54. Zabalgoitia M, Halperin JL, Pearce LA, Blackshear JL, Asinger RW, Hart RG. Transesophageal echocardiographic correlates of clinical risk of thromboembolism in nonvalvular atrial fibrillation. Stroke Prevention in Atrial Fibrillation III Investigators. J Am Coll Cardiol. 1998;31(7):1622–6.
55. The Stroke Prevention in Atrial Fibrillation (SPAF) Investigators. Predictors of thromboembolism in atrial fibrillation: I. Clinical features of patients at risk. Ann Intern Med. 1992;116(1):1–5.
56. Patti G, Lucerna M, Cavallari I, et al. Insulin-requiring versus noninsulin-requiring diabetes and thromboembolic risk in patients with atrial fibrillation: PREFER in AF. J Am Coll Cardiol. 2017;69(4):409–19.
57. De Caterina R, Patti G, Westerbergh J, et al. Heterogeneity of diabetes as a risk factor for major adverse cardiovascular events in anticoagulated patients with atrial fibrillation: an analysis of the ARISTOTLE trial. Eur Heart J Cardiovasc Pharmacother. 2022;8(3):227–35.
58. Stroke Risk in Atrial Fibrillation Working Group. Independent predictors of stroke in patients with atrial fibrillation: a systematic review. Neurology. 2007;69(6):546–54.
59. Hughes M, Lip GY, Guideline Development Group, National Clinical Guideline for Management of Atrial Fibrillation in Primary and Secondary Care, National Institute for Health and Clinical Excellence. Stroke and thromboembolism in atrial fibrillation: a systematic review of stroke risk factors, risk stratification schema and cost effectiveness data. Thromb Haemost. 2008;99(2):295–304.
60. Camm AJ, Kirchhof P, Lip GY, et al. Guidelines for the management of atrial fibrillation: the Task Force for the Management of Atrial Fibrillation of the European Society of Cardiology (ESC). Eur Heart J. 2010;31(19):2369–429.
61. Darby AE, Dimarco JP. Management of atrial fibrillation in patients with structural heart disease. Circulation. 2012;125(7):945–57.
62. Szekely P. Systemic embolism and anticoagulant prophylaxis in rheumatic heart disease. Br Med J. 1964;1(5392):1209–12.
63. Philippart R, Brunet-Bernard A, Clementy N, et al. Prognostic value of CHA2DS2-VASc score in patients with 'non-valvular atrial fibrillation' and valvular heart disease: the Loire Valley Atrial Fibrillation Project. Eur Heart J. 2015;36(28):1822–30.
64. Philippart R, Brunet-Bernard A, Clementy N, et al. Oral anticoagulation, stroke and thromboembolism in patients with atrial fibrillation and valve bioprosthesis. The Loire Valley Atrial Fibrillation Project. Thromb Haemost. 2016;115(5):1056–63.
65. Renda G, Ricci F, Giugliano RP, De Caterina R. Non-vitamin K antagonist oral anticoagulants in patients with atrial fibrillation and valvular heart disease. J Am Coll Cardiol. 2017;69(11):1363–71.
66. Kim JY, Kim SH, Myong JP, et al. Outcomes of direct oral anticoagulants in patients with mitral stenosis. J Am Coll Cardiol. 2019;73(10):1123–31.
67. Sadeghipour P, Pouraliakbar H, Parsaee M, et al. RIvaroxaban in mitral stenosis (RISE MS): A pilot randomized clinical trial. Int J Cardiol. 2022;356:83–6.
68. Friberg L, Benson L, Rosenqvist M, Lip GY. Assessment of female sex as a risk factor in atrial fibrillation in Sweden: nationwide retrospective cohort study. BMJ. 2012;344:e3522.
69. Overvad TF, Potpara TS, Nielsen PB. Stroke risk stratification: CHA2DS2-VA or CHA2DS2-VASc? Heart Lung Circ. 2019;28(2):e14–e5.

70. Nielsen PB, Overvad TF. Female sex as a risk modifier for stroke risk in atrial fibrillation: using CHA2DS2-VASc versus CHA2DS2-VA for stroke risk stratification in atrial fibrillation: a note of caution. Thromb Haemost. 2020;120(6):894–8.
71. Singer DE, Chang Y, Borowsky LH, et al. A new risk scheme to predict ischemic stroke and other thromboembolism in atrial fibrillation: the ATRIA study stroke risk score. J Am Heart Assoc. 2013;2(3):e000250.
72. Piccini JP, Stevens SR, Chang Y, et al. Renal dysfunction as a predictor of stroke and systemic embolism in patients with nonvalvular atrial fibrillation: validation of the R(2)CHADS(2) index in the ROCKET AF (Rivaroxaban Once-daily, oral, direct factor Xa inhibition Compared with vitamin K antagonism for prevention of stroke and Embolism Trial in Atrial Fibrillation) and ATRIA (AnTicoagulation and Risk factors In Atrial fibrillation) study cohorts. Circulation. 2013;127(2):224–32.
73. Hijazi Z, Lindbäck J, Alexander JH, et al. The ABC (age, biomarkers, clinical history) stroke risk score: a biomarker-based risk score for predicting stroke in atrial fibrillation. Eur Heart J. 2016;37(20):1582–90.
74. Benz AP, Hijazi Z, Lindbäck J, et al. Biomarker-based risk prediction with the ABC-AF scores in patients with atrial fibrillation not receiving oral anticoagulation. Circulation. 2021;143(19):1863–73.
75. Andrade JG, Aguilar M, Atzema C, et al. The 2020 Canadian Cardiovascular Society/Canadian Heart Rhythm Society comprehensive guidelines for the management of atrial fibrillation. Can J Cardiol. 2020;36(12):1847–948.
76. Morrone D, Kroep S, Ricci F, et al. Mortality prediction of the CHA(2)DS(2)-VASc Score, the HAS-BLED score, and their combination in anticoagulated patients with atrial fibrillation. J Clin Med. 2020;9(12):3987.
77. Pisters R, Lane DA, Nieuwlaat R, de Vos CB, Crijns HJ, Lip GY. A novel user-friendly score (HAS-BLED) to assess 1-year risk of major bleeding in patients with atrial fibrillation: the Euro Heart Survey. Chest. 2010;138(5):1093–100.
78. Chao TF, Lip GYH, Lin YJ, et al. Incident risk factors and major bleeding in patients with atrial fibrillation treated with oral anticoagulants: a comparison of baseline, follow-up and delta HAS-BLED scores with an approach focused on modifiable bleeding risk factors. Thromb Haemost. 2018;118(4):768–77.
79. Man-Son-Hing M, Nichol G, Lau A, Laupacis A. Choosing antithrombotic therapy for elderly patients with atrial fibrillation who are at risk for falls. Arch Intern Med. 1999;159(7):677–85.
80. Morrone D, De Caterina R. Bleeding risk score: limits and practicability. Heart. 2022;108(4):246–8.
81. Hijazi Z, Oldgren J, Lindbäck J, et al. The novel biomarker-based ABC (age, biomarkers, clinical history)-bleeding risk score for patients with atrial fibrillation: a derivation and validation study. Lancet. 2016;387(10035):2302–11.
82. De Caterina R, Husted S, Wallentin L, et al. Vitamin K antagonists in heart disease: current status and perspectives (Section III). Position paper of the ESC Working Group on Thrombosis—Task Force on Anticoagulants in Heart Disease. Thromb Haemost. 2013;110(6):1087–107.
83. Hart RG, Pearce LA, Aguilar MI. Meta-analysis: antithrombotic therapy to prevent stroke in patients who have nonvalvular atrial fibrillation. Ann Intern Med. 2007;146(12):857–67.
84. Albers GW, Dalen JE, Laupacis A, Manning WJ, Petersen P, Singer DE. Antithrombotic therapy in atrial fibrillation. Chest. 2001;119(1 Suppl):194S–206S.
85. Connolly SJ, Laupacis A, Gent M, Roberts RS, Cairns JA, Joyner C. Canadian Atrial Fibrillation Anticoagulation (CAFA) study. J Am Coll Cardiol. 1991;18(2):349–55.
86. Giugliano RP, Ruff CT, Braunwald E, et al. Edoxaban versus warfarin in patients with atrial fibrillation. N Engl J Med. 2013;369(22):2093–104.
87. Palareti G, Leali N, Coccheri S, et al. Bleeding complications of oral anticoagulant treatment: an inception-cohort, prospective collaborative study (ISCOAT). Italian Study on Complications of Oral Anticoagulant Therapy. Lancet. 1996;348(9025):423–8.
88. Levine MN, Raskob G, Landefeld S, Kearon C. Hemorrhagic complications of anticoagulant treatment. Chest. 1998;114(5 Suppl):511S–23S.
89. Petersen P, Boysen G, Godtfredsen J, Andersen ED, Andersen B. Placebo-controlled, randomised trial of warfarin and aspirin for prevention of thromboembolic complications in chronic atrial fibrillation. The Copenhagen AFASAK study. Lancet. 1989;1(8631):175–9.
90. The Boston Area Anticoagulation Trial for Atrial Fibrillation Investigators, Singer DE, Hughes RA, et al. The effect of low-dose warfarin on the risk of stroke in patients with nonrheumatic atrial fibrillation. N Engl J Med. 1990;323(22):1505–11.
91. Stroke Prevention in Atrial Fibrillation Study. Final results. Circulation. 1991;84(2):527–39.
92. Ezekowitz MD, Bridgers SL, James KE, et al. Warfarin in the prevention of stroke associated with nonrheumatic atrial fibrillation. Veterans Affairs Stroke Prevention in Nonrheumatic Atrial Fibrillation Investigators. N Engl J Med. 1992;327(20):1406–12.
93. Rieder MJ, Reiner AP, Gage BF, et al. Effect of VKORC1 haplotypes on transcriptional regulation and warfarin dose. N Engl J Med. 2005;352(22):2285–93.
94. Aithal GP, Day CP, Kesteven PJ, Daly AK. Association of polymorphisms in the cytochrome P450 CYP2C9 with warfarin dose requirement and risk of bleeding complications. Lancet. 1999;353(9154):717–19.
95. McDonald MG, Rieder MJ, Nakano M, Hsia CK, Rettie AE. CYP4F2 is a vitamin K1 oxidase: an explanation for altered warfarin dose in carriers of the V433M variant. Mol Pharmacol. 2009;75(6):1337–46.
96. Wang L, McLeod HL, Weinshilboum RM. Genomics and drug response. N Engl J Med. 2011;364(12):1144–53.
97. Frykman V, Beerman B, Ryden L, Rosenqvist M, Medical Products Agency, Swedish Society of Cardiology. Management of atrial fibrillation: discrepancy between guideline recommendations and actual practice exposes patients to risk for complications. Eur Heart J. 2001;22(20):1954–9.
98. Connolly SJ, Ezekowitz MD, Yusuf S, et al. Dabigatran versus warfarin in patients with atrial fibrillation. N Engl J Med. 2009;361(12):1139–51.
99. Patel MR, Mahaffey KW, Garg J, et al. Rivaroxaban versus warfarin in nonvalvular atrial fibrillation. N Engl J Med. 2011;365(10):883–91.
100. Granger CB, Alexander JH, McMurray JJ, et al. Apixaban versus warfarin in patients with atrial fibrillation. N Engl J Med. 2011;365(11):981–92.
101. Ruff CT, Giugliano RP, Braunwald E, et al. Comparison of the efficacy and safety of new oral anticoagulants with warfarin in patients with atrial fibrillation: a meta-analysis of randomised trials. Lancet. 2014;383(9921):955–62.
102. Stangier J. Clinical pharmacokinetics and pharmacodynamics of the oral direct thrombin inhibitor dabigatran etexilate. Clin Pharmacokinet. 2008;47(5):285–95.
103. Eikelboom JW, Connolly SJ, Brueckmann M, et al. Dabigatran versus warfarin in patients with mechanical heart valves. N Engl J Med. 2013;369(13):1206–14.
104. Aimo A, Giugliano RP, De Caterina R. Non-vitamin K antagonist oral anticoagulants for mechanical heart valves: is the door still open? Circulation. 2018;138(13):1356–65.

105. Perzborn E, Strassburger J, Wilmen A, et al. In vitro and in vivo studies of the novel antithrombotic agent BAY 59-7939—an oral, direct factor Xa inhibitor. J Thromb Haemost. 2005;3(3):514–21.
106. Kubitza D, Becka M, Voith B, Zuehlsdorf M, Wensing G. Safety, pharmacodynamics, and pharmacokinetics of single doses of BAY 59-7939, an oral, direct factor Xa inhibitor. Clin Pharmacol Ther. 2005;78(4):412–21.
107. Carreiro J, Ansell J. Apixaban, an oral direct factor Xa inhibitor: awaiting the verdict. Expert Opin Investig Drugs. 2008;17(12):1937–45.
108. Connolly SJ, Eikelboom J, Joyner C, et al. Apixaban in patients with atrial fibrillation. N Engl J Med. 2011;364(9):806–17.
109. Zafar MU, Vorchheimer DA, Gaztanaga J, et al. Antithrombotic effects of factor Xa inhibition with DU-176b: phase-I study of an oral, direct factor Xa inhibitor using an ex-vivo flow chamber. Thromb Haemost. 2007;98(4):883–8.
110. Ruff CT, Giugliano RP, Antman EM, et al. Evaluation of the novel factor Xa inhibitor edoxaban compared with warfarin in patients with atrial fibrillation: design and rationale for the Effective aNticoaGulation with factor xA next GEneration in Atrial Fibrillation-Thrombolysis In Myocardial Infarction study 48 (ENGAGE AF-TIMI 48). Am Heart J. 2010;160(4):635–41.
111. Huisman MV, Rothman KJ, Paquette M, et al. Two-year follow-up of patients treated with dabigatran for stroke prevention in atrial fibrillation: Global Registry on Long-Term Antithrombotic Treatment in Patients with Atrial Fibrillation (GLORIA-AF) registry. Am Heart J. 2018;198:55–63.
112. Camm AJ, Amarenco P, Haas S, et al. XANTUS: a real-world, prospective, observational study of patients treated with rivaroxaban for stroke prevention in atrial fibrillation. Eur Heart J. 2016;37(14):1145–53.
113. Martinez CAA, Lanas F, Radaideh G, et al. XANTUS-EL: a real-world, prospective, observational study of patients treated with rivaroxaban for stroke prevention in atrial fibrillation in Eastern Europe, Middle East, Africa and Latin America. Egypt Heart J. 2018;70(4):307–13.
114. Li XS, Deitelzweig S, Keshishian A, et al. Effectiveness and safety of apixaban versus warfarin in non-valvular atrial fibrillation patients in 'real-world' clinical practice. A propensity-matched analysis of 76,940 patients. Thromb Haemost. 2017;117(6):1072–82.
115. De Caterina R, Kim YH, Koretsune Y, et al. Safety and Effectiveness of Edoxaban in Atrial Fibrillation Patients in Routine Clinical Practice: One-Year Follow-Up from the Global Noninterventional ETNA-AF Program. J Clin Med. 2021;10(4):573.
116. de Groot JR, Weiss TW, Kelly P, et al. Edoxaban for stroke prevention in atrial fibrillation in routine clinical care: 1-year follow-up of the prospective observational ETNA-AF-Europe study. Eur Heart J Cardiovasc Pharmacother. 2021;7(FI1):f30–9.
117. Stanton BE, Barasch NS, Tellor KB. Comparison of the safety and effectiveness of apixaban versus warfarin in patients with severe renal impairment. Pharmacotherapy. 2017;37(4):412–19.
118. Siontis KC, Yao X, Gersh BJ, Noseworthy PA. Direct oral anticoagulants in patients with atrial fibrillation and valvular heart disease other than significant mitral stenosis and mechanical valves: a meta-analysis. Circulation. 2017;135(7):714–16.
119. Steinberg BA, Shrader P, Thomas L, et al. Off-label dosing of non-vitamin k antagonist oral anticoagulants and adverse outcomes: the ORBIT-AF II Registry. J Am Coll Cardiol. 2016;68(24):2597–604.
120. Yao X, Shah ND, Sangaralingham LR, Gersh BJ, Noseworthy PA. Non-vitamin K antagonist oral anticoagulant dosing in patients with atrial fibrillation and renal dysfunction. J Am Coll Cardiol. 2017;69(23):2779–90.
121. Hirsh J, Fuster V. Guide to anticoagulant therapy. Part 1: heparin. American Heart Association. Circulation. 1994;89(3):1449–68.
122. Greinacher A. Heparin-induced thrombocytopenia. Ne Engl J Med. 2015;373(3):252–61.
123. Hirsh J, Raschke R. Heparin and low-molecular-weight heparin: the Seventh ACCP Conference on Antithrombotic and Thrombolytic Therapy. Chest. 2004;126(3 Suppl):188s–203s.
124. Kristensen SD, Knuuti J, Saraste A, et al. 2014 ESC/ESA Guidelines on non-cardiac surgery: cardiovascular assessment and management: the Joint Task Force on non-cardiac surgery: cardiovascular assessment and management of the European Society of Cardiology (ESC) and the European Society of Anaesthesiology (ESA). Eur Heart J. 2014;35(35):2383–431.
125. Greer IA, Nelson-Piercy C. Low-molecular-weight heparins for thromboprophylaxis and treatment of venous thromboembolism in pregnancy: a systematic review of safety and efficacy. Blood. 2005;106(2):401–7.
126. Connolly SJ, Pogue J, Hart RG, et al. Effect of clopidogrel added to aspirin in patients with atrial fibrillation. N Engl J Med. 2009;360(20):2066–78.
127. Sjalander S, Sjalander A, Svensson PJ, Friberg L. Atrial fibrillation patients do not benefit from acetylsalicylic acid. Europace. 2014;16(5):631–8.
128. Active Writing Group of the ACTIVE Investigators, Connolly S, Pogue J, et al. Clopidogrel plus aspirin versus oral anticoagulation for atrial fibrillation in the Atrial fibrillation Clopidogrel Trial with Irbesartan for prevention of Vascular Events (ACTIVE W): a randomised controlled trial. Lancet. 2006;367(9526):1903–12.
129. Mant J, Hobbs FD, Fletcher K, et al. Warfarin versus aspirin for stroke prevention in an elderly community population with atrial fibrillation (the Birmingham Atrial Fibrillation Treatment of the Aged Study, BAFTA): a randomised controlled trial. Lancet. 2007;370(9586):493–503.
130. Verheugt FWA, Gao H, Al Mahmeed W, et al. Characteristics of patients with atrial fibrillation prescribed antiplatelet monotherapy compared with those on anticoagulants: insights from the GARFIELD-AF registry. Eur Heart J. 2018;39(6):464–73.
131. Yasuda S, Kaikita K, Akao M, et al. Antithrombotic therapy for atrial fibrillation with stable coronary disease. N Engl J Med. 2019;381(12):1103–13.
132. Blackshear JL, Odell JA. Appendage obliteration to reduce stroke in cardiac surgical patients with atrial fibrillation. Ann Thorac Surg. 1996;61(2):755–9.
133. Klein AL, Grimm RA, Murray RD, et al. Use of transesophageal echocardiography to guide cardioversion in patients with atrial fibrillation. N Engl J Med. 2001;344(19):1411–20.
134. Al-Saady NM, Obel OA, Camm AJ. Left atrial appendage: structure, function, and role in thromboembolism. Heart. 1999;82(5):547–54.
135. Sakellaridis T, Argiriou M, Charitos C, et al. Left atrial appendage exclusion—where do we stand? J Thorac Dis. 2014;6 Suppl 1(Suppl 1):S70–7.
136. Ding WY, Mandrola J, Gupta D. Left atrial appendage occlusion: past, present and future. Thromb Haemost. 2020;120(11):1484–91.
137. Lakkireddy D, Thaler D, Ellis CR, et al. Amplatzer Amulet left atrial appendage occluder versus watchman device for stroke prophylaxis (Amulet IDE): a randomized, controlled trial. Circulation. 2021;144(19):1543–52.
138. Cruz-Gonzalez I, Fuertes-Barahona M, Moreno-Samos JC, Gonzalez-Ferreiro R, Lam YY, Sanchez PL. Left atrial appendage occlusion: the current device landscape and future perspectives. Interv Cardiol Clin. 2018;7(2):253–65.

139. Lam YY. A new left atrial appendage occluder (Lifetech LAmbre Device) for stroke prevention in atrial fibrillation. Cardiovasc Revasc Med. 2013;14(3):134–6.
140. Deegan R, Ellis CR, Bennett JM. The left atrial appendage, including LAA Occlusion Devices Line Watchman, Amulet, and Lariat. Semin Cardiothorac Vasc Anesth. 2019;23(1):70–87.
141. Glikson M, Wolff R, Hindricks G, et al. EHRA/EAPCI expert consensus statement on catheter-based left atrial appendage occlusion—an update. Europace. 2020;22(2):184.
142. Osmancik P, Herman D, Neuzil P, Hala P, Taborsky M, Kala P, et al. Left Atrial appendage closure versus direct oral anticoagulants in high-risk patients with atrial fibrillation. J Am Coll Cardiol. 2020;75(25):3122–35.
143. Li F, Sun JY, Wu LD, Hao JF, Wang RX. The long-term efficacy and safety of combining ablation and left atrial appendage closure: a systematic review and meta-analysis. J Cardiovasc Electrophysiol. 2021;32(11):3068–81.
144. Akella K, Murtaza G, Turagam M, et al. Evaluating the role of transesophageal echocardiography (TEE) or intracardiac echocardiography (ICE) in left atrial appendage occlusion: a meta-analysis. J Interv Card Electrophysiol. 2021;60(1):41–8.
145. Kar S, Doshi SK, Sadhu A, et al. Primary outcome evaluation of a next-generation left atrial appendage closure device: results from the PINNACLE FLX trial. Circulation. 2021;143(18):1754–62.
146. Darden D, Duong T, Du C, et al. Sex differences in procedural outcomes among patients undergoing left atrial appendage occlusion: insights from the NCDR LAAO Registry. JAMA Cardiol. 2021;6(11):1275–84.
147. Ates I, Marmagkiolis K, Kose G, Iliescu C, Cilingiroglu M. Evaluation of effectiveness and safety of left atrial appendage closure under moderate conscious sedation. J Invasive Cardiol. 2020;32(9):358–62.
148. Marmagkiolis K, Ates I, Kose G, Iliescu C, Cilingiroglu M. Effectiveness and safety of same day discharge after left atrial appendage closure under moderate conscious sedation. Catheter Cardiovasc Interv. 2021;97(5):912–16.
149. Whitlock RP, Belley-Cote EP, Paparella D, et al. Left atrial appendage occlusion during cardiac surgery to prevent stroke. N Engl J Med. 2021;384(22):2081–91.
150. Page RL. The closing argument for surgical left atrial appendage occlusion. N Engl J Med. 2021;384(22):2154–5.
151. Lip GYH, Collet JP, de Caterina R, et al. Antithrombotic therapy in atrial fibrillation associated with valvular heart disease: executive summary of a Joint Consensus Document from the European Heart Rhythm Association (EHRA) and European Society of Cardiology Working Group on Thrombosis, Endorsed by the ESC Working Group on Valvular Heart Disease, Cardiac Arrhythmia Society of Southern Africa (CASSA), Heart Rhythm Society (HRS), Asia Pacific Heart Rhythm Society (APHRS), South African Heart (SA Heart) Association and Sociedad Latinoamericana de Estimulacion Cardiaca y Electrofisiologia (SOLEACE). Thromb Haemost. 2017;117(12):2215–36.
152. Skurk C, Landmesser U. Left atrial appendage occlusion for stroke prevention—state of the art as provided in an updated EHRA/EAPCI consensus statement and future perspectives. EuroIntervention. 2020;15(13):1117–19.
153. Park JW, Bethencourt A, Sievert H, et al. Left atrial appendage closure with Amplatzer cardiac plug in atrial fibrillation: initial European experience. Catheter Cardiovasc Interv. 2011;77(5):700–6.
154. Landmesser U, Schmidt B, Nielsen-Kudsk JE, et al. Left atrial appendage occlusion with the AMPLATZER Amulet device: periprocedural and early clinical/echocardiographic data from a global prospective observational study. EuroIntervention. 2017;13(7):867–76.
155. Korsholm K, Nielsen KM, Jensen JM, Jensen HK, Andersen G, Nielsen-Kudsk JE. Transcatheter left atrial appendage occlusion in patients with atrial fibrillation and a high bleeding risk using aspirin alone for post-implant antithrombotic therapy. EuroIntervention. 2017;12(17):2075–82.
156. Freeman JV, Varosy P, Price MJ, et al. The NCDR Left Atrial Appendage Occlusion Registry. J Am Coll Cardiol. 2020;75(13):1503–18.

CHAPTER 21

Venous thromboembolism: prophylaxis and treatment

Chaozer Er, Walter Ageno, and Alexander T. Cohen

Contents

Summary

Venous thromboembolism (VTE) is the third most frequent cardiovascular disease following myocardial infarction and stroke. Many VTE cases can be attributed to recent hospital admissions and are therefore preventable. As not all hospitalized patients have high VTE risk, performing VTE risk assessment using validated risk assessment models to identify patients who would benefit from thromboprophylaxis is advised. Other than the conventional agents, non-vitamin K antagonist oral anticoagulants can also be used in some settings. High-risk pulmonary embolism is generally treated with systemic thrombolysis while low-risk pulmonary embolism can be treated in the outpatient setting. Patients with intermediate-risk pulmonary embolism should be treated as inpatients for the first few days. Deep vein thrombosis is mostly treated with anticoagulation. Catheter-directed therapy can be considered in highly selected VTE cases. Non-vitamin K antagonist oral anticoagulants are the preferred agents, but special considerations should be given in patients who have advanced liver disease or kidney disease, antiphospholipid syndrome, or had bariatric surgery.

Introduction

Thrombosis results in significant mortality worldwide. Following myocardial infarction and stroke, venous thromboembolism (VTE) is the third most frequent cardiovascular disease.[1] VTE is comprised of deep vein thrombosis (DVT) and pulmonary embolism (PE). DVT frequently happens in the leg veins, but can also occur in abdominopelvic, cerebral, neck, and veins of the upper limbs.

Epidemiology of venous thromboembolism

The annual incidence rates for PE and DVT range from 39 to 115 and 53 to 162 per 100,000 people, respectively.[2] The incidence increases exponentially with age.[2,3] One study in the US estimated the incidence of VTE to be 143 per 100,000 for those aged 40 to 49, rising to 1134 per 100,000 among those aged 80 years and older.[2] Among all ethnicities, Black persons have higher VTE incidence than White persons, while Asian persons have the lowest incidence.[4–7] Men and women have a similar lifetime risk of developing VTE, but the risk for women is higher when they are 20–40 years old due to sex-specific risk factors.[3] VTE causes significant healthcare expenditure in the US and the European Union,[8–10] and its related healthcare burden is expected to rise in the years to come.[1]

Predisposing factors for venous thromboembolism

VTE occurs when the 'thrombosis threshold' is reached via the interactions of various predisposing factors.[1,3] The risk factors are classified as strong, moderate, or weak by the European Society of Cardiology (ESC)[1] (➔ Table 21.1). They can also be persistent or transient.[1,11]

Cancer is a major risk factor for VTE, and the VTE risk varies with cancer types.[1,3] The annual incidence of a first VTE is 3% for bladder and breast cancers, 4–7% for colon and prostate cancers, 10–12% for lung, stomach, ovary, and brain cancers, and 15% for pancreatic cancer.[12]

Prevention of venous thromboembolism

Recent hospital admissions for surgery or acute medical illness are responsible for about 50% of VTEs in the community.[13] VTE may be clinically silent and present as fatal PE.[14,15] Primary prevention by providing thromboprophylaxis in high-risk groups is more cost-effective than performing screening for subclinical DVT (secondary prevention).[14]

The modalities of thromboprophylaxis include mechanical methods [graded compression stocking (GCS) and intermittent pneumatic compressor (IPC)] and pharmacological agents like low-molecular-weight heparins (LMWHs), unfractionated heparin (UFH), fondaparinux, non-vitamin K antagonist oral anticoagulants (NOACs), and aspirin.

Over-prophylaxis of low-risk groups and under-prophylaxis of high-risk groups may result in harm and reduced benefits.[13] It is therefore important to carefully assess the thrombosis and bleeding risk of each individual patient before prescribing thromboprophylaxis (➔ Figure 21.1). Various risk assessment models (RAMs) have been developed in both surgical and medical patients.

Table 21.1 Risk factors for venous thromboembolism

Strong risk factors (odds ratio >10)	Moderate risk factors (odds ratio 2–9)	Weak risk factors (odds ratio <2)
Transient: ◆ Lower limb fracture ◆ Hospitalization for heart failure or atrial fibrillation/flutter (within previous 3 months) ◆ Hip or knee replacement ◆ Myocardial infarction (within previous 3 months)	Transient: ◆ Arthroscopic knee surgery ◆ Central venous lines ◆ Intravenous catheters ◆ Chemotherapy ◆ Congestive heart failure or respiratory failure ◆ Hormone replacement therapy ◆ Oral contraceptive therapy ◆ Postpartum period ◆ Infection (pneumonia, urinary tract infection)	Transient: ◆ Bed rest >3 days ◆ Seated immobility ◆ Pregnancy ◆ Laparoscopic surgery
Persistent: ◆ Previous venous thromboembolism ◆ Spinal cord injury	Persistent: ◆ Autoimmune disease ◆ Inflammatory bowel disease ◆ Cancer ◆ Paralytic stroke ◆ Thrombophilia	Persistent: ◆ Diabetes mellitus ◆ Arterial hypertension ◆ Increasing age ◆ Obesity ◆ Varicose veins

Source data from Konstantinides SV, Meyer G, Becattini C, et al; ESC Scientific Document Group. 2019 ESC Guidelines for the diagnosis and management of acute pulmonary embolism developed in collaboration with the European Respiratory Society (ERS). Eur Heart J. 2020 Jan 21;41(4):543–603. doi: 10.1093/eurheartj/ehz405. PMID: 31504429.

Thromboprophylaxis in medical patients

The Padua Prediction Score (PPS), International Medical Prevention Registry on Venous Thromboembolism (IMPROVE) score, and the UK Department of Health VTE RAM score are useful tools for VTE risk assessment for acutely ill medical patients. PPS and IMPROVE RAM assigned different points to various VTE risk factors such as old age, reduced mobility, active cancer, previous VTE, and known thrombophilia.[16,17] The PPS also included recent trauma or surgery, obesity, hormonal treatment, and the underlying medical conditions (infection, stroke, heart or respiratory failures), whereas IMPROVE factored in intensive care unit (ICU) stay.[16,17] In the Padua study, VTE occurred in 7.5% of patients with Padua score of 4 or higher, while only 0.3% in the group with a low score had VTE.[16] In the original study, the IMPROVE VTE score of 2 or higher correlated with a 3-month VTE risk of at least 2%, whereas a score of 0–1 predicted 1% or less of the VTE risk.[17] The IMPROVE VTE score has been subsequently externally validated.[18,19] The IMPROVE investigators have also developed the IMPROVE bleeding score to identify acutely ill medical patients with high bleeding risk (IMPROVE bleeding score ≥7),[13] and use of pharmacological thromboprophylaxis in this group needs to be weighed against the bleeding risk. Both the Padua and the IMPROVE models were endorsed by the American Society of Haematology (ASH) 2018 guideline on VTE prophylaxis.[13] The UK National Institute for Health and Care Excellence (NICE) guideline recommended using the UK Department of Health VTE RAM for VTE risk assessment.[20,21] This RAM requires the users to assess patients' level of mobility, thrombosis, and bleeding risk factors.[20] The presence of any thrombosis risk factor should prompt thromboprophylaxis, whereas any bleeding risk factor should prompt clinical staff to consider whether the bleeding risk is sufficient to preclude pharmacological prophylaxis.[20,21]

The MEDENOX, PREVENT, and ARTEMIS studies have shown enoxaparin, dalteparin, and fondaparinux safely reduce VTE in medical patients.[22–24] NOAC use as thromboprophylaxis in medical patients has also been studied. In the MAGELLAN trial patients were randomized to receive rivaroxaban 10 mg

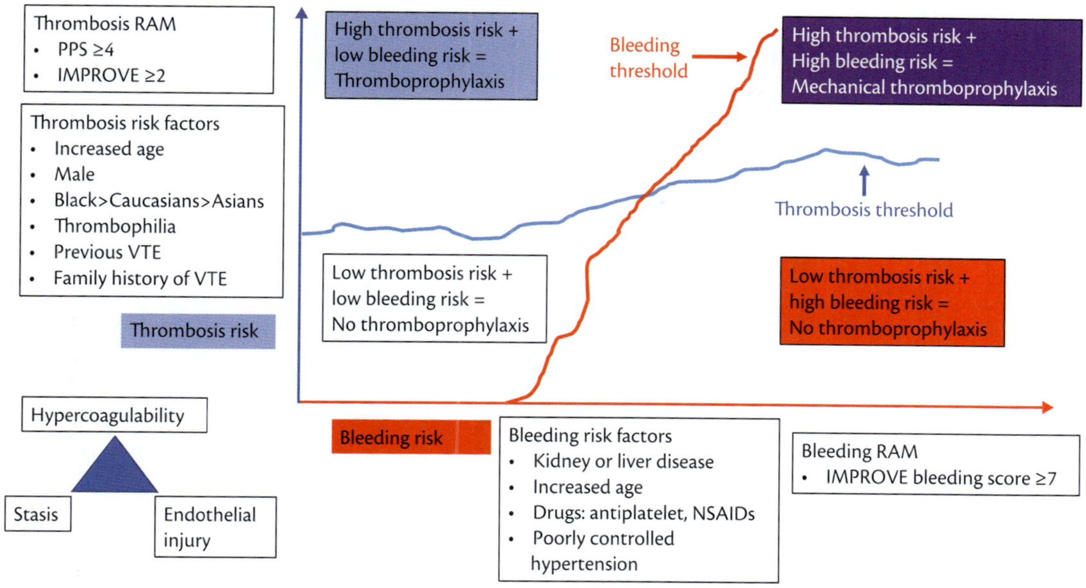

Figure 21.1 Illustration of pathophysiology of venous thromboembolism (VTE) and the rationale of thromboprophylaxis. VTE forms when a thrombosis threshold is reached via the interactions of various risk factors leading to any of the Virchow's triad. Each individual has a different thrombosis threshold as determined by their age, sex, race, history of prior VTE, presence of thrombophilia, and family history of VTE. Bleeding risk differs in every patient and is related to the comorbidities (e.g. liver or kidney disease), medications, and age. Thromboprophylaxis should be prescribed to patients who have high VTE risk and in whom the bleeding risk is also high, mechanical thromboprophylaxis should be considered. Risk assessment models (RAMs) such as the Padua Prediction Score (PPS) or IMPROVE should be used for VTE risk assessment. NSAIDs, non-steroidal anti-inflammatory drugs.

once daily or enoxaparin 40 mg subcutaneously once daily for standard-duration prophylaxis (10 ± 4 days following admission). Rivaroxaban was non-inferior to enoxaparin for standard-duration thromboprophylaxis, but was associated with a twofold increase in clinically relevant bleeding and in major bleeding.[25]

Thromboprophylaxis was given for 6–14 days in the earlier trials,[22–24] but VTE risk in medical patients remains high for 45–60 days after discharge.[13,26] Extended thromboprophylaxis (continuation of thromboprophylaxis after hospital discharge) using NOACs was studied. Extended thromboprophylaxis with rivaroxaban 10 mg daily and apixaban 2.5 mg twice daily were associated with higher bleeding risk than enoxaparin in the MAGELLAN and ADOPT studies.[25,27] Rivaroxaban extended thromboprophylaxis failed to significantly reduce VTE in the MARINER study.[28] Betrixaban extended thromboprophylaxis was compared with standard enoxaparin thromboprophylaxis in the APEX study, and the exploratory analysis suggested betrixaban may be beneficial in thromboprophylaxis without resulting in higher major bleeding risk.[29] Extended thromboprophylaxis is currently not recommended by the major guidelines.[13,30]

The ASH, American College of Chest Physicians (ACCP), and NICE guidelines on thromboprophylaxis in medical patients are summarized in ➔ Table 21.2.[13,21,30] It is recommended that VTE and bleeding risk are assessed using structured RAM, such as the IMPROVE VTE, and bleeding scores when medically ill patients are admitted. LMWH thromboprophylaxis should be prescribed if there are no contraindications and can be stopped after 6–14 days or at discharge in patients with longer admissions or when medical issues have resolved or stabilized. In patients who have a high bleeding risk, IPC can be used as thromboprophylaxis.

Thromboprophylaxis in non-orthopaedic surgical patients

More than 60% of hospitalized patients who are at risk of VTE are surgical patients.[31,32] Even with thromboprophylaxis, approximately 25% of VTE in the community is related to surgery.[33] Surgical patients have a high VTE risk due to all elements of Virchow's triad; postoperative reduced mobility, venous endothelial injury caused by surgeries, hypercoagulability (e.g. reduced antithrombin) following surgical trauma.[34]

Every surgical patient has a different VTE risk due to various surgery and patient-related factors.[33] For example, hip and knee arthroplasty, vascular surgery, and neurosurgical procedures imply a high VTE risk.[33] Patients who have had a previous VTE (particularly unprovoked VTE) or cancer also have a high VTE risk post operation.[33] It is therefore important to have a RAM in stratifying VTE risk in surgical patients.

The ACCP 2012 guideline on prevention of VTE in non-orthopaedic surgical patients recommends using the Rogers score or the Caprini score to risk stratify VTE risk of surgical patients.[35] Unlike the Caprini score, the Rogers score does not include personal history or family history of VTE and thrombophilia in the risk assessment.[36] The original study also did not provide the proportion of patients who had received thromboprophylaxis, which may help to explain the relatively low VTE risk observed.[35] The UK NICE guideline recommends using the UK Department of Health VTE RAM to assess VTE risk for both medical and surgical patients.[21]

➔ Table 21.2 provides a summary of the major guidelines on thromboprophylaxis in surgical patients.[21,33,35] The ACCP

Table 21.2 Summary of ACCP, ASH, NICE, ASCO thromboprophylaxis guidelines in medical, surgical, orthopaedic, and cancer patients

Patient groups			
Medical	**ACCP 2012**	**ASH 2018**	**NICE 2018**
Acutely ill	LMWHs, UFH, or fondaparinux if increased thrombosis risk and no high bleeding risk	LMWHs or fondaparinux > UFH > mechanical (IPC or GCS) > no prophylaxis	Perform VTE risk assessment using the UK Department of Health VTE risk assessment tool Thromboprophylaxis if VTE risk outweighs bleeding risk for a minimum of 7 days
	High thrombosis and bleeding risk, use GCS or IPC rather than no prophylaxis	Those who do not receive pharmacological prophylaxis, use IPC or GCS > no prophylaxis	LMWHs > fondaparinux
Critically ill	LMWHs or UFH rather than no prophylaxis	LMWHs > UFH > mechanical (IPC or GCS) > no prophylaxis	Assess VTE and bleeding risk using the same tool
	Use IPC or GCS if high bleeding risk rather than no prophylaxis	Those who do not receive pharmacological prophylaxis, use IPC or GCS > no prophylaxis	LMWHs first line Use mechanical prophylaxis (IPC or antiembolic stocking) if pharmacological agent contraindicated
Chronically ill patients in nursing home	No prophylaxis	No prophylaxis	Not mentioned
Extended thromboprophylaxis	Not recommended	Not recommended	Not mentioned
Surgical	**ACCP 2012**	**ASH 2019**	**NICE 2018**
Abdominal or pelvic surgeries	*Very low VTE risk* (Rogers score <7, Caprini score 0): no thromboprophylaxis other than early ambulation *Low VTE risk* (Rogers score 7–10, Caprini score 1–2): IPC over no prophylaxis *Moderate VTE risk* (Rogers score >10, Caprini score 3–4): 1. LMWHs, UFH, or IPC over no prophylaxis 2. If high bleeding risk → IPC *High VTE risk* (Caprini score ≥5): 1. LMWHs or UFH over no prophylaxis 2. IPC or GCS should be added to pharmacological prophylaxis 3. If high bleeding risk → IPC until pharmacological prophylaxis can be initiated 4. If LMWHs and UFH are not available or contraindicated → low-dose aspirin, fondaparinux or IPC	Use pharmacological (LMWHs or UFH) or mechanical prophylaxis rather than no prophylaxis Those who receive pharmacological prophylaxis, suggest combining with mechanical prophylaxis Mechanical prophylaxis may be preferred for those with high bleeding risk	Assess all surgical and trauma patients' VTE and bleeding risk after using the UK Department of Health VTE risk assessment tool Start mechanical prophylaxis (GPS or IPC) upon admission and continue until the person no longer has significantly reduced mobility Add pharmacological prophylaxis (LMWHs or fondaparinux) for a minimum of 7 days for people undergoing abdominal surgery whose risk of VTE outweighs their risk of bleeding
Extended prophylaxis	For high-VTE-risk patients undergoing abdominal or pelvic surgery for cancer who are not otherwise at high risk for major bleeding complications, extended duration of pharmacological prophylaxis (4 weeks) with a LMWH over limited-duration prophylaxis is recommended	Extended prophylaxis (over 3 weeks) is suggested	Consider extending pharmacological VTE prophylaxis to 28 days postoperatively for people who have had major cancer surgery in the abdomen
Orthopaedic	**ACCP 2012**	**ASH 2019**	**NICE 2018**
Total knee arthroplasty	Minimum 10–14 days of a LMWH (preferred), fondaparinux, apixaban, dabigatran, rivaroxaban, or UFH, vitamin K antagonists (VKAs), aspirin, or IPC	Aspirin or anticoagulants (in order of preference NOAC > LMWHs > warfarin if anticoagulant is used)	Aspirin (75 or 150 mg) for 14 days or a LMWH for 14 days + antiembolic stocking until discharge or rivaroxaban Use apixaban or dabigatran if other options not available Use IPC if pharmacological prophylaxis is contraindicated

Total hip arthroplasty	Same as total knee arthroplasty	Same as total knee arthroplasty	LMWHs for 10 days followed by aspirin (75 mg or 150 mg) for a further 28 days or LMWHs for 28 days + antiembolic stocking until discharge or rivaroxaban Use apixaban or dabigatran if other options not available Use antiembolic stocking if pharmacological prophylaxis is contraindicated
Hip fracture surgery	Minimum 10–14 days of LMWHs (preferred), fondaparinux, UFH, VKAs, aspirin, or IPC	LMWHs or UFH	LMWHs or fondaparinux for a month Use IPC if pharmacological prophylaxis is contraindicated
Distal lower limb injuries	No prophylaxis in patients with isolated lower-leg injuries requiring leg immobilization	NA	Pharmacological prophylaxis for foot or ankle surgery: ◆ That requires immobilization ◆ When total anaesthesia time is >90 minutes ◆ The person's VTE risk outweighs their bleeding risk
Extended thromboprophylaxis	Patients undergoing major orthopaedic surgery: IPC + antithrombotic during hospital stay + extended prophylaxis in the outpatient period for up to 35 days from the day of surgery	Extended prophylaxis beyond 3 weeks for patients undergoing major surgery	As above
Cancer	**ACCP 2012 (medical)**	**ASCO 2019**	**NICE 2018**
Outpatients	Without additional VTE risk factors: no prophylaxis With additional VTE risk factors such as previous VTE, immobilization, hormonal therapy, angiogenesis inhibitors, thalidomide, and lenalidomide): LMWH or UFH prophylaxis over no prophylaxis With indwelling central venous catheters: against routine prophylaxis	No routine prophylaxis for all outpatients High-risk outpatients with cancer (Khorana score of ≥2 prior to starting a new systemic chemotherapy regimen): may be offered thromboprophylaxis with apixaban, rivaroxaban, or a LMWH	No routine prophylaxis to people with cancer who are receiving cancer modifying treatments and who are mobile unless they are also at increased risk of VTE because of something other than the cancer
Inpatients		Hospitalized patients who have active malignancy and acute medical illness or reduced mobility: pharmacological thromboprophylaxis Patients admitted for the sole purpose of minor procedures or chemotherapy infusion: no prophylaxis	As above
Myeloma patients		Receiving thalidomide- or lenalidomide-based regimens with chemotherapy and/or dexamethasone: aspirin or LMWHs for lower-risk patients and LMWHs for higher-risk patients	Receiving chemotherapy with thalidomide, pomalidomide, or lenalidomide with steroids: aspirin, or LMWHs

ACCP, American College of Chest Physicians; ASCO, American Society of Clinical Oncology; ASH, American Society of Haematology; GCS, graded compression stocking; IPC, intermittent pneumatic compressor; LMWH, low-molecular-weight heparin; NICE, National Institute for Health and Care Excellence; NOAC, non-vitamin K antagonist oral anticoagulant; UFH, unfractionated heparin; VKA, vitamin K antagonist; VTE, venous thromboembolism.

Source data from Gould MK, Garcia DA, Wren SM, Ket al. Prevention of VTE in nonorthopedic surgical patients: Antithrombotic Therapy and Prevention of Thrombosis, 9th ed: American College of Chest Physicians Evidence-Based Clinical Practice Guidelines. Chest. 2012 Feb;141(2 Suppl):e227S–e277S. doi: 10.1378/chest.11-2297; and Schünemann HJ, Cushman M, Burnett AE, et al. American Society of Hematology 2018 guidelines for management of venous thromboembolism: prophylaxis for hospitalized and nonhospitalized medical patients. Blood Adv. 2018 Nov 27;2(22):3198–3225. doi: 10.1182/bloodadvances.2018022954; and Anderson DR, Morgano GP, Bennett C, et al. American Society of Hematology 2019 guidelines for management of venous thromboembolism: prevention of venous thromboembolism in surgical hospitalized patients. Blood Adv. 2019 Dec 10;3(23):3898–3944. doi: 10.1182/bloodadvances.2019000975; and National Guideline Centre (UK). Venous thromboembolism in over 16s: Reducing the risk of hospital-acquired deep vein thrombosis or pulmonary embolism. London: National Institute for Health and Care Excellence (NICE); 2018 Mar; and Key NS, Khorana AA, Kuderer NM, et al. Venous Thromboembolism Prophylaxis and Treatment in Patients With Cancer: ASCO Clinical Practice Guideline Update. J Clin Oncol. 2020 Feb 10;38(5):496–520. doi: 10.1200/JCO.19.01461.

guideline suggests stratifying surgical patients using the Caprini score into high, moderate, low, and very low VTE risks.[35] No prophylaxis is recommended for very-low-risk patients, IPC for low risk, LMWHs for moderate risk, and a combination of a LMWH and IPC is recommended for the high-risk group.[35] Surgeons or interventionists should be consulted before pharmacological prophylaxis is prescribed. Both patient-related and procedure-related factors must be considered when undertaking risk assessment for bleeding and VTE. A LMWH as VTE prophylaxis should be prescribed after surgery when haemostasis is achieved (usually within 12 hours). Thromboprophylaxis can be stopped prior to discharge or when the patient's mobility has returned to normal in many moderate-risk surgical patients. A longer prophylaxis should be considered in high-risk patients who have a history of VTE or cancer.

Thromboprophylaxis in orthopaedic surgery patients

Total joint arthroplasty for knee and hip replacements as well as hip fracture surgery have a high VTE risk.[33,37] Other than endothelial injury caused by surgery, positioning of the lower limb and application of the tourniquet during total joint arthroplasty can lead to femoral vein occlusion, hypercoagulability, and hence increase the risk of VTE.[38–40]

➲ Table 21.2 summarizes the recommendations of various guidelines on VTE prophylaxis in total joint arthroplasty and hip fracture surgery.[21,33,37]

The evidence of thromboprophylaxis for distal lower limb injuries is less clear. The DVT risk is directly proportional to the proximity of the fracture to the knee.[37] The 2012 ACCP guideline suggested no prophylaxis in patients with isolated lower-leg injuries requiring leg immobilization.[37] Fractures below the knee, tendon ruptures, and cartilage injuries to the knee and ankle were included as lower-leg injuries in the guideline. More evidence became available after that. A meta-analysis that included 13 studies published from 1993 to 2017 concluded that thromboprophylaxis with a LMWH or fondaparinux for patients with lower limb immobilization after injury approximately halves the VTE risk, and there were only four major bleeding events across all studies.[41] All studies included had a risk of bias and patients included were heterogeneous, with some studies including fractures only while others included tendon ruptures and mixed pathologies.[41] The reported VTE incidence following lower limb immobilization without thromboprophylaxis had a wide range of 4.3–40%, while symptomatic or clinically important VTE occurred in 1.8–5.5% of patients without thromboprophylaxis.[42] Without a good gauge of the baseline risk it would be hard to estimate the number needed to treat, but a decision-analytic modelling suggested that thromboprophylaxis in this group of patients is cost-effective.[42,43] Two randomized controlled trials and a study in Edinburgh, UK, however, showed that thromboprophylaxis was ineffective.[44–46] Though there is no universal consensus so far, it is agreed that patients with lower limb immobilization following an injury should have their VTE risk assessed and be prescribed thromboprophylaxis if the risk is high (e.g. personal or family history of VTE).[41,42,46] This is in keeping with the NICE guideline suggesting that patients with reduced mobility should have thrombosis and bleeding risk assessed.[21] If the patient has other risk factors, such as age over 60 years, obesity, active cancer, or previous VTE, thromboprophylaxis will be advised.

Thromboprophylaxis in cancer patients

VTE risk is four- to sevenfold higher in cancer patients.[47] The annual incidence varies from 0.5% to 20%.[47] The rate differs in relationship to the cancer site and type, the presence or absence of metastases, surgical procedures, anticancer therapy (chemotherapy, radiotherapy, hormonal therapy, and immunotherapy), the use of intravascular catheters, hospitalization, and patient-related factors such as age, comorbidities, and a history of previous VTE.[47] Cancer patients receiving chemotherapy have a particularly high VTE risk.[48]

Patients with cancer-associated thrombosis (CAT) have higher VTE recurrence rates, bleeding complications from anticoagulation, and mortality compared with cancer patients without VTE.[48–50] The Khorana score was developed to identify cancer patients with a high VTE risk and hence those who may benefit from thromboprophylaxis.[48–51] In the original study, the high-risk group had a nearly 7% risk of developing VTE over a period of 2.5 months, and this was comparable to the risk of hospitalized patients for whom thromboprophylaxis has been shown to be effective.[48] The Khorana score was used by the American Society of Clinical Oncology (ASCO) to risk stratify VTE risk of cancer patients in the outpatient setting.[52] Cancer site, pre-chemotherapy full blood counts, and body mass index (BMI) were included in the scoring system, and a score of 3 or more is considered high risk, 1–2 is considered intermediate risk, and 0 is considered low risk.

See ➲ Table 21.2 for a summary of thromboprophylaxis guidelines on cancer patients.[21,30,52]

Thromboprophylaxis in COVID-19 patients

The true VTE incidence in hospitalized COVID-19 patients remains unclear, but a meta-analysis including more than 11,000 patients showed a pooled incidence of VTE in COVID-19 patients to be 17% (12% for DVT, 7.1% for PE).[53,54] COVID-19 causes VTE via two mechanisms—hypercoagulability and endothelial injury—which are responsible for large vessel and microvascular thrombosis, respectively.[53] The alterations in various haematological parameters, such as increased D-dimer, thrombin production, and factor V and VIII levels in COVID-19 patients, contribute to the prothrombotic state.[53]

Critically ill COVID-19 patients are those who require ICU care or organ support, while acutely ill COVID-19 patients refer to those who require hospital admission without ICU support (i.e. general medical ward-type of patients). There are three types of thromboprophylaxis strategies: prophylactic (standard-dose thromboprophylaxis used in medical patients, such as low-dose LMWHs, e.g. enoxaparin 40 mg once daily), intermediate (twice-daily LMWHs/double the standard dose for medical patients, e.g. enoxaparin 40 mg twice daily), and therapeutic intensity (e.g. enoxaparin 1 mg/kg twice daily). Intermediate-dose thromboprophylaxis is generally discouraged,[55–58] as there is a lack of supportive evidence from randomized controlled trials and it may be confusing and error-prone in clinical practice.[57] LMWHs are the preferred agents, and all hospitalized COVID-19 patients should receive at least standard-dose thromboprophylaxis.[55–58]

➔ Table 21.3 provides a summary of a few of the many published guidelines on thromboprophylaxis in COVID-19 patients.

Treatment of venous thromboembolism

The management of acute VTE is a medical emergency. Prompt and appropriate treatment of VTE is important and the aim of VTE treatment is to prevent thrombus extension, embolization, cardiopulmonary collapse, death, recurrence of VTE, and long-term complications.[3]

Phases in anticoagulation

Anticoagulation in VTE is split into an initiation, a treatment, and an extended phase.[59] The initiation phase refers to provision of anticoagulants (parenteral or high-dose oral form) following VTE diagnosis, and lasts from 5 to 21 days depending on the anticoagulant choice.[59] The treatment phase is the period where standard doses of anticoagulants are used after the initiation phase, and typically lasts for 3–6 months.[59] The extended phase follows the treatment phase and aims at reducing VTE recurrence (secondary prevention) by using full or reduced doses of anticoagulants.[59] It has no pre-planned stop date.[59]

The ASH guideline used 'initial treatment' to describe the first 5–21 days following VTE diagnosis, 'primary treatment' to refer to the minimal length of time a patient must be on therapeutic anticoagulation to treat the initial VTE (generally 3–6 months), and 'secondary prevention' as the period following completion of primary treatment when a decision to continue long-term anticoagulation to prevent recurrence needs to be made.[60]

Pulmonary embolism

Classification of pulmonary embolism

The ESC classified PE into low, intermediate, and high risk[1] (➔ Table 21.4). The presence of haemodynamic instability defines high-risk PE.[1] Haemodynamic instability is defined by the presence of any of the following[1]:

1. Cardiac arrest or need for cardiopulmonary resuscitation.
2. Obstructive shock [(a) and (b) are both present]:
   a. Systolic blood pressure (SBP) less than 90 mmHg or vasopressors required to achieve a SBP of at least 90 mmHg despite adequate filling status.
   b. End-organ hypoperfusion (oliguria, altered mental status, raised serum lactate).
3. Persistent hypotension: SBP less than 90 mmHg or SBP drop of at least 40 mmHg, lasting longer than 15 minutes and not caused by new-onset arrhythmia, hypovolaemia, or sepsis.

Patients who have no haemodynamic instability are further risk stratified based on their clinical features (e.g. heart rate, oxygenation), imaging (presence of right ventricular dysfunction),

Table 21.3 Summary of major guidelines on thromboprophylaxis in COVID-19 patients

COVID-19 patients	ACCP 2022	ASH 2021	NICE 2022	Anticoagulation Forum 2022
Acutely ill	Therapeutic LMWHs or UFH > standard > intermediate dose	Prophylactic > intermediate or therapeutic intensity	Standard dose for minimum 7 days for anyone on oxygen Consider therapeutic dose in those requiring low-flow oxygen if no increased bleeding risk	At least standard dose LWMH or UFH, consider therapeutic dose if increased risk of progression or VTE (patients admitted for COVID-19 infection on supplemental oxygen + D-dimer 2–4 times of upper limit of normal) and have not high bleeding risk
Critically ill	Standard dose LMWHs or UFH > therapeutic or intermediate dose	Prophylactic > intermediate or therapeutic intensity	Standard dose for minimum 7 days for anyone on non-invasive ventilation or mechanical ventilation	Standard dose instead of intermediate or therapeutic
Patients in the community	Not mentioned	Not mentioned	For patients managed in hospital-led acute care in the community setting, assess bleeding and VTE risk, consider pharmacological prophylaxis if the VTE risk > bleeding risk	Against antithrombotic for non-hospitalized, ambulatory patients with mild COVID-19

ACCP, American College of Chest Physicians; ASH, American Society of Haematology; LMWH, low-molecular-weight heparin; NICE, National Institute for Health and Care Excellence; UFH, unfractionated heparin; VTE, venous thromboembolism.

Source data from Moores LK, Tritschler T, Brosnahan S, et al. Thromboprophylaxis in Patients With COVID-19: A Brief Update to the CHEST Guideline and Expert Panel Report. Chest. 2022 Jul;162(1):213–225. doi: 10.1016/j.chest.2022.02.006; and Cuker A, Tseng EK, Nieuwlaat R, et al. American Society of Hematology living guidelines on the use of anticoagulation for thromboprophylaxis in patients with COVID-19: May 2021 update on the use of intermediate-intensity anticoagulation in critically ill patients. Blood Adv. 2021 Oct 26;5(20):3951–3959. doi: 10.1182/bloodadvances.2021005493; and Barnes GD, Burnett A, Allen A, et al. Thromboembolic prevention and anticoagulant therapy during the COVID-19 pandemic: updated clinical guidance from the anticoagulation forum. J Thromb Thrombolysis. 2022 Aug;54(2):197–210. doi: 10.1007/s11239-022-02643-3; and COVID-19 rapid guideline: managing COVID-19. London: National Institute for Health and Care Excellence (NICE); 2022 Jun 15.

Table 21.4 Summary of pulmonary embolism severity

PE severity	Haemodynamic instability	PESI class III–V	Right ventricular dysfunction on TTE or CTPA	Raised cardiac troponin
High risk	+	+	+	+
Intermediate–high risk	–	+	+	+
Intermediate–low risk	–	+	One or none positive	
Low risk	–	–	–	Assessment optional, if assessed negative

CTPA, computed tomography pulmonary angiogram; PE, pulmonary embolism; PESI, Pulmonary Embolism Severity Index; TTE, transthoracic echocardiography.
Source data from Konstantinides SV, Meyer G, Becattini C, et al; ESC Scientific Document Group. 2019 ESC Guidelines for the diagnosis and management of acute pulmonary embolism developed in collaboration with the European Respiratory Society (ERS). Eur Heart J. 2020 Jan 21;41(4):543–603. doi: 10.1093/eurheartj/ehz405. PMID: 31504429.

cardiac biomarkers (e.g. troponin and N-terminal pro B-type natriuretic peptide, NT-proBNP), and the presence of comorbidities.[1] The Pulmonary Embolism Severity Index (PESI) and its simplified version (sPESI) have been shown to be reliable in identifying low-risk PE (PESI class I to II or sPESI 0) patients who have a low 30-day mortality.[1] Patients who are PESI class I or II but have right ventricular dysfunction or raised cardiac laboratory markers are considered as having intermediate risk PE.[1]

The remaining patients who do not have low PESI class (I or II) or haemodynamic instability are classified as having intermediate risk PE.[1] Those who have right ventricular dysfunction as evident in the transthoracic echocardiography or computed tomography pulmonary angiogram and elevated cardiac biomarkers (troponin or NT-proBNP) are subclassified as intermediate–high-risk PE.[1] Those who have no right ventricular dysfunction and/or raised cardiac markers belong to intermediate-low risk PE.[1]

Treatment of pulmonary embolism

Anticoagulation is the cornerstone of VTE treatment, but it does not reduce the clot burden as quickly as thrombolysis in the acute setting.[61] There are two ways of administering thrombolytic agents: systemic thrombolysis and catheter-directed therapy (CDT). Systemic thrombolysis involves the direct administration of a thrombolytic agent [e.g. alteplase 100 mg over 2 hours (refer to the ESC 2019 PE guidelines,[1] Table 10, for thrombolytic regimens, doses, and contraindications)] via peripheral intravenous catheter into the systemic circulation. CDT involves the percutaneous placement of an intravascular catheter, usually via the femoral vein route, into the thrombosed pulmonary vessels to fragment or aspirate the thrombus directly (catheter-directed thrombectomy).[61] The thrombolytic agent can be directly administered via the intravascular catheter into the pulmonary arteries (catheter-directed thrombolysis) and, due to its direct delivery, the dose of the thrombolytic agent is usually much lower and hence is believed to entail a lower bleeding risk.[61] Depending on the scenario, the interventionist may choose to perform either catheter-directed thrombectomy or catheter-directed thrombolysis, or both, in the same setting.

High-risk PE should be treated with systemic thrombolysis in the absence of high bleeding risk.[1,59,60] Surgical pulmonary embolectomy or CDT should be considered if systemic thrombolysis is contraindicated (e.g. in the presence of high bleeding risk) or has failed.[1,59] In cases where high-risk PE is causing a shock that is likely to lead to death before systemic thrombolysis can take effect (e.g. within hours), CDT may be considered.[59] One meta-analysis showed that systemic thrombolysis reduces mortality in patients with high-risk PE, but is associated with a 9.9% risk of severe bleeding and a 1.7% risk of intracranial bleeding.[62]

Patients with low-risk PE can safely be discharged early and treated as outpatients, provided that there are no other reasons for hospitalization, there is family or social support, and early access to medical care.[1,60] Other than PESI and sPESI, the Hestia exclusion criteria consist of aspects of PE severity, comorbidity, and feasibility of outpatient treatment; this is an alternative checklist that can be used to determine the suitability for outpatient treatment.[1,63] All answers must be 'negative' for patients to be treated as outpatients.[1,63] The Hestia rule was compared with sPESI in the HOME-PE study and found to have similar safety and effectiveness.[64]

The mainstay of treatment of intermediate-risk PE is anticoagulation.[1,59,60] Patients should initially be admitted for close monitoring for a minimum of 3 days.[1,60] Routine systemic thrombolysis is not recommended, as bleeding risk here outweighs the expected benefits.[1,59,60] Thrombolysis (systemic or catheter directed) should be reserved for patients who deteriorate and develop haemodynamic compromise while on anticoagulation,[1] but this therapy may be considered in selected patients who deteriorate after starting anticoagulation but have yet to develop hypotension and who have an acceptable bleeding risk (intermediate-risk PE with low bleeding risk and at high risk of decompensation).[59,60]

Deep vein thrombosis

Isolated distal deep vein thrombosis

Isolated distal DVT refers to DVT confined to the calf veins below the knee level and the popliteal vein is not involved.[59] As the risk of recurrence and progression (10–15%) is lower compared to proximal DVT, serial monitoring with repeat compressive ultrasonography once weekly for 2 weeks is suggested in the absence of severe symptoms or other risk factors for extension.[59] Factors that may favour anticoagulation include a positive D-dimer without alternative reasons, extensive thrombosis (i.e. >5 cm in length, involvement of multiple veins), cancer, history of VTE, in-patient status, COVID-19 infection, highly symptomatic, thrombosis close to proximal veins, or patient preference to avoid repeat imaging.[59] Factors favouring serial imaging are thrombus confined to muscular veins (e.g. soleus or gastrocnemius), high or moderate bleeding risk, and patient preference to avoid anticoagulation.[59] If repeat compressive ultrasonography demonstrates extension of the DVT (either this remains as distal DVT or extends into proximal veins above the knee), anticoagulation as for proximal DVT is advised.[59] In clinical practice, the large majority of patients with isolated distal DVT receive a short course (6–12 weeks) of anticoagulant treatment.[65]

Proximal deep vein thrombosis

Acute proximal DVT should be treated with anticoagulation. Routine thrombolytic treatment is not recommended other than in patients who have limb-threatening DVT.[59,60] When thrombolytic treatment is considered for extensive proximal DVT (involving the iliac veins), CDT is preferred over systemic thrombolysis.[60] The CaVent trial showed that CDT reduced post-thrombotic syndrome (PTS), appeared to be cost-effective, but did not alter quality of life.[59,66–70] The ATTRACT and CAVA studies found that CDT was associated with higher bleeding risk and did not reduce PTS.[71–73] Subgroup analysis of the ATTRACT study, however, showed that patients who have acute iliofemoral DVT treated with CDT may have a reduced risk of moderate-to-severe PTS.[3,73] This raised the question whether selected young patients who have acute iliofemoral DVT, low bleeding risk, and severe symptoms from the DVT may benefit from CDT.[60] This may be especially true if they value rapid symptoms resolution and are averse to the possibility of PTS.[60]

Choice of anticoagulants

For patients with high-risk PE or with imminent haemodynamic instability in whom thrombolytic treatment will be required, UFH may be preferred as the initial anticoagulant.[1] Once patients have stabilized after thrombolytic therapy, anticoagulants can be switched to oral form.[1]

For patients with intermediate-risk PE, LMWHs or fondaparinux are preferred over UFH as the initial anticoagulants due to their lower risk of inducing bleeding and heparin-induced thrombocytopaenia.[1] As shown in the PEITHO trial, the deterioration of intermediate-risk PE patients most often occurs in the first 2–3 days following diagnosis, therefore it may be reasonable to use LWMH for the first 2–3 days before switching to oral anticoagulants.[1]

Many patients with low-risk PE can be treated as outpatients. NOACs are the treatment of choice because of their superior safety profile and convenience. NOACs have predictable bioavailability and pharmacokinetics, and no need for routine monitoring.[1] Rivaroxaban and apixaban are initiated at higher doses before switching to the standard dose (➔ Drug dosing).[1] This approach obviates the need for parenteral anticoagulants in the initial phase, is proven to be effective, and has a good safety profile.[1]

Patients who have uncomplicated DVT with no other reasons for hospital admission can also be treated as outpatients safely.[60] NOACs that require no parenteral anticoagulant bridging are preferred.

Heparin followed by a vitamin K antagonist (VKA) was the standard therapy until NOACs came into the picture. NOACs have been shown to be non-inferior to parenteral therapy overlapped with VKAs in both the treatment and the extended phases. NOACs are associated with lower bleeding rates compared with conventional therapy.[1] The ASH and ACCP guidelines now advocate using NOACs over VKAs in VTE patients.[59,60]

Anticoagulation duration

All VTE patients should complete at least 3 months of anticoagulation (treatment phase) in the absence of contraindications and then should be assessed for the need for extended therapy (➔ Figure 21.2).[59] Extended anticoagulation is suggested for unprovoked VTE (VTE diagnosed in the absence of

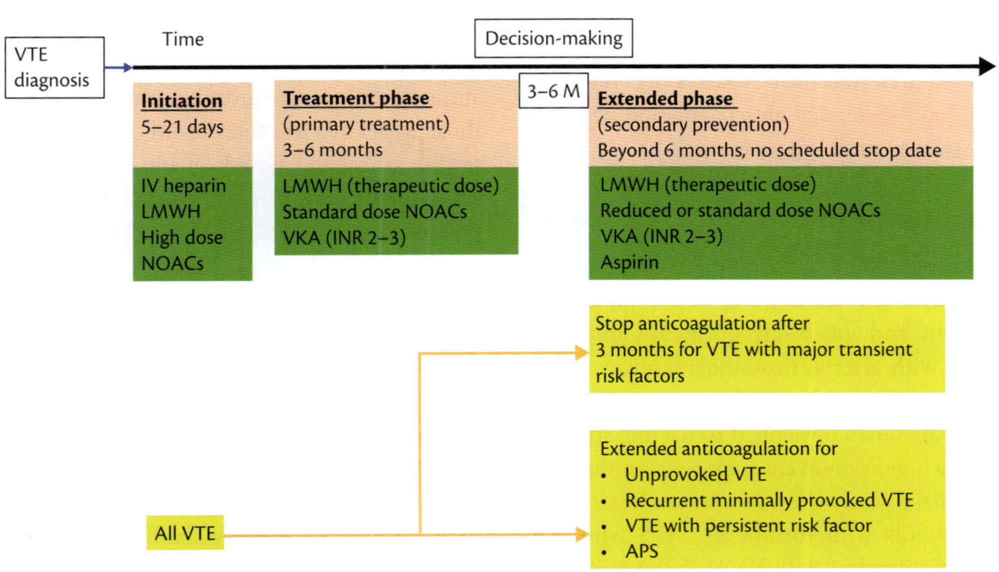

Figure 21.2 Summary of VTE treatment: anticoagulation phases, anticoagulant types, and duration of anticoagulation. APS, antiphospholipid syndrome.

provocation), recurrent unprovoked VTE, or VTE provoked by a chronic risk factor.[59,60] NOACs are preferred over VKAs in the extended phase.[59] Standard or reduced dose NOACs can be used for the extended phase,[60] but a reduced dose may be preferred for many patients, particularly those with a significant, but not very high risk of recurrence.[1,59] VTE diagnosed in the presence of a major (e.g. surgery with general anaesthesia >30 minutes' duration or major trauma) or minor transient risk factors (e.g. hospital admission of <3 days for acute illness) do not require extended anticoagulation after completing the treatment phase.[59] Patients who receive extended therapy should be assessed periodically for their bleeding risk, therapy burdens, and change in values or preferences.[59] Aspirin has been shown to be effective in reducing recurrent VTE, but is much less effective in preventing recurrences compared to reduced-dose NOACs.[59] Some anticoagulants have a bleeding risk similar to aspirin; therefore, aspirin should not be considered as an alternative for secondary VTE prevention.[59] For patients who are stopping anticoagulation, aspirin can, however, be considered for VTE prevention.[59]

Cancer-associated thrombosis

LMWHs are superior to VKAs in terms of efficacy and safety in treating CAT.[74] NOACs have been shown to be an effective or more effective option in CAT treatment when compared to LMWHs; however, a trend to higher bleeding rates was reported in the meta-analyses.[75] Some guidelines suggest that NOACs should be avoided in patients with high bleeding risk.[75] The ACCP 2021 guideline recommends an oral anti-Xa inhibitor (apixaban, edoxaban, or rivaroxaban) over LMWHs for the initiation and treatment phase.[59] The UK NICE guideline suggests considering NOACs for CAT treatment and use of LMWHs if NOACs are unsuitable.[76] In patients with a luminal gastrointestinal tract (GIT) cancer, edoxaban and rivaroxaban therapy appear to be associated with higher risk of GIT bleeding while apixaban does not.[59] Apixaban or LWMH may therefore be the preferred option for luminal GIT cancer-associated VTE.[59] In patients who have nausea, mucositis, or chemotherapy-related thrombocytopaenia, a LMWH may be preferred, as it bypasses the GIT and is more easily dose adjusted.[59] Extended anticoagulation beyond 6 months should be considered until cancer is cured.[1,76]

Antiphospholipid syndrome

In patients with antiphospholipid syndrome (APS), VKAs are preferred for patients who are 'triple positive' for lupus anticoagulant, anticardiolipin, and anti-β_2-glycoprotein I antibodies or have APS associated with arterial thromboembolism. In one study that included only triple-positive APS patients, 12% of the patients treated with rivaroxaban developed ischaemic stroke or myocardial infarction, whereas no event happened in the VKA arm.[77] Another randomized study showed that stroke occurred more commonly in patients with thrombotic APS who were treated with rivaroxaban compared with VKAs.[78] The ACCP and ESC Guidelines therefore recommended VKAs over NOACs for patients with confirmed APS.[1,59] The International Society on Thrombosis and Haemostasis (ISTH) guideline recommended that VKAs should be used for high-risk APS, which includes APS patients with triple positivity, arterial thrombosis, small vessel thrombosis/organ involvement, or heart valve disease according to the Sydney criteria.[79] It mentioned, however, single- or double-positive non-high-risk APS patients who have been on NOACs with good adherence for several months for a first episode of VTE, for whom a patient-centred and well-informed decision of whether to continue a NOAC is appropriate.[79] The European League Against Rheumatism guideline advocated VKAs as first-line treatment for APS patients with VTE, but mentioned that NOACs could be considered in patients who are not able to achieve a target international normalized ratio (INR) despite good adherence or those with contraindications to VKAs.[80] The British Society for Haematology guideline recommended to change a NOAC to a VKA for those triple-positive APS patients currently on NOACs, and to continue a NOAC over no anticoagulation if patients do not wish to switch.[81] It also suggested against the initiation of a NOAC for VTE treatment in non-triple-positive APS patients, but also say that patients who are already on a NOAC may continue or switch to a VKA after discussion between the patient and the specialist.[81] Extended anticoagulation is recommended for APS patients.[1] A systematic review has shown that safety and efficacy of NOACs may be highly dependent on clinical and immunological phenotype of APS patients and that, although VKAs are the first-choice treatment in APS patients with VTE, NOACs may be a reasonable option in some specific situations after a well-informed discussion with the patient.[79–82]

Chronic kidney disease

The NOACs have variable renal elimination rates with 80%, 50%, 35%, and 27% of dabigatran, edoxaban, rivaroxaban, and apixaban being metabolized by the kidneys, respectively.[83] Renal function assessment for NOAC dosing is best estimated by applying the Cockcroft–Gault equation to calculate the estimated creatinine clearance (CrCl).[71] In the original trials, VTE patients with CrCl less than 30 mL/min were excluded from the studies looking at rivaroxaban, edoxaban, and dabigatran, while those with CrCl less than 25 mL/min were not included in those testing apixaban.[1] Based on modelling and clinical experience, rivaroxaban, apixaban, and edoxaban can be used with caution in patients who have a CrCl of 15–30 mL/min.[3]

Observational data, however, showed that apixaban, rivaroxaban, and edoxaban had a good safety profile and were effective in patients with severe kidney disease, though most data were from patients on anticoagulation for atrial fibrillation (AF).[83–87] One retrospective cohort study using data from medical insurance sources looked at apixaban use for VTE treatment in patients with chronic kidney disease. It showed that apixaban was associated with lower VTE recurrence and major bleeding than warfarin in patients with all stages of chronic kidney disease, including end-stage renal disease.[88] More studies are needed to confirm this finding.[88]

In 2014, the US Food and Drug Administration approved apixaban for patients with end-stage renal disease with AF based on pharmacokinetic data,[87] but high-quality prospective studies are lacking.[1] Retrospective studies seem to indicate that apixaban use for patients with end-stage renal disease on haemodialysis with VTE and AF is safe and effective.[88–90] Until more prospective data are available, the use of NOACs to treat VTE in patients with end-stage renal disease should be individualized, and patients need to be well informed about the lack of evidence of such practice.[83]

The UK NICE guideline published in 2020 shared the consensus with the ESC that UFH, LMWHs, or NOACs are all suitable options for VTE treatment in renal impairment and recommended using UFH, LWMHs, or VKAs for VTE patients with CrCl less than 15 mL/min and not using dabigatran for patients with CrCl less than 30 mL/min.[76]

Liver disease

Advanced liver disease is a risk factor for both bleeding and thrombosis.[83,91] It can affect drug metabolism and cause an elevated baseline INR, which can be challenging in managing warfarin titration.[83,91] Patients with cirrhosis were generally excluded from all original NOAC trials.[83,91] A small observational study that included only 20 patients with Child class A and B cirrhosis showed that NOACs have similar bleeding rates compared with LMWHs/VKAs.[92] Another retrospective cohort study that included 27 patients with cirrhosis (including six with Child class C cirrhosis) showed that NOACs were as effective as LMWHs/VKAs, and may be associated with a lower bleeding risk.[93] The European Heart Rhythm Association 2021 guideline recommends against using NOACs in patients with Child class C cirrhosis, the avoidance of rivaroxaban, and the use of other NOACs with caution in Child class B cirrhosis, and the use of standard dose NOACs for Child class A cirrhosis.[83] This approach is probably the best until more data are available.

Obesity

As NOACs are administered at a fixed dose, there is concern of under-dosing in obese patients due to various factors such as increased volume of distribution, renal blood flow, CrCl, and drug clearance.[1,94] The ISTH 2016 guideline, that has by now been reversed, suggested that NOACs should not be used in patients with a BMI greater than 40 kg/m^2 or a weight greater than 120 kg due to limited clinical data available until at that time.[95] Since then, more data have become available. A retrospective single-centre cohort study that included 128 patients showed that rivaroxaban and apixaban were safe alternatives to warfarin for AF in morbidly obese patients.[96] A systematic review showed that NOAC use in AF patients with BMI of at least 30 kg/m^2 and at least 40 kg/m^2 was associated with lower thrombotic risk and similar-to-lower bleeding risk.[94] A US healthcare claims database analysis showed that apixaban use in obese and morbidly obese patients was associated with lower VTE recurrence, major bleeding, and clinically relevant non-major bleeding when compared with warfarin.[97] Another retrospective study that included 795 patients showed that apixaban and rivaroxaban use have similar efficacy and safety when compared with warfarin in both AF and VTE patients.[98] The ISTH has reissued a new guidance in 2021 suggesting that standard-dose rivaroxaban or apixaban are among appropriate anticoagulant options for VTE treatment regardless of high BMI and weight, and that routine monitoring of NOAC peak or trough level is not necessary.[99] VKAs, LMWHs, and fondaparinux are other viable options in this group of patients.[99] Use of dabigatran, edoxaban, or betrixaban for VTE treatment is not recommended in patients with BMI greater than 40 kg/m^2 or weight greater than 120 kg.[99]

Bariatric surgery

Bariatric surgeries primarily involve the stomach (gastrectomy, gastric banding) and/or small bowels (Roux-en-Y gastric bypass), which are the absorption sites of NOACs and therefore have important effect on NOAC levels.[83,99] The post-surgery restrictive diet may have an impact on rivaroxaban bioavailability, which is increased with food.[83,99] A systematic review that looked at NOAC use in the post-bariatric surgery setting showed that there was no increased risk of bleeding or systemic embolism when compared with enoxaparin or warfarin, and about 78% of patients achieved adequate maximum serum concentration (Cmax).[100] The EHRA 2021 guideline on NOACs suggested to choose post-bariatric surgery an anticoagulant on a case-by-case basis, as strong clinical evidence is lacking for NOACs, and VKAs are a valid alternative with the possibility of INR monitoring.[83] Drug level monitoring should be considered if NOACs are used.[83] The ISTH 2021 guideline suggested to use parenteral anticoagulation and not to use NOACs for VTE treatment or prevention in the acute setting after bariatric surgery.[99] Switching to VKAs or NOACs may be considered after at least 4 weeks of parenteral anticoagulation; it was suggested to obtain a NOAC trough level.[100]

What's new

- Rivaroxaban is licensed for thromboprophylaxis in medical patients.
- Hospitalized COVID-19 patients should receive at least a prophylactic dose of a LMWH as thromboprophylaxis while some patients admitted to the general wards (non-critically ill) may benefit from a therapeutic dose of LMWHs.
- VKAs are the anticoagulants of choice in patients with APS but NOACs may be used in some patients (non-triple positive and non-high-risk APS) after discussing with patients about the available evidence.
- NOACs are the preferred choice of treatment in most CATs.
- Rivaroxaban and apixaban are appropriate anticoagulants in patients who have a BMI greater than 40 kg/m^2 or weight greater than 120 kg.

Guideline recommendations

- Systemic thrombolysis is recommended in high-risk PE, surgical embolectomy, or CDT should be considered if thrombolysis is contraindicated or has failed.[1]

- NOACs are preferred to VKAs but are not recommended in patients with severe renal impairment, during pregnancy and lactation, and in patients with APS.[1]
- Carefully selected patients with low-risk PE can be discharged early and be treated as outpatients.[1]
- VTE secondary to a major or transient risk factor is treated with 3 months of anticoagulation.[1]
- Extended anticoagulation is recommended in patients with recurrent VTEs with at least one VTE not related to a major transient risk factor or APS patients.[1]
- Extended anticoagulation should be considered in patients with a first episode of VTE not related to any identifiable risk factor or when the VTE is associated with a persistent risk factor other than APS.[1]
- When using extended anticoagulation, reduced-dose NOACs should be considered after 6 months of therapeutic anticoagulation in PE patients without cancer.[1]

What's next

- Extended thromboprophylaxis with NOACs may be beneficial in particular groups of medical patients; a useful tool to help with patient selection needs to be devised.
- CDT is gaining an increasing role in managing intermediate-risk PE; more prospective data are required.
- There is much research looking into the balance of risk and benefit for extending anticoagulation in non-cancer and cancer-associated VTE.
- Factor XIa inhibitors are being investigated for VTE therapy. These drugs may have a good safety profile.

Drug dosing

Drug dosing for venous thromboembolism

Anticoagulants	Therapeutic dose	Thromboprophylaxis dose	Renally adjusted dose
Anti Xa			
Apixaban (oral)	10 mg BD for 7 days, then 5 mg BD Consider reduced dose of 2.5 mg BD after 6 months of anticoagulation	2.5 mg BD	CrCl <15mL/min: avoid use CrCl 15–29 mL/min: use with caution
Edoxaban (oral)	Start after at least 5 days of parenteral anticoagulant Weight >60 kg: 60 mg OD Weight ≤60 kg: 30 mg OD	NA	CrCl <15 mL/min: avoid use CrCl 15–50 mL/min: 30 mg OD
Rivaroxaban (oral)	15 mg BD for 21 days, then 20 mg OD Consider reduced dose of 10 mg OD after 6 months of anticoagulation	10 mg OD	CrCl <15mL/min: avoid use CrCl 15-29 mL/min: use with caution
Fondaparinux (SC: subcutaneous)	<50 kg: 5 mg OD 50–100 kg: 7.5 mg OD >100 kg: 10 mg OD	2.5 mg OD	CrCl 30-50 mL/min: use with caution CrCl <30 mL/min: contraindicated
Direct thrombin inhibitor			
Dabigatran (oral)	Start after at least 5 days of parenteral anticoagulant 150 mg BD	220 mg OD	CrCl <30 mL/min: avoid use
LMWHs			
Enoxaparin (SC)	1 mg/kg every 12 hours	40 mg OD	CrCl <30 mL/min: 1 mg/kg OD (VTE treatment) 30 mg OD (VTE prophylaxis)
Dalteparin (SC)	100 units/kg every 12 hours or 200 units/kg OD	5000 units OD	CrCl <30 mL/min: use not recommended

OD, once daily; BD, twice daily; SC, subcutaneous.

References

1. Konstantinides SV, Meyer G, Bueno H, et al. 2019 ESC Guidelines for the diagnosis and management of acute pulmonary embolism developed in collaboration with the European respiratory society (ERS). Eur Heart J. 2020;41(4):543–603.
2. Wendelboe AM, Raskob GE. Global burden of thrombosis: epidemiologic aspects. Circ Res. 2016;118(9):1340–7.
3. Khan F, Tritschler T, Kahn SR, Rodger MA. Venous thromboembolism. Lancet. 2021:398(10294):64–77.

4. Zakai NA, McClure LA, Judd SE, et al. Racial and regional differences in venous thromboembolism in the United States in 3 cohorts. Circulation. 2014;129(14):1502–9.
5. White RH, Zhou H, Romano PS. Incidence of idiopathic deep venous thrombosis and secondary thromboembolism among ethnic groups in California. Ann Intern Med. 1998;128(9):737–40.
6. Klatsky AL, Armstrong MA, Poggi J. Risk of pulmonary embolism and/or deep venous thrombosis in Asian-Americans. Am J Cardiol. 2000;85(11):1334–7.
7. Lee LH, Gallus A, Jindal R, Wang C, Wu CC. Incidence of venous thromboembolism in Asian populations: a systematic review. Thromb Haemost. 2017;117(12):2243–60.
8. Barco S, Woersching AL, Spyropoulos AC, Piovella F, Mahan CE. European Union-28: an annualised cost-of-illness model for venous thromboembolism. Thromb Haemost. 2016;115(4):800–8.
9. Beckman MG, Hooper WC, Critchley SE, Ortel TL. Venous thromboembolism. A public health concern. Am J Prevent Med. 2010;38(4):S495–501.
10. Grosse SD, Nelson RE, Nyarko KA, Richardson LC, Raskob GE. The economic burden of incident venous thromboembolism in the United States: a review of estimated attributable healthcare costs. Thromb Res. 2016;137:3–10.
11. Kearon C, Ageno W, Cannegieter SC, Cosmi B, Geersing GJ, Kyrle PA. Categorization of patients as having provoked or unprovoked venous thromboembolism: guidance from the SSC of ISTH. J Thromb Haemost. 2016;14(7):1480–3.
12. Cohen AT, Katholing A, Rietbrock S, Bamber L, Martinez C. Epidemiology of first and recurrent venous thromboembolism in patients with active cancer. A population-based cohort study. Thromb Haemost. 2017;117(1):57–65.
13. Schünemann HJ, Cushman M, Burnett AE, et al. American Society of Hematology 2018 guidelines for management of venous thromboembolism: prophylaxis for hospitalized and nonhospitalized medical patients. Blood Adv. 2018;2(22):3198–225.
14. Kelly J, Rudd A, Lewis RR, Hunt BJ. Screening for subclinical deep-vein thrombosis. QJM. 2001;94(10):511–19.
15. Sandler DA, Martin JF. Autopsy proven pulmonary embolism in hospital patients: are we detecting enough deep vein thrombosis? J R Soc Med. 1989;82(4):203–5.
16. Barbar S, Noventa F, Rossetto V, et al. A risk assessment model for the identification of hospitalized medical patients at risk for venous thromboembolism: the Padua Prediction Score. J Thromb Haemost. 2010;8(11):2450–7.
17. Spyropoulos AC, Anderson FA, FitzGerald G, et al. Predictive and associative models to identify hospitalized medical patients at risk for VTE. Chest. 2011;140(3):706–14.
18. Mahan CE, Liu Y, Turpie AG, et al. External validation of a risk assessment model for venous thromboembolism in the hospitalised acutely-ill medical patient (VTE-VALOURR). Thromb Haemost. 2014;112(4):692–9.
19. Rosenberg D, Eichorn A, Alarcon M, McCullagh L, McGinn T, Spyropoulos AC. External validation of the risk assessment model of the international medical prevention registry on venous thromboembolism (IMPROVE) for medical patients in a tertiary health system. J Am Heart Assoc. 2014;3(6):e001152.
20. National Institute for Health and Care Excellence. Venous thromboembolism: reducing the risk for patients in hospital. Clinical guideline [CG92]. 2010 (updated 2015). Available from: http://www.nice.org.uk/guidance/CG92
21. National Institute for Health and Care Excellence. Venous Thromboembolism in Over 16s: Reducing the Risk of Hospital-Acquired Deep Vein Thrombosis or Pulmonary Embolism. London: National Institute for Health and Care Excellence; 2018.
22. Samama MM, Cohen AT, Darmon JY, et al. A comparison of enoxaparin with placebo for the prevention of venous thromboembolism in acutely ill medical patients. Prophylaxis in Medical Patients with Enoxaparin Study Group. N Engl J Med. 1999;341(11):793–800.
23. Leizorovicz A, Cohen AT, Turpie AGG, Olsson CG, Vaitkus PT, Goldhaber SZ. Randomized, placebo-controlled trial of dalteparin for the prevention of venous thromboembolism in acutely ill medical patients. Circulation. 2004;110(7):874–9.
24. Cohen AT, Davidson BL, Gallus AS, et al. Efficacy and safety of fondaparinux for the prevention of venous thromboembolism in older acute medical patients: randomised placebo controlled trial. BMJ. 2006;332(7537):325–7.
25. Cohen AT, Spiro TE, Büller HR, et al. Rivaroxaban for thromboprophylaxis in acutely ill medical patients. N Engl J Med. 2013;368(6):513–23.
26. Hull RD, Merali T, Mills A, Stevenson AL, Liang J. Venous thromboembolism in elderly high-risk medical patients: time course of events and influence of risk factors. Clin Appl Thromb Hemost. 2013;19(4):357–62.
27. Goldhaber SZ, Leizorovicz A, Kakkar AK, et al. Apixaban versus enoxaparin for thromboprophylaxis in medically ill patients. N Engl J Med. 2011;365(23):2167–77.
28. Spyropoulos AC, Ageno W, Albers GW, et al. Rivaroxaban for thromboprophylaxis after hospitalization for medical illness. N Engl J Med. 2018;379(12):1118–27.
29. Cohen AT, Harrington RA, Goldhaber SZ, et al. Extended thromboprophylaxis with betrixaban in acutely ill medical patients. N Engl J Med. 2016;375(6):534–44.
30. Kahn SR, Lim W, Dunn AS, et al. Prevention of VTE in nonsurgical patients. Antithrombotic therapy and prevention of thrombosis, 9th ed: American College of Chest Physicians evidence-based clinical practice guidelines. Chest. 2012;141(2 Suppl):e195S–226S.
31. Cohen AT, Tapson VF, Bergmann JF, et al. Venous thromboembolism risk and prophylaxis in the acute hospital care setting (ENDORSE study): a multinational cross-sectional study. Lancet. 2008;371(9610):387–94.
32. Pinjala R, ENDORSE-India investigators. Venous thromboembolism risk & prophylaxis in the acute hospital care setting (ENDORSE), a multinational cross-sectional study: results from the Indian subset data. Indian J Med Res. 2012;136(1):60–7.
33. Anderson DR, Morgano GP, Bennett C, et al. American Society of Hematology 2019 guidelines for management of venous thromboembolism: Prevention of venous thromboembolism in surgical hospitalized patients. Blood Adv. 2019;3(23):3898–944.
34. Edeer AD, Comez S, Damar HT, Savci A. Prevalence and risk factors of venous thromboembolism in postoperative patients: a retrospective study. Pak J Med Sci. 2018;34(6):1539–44.
35. Gould MK, Garcia DA, Wren SM, et al. Prevention of VTE in nonorthopedic surgical patients: Antithrombotic Therapy and Prevention of Thrombosis, 9th ed: American College of Chest Physicians Evidence-Based Clinical Practice Guidelines. Chest. 2012;141(2 Suppl):e227S–77S.
36. Cronin MA, Dengler N, Krauss ES, et al. Completion of the updated Caprini risk assessment model (2013 version). Clin Appl Thromb Hemost. 2019;25:1076029619838052.
37. Falck-Ytter Y, Francis CW, Johanson NA, et al. Prevention of VTE in orthopedic surgery patients: Antithrombotic Therapy and Prevention of Thrombosis, 9th ed: American College of Chest Physicians evidence-based clinical practice guidelines. Chest. 2012;141(2 Suppl):e278S–325S.
38. Stamatakis JD, Kakkar V v, Sagar S, Lawrence D, Nairn D, Bentley PG. Femoral vein thrombosis and total hip replacement. Br Med J. 1977;2(6081):223–5.

39. Binns M, Pho R. Femoral vein occlusion during hip arthroplasty. Clin Orthop Relat Res. 1990;255:168–72.
40. Sharrock NE, Go G, Sculco TP, Ranawat CS, Maynard MJ, Harpel PC. Changes in circulatory indices of thrombosis and fibrinolysis during total knee arthroplasty performed under tourniquet. J Arthroplasty. 1995;10(4):523–8.
41. Horner D, Stevens JW, Pandor A, et al. Pharmacological thromboprophylaxis to prevent venous thromboembolism in patients with temporary lower limb immobilization after injury: systematic review and network meta-analysis. J Thromb Haemost. 2020;18(2):422–38.
42. Horner D, Goodacre S, Pandor A, et al. Thromboprophylaxis in lower limb immobilisation after injury (TiLLI). Emerg Med J. 2020;37(1):36–41.
43. Pandor A, Horner D, Davis S, et al. Different strategies for pharmacological thromboprophylaxis for lower-limb immobilisation after injury: systematic review and economic evaluation. Health Technol Assess. 2019;23(63):1–190.
44. van Adrichem RA, Nemeth B, Algra A, et al. Thromboprophylaxis after knee arthroscopy and lower-leg casting. N Engl J Med. 2017;376(6):515–25.
45. Selby R, Geerts WH, Kreder HJ, et al. A double-blind, randomized controlled trial of the prevention of clinically important venous thromboembolism after isolated lower leg fractures. J Orthop Trauma. 2015;29(5):224–30.
46. Ricci WM, Broekhuyse H, Keating JF, Teague DC, White TO. Thromboprophylaxis an update of current practice. OTA Int. 2019;2(4):e027.
47. Mazzolai L, Aboyans V, Ageno W, et al. Diagnosis and management of acute deep vein thrombosis: a joint consensus document from the European Society of Cardiology working groups of aorta and peripheral vascular diseases and pulmonary circulation and right ventricular function. Eur Heart J. 2018;39(47):4208–18.
48. Khorana A, Kuderer NM, Culakova E, Lyman GH, Francis CW. Development and validation of a predictive model for chemotherapy-associated thrombosis. Blood. 2008;111(10):4902–7.
49. Sørensen HT, Mellemkjaer L, Olsen JH, Baron JA. Prognosis of cancers associated with venous thromboembolism. N Engl J Med. 2000;343(25):1846–50.
50. Chew HK, Wun T, Harvey D, Zhou H, White RH. Incidence of venous thromboembolism and its effect on survival among patients with common cancers. Arch Intern Med. 2006;166(4):458–64.
51. Prandoni P, Lensing AWA, Piccioli A, et al. Recurrent venous thromboembolism and bleeding complications during anticoagulant treatment in patients with cancer and venous thrombosis. Blood. 2002;100(10):3484–8.
52. Key NS, Chb MB, Khorana AA, et al. Venous thromboembolism prophylaxis and treatment in patients with cancer: ASCO Clinical Practice Guideline Update. J Clin Oncol. 2019;38(5):496–520.
53. Poor HD. Pulmonary thrombosis and thromboembolism in COVID-19. Chest. 2021;160(4):1471–80.
54. Jiménez D, García-Sanchez A, Rali P, et al. Incidence of VTE and bleeding among hospitalized patients with coronavirus disease 2019: a systematic review and meta-analysis. Chest. 2021;159(3):1182–96.
55. Barnes GD, Burnett A, Allen A, et al. Thromboembolic prevention and anticoagulant therapy during the COVID-19 pandemic: updated clinical guidance from the anticoagulation forum. J Thromb Thrombolysis. 2022;54(2):197–210.
56. Cuker A, Tseng EK, Nieuwlaat R, et al. American Society of Hematology 2021 guidelines on the use of anticoagulation for thromboprophylaxis in patients with COVID-19. Blood Adv. 2021;5(3):872–88.
57. Moores LK, Tritschler T, Brosnahan S, et al. Thromboprophylaxis in patients with COVID-19. Chest. 2022;162(1):213–25.
58. National Institute for Health and Care Excellence. COVID-19 Rapid Guideline: Managing COVID-19. London: National Institute for Health and Care Excellence.
59. Stevens SM, Woller SC, Baumann Kreuziger L, et al. Executive summary: antithrombotic therapy for VTE disease: second update of the CHEST Guideline and Expert Panel Report. Chest. 2021;160(6):2247–59.
60. Ortel TL, Neumann I, Ageno W, et al. American Society of Hematology 2020 guidelines for management of venous thromboembolism: treatment of deep vein thrombosis and pulmonary embolism. Blood Adv. 2020;4(19):4693–738.
61. Naidu SG, Knuttinen MG, Kriegshauser JS, Eversman WG, Oklu R. Rationale for catheter directed therapy in pulmonary embolism. Cardiovasc Diagn Ther. 2017;7(Suppl 3):S320–8.
62. Marti C, John G, Konstantinides S, et al. Systemic thrombolytic therapy for acute pulmonary embolism: a systematic review and meta-analysis. Eur Heart J. 2015;36(10):605–14.
63. Zondag W, Mos ICM, Creemers-Schild D, et al. Outpatient treatment in patients with acute pulmonary embolism: the Hestia Study. J Thromb Haemost. 2011;9(8):1500–7.
64. Roy PM, Penaloza A, Hugli O, et al. Triaging acute pulmonary embolism for home treatment by Hestia or simplified PESI criteria: the HOME-PE randomized trial. Eur Heart J. 2021;42(33):3146–57.
65. Schellong SM, Goldhaber SZ, Weitz JI, et al. Isolated distal deep vein thrombosis: perspectives from the GARFIELD-VTE Registry. Thromb Haemost. 2019;119(10):1675–85.
66. Enden T, Haig Y, Kløw NE, et al. Long-term outcome after additional catheter-directed thrombolysis versus standard treatment for acute iliofemoral deep vein thrombosis (the CaVenT study): a randomised controlled trial. Lancet. 2012;379(9810):31–8.
67. Haig Y, Enden T, Slagsvold CE, Sandvik L, Sandset PM, Kløw NE. Determinants of early and long-term efficacy of catheter-directed thrombolysis in proximal deep vein thrombosis. J Vasc Interv Radiol. 2013;24(1):17–24.
68. Enden T, Resch S, White C, Wik HS, Kløw NE, Sandset PM. Cost-effectiveness of additional catheter-directed thrombolysis for deep vein thrombosis. J Thromb Haemost. 2013;11(6):1032–42.
69. Watson L, Broderick C, Armon MP. Thrombolysis for acute deep vein thrombosis. Cochrane Database Syst Rev. 2016;11:CD002783.
70. Haig Y, Enden T, Grøtta O, et al. Post-thrombotic syndrome after catheter-directed thrombolysis for deep vein thrombosis (CaVenT): 5-year follow-up results of an open-label, randomised controlled trial. Lancet Haematol. 2016;3(2):e64–71.
71. Notten P, ten Cate-Hoek AJ, Arnoldussen CWKP, et al. Ultrasound-accelerated catheter-directed thrombolysis versus anticoagulation for the prevention of post-thrombotic syndrome (CAVA): a single-blind, multicentre, randomised trial. Lancet Haematol. 2020;7(1):e40–9.
72. Kearon C, Gu CS, Julian JA, et al. Pharmacomechanical catheter-directed thrombolysis in acute femoral-popliteal deep vein thrombosis: analysis from a stratified randomized trial. Thromb Haemost. 2019;119(4):633–44.
73. Vedantham S, Goldhaber SZ, Julian JA, et al. Pharmacomechanical catheter-directed thrombolysis for deep-vein thrombosis. N Engl J Med. 2017;377(23):2240–52.
74. Posch F, Königsbrügge O, Zielinski C, Pabinger I, Ay C. Treatment of venous thromboembolism in patients with cancer: a network meta-analysis comparing efficacy and safety of anticoagulants. Thromb Res. 2015;136(3):582–9.

75. Mulder FI, Bosch FTM, Young AM, et al. Direct oral anticoagulants for cancer-associated venous thromboembolism: a systematic review and meta-analysis. Blood. 2020;136(12):1433–41.
76. National Institute for Health and Care Excellence. Venous thromboembolic diseases: diagnosis, management and thrombophilia testing. NICE Guideline [NG158]. 2020. Available from: https://www.nice.org.uk/guidance/ng158
77. Pengo V, Denas G, Zoppellaro G, et al. Rivaroxaban vs warfarin in high-risk patients with antiphospholipid syndrome. Blood. 2018;132(13):1365–71.
78. Ordi-Ros J, Sáez-Comet L, Pérez-Conesa M, et al. Rivaroxaban versus vitamin K antagonist in antiphospholipid syndrome: a randomized noninferiority trial. Ann Intern Med. 2019;171(10):685–94.
79. Zuily S, Cohen H, Isenberg D, et al. Use of direct oral anticoagulants in patients with thrombotic antiphospholipid syndrome: guidance from the Scientific and Standardization Committee of the International Society on Thrombosis and Haemostasis. J Thromb Haemost. 2020;18(9):2126–37.
80. Tektonidou MG, Andreoli L, Limper M, et al. EULAR recommendations for the management of antiphospholipid syndrome in adults. Ann Rheum Dis. 2019;78(10):1296–304.
81. Arachchillage DRJ, Gomez K, Alikhan R, Anderson JAM, Lester W, Laffan M. Addendum to British Society for Haematology Guidelines on Investigation and Management of Antiphospholipid syndrome, 2012 (Br. J. Haematol. 2012; 157: 47–58): use of direct acting oral anticoagulants. Br J Haematol. 2020;189(2):212–15.
82. Pastori D, Menichelli D, Cammisotto V, Pignatelli P. Use of direct oral anticoagulants in patients with antiphospholipid syndrome: a systematic review and comparison of the international guidelines. Front Cardiovasc Med. 2021;8:715878.
83. Steffel J, Collins R, Antz M, et al. 2021 European Heart Rhythm Association practical guide on the use of non-vitamin K antagonist oral anticoagulants in patients with atrial fibrillation. Europace. 2021;23(10):1612–76.
84. Fazio G, Dentamaro I, Gambacurta R, Alcamo P, Colonna P. Safety of edoxaban 30 mg in elderly patients with severe renal impairment. Clin Drug Investig. 2018;38(11):1023–30.
85. Weir MR, Ashton V, Moore KT, Shrivastava S, Peterson ED, Ammann EM. Rivaroxaban versus warfarin in patients with nonvalvular atrial fibrillation and stage IV-V chronic kidney disease. Am Heart J. 2020;223:3–11.
86. Schafer JH, Casey AL, Dupre KA, Staubes BA. Safety and efficacy of apixaban versus warfarin in patients with advanced chronic kidney disease. Ann Pharmacother. 2018;52(11):1078–84.
87. Hanni C, Petrovitch E, Ali M, et al. Outcomes associated with apixaban vs warfarin in patients with renal dysfunction. Blood Adv. 2020;4(11):2366–71.
88. Cohen AT, Sah J, Dhamane AD, et al. Effectiveness and safety of apixaban versus warfarin in venous thromboembolism patients with chronic kidney disease. Thromb Haemost. 2022;122(6):926–38.
89. Murtaza G, Turagam MK, Garg J, et al. Safety and efficacy of apixaban versus warfarin in patients with atrial fibrillation or venous thromboembolism and end-stage renal disease on hemodialysis: a systematic review and meta-analysis. Indian Pacing Electrophysiol J. 2021;21(4):221–6.
90. Reed D, Palkimas S, Hockman R, Abraham S, Le T, Maitland H. Safety and effectiveness of apixaban compared to warfarin in dialysis patients. Res Pract Thromb Haemost. 2018;2(2):291–8.
91. Elhosseiny S, al Moussawi H, Chalhoub JM, Lafferty J, Deeb L. Direct oral anticoagulants in cirrhotic patients: current evidence and clinical observations. Can J Gastroenterol Hepatol. 2019;2019:4383269.
92. Intagliata NM, Henry ZH, Maitland H, et al. Direct oral anticoagulants in cirrhosis patients pose similar risks of bleeding when compared to traditional anticoagulation. Dig Dis Sci. 2016;61(6):1721–7.
93. Hum J, Shatzel JJ, Jou JH, Deloughery TG. The efficacy and safety of direct oral anticoagulants vs traditional anticoagulants in cirrhosis. Eur J Haematol. 2017;98(4):393–7.
94. Grymonprez M, de Backer TL, Steurbaut S, Boussery K, Lahousse L. Non-vitamin K antagonist oral anticoagulants (NOACs) versus warfarin in patients with atrial fibrillation and (morbid) obesity or low body weight: a systematic review and meta-analysis. Cardiovasc Drugs Ther. 2022;36(4):749–61.
95. Martin K, Beyer-Westendorf J, Davidson BL, Huisman MV, Sandset PM, Moll S. Use of the direct oral anticoagulants in obese patients: guidance from the SSC of the ISTH. J Thromb Haemost. 2016;14(6):1308–13.
96. Kido K, Ngorsuraches S. Comparing the efficacy and safety of direct oral anticoagulants with warfarin in the morbidly obese population with atrial fibrillation. Ann Pharmacother. 2019;53(2):165–70.
97. Cohen A, Sah J, Lee T, et al. Effectiveness and safety of apixaban vs. warfarin in venous thromboembolism patients with obesity and morbid obesity. J Clin Med. 2021;10(2):200.
98. Kushnir M, Choi Y, Eisenberg R, et al. Efficacy and safety of direct oral factor Xa inhibitors compared with warfarin in patients with morbid obesity: a single-centre, retrospective analysis of chart data. Lancet Haematol. 2019;6(7):e359–65.
99. Martin KA, Beyer-Westendorf J, Davidson BL, Huisman MV, Sandset PM, Moll S. Use of direct oral anticoagulants in patients with obesity for treatment and prevention of venous thromboembolism: updated communication from the ISTH SSC Subcommittee on Control of Anticoagulation. J Thromb Haemost. 2021;19(8):1874–82.

CHAPTER 22

Biomarker-based risk stratification in cardiovascular disease

Ziad Hijazi, Gorav Batra, Johan Lindbäck, and Lars Wallentin

Contents

Summary

Biomarkers provide incremental prognostic information on major clinical outcomes and might be integrated in decision support tools for patients with acute and chronic cardiovascular diseases. The development of decision support tools should follow statistical guidelines to be robust and externally valid, allowing them to be used in different settings outside the dataset where they were developed. The ABC (Age, Biomarkers, Clinical history) risk score in atrial fibrillation and coronary heart disease are examples of well-documented, externally validated, and calibrated, biomarker-based risk scores performing better than conventional risk scores. These scores may be used as tools for integrated risk assessment. Before clinical implementation, the incremental clinical utility of novel biomarkers should be demonstrated in prospective clinical cohorts. Risk scores incorporating biomarkers and/or artificial intelligence might be the future for prediction of cardiovascular events and provide decision support on selection of treatment.

Introduction

Specific diagnosis and evaluation of risk is necessary to initiate appropriate triage and optimal treatment in patients with symptoms suggestive of cardiovascular disease (CVD). The likelihood of CVD and the subsequent risk of adverse events, including death, is not binary, but rather a continuum from low to high risk. Atrial fibrillation (AF) and coronary heart disease (CHD), including acute coronary syndrome (ACS) and chronic coronary syndrome, have in common a prothrombotic state that may cause harm in the form of thromboembolic complications.

With better evidence-based care, outcomes for patients with CVD have dramatically improved. In patients with CHD the availability of early routine coronary revascularization and better secondary preventive treatment, including intense platelet inhibition, has substantially reduced the risk of fatal events, incapacitating consequences, and recurrent events.[1] Likewise, in AF the increased utilization of catheter-based procedures and stroke prevention with the non-vitamin K oral anticoagulants has improved event-free survival and quality of life. Still, many patients with these and other cardiovascular conditions remain at high risk for recurrent coronary events, stroke, and mortality.[2] The average effectiveness of novel antithrombotic treatments, which inherently increase risk of bleeding, reflects population-level data and cannot always be extrapolated to the individual patient. The assessment of the individual patient-level risk/benefit is therefore essential before selecting treatment, its intensity, and duration. This is particularly important since healthcare providers, based on clinical judgement, tend to treat low-risk individuals more optimally while higher-risk patients who might actually benefit the most from guideline-directed therapy tend to be undertreated—the so-called treatment-risk paradox.[3,4]

Biomarkers

Circulating biomarkers play an important role in the diagnosis and management of patients with CVD. Measurement of cardiac troponin (cTn) is now routine of care in many patients with CVD (➔ Figure 22.1).[5] Upon myocardial cell damage, cTn is released into the bloodstream. Elevated levels of cTn, that have both a diagnostic and prognostic impact, can be found in both cardiac and non-cardiac conditions, such as myocardial infarction (MI), heart failure, AF, and renal failure.[6]

Natriuretic peptides, measured as brain natriuretic peptide (BNP) or N-terminal prohormone of BNP (NT-proBNP), are involved in regulating volume homeostasis and cardiovascular remodelling and are released into the bloodstream in response to increased ventricular stretch or wall stress.[7] BNP is synthesized as a prohormone (proBNP) and cleaved into BNP and NT-proBNP. Currently, BNP and NT-proBNP are mainly used for diagnosis of heart failure and myocardial dysfunction.[7] Independent of its diagnostic utility, several studies have shown that levels of natriuretic peptides provide strong prognostic information in patients with various cardiac conditions, including heart failure, CHD and AF.[8–10]

During recent years, novel biomarkers have been investigated as potential useful risk markers in CVD. Growth differentiation factor 15 (GDF-15) is expressed in low concentrations across most cell types under normal physiological conditions.[11] Expression of GDF-15 is induced in response to unfavourable milieus with oxidative stress such as pro-inflammatory states and cellular stress

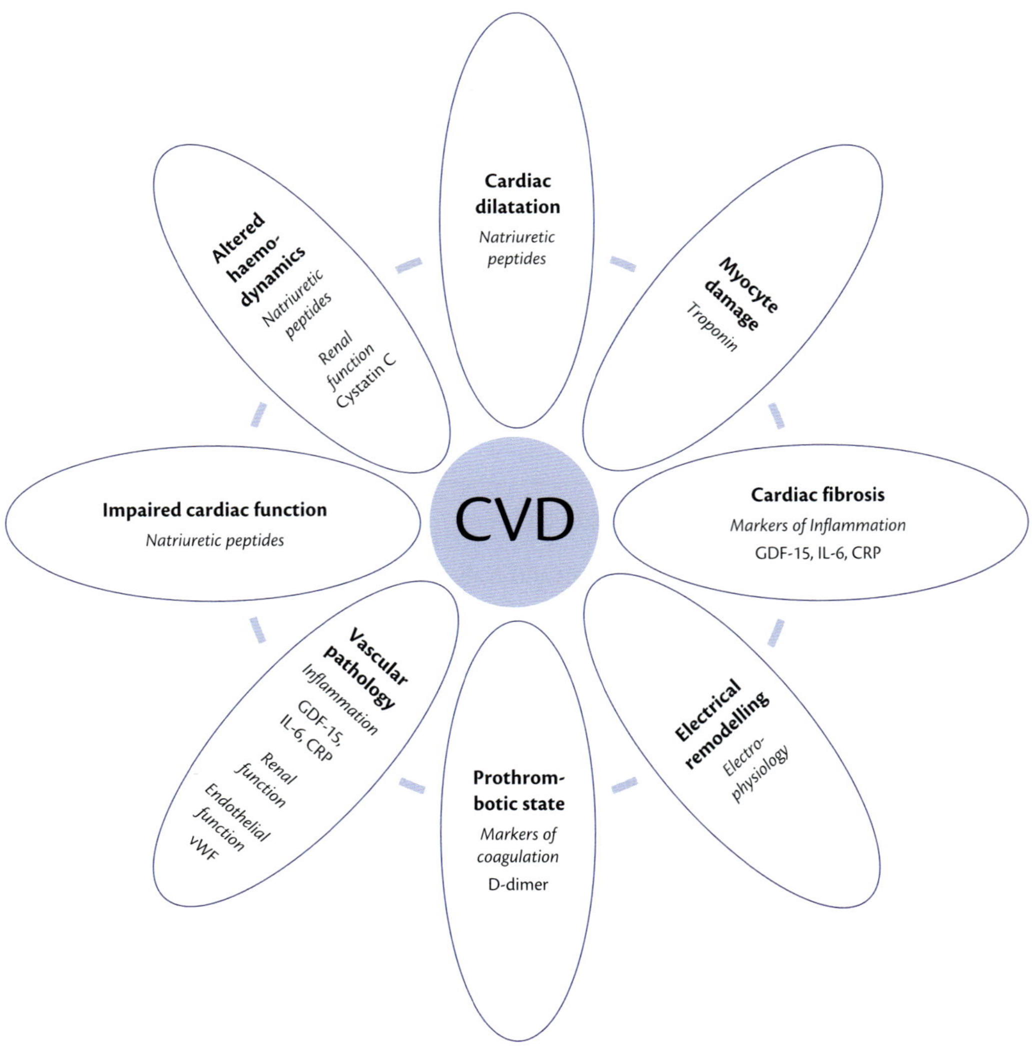

Figure 22.1 Illustration of the pathophysiological mechanisms in cardiovascular disease (CVD) and associated biomarkers. CRP, C-reactive protein; vWF, von Willebrand factor.

(e.g. myocardial stretch and ischaemia). The levels of GDF-15 also increase with age and in patients with diabetes mellitus and renal dysfunction. GDF-15 levels are correlated with levels of other biomarkers associated with the same conditions, such as NT-proBNP, cTn, cystatin C, and C-reactive protein (CRP).[11] Although GDF-15 is an unspecific biomarker, it is documented as an important incremental indicator of risk for both fatal and non-fatal events including bleeding events in various cardiovascular conditions.[12,13]

Several other biomarkers [e.g. creatinine, cystatin-C, glucose, haemoglobin A1c (HbA1c), low-density lipoprotein cholesterol, and CRP] are routinely used for diagnosis of underlying comorbidities and decision support in patients with CVD.[14–16] Therefore, the utility of additional biomarkers such as NT-proBNP, cTn, and GDF-15, need to be based on evidence of their incremental diagnostic and prognostic value after adjustment for already established clinical and biomarker-based information.

Biomarkers and biomarker-based risk stratification in acute coronary syndrome

Biomarkers in coronary heart disease

High-sensitivity (hs)-cTn has an integral part in the diagnostic criteria for ACS.[17] In addition, initial and serial measurements of cTn provide prognostic utility in patients with CHD.[18–21] The association between cTn and ischaemic events and mortality is most prominent in patients with ACS managed non-invasively and seems to diminish in revascularized patients, most likely due to substantial risk reduction caused by restoration of coronary blood flow.[18–21] In contrast, elevated levels of cTn are associated with increased risk of cardiac mortality and morbidity in patients with chronic coronary syndrome, irrespective of initial management (➔ Figure 22.2).[22,23]

In patients with CHD, several studies have consistently shown that elevated levels of BNP and NT-proBNP are associated with adverse outcome independently of other biomarkers, and irrespective of non-invasive or invasive management.[20,21] In patients with chronic coronary syndrome, studies have shown BNP and NT-proBNP to be related to extent of CHD and to provide prognostic information for risk of mortality and adverse cardiovascular events (➔ Figure 22.2), superior to clinical factors.[23,24] The underlying pathophysiological processes for these associations are unknown, but it is believed that increased concentrations of BNP and NT-proBNP reflect left ventricular dysfunction caused by myocardial ischaemia leading to an increased wall stress.

Evidence suggests that GDF-15 might be used as a prognostic marker in patients with ACS and chronic coronary syndrome. Several studies have shown that GDF-15 is independently associated with cardiovascular outcomes, including spontaneous MI, heart failure, stroke, cardiovascular death, as well as with non-cardiovascular and cancer-related death (➔ Figure 22.2).[20,21,25] In addition, GDF-15 is associated with the risk of bleeding in patients with CHD treated with antithrombotic agents, independently of other clinical factors and other biomarkers associated with a raised risk of bleeding (e.g. haemoglobin and creatinine).[26]

Biomarker-based risk scores in coronary heart disease

Risk stratification for ischaemic events in coronary heart disease

Patients with acute and stable CHD are heterogeneous and have a variable prognosis that is dependent on patient characteristics, comorbidities, disease presentation, and treatments that might modify the course of the disease. Risk stratification tools might better capture the individual patient's risk of subsequent cardiovascular events, thereby allowing tailoring of treatment and more effective utilization of available resources.

Incorporating the previously mentioned natriuretic peptides, cTn, and GDF-15 into multimarker risk scores can contribute to estimation of ischaemic risk. As an example, the ABC (Age, Biomarkers, Clinical history)-CHD risk score is a biomarker-based tool that provides stratification for cardiovascular mortality in patients with chronic coronary syndrome for whom there are very few validated risk scores (➔ Figure 22.3).[23] After screening a large number of variables, two biomarkers (NT-proBNP and hs-cTn) in the ABC-CHD model provided stronger prognostic

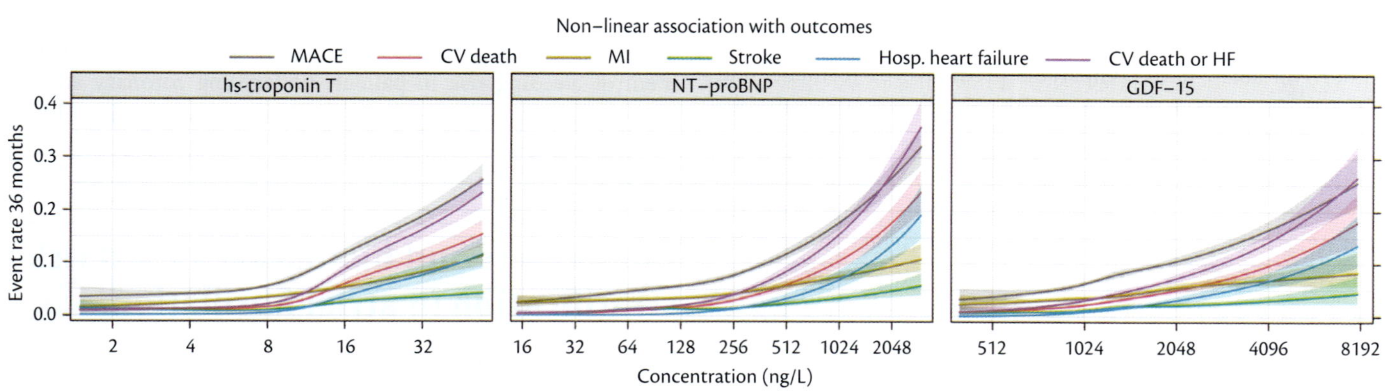

Figure 22.2 Associations between biomarker levels and clinical outcomes in chronic coronary syndrome. CV, cardiovascular; HF, heart failure; MACE, major adverse cardiovascular events.

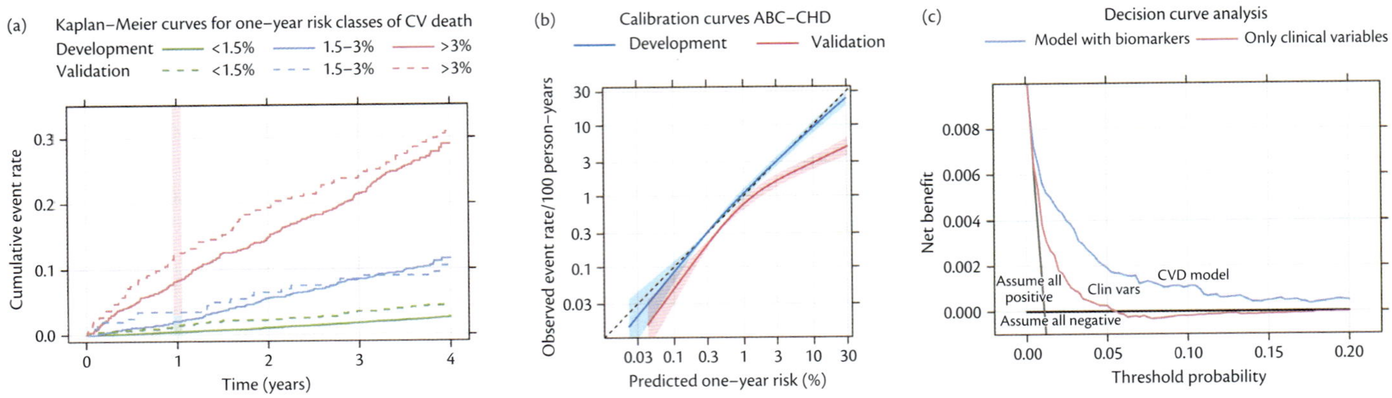

Figure 22.3 (a) Cumulative risk of cardiovascular death by predicted 1-year ABC-CHD risk groups. (b) Calibration and (c) clinical utility of the ABC-CHD risk score.

information than any other clinical and biomarker variables. The final ABC-CHD risk model included age, these two biomarkers, and the clinical variables smoking, diabetes mellitus, peripheral arterial disease, and low-density lipoprotein cholesterol. The ABC-CHD score showed in internal and external validation high discrimination [concordance index (c-index) 0.81] and good calibration for cardiovascular death (➔ Figure 22.3). Given that the model included NT-proBNP and hs-cTn, the model performed even better for prediction of heart failure, but less well for other non-fatal endpoints such as MI. Decision curve analyses also showed an added clinical value of having biomarkers in the score rather than only clinical variables (➔ Figure 22.3).

In patients with ACS, numerous risk scores have been developed for prediction of mortality and recurrent cardiovascular events both on admission and at discharge. The GRACE risk score, recommended by the European Society of Cardiology (ESC) Guidelines for ST elevation myocardial infarction (STEMI) and non-STEMI, was developed in 2006 to primarily guide physicians about early therapeutic strategies on admission, including decision-making about urgent revascularization.[27,28] The subsequently updated version, the GRACE 2.0 risk score, was developed to estimate the risk of mortality while in hospital and up to 3 years after discharge.[29] Variables in the GRACE 2.0 risk score include age, heart rate, systolic blood pressure, cardiac arrest, Killip class, ST-segment deviation on electrocardiography, and two biomarkers (elevated cTn as a dichotomous variable and creatinine as a continuous variable). Other risk scores, incorporating mainly clinical variables, have comparable predictive performance but have not been implemented in clinical practice. Recently, the biomarker-based ABC-ACS ischaemia score was developed as a complement to the GRACE score and provides risk stratification for cardiovascular mortality and spontaneous MI at discharge after ACS.[30] The model, which incorporates two biomarkers (NT-proBNP and GDF-15) and six clinical factors (age, extent of coronary artery disease, prior vascular disease, Killip class, type of ACS, and type of $P2Y_{12}$ inhibitor), showed good discrimination (c-index 0.71) and calibration, and might be useful for decision support and for dialogue with the patient on secondary preventive treatments at discharge after ACS.

Risk stratification for major bleeding in coronary heart disease

Antithrombotic drugs, such as acetylsalicylic acid and $P2Y_{12}$ inhibitors, are recommended by the ESC Guidelines to reduce rates of recurrent cardiovascular ischaemic events after a recent ACS.[28,31] However, antithrombotic drugs come with the risk of bleeding.[32–34] Major bleeding events are also associated with increased mortality and worse health-related quality of life. Currently, no bleeding risk score has been implemented in routine clinical practice. Most available bleeding scores have focused on predicting in-hospital and early bleeds rather than long-term risks, and have moderate predictive performance. For instance, the ACUITY-HORIZONS-AMI and the CRUSADE scores showed a reasonable predictive value for in-hospital and 30-day major bleeding in patients with ACS.[35,36] The moderate performance might to some extent be explained by the fact that many bleeding scores utilize only clinical variables for risk prediction. For long-term risk, the DAPT, PRECISE-DAPT, and PARIS bleeding scores provide clinicians with structured tools for risk assessment of bleeding following coronary revascularization, but again with moderate performance.[37–39] The PRECISE-DAPT score includes three biomarkers (haemoglobin, white blood cells, and renal clearance based on creatinine) and showed moderate discriminative performance (c-index 0.73).[39] Many variables associated with bleeding risk are also associated with increased ischaemic risk, thus, raising concerns about the clinical utility of currently available bleeding scores. While the ESC Guidelines recommend considering the assessment of bleeding risk in patients undergoing coronary angiography, it remains challenging to implement this recommendation due to the absence of reliable risk scores for individual patients.[28]

Biomarkers and biomarker-based risk stratification in atrial fibrillation

Risk stratification in atrial fibrillation

The AF population is heterogeneous regarding risk of stroke and major bleeding. To address these observations, AF risk stratification schemes were created in the 1990s.[40,41] Development of predictive risk score models in AF soon followed, with the derivation of the $CHADS_2$ risk score in 2001[42] and additional risk scores thereafter.[43–45] The overall advantage with the scores was to provide clinicians with structured and rather uncomplicated tools for risk assessment of stroke and the indication for anticoagulant treatment in AF. Several of these scores were rather comparable in regard to the predictive performance. Due to a more complicated formula the use of some did not become widespread and thus underlined the importance of practicality and utility regarding clinical risk scores.[43,46] The CHA_2DS_2-VASc score managed to provide a more accurate identification of low-risk patients as compared with the previous $CHADS_2$, and has since 2010 been the primarily recommended stroke risk score in the European guidelines of AF management.[43,47] Nonetheless, there remains considerable differences between risk score performances, for example, regarding the proportion of patients classified as low or high risk, respectively, as well as substantial variability in the predictive power concerning stroke outcomes.[46,48–50] Also, calibration remains a concern, as observed stroke rates for those categorized as low risk may range from 0% to 2.3% per year and those categorized as high risk from 2.5% to 7.9% per year. Recently, an additional complexity was brought to light, showing that also geographic variation may hamper global generalizability of some clinical risk scores and again indicating potential concerns regarding calibration.[51]

Due to the inherent increased risk of bleeding with antithrombotic treatment, several risk stratification models in AF for major bleeding risk have been proposed such as the $HEMORR_2HAGES$, HAS-BLED, ATRIA, and ORBIT scores.[47,50,52–55] Most of the bleeding risk scores have a rather similar predictive performance, with some discriminatory advantages for the ORBIT score. However, since 2010 the HAS-BLED score has been suggested in the European guidelines for management of AF. The bleeding risk scores share several of the limitations detailed for the AF stroke scores regarding performance and calibration.

Biomarkers of stroke and bleeding in atrial fibrillation

Circulating biomarkers provide an opportunity to gain otherwise unknown information concerning risk as the levels often reflect some of the key pathways involved in the risk for thromboembolism (➔ Figure 22.1). In the past decade, several biomarkers have shown an independent added value for risk stratification and prognostication in patients with AF based on a multitude of data from registry cohorts as well as retrospective randomized controlled trial cohorts. The associations with outcomes for the most established biomarkers are presented in ➔ Table 22.1.[56] NT-proBNP has consistently been associated with the risk of stroke, but does not have an independent association with major bleeding events in patients with AF, which makes it a useful marker specifically for thromboembolic events (➔ Table 22.1). On the other hand, the biomarker GDF-15 is strongly associated with major bleeding events in AF, but less so with ischaemic stroke (➔ Table 22.1). Furthermore, cTn provides incremental information on both of these outcomes in AF (➔ Table 22.1).

Table 22.1 Schematic presentation of the strength of association of different biomarkers with outcomes in patients with atrial fibrillation

Biomarker	Stroke/ embolism	Mortality	Major bleeding
Cardiac biomarkers			
NT-proBNP	+++	+++	+
cTn	+++	+++	+++
Renal dysfunction	+/++	++	++
Inflammation/fibrosis			
GDF-15	++	+++	+++
IL-6	++	+++	++
CRP	+	+++	+
Endothelial function			
vWF	+	++	++
Coagulation			
D-dimer	++	++	++

Association with outcomes in analyses unadjusted (+), adjusted for clinical risk factors (++), or adjusted for clinical risk factors and other biomarkers (+++).

CRP, C-reactive protein; cTn, cardiac troponin; GDF-15, growth differentiation factor 15; IL-6, interleukin 6; NT-proBNP, N-terminal prohormone of brain natriuretic peptide; vWF, von Willebrand factor.

Source data from Hijazi Z, Oldgren J, Siegbahn A, Wallentin L. Application of biomarkers for risk stratification in patients with atrial fibrillation. Clin Chem. 2017;63(1):152–64. doi: 10.1373/clinchem.2016.255182.

In patients with AF and high levels of a biomarker, such as NT-proBNP or cTn, the risk of thromboembolic events may be more than doubled, and the risk of death increased more than fivefold, as compared with patients with lower biomarker levels.[10] Similarly, for GDF-15 and the risk of bleeding, a high concentration indicates a doubled risk as compared with low concentrations.[12] However, the risk implied with elevated levels of these biomarkers may be even greater, as the association with outcomes usually is non-linear (➔ Figure 22.4). The information provided by the biomarkers is incremental to and independent of other common risk indicators, such as age, sex, comorbidities, and so on. Despite incomplete knowledge of the precise mechanism, the evidence and the general availability to measure these biomarkers makes them attractive tools for decision support in patients with AF.

Biomarker-based risk scores for stroke and major bleeding in atrial fibrillation

Based on the robust advances provided by blood biomarkers regarding risk stratification in AF, as outlined previously in this chapter (➔ Biomarkers of stroke and bleeding in atrial fibrillation), coupled with the limitations of the clinical risk scores of stroke and major bleeding, biomarker-based risk scores of stroke and bleeding in AF were developed.[57,58] At present, the best validated biomarker-based risk scores in AF are the ABC-AF stroke and the ABC-AF bleeding risk scores.[57–66] The ABC-AF stroke score consists of the

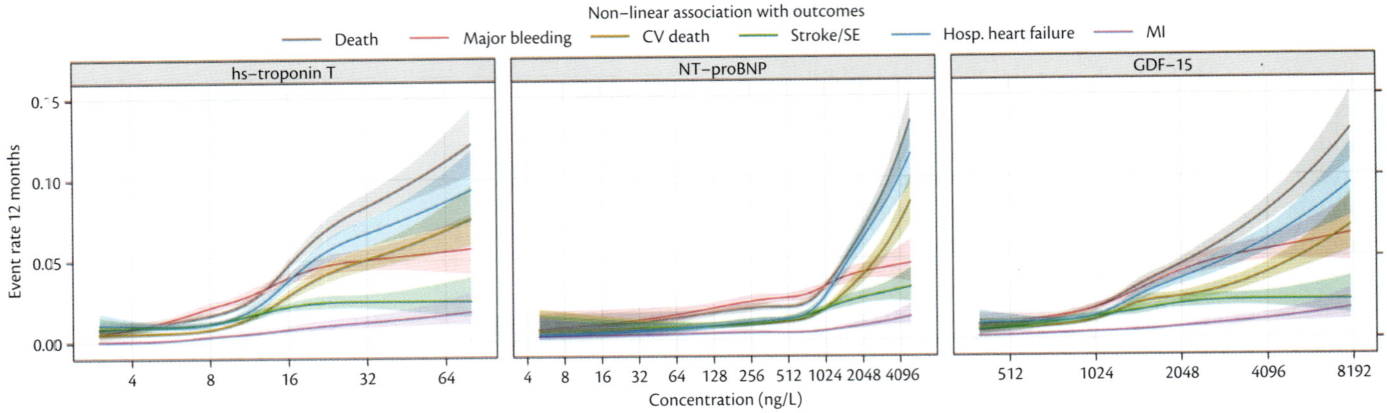

Figure 22.4 Associations between biomarker levels and clinical outcomes in atrial fibrillation.

variables age, biomarkers (NT-proBNP, hs-cTn), and clinical history of previous stroke/transient ischaemic attack. The ABC-AF bleeding score, consists of age, biomarkers (GDF-15, haemoglobin, and hs-cTn), and clinical history of previous bleeding. Both ABC-AF scores have been shown to outperform the clinical risk scores recommended by current guidelines and thus provide an option for a more precise risk assessment of stroke and major bleeding in AF. The results from several validation studies, based on large clinical cohorts, from both randomized trials and less-selected registry cohorts, are presented in ➲ Table 22.2.

The ABC-AF scores have also been consistent in important subgroups, such as previous stroke, and irrespective of concurrent, or type of, oral anticoagulation therapy and have similar performance in different regions and countries. In addition to the discriminatory performance, the ABC-AF scores are well calibrated (➲ Figure 22.5). Based on such properties, the ABC-AF scores are able to stratify patients within the non-biomarker-based risk scores and thereby provide a substantial reclassification of risk in around 25% of patients.[64] Decision curve analyses also show an important clinical value of the scores (➲ Figure 22.5). These findings highlight the improvements gained by the inclusion of robust biomarkers in clinical risk scores as they often provide more prognostic information than other variables. Such characteristics make the scores better calibrated and thus improve the generalizability of the scores. Accordingly, the ABC-AF scores offer the advantage to compare quantitative estimates of the annual stroke and bleeding risks with different treatment alternatives for individual patients.[66a] By including the scores in web calculators, smartphone applications, or potential easily available point-of-care tools, an integrated risk assessment and decision support for the individual patient with AF is possible.

Statistical considerations in development of biomarker-based risk scores

There are probably as many ways of developing a risk score (prognostic score, predictive score, prediction model) as there are researchers trying to develop them, and there is no consensus of a single best way to develop a risk score. However, there are pitfalls that can be avoided by following a few statistical recommendations.[67–70]

The ultimate goal when developing a risk score is to end up with a tool that supports clinical decision-making. The score should be robust and externally valid, meaning that it can be used in different settings outside the data where it was developed.[71] Contrary to some belief, the result of the prediction is not a classification. Rather, the prediction should be continuous, such as the probability of having a stroke within 1 year, and can thereafter be used together with other information for making a decision.

Table 22.2 Discriminatory performance (c-indices) of the biomarker-based ABC-AF risk scores

Study population	ABC-AF-stroke vs CHA_2DS_2-VASc	ABC-AF-bleeding vs HAS-BLED
ARISTOTLE cohort (n = 14,701)[58]	0.68 vs 0.62	0.68 vs 0.61
STABILITY AF cohort (n = 1400)[58]	0.66 vs 0.58	NA
RE-LY cohort (n = 8356)[66]	0.65 vs 0.60	0.71 vs 0.62
Murcia AF registry (n = 1125)[65]	0.66 vs 0.60	NA
ENGAGE AF cohort (n = 8705)[64]	0.67 vs 0.59	0.69 vs 0.62
ACTIVE A/AVERROES (n = 4305)[62]	0.70 vs 0.63	0.73 vs 0.60
Vienna ER registry (n = 2108)[59]	0.64 vs 0.55	NA

NA, GDF-15 not available or ABC-AF-bleeding score not calculated. The number of patients in each cohort may differ slightly for the ABC-AF-bleeding results.

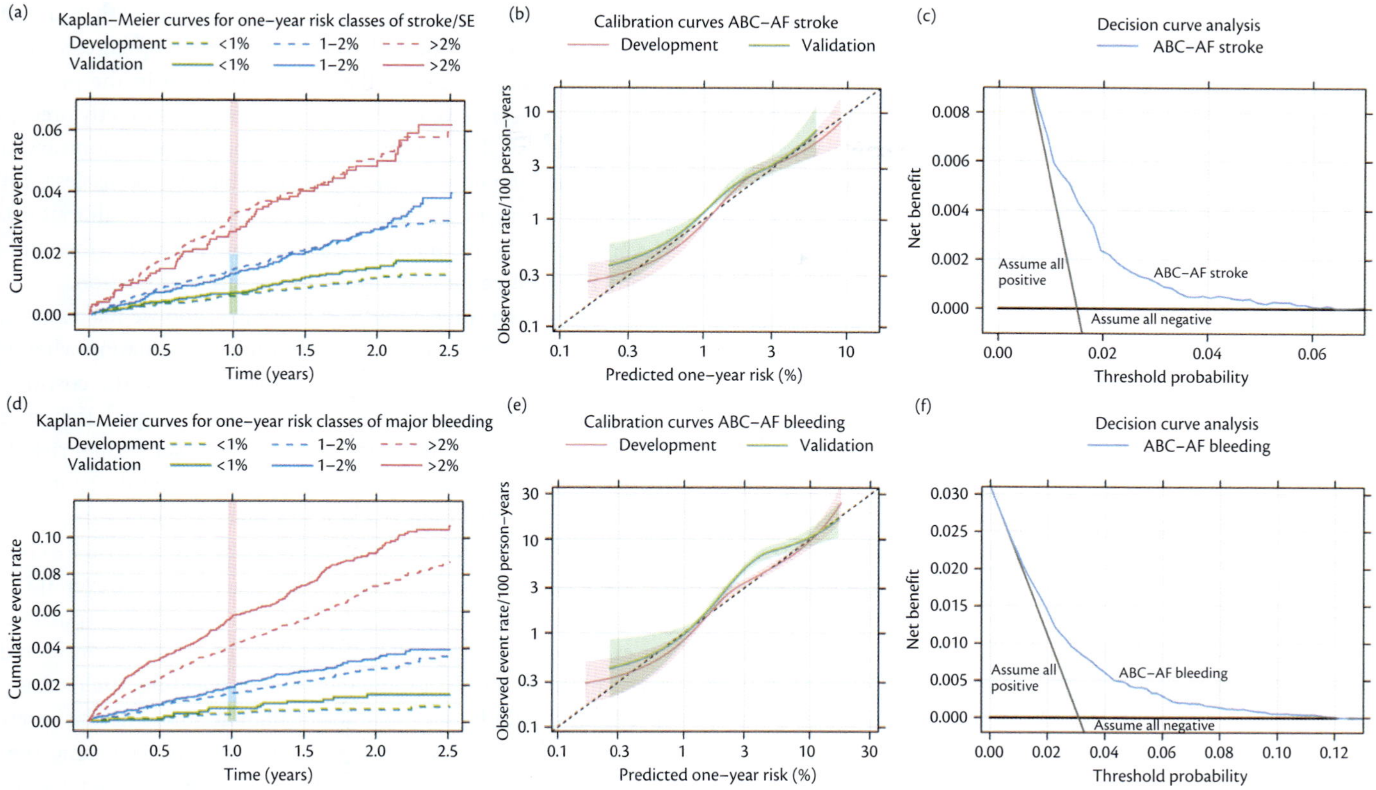

Figure 22.5 Calibration and utility of the ABC-AF stroke score (a–c) and the ABC-AF bleeding score (d–f) in patients with atrial fibrillation. Cumulative risk of cardiovascular death by predicted 1-year ABC-AF risk groups (a, d). Calibration (b, e), and clinical utility (c, f) of the ABC-AF risk scores.

Selection of target populations and events of interest

When developing a risk score for predicting future events, it is important that both the target populations and events are well defined. The target population should include anyone the risk score would be eligible for, such as patients with a particular diagnosis anywhere in the world or maybe only patients presenting with specific symptoms at the local clinic. The data used for the development should therefore be representative of the target population.

When considering the event of interest, a broad definition of, for example, bleeding events, leads to higher event rates and consequently larger predicted risks on average than a narrower definition. If the intended use is to predict the risk of a *major* bleed, including *all* kinds of bleeds as outcome when developing the score may consequently lead to a score that consistently overestimates the target risk. The time frame of the predictions is also important, for example, in-hospital, within 30 days from admission, or 1-year post discharge.

Many published risk scores have been developed using too small sample sizes with the consequence of having a poor chance to be externally valid. It is important to make sure that the sample size is large enough before starting the development. The effective sample size depends on the information level of the outcome event, with highest information achieved when the outcome is continuous and lowest when the outcome is binary and rare. For a time-to-event or rare binary outcome, it is the number of events that defines the effective sample size. A larger sample size is required when there are more variables in the score. A popular rule of thumb suggests that at least ten events per variable in the model is needed. However, recent research has shown that this rule is situation dependent and often at least 20 events per variable are needed.[72,73] More elaborate sample size recommendations for prognostic models have recently been published.[73–75]

Selection of predictor variables

An early step in the development of a risk score is to choose which variables to include. The current recommended approach is to a priori make the decision based on subject matter knowledge (e.g. from published sources like systematic reviews or meta-analyses). So-called univariable screening, using the development dataset to select variables based on their strength of association with the outcome, is not recommended since it is known to lead to overfitting, decreasing the chance for the score to be externally valid.[68,69,76,77] Although historically popular, stepwise variable selection methods are not recommended since they have been shown to have many problems.[68–70] One problem is that the subject expert is excluded from the decision. Another problem is that the regression coefficients in the final model will be biased away from zero due to overfitting the model to the current data. To increase the potential use of the risk score, consider including only variables that are routinely available. When biomarkers are included, make sure the laboratory methods are reproducible and measure absolute concentrations.

Similar to clinical variables (e.g. age and blood pressure), biomarkers are continuous and often include more information than categorical variables. To fully use their information it is important to keep them continuous in the score.[78] Splitting a continuous variable into categories will reduce information and likely require another variable to make up for lost information. Also, apart from very rare occasions, biology is not split according to arbitrary cut-offs. It is sometimes argued that categorization is needed for clinical decision-making but that is only true at the final step when the decision is made.

One trait that is characteristic for biomarkers is an often right-skewed concentration distribution. This is not a problem per se but can indicate that it is more appropriate to consider a multiplicative rather than an additive scale to represent the concentration. A logarithmic transformation can be useful as it makes differences on the log-scale correspond to ratios on the original scale. Sometimes it is difficult to measure very low concentrations with adequate accuracy. Any method replacing values below the lower reporting limit (RL) with a single arbitrarily chosen value, like the RL or RL/2, is known to be biased,[79,80] although one recommendation when the distribution is log-normal is to replace the censored values with the RL divided by the square root of 2.[81] Optimally one should use a statistical method that is able to handle the values correctly as censored observations.[82,83] Often, but not always, the association between an outcome and a continuous variable is monotonically increasing or decreasing but not necessarily linear. One way to model the non-linearity is to use restricted cubic splines which are flexible and can capture almost any non-linear association (➔ Figures 22.2 and 22.4)[68,69,76]

Prediction performance

How do we decide if the risk score is good? Ideally, the implementation of the score should be tested in the intended clinical setting to evaluate whether using the score actually improves decision-making and thereby results in less adverse events and/or reduced medical costs.[71] This requires additional studies that can be time-consuming and expensive. Before designing such a trial, it is advantageous to know if the score at least can perform its first task of producing the underlying probabilities. Three commonly used performance concepts that should be fulfilled are calibration, discrimination, and clinical utility.

Calibration is the concept of making correct predictions on average. If a risk score claims that, for a certain group of patients with the same risk profile, the yearly risk of a thrombotic event is 2%, we should expect that approximately 2% of those patients will experience the event within a year. Point-based scores typically do not produce absolute probabilities making it impossible to evaluate their calibration. A good way to evaluate calibration is graphically by producing a smooth calibration curve (➔ Figures 22.3 and 22.5).[68,69,84,85]

Discrimination is the risk score's ability to rank patients according to their risk of event. The c-index is one of the most commonly used measures for evaluating risk scores with binary or time-to-event outcomes.[68,86] It is defined as the probability that between two randomly selected patients, one with and one without an event, the one with the event has higher predicted risk. It is strongly dependent on the risk distribution in the population.[86] A score can have poor discrimination but correctly predict the average risk if the population is homogeneous. Contrary, a risk score can be good at discriminating but still be useless if it produces incorrect risk estimates for everyone (poor calibration). Nevertheless, discriminative measures can be useful for comparing two well-calibrated models in the same population.

The risk score is only a tool and every decision we make, using the tool or not, comes with a cost. In the naïve situation when it is assumed that there are no costs involved or that the cost of a false-positive and a false-negative prediction are equal, the score can be used directly with a decision threshold set to 50% risk. If the risk score indicates higher than 50% risk, the decision will be according to the 'high risk', for example, initiate treatment or increase the frequency of follow-up visits, and otherwise we consider the risk as low with corresponding actions. However, if the cost of a false negative is much higher than that of a false positive, for example, if missing a potential ischaemic stroke is considered much more severe than inducing a major bleeding, the decision threshold should be set much lower than at 50%. There is rarely one single threshold that applies to all patients. The same predicted score can lead to different decisions based on the personal cost of a wrong decision. Therefore, the treatment decision should be made together with the patient and incorporate the cost and benefit of the decision. Decision curves can help with assessing the net benefit of using the risk score for assigning patients to high or low risk for a range of decision thresholds while incorporating the cost of a wrong decision (➔ Figures 22.3 and 22.5).[87]

Internal and external validation

The performance measures evaluated in the development data indicate the apparent performance of the risk score. It is more likely that a score fits the data used for development than data from external sources. Overfitting simply means that the model is overly fitted to the current data and that the apparent performance measures are likely too good to be true. A thorough internal validation is therefore mandatory and can save money as poor internal validity can deter us from performing an expensive external validation with even less hope of validating the score. In some fields, especially machine learning, it is popular to split the development data into a training dataset and a test dataset. It is claimed that holding out data gives the opportunity to independently validate the risk score, developed in the training dataset, using the test dataset. However, this is only a chimera and, in fact, wastes valuable data that could have been used for better development of the risk score. It is better to use all data for development and use cross-validation or bootstrap methods for internal validation.[68,69,72,88] External validation means that the developed score is evaluated in a different setting.[89,90] Typical examples include different geographical locations or a different time period, preferably performed by different researchers. The most important property to externally assess is calibration (➔ Figures 22.3 and

22.5). The score might be equally good at discriminating, but if all estimated probabilities are systematically wrong the score cannot be trusted. Nevertheless, by thoroughly assessing the calibration it might be possible to recalibrate the score for the new setting.[69] An important but sometimes neglected fact is that external validation means that the score is evaluated by calculating predictions for the new patients using the originally developed regression equation and comparing them with the observed outcome and not by re-fitting the same variables to the outcome. The latter would not evaluate the score but rather estimate a new score that in turn would need to be externally validated.

Presentation of the model and reporting the results

When the developed and/or validated score is to be published, all steps in the process should be reported. In particular, include a detailed algorithm (e.g. the full regression equation) on how to produce predicted probabilities for new patients so others can use, and validate, the score. Nomograms can help with interpretation of the model as well as being a tool for rough estimation of risks. Optimally, a readily available web-based application can aid the calculation of more precise risk estimates. A strong recommendation is to follow the Transparent Reporting of a multivariable prediction model for Individual Prognosis Or Diagnosis (TRIPOD) statement.[91]

Future perspectives

So far, the clinical utility of biomarkers and biomarker-based risk scores have mainly been documented in retrospective clinical materials. Currently, there are ongoing prospective randomized controlled trials evaluating their utility in comparison to routine care. In a few years from now, these novel tools might therefore be implemented for further improvement of outcomes in individual patients. Future measurements of predictive biomarkers might also be incorporated into point-of-care and/or multiplex analytical tools. Currently, an array of novel prognostic biomarkers is being discovered through proteomic and genomic analyses and/or artificial intelligence which might lead to further development of biomarker-based risk prediction providing additional information. However, before clinical implementation, the increment clinical utility of novel biomarkers needs to be demonstrated in prospective clinical cohorts.

What's new

- Biomarkers provide unique and incremental prognostic information on major clinical outcomes in patients with CVD.
- Biomarkers, when combined into risk scores, might facilitate decision-making at the individual level balancing the benefits and risks with secondary preventive treatment.
- The ABC risk score in AF and in CHD are biomarker-based risk scores performing better than traditional risk scores and may be combined into an easily available tool for integrated risk assessment.

Guideline recommendations

- Clinical risk scores offer tools for systematic risk stratification and decision support in both AF and CHD and are recommended by the ESC Guidelines for risk stratification of ischaemic and major bleeding events, respectively.
- Biomarkers may be used in order to further refine the risk prediction of these events.
- Systematic evaluation of biomarkers and risk scores is recommended.

What's next

- An integrated approach to risk assessment that incorporates both risk for thromboembolism and risk for major bleeding provides an improved basis for the decision on antithrombotic therapy in patients with CVD.
- Prospective randomized trials to evaluate the biomarker-based strategies.
- Search for potentially more disease- and outcome-specific biomarkers.
- Novel risk scores incorporating biomarkers and/or artificial intelligence for prediction of cardiovascular events.

References

1. Roe MT, Ohman EM. A new era in secondary prevention after acute coronary syndrome. N Engl J Med. 2012;366(1):85–7.
2. Reed GW, Rossi JE, Cannon CP. Acute myocardial infarction. Lancet. 2017;389(10065):197–210.
3. Fox KAA, Anderson FA, Dabbous OH, et al. Intervention in acute coronary syndromes: do patients undergo intervention on the basis of their risk characteristics? The Global Registry of Acute Coronary Events (GRACE). Heart. 2005;93(2):177–82.
4. Hsu JC, Maddox TM, Kennedy KF, et al. Oral anticoagulant therapy prescription in patients with atrial fibrillation across the spectrum of stroke risk: insights from the NCDR PINNACLE Registry. JAMA Cardiol. 2016;1(1):55–62.
5. Hijazi Z, Oldgren J, Siegbahn A, Granger CB, Wallentin L. Biomarkers in atrial fibrillation: a clinical review. Eur Heart J. 2013;34(20):1475–80.
6. Roongsritong C, Warraich I, Bradley C. Common causes of troponin elevations in the absence of acute myocardial infarction: incidence and clinical significance. Chest. 2004;125(5):1877–84.
7. de Lemos JA, McGuire DK, Drazner MH. B-type natriuretic peptide in cardiovascular disease. Lancet. 2003;362(9380):316–22.
8. Anand IS, Fisher LD, Chiang Y-T, et al. Changes in brain natriuretic peptide and norepinephrine over time and mortality and morbidity in the Valsartan Heart Failure Trial (Val-HeFT). Circulation. 2003;107(9):1278–83.

9. Heeschen C, Hamm CW, Mitrovic V, Lantelme N-H, White HD. N-terminal pro-B-type natriuretic peptide levels for dynamic risk stratification of patients with acute coronary syndromes. Circulation. 2004;110(20):3206–12.
10. Hijazi Z, Oldgren J, Andersson U, et al. Cardiac biomarkers are associated with an increased risk of stroke and death in patients with atrial fibrillation: a Randomized Evaluation of Long-term Anticoagulation Therapy (RE-LY) substudy. Circulation. 2012;125(13):1605–16.
11. Kempf T, Horn-Wichmann Rd, Brabant G, et al. Circulating concentrations of growth-differentiation factor 15 in apparently healthy elderly individuals and patients with chronic heart failure as assessed by a new immunoradiometric sandwich assay. Clin Chem. 2007;53(2):284–91.
12. Wallentin L, Hijazi Z, Andersson U, et al. Growth differentiation factor 15, a marker of oxidative stress and inflammation, for risk assessment in patients with atrial fibrillation: insights from the Apixaban for Reduction in Stroke and Other Thromboembolic Events in Atrial Fibrillation (ARISTOTLE) trial. Circulation. 2014;130(21):1847–58.
13. Wollert KC, Kempf T, Wallentin L. Growth differentiation factor 15 as a biomarker in cardiovascular disease. Clin Chem. 2017;63(1):140–51.
14. Jernberg T, Lindahl B, James S, et al. Cystatin C: a novel predictor of outcome in suspected or confirmed non–ST-elevation acute coronary syndrome. Circulation. 2004;110(16):2342–48.
15. Pan W, Lu H, Lian B, et al. Prognostic value of HbA1c for in-hospital and short-term mortality in patients with acute coronary syndrome: a systematic review and meta-analysis. Cardiovasc Diabetol. 2019;18(1):169.
16. Ray KK, Cannon CP, Cairns R, et al. Prognostic utility of ApoB/AI, total cholesterol/HDL, non-HDL cholesterol, or hs-CRP as predictors of clinical risk in patients receiving statin therapy after acute coronary syndromes. Arterioscler Thromb Vasc Biol. 2009;29(3):424–30.
17. Thygesen K, Alpert JS, Jaffe AS, et al. Fourth universal definition of myocardial infarction (2018). Eur Heart J. 2019;40(3):237–69.
18. Antman EM, Tanasijevic MJ, Thompson B, et al. Cardiac-specific troponin I levels to predict the risk of mortality in patients with acute coronary syndromes. N Engl J Med. 1996;335(18):1342–9.
19. Ohman EM, Armstrong PW, Christenson RH, et al. Cardiac troponin T levels for risk stratification in acute myocardial ischemia. N Engl J Med. 1996;335(18):1333–42.
20. Wallentin L, Lindholm D, Siegbahn A, et al. Biomarkers in relation to the effects of ticagrelor in comparison with clopidogrel in non-ST-elevation acute coronary syndrome patients managed with or without in-hospital revascularization. Circulation. 2014;129(3):293–303.
21. Lindholm D, James SK, Bertilsson M, et al. Biomarkers and coronary lesions predict outcomes after revascularization in non–ST-elevation acute coronary syndrome. Clin Chem. 2017;63(2):573–84.
22. Giannitsis E, Spanuth E, Horsch A, et al. High-sensitivity cardiac troponin T and N-terminal pro-B-type natriuretic peptide predict mortality in stable coronary artery disease: results from the Ludwigshafen Risk and Cardiovascular Health (LURIC) study. Clin Chem Lab Med. 2013;51(10):2019–28.
23. Lindholm D, Lindbäck J, Armstrong PW, et al. Biomarker-based risk model to predict cardiovascular mortality in patients with stable coronary disease. J Am Coll Cardiol. 2017;70(7):813–26.
24. Omland T, Sabatine MS, Jablonski KA, et al. Prognostic value of B-type natriuretic peptides in patients with stable coronary artery disease: the PEACE trial. J Am Coll Cardiol. 2007;50(3):205–14.
25. Hagström E, Held C, Stewart RAH, et al. Growth differentiation factor 15 predicts all-cause morbidity and mortality in stable coronary heart disease. Clin Chem. 2017;63(1):325–33.
26. Hagström E, James SK, Bertilsson M, et al. Growth differentiation factor-15 level predicts major bleeding and cardiovascular events in patients with acute coronary syndromes: results from the PLATO study. Eur Heart J. 2016;37(16):1325–33.
27. Fox KAA, Dabbous OH, Goldberg RJ, et al. Prediction of risk of death and myocardial infarction in the six months after presentation with acute coronary syndrome: prospective multinational observational study (GRACE). BMJ. 2006;333(7578):1091.
28. Collet J-P, Thiele H, Barbato E, et al. 2020 ESC Guidelines for the management of acute coronary syndromes in patients presenting without persistent ST-segment elevation: the Task Force for the management of acute coronary syndromes in patients presenting without persistent ST-segment elevation of the European Society of Cardiology (ESC). Eur Heart J. 2020;42(14):1289–367.
29. Fox KAA, FitzGerald G, Puymirat E, et al. Should patients with acute coronary disease be stratified for management according to their risk? Derivation, external validation and outcomes using the updated GRACE risk score. BMJ Open. 2014;4(2):e004425.
30. Batra G, Lindbäck J, Becker RC, et al. The biomarker-based ABC score for prediction of ischemic events in patients with acute coronary syndrome. J Am Coll Cardiol. 2022;80(18):1735–47.
31. Ibanez B, James S, Agewall S, et al. 2017 ESC Guidelines for the management of acute myocardial infarction in patients presenting with ST-segment elevation: the Task Force for the management of acute myocardial infarction in patients presenting with ST-segment elevation of the European Society of Cardiology (ESC). Eur Heart J. 2017;39(2):119–77.
32. Yusuf S, Zhao F, Mehta SR, et al. Effects of clopidogrel in addition to aspirin in patients with acute coronary syndromes without ST-segment elevation. N Engl J Med. 2001;345(7):494–502.
33. Wallentin L, Becker RC, Budaj A, et al. Ticagrelor versus clopidogrel in patients with acute coronary syndromes. N Engl J Med. 2009;361(11):1045–57.
34. Wiviott SD, Braunwald E, McCabe CH, et al. Prasugrel versus clopidogrel in patients with acute coronary syndromes. N Engl J Med. 2007;357(20):2001–15.
35. Subherwal S, Bach RG, Chen AY, et al. Baseline risk of major bleeding in non-ST-segment–elevation myocardial infarction. Circulation. 2009;119(14):1873–82.
36. Mathews R, Peterson ED, Chen AY, et al. In-hospital major bleeding during ST-elevation and non–ST-elevation myocardial infarction care: derivation and validation of a model from the ACTION Registry®-GWTG. Am J Cardiol. 2011;107(8):1136–43.
37. Yeh RW, Secemsky EA, Kereiakes DJ, et al. Development and validation of a prediction rule for benefit and harm of dual antiplatelet therapy beyond 1 year after percutaneous coronary intervention. JAMA. 2016;315(16):1735–49.
38. Costa F, van Klaveren D, James S, et al. Derivation and validation of the predicting bleeding complications in patients undergoing stent implantation and subsequent dual antiplatelet therapy (PRECISE-DAPT) score: a pooled analysis of individual-patient datasets from clinical trials. Lancet. 2017;389(10073):1025–34.
39. Baber U, Mehran R, Giustino G, et al. Coronary thrombosis and major bleeding after PCI with drug-eluting stents: risk scores from PARIS. J Am Coll Cardiol. 2016;67(19):2224–34.
40. Risk factors for stroke and efficacy of antithrombotic therapy in atrial fibrillation. Analysis of pooled data from five randomized controlled trials. Arch Intern Med. 1994;154(13):1449–57.
41. The SPAF III Writing Committee for the Stroke Prevention in Atrial Fibrillation Investigators. Patients with nonvalvular atrial fibrillation at low risk of stroke during treatment with aspirin: Stroke Prevention in Atrial Fibrillation III Study. JAMA. 1998;279(16):1273–77.

42. Gage BF, Waterman AD, Shannon W, et al. Validation of clinical classification schemes for predicting stroke: results from the National Registry of Atrial Fibrillation. JAMA. 2001;285(22):2864–70.
43. Lip GY, Nieuwlaat R, Pisters R, Lane DA, Crijns HJ. Refining clinical risk stratification for predicting stroke and thromboembolism in atrial fibrillation using a novel risk factor-based approach: the euro heart survey on atrial fibrillation. Chest. 2010;137(2):263–72.
44. Singer DE, Albers GW, Dalen JE, et al. Antithrombotic therapy in atrial fibrillation: American College of Chest Physicians Evidence-Based Clinical Practice Guidelines (8th Edition). Chest. 2008;133(6 Suppl):546S–92S.
45. Wang TJ, Massaro JM, Levy D, et al. A risk score for predicting stroke or death in individuals with new-onset atrial fibrillation in the community: the Framingham Heart Study. JAMA. 2003;290(8):1049–56.
46. Fang MC, Go AS, Chang Y, et al. Comparison of risk stratification schemes to predict thromboembolism in people with nonvalvular atrial fibrillation. J Am Coll Cardiol. 2008;51(8):810–15.
47. Camm AJ, Kirchhof P, Lip GY, et al. Guidelines for the management of atrial fibrillation: the Task Force for the Management of Atrial Fibrillation of the European Society of Cardiology (ESC). Eur Heart J. 2010;31(19):2369–429.
48. Hart R. Comparison of 12 risk stratification schemes to predict stroke in patients with nonvalvular atrial fibrillation. Stroke. 2008;39(6):1901–10.
49. Van Staa TP, Setakis E, Di Tanna GL, Lane DA, Lip GY. A comparison of risk stratification schemes for stroke in 79,884 atrial fibrillation patients in general practice. J Thromb Haemost. 2011;9(1):39–48.
50. Friberg L, Rosenqvist M, Lip GY. Evaluation of risk stratification schemes for ischaemic stroke and bleeding in 182 678 patients with atrial fibrillation: the Swedish Atrial Fibrillation cohort study. Eur Heart J. 2012;33(12):1500–10.
51. Quinn GR, Severdija ON, Chang Y, Singer DE. Wide variation in reported rates of stroke across cohorts of patients with atrial fibrillation. Circulation. 2017;135(3):208–19.
52. Apostolakis S, Lane DA, Guo Y, Buller H, Lip GY. Performance of the HEMORR(2)HAGES, ATRIA, and HAS-BLED bleeding risk-prediction scores in patients with atrial fibrillation undergoing anticoagulation: the AMADEUS (evaluating the use of SR34006 compared to warfarin or acenocoumarol in patients with atrial fibrillation) study. J Am Coll Cardiol. 2012;60(9):861–7.
53. Fang MC, Go AS, Chang Y, et al. A new risk scheme to predict warfarin-associated hemorrhage: the ATRIA (Anticoagulation and Risk Factors in Atrial Fibrillation) Study. J Am Coll Cardiol. 2011;58(4):395–401.
54. O'Brien EC, Simon DN, Thomas LE, et al. The ORBIT bleeding score: a simple bedside score to assess bleeding risk in atrial fibrillation. Eur Heart J. 2015;36(46):3258–64.
55. Pisters R, Lane DA, Nieuwlaat R, et al. A novel user-friendly score (HAS-BLED) to assess one-year risk of major bleeding in atrial fibrillation patients: the Euro Heart Survey. Chest. 2010;138(5):1093–100.
56. Hijazi Z, Oldgren J, Siegbahn A, Wallentin L. Application of biomarkers for risk stratification in patients with atrial fibrillation. Clin Chem. 2017;63(1):152–64.
57. Hijazi Z, Oldgren J, Lindbäck J, et al. The novel biomarker-based ABC (age, biomarkers, clinical history)-bleeding risk score for patients with atrial fibrillation: a derivation and validation study. Lancet. 2016;387(10035):2302–11.
58. Hijazi Z, Lindbäck J, Alexander JH, et al. The ABC (age, biomarkers, clinical history) stroke risk score: a biomarker-based risk score for predicting stroke in atrial fibrillation. Eur Heart J. 2016;37(20):1582–90.
59. Niederdöckl J, Oppenauer J, Schnaubelt S, et al. The ABC-stroke score refines stroke risk stratification in patients with atrial fibrillation at the emergency department. Front Med. 2022;9:830580.
60. Pol T, Hijazi Z, Lindbäck J, et al. Evaluation of the prognostic value of GDF-15, ABC-AF-bleeding score and ABC-AF-death score in patients with atrial fibrillation across different geographical areas. Open Heart. 2021;8(1):e001471.
61. Oyama K, Giugliano RP, Berg DD, et al. Serial assessment of biomarkers and the risk of stroke or systemic embolism and bleeding in patients with atrial fibrillation in the ENGAGE AF-TIMI 48 trial. Eur Heart J. 2021;42(17):1698–706.
62. Benz AP, Hijazi Z, Lindbäck J, et al. Biomarker-based risk prediction with the ABC-AF scores in patients with atrial fibrillation not receiving oral anticoagulation. Circulation. 2021;143(19):1863–73.
63. Hijazi Z, Oldgren J, Lindbäck J, et al. Evaluation of the age, biomarkers, and clinical history-bleeding risk score in patients with atrial fibrillation with combined aspirin and anticoagulation therapy enrolled in the ARISTOTLE and RE-LY Trials. JAMA Netw Open. 2020;3(9):e2015943.
64. Berg DD, Ruff CT, Jarolim P, et al. Performance of the ABC scores for assessing the risk of stroke or systemic embolism and bleeding in patients with atrial fibrillation in ENGAGE AF-TIMI 48. Circulation. 2019;139(6):760–71.
65. Rivera-Caravaca JM, Roldán V, Esteve-Pastor MA, et al. Long-term stroke risk prediction in patients with atrial fibrillation: comparison of the ABC-Stroke and CHA2DS2-VASc scores. J Am Heart Assoc. 2017;6(7):e006490.
66. Oldgren J, Hijazi Z, Lindbäck J, et al. Performance and validation of a novel biomarker-based stroke risk score for atrial fibrillation. Circulation. 2016;134(22):1697–707.
66a. Ziad Hijazi, Lindbäck J, Oldgren J, et al. Individual net clinical outcome with oral anticoagulation in atrial fibrillation using the ABC-AF risk scores. Am Heart J. 2023;261:55–63.
67. Gerds TA, Kattan MW. Medical Risk Prediction Models. 1st edition. Boca Raton, FL: Routledge; 2021.
68. Harrell Jr FE. Regression Modeling Strategies: With Applications to Linear Models, Logistic and Ordinal Regression, and Survival Analysis. 2nd edition. New York: Springer; 2015.
69. Steyerberg EW. Clinical Prediction Models: A Practical Approach to Development, Validation, and Updating. 2nd edition. Cham: Springer; 2019.
70. Steyerberg EW, Vergouwe Y. Towards better clinical prediction models: seven steps for development and an ABCD for validation. Eur Heart J. 2014;35(29):1925–31.
71. Altman DG, Royston P. What do we mean by validating a prognostic model? Stat Med. 2000;19(4):453–73.
72. Austin PC, Steyerberg EW. Events per variable (EPV) and the relative performance of different strategies for estimating the out-of-sample validity of logistic regression models. Stat Methods Med Res. 2017;26(2):796–808.
73. Riley RD, Snell KI, Ensor J, et al. Minimum sample size for developing a multivariable prediction model: PART II—binary and time-to-event outcomes. Stat Med. 2019;38(7):1276–96.
74. Collins GS, Ogundimu EO, Altman DG. Sample size considerations for the external validation of a multivariable prognostic model: a resampling study: sample size considerations for validating a prognostic model. Stat Med. 2016;35(2):214–26.
75. Riley RD, Debray TPA, Collins GS, et al. Minimum sample size for external validation of a clinical prediction model with a binary outcome. Stat Med. 2021;40(19):4230–51.
76. Sauerbrei W, Perperoglou A, Schmid M, et al. State of the art in selection of variables and functional forms in multivariable analysis—outstanding issues. Diagn Progn Res. 2020;4(1):3.

77. Sun G-W, Shook TL, Kay GL. Inappropriate use of bivariable analysis to screen risk factors for use in multivariable analysis. J Clin Epidemiol. 1996;49(8):907–16.
78. Royston P, Altman DG, Sauerbrei W. Dichotomizing continuous predictors in multiple regression: a bad idea. Stat Med. 2006;25(1):127–41.
79. Arunajadai SG, Rauh VA. Handling covariates subject to limits of detection in regression. Environ Ecol Stat. 2012;19:369–91.
80. Nie L, Chu H, Liu C, et al. Linear regression with an independent variable subject to a detection limit. Epidemiology. 2010;21(4):S17–S24.
81. Hornung RW, Reed LD. Estimation of average concentration in the presence of nondetectable values. Appl Occup Environ Hyg. 1990;5(1):46–51.
82. Chiou SH, Betensky RA, Balasubramanian R. The missing indicator approach for censored covariates subject to limit of detection in logistic regression models. Ann Epidemiol. 2019;38:57–64.
83. Ortega-Villa AM, Liu D, Ward MH, Albert PS. New insights into modeling exposure measurements below the limit of detection. Environ Epidemiol. 2021;5(1):e116.
84. Austin PC, Harrell Jr FE, van Klaveren D. Graphical calibration curves and the integrated calibration index (ICI) for survival models. Stat Med. 2020;39(21):2714–42.
85. Austin PC, Steyerberg EW. Graphical assessment of internal and external calibration of logistic regression models by using loess smoothers. Stat Med. 2014;33(3):517–35.
86. Austin PC, Steyerberg EW. Interpreting the concordance statistic of a logistic regression model: relation to the variance and odds ratio of a continuous explanatory variable. BMC Med Res Methodol. 2012;12(1):82.
87. Vickers AJ, Elkin EB. Decision curve analysis: a novel method for evaluating prediction models. Med Decis Making. 2006;26(6):565–74.
88. Steyerberg EW. Validation in prediction research: the waste by data splitting. J Clin Epidemiol. 2018;103:131–3.
89. Altman DG, Vergouwe Y, Royston P, Moons KGM. Prognosis and prognostic research: validating a prognostic model. BMJ. 2009;338:b605.
90. Royston P, Altman DG. External validation of a Cox prognostic model: principles and methods. BMC Med Res Methodol. 2013;13(1):33.
91. Collins GS, Reitsma JB, Altman DG, Moons KGM. Transparent Reporting of a multivariable prediction model for Individual Prognosis Or Diagnosis (TRIPOD): the TRIPOD statement. Ann Intern Med. 2015;162(1):55–63.

SECTION 4

Special situations

CHAPTER 23

Antithrombotic therapies in inherited or acquired thrombophilia

Vittorio Pengo and Gentian Denas

Contents

Summary

The treatment of thrombophilias and their related clinical events is based on antithrombotic agents. Testing for inherited thrombophilia generally does not alter the clinical management of patients with venous or arterial thrombosis or pregnancy complications. An exception may be the presence of severe inherited thrombophilia that is usually rare and comprises deficiency of natural coagulation inhibitors (antithrombin, protein C, and protein S) or homozygosity and compound heterozygosity of factor V Leiden and prothrombin variant G20210A. In contrast, the presence of acquired thrombophilia guides antithrombotic treatment in affected patients. Appropriate treatment is important in patients with the antiphospholipid syndrome, heparin-induced thrombocytopenia, paroxysmal nocturnal haemoglobinuria, polycythaemia vera/essential thrombocythaemia, and sickle cell disease. Other common conditions of acquired thrombophilia, such as combined oral contraceptives and cancer-associated thrombosis, deserve special attention. Finally, the correct differential diagnosis of thrombotic microangiopathies is the basis of correct antithrombotic treatment.

Introduction

Disruption of the physiological coagulation–fibrinolysis balance in favour of coagulation causes a hypercoagulable state called thrombophilia. Factors leading to thrombophilia are inherited or acquired. The identification of thrombophilia has a number of potential clinical implications, including increased risk of a first episode of venous thromboembolism (VTE), increased risk of arterial thrombosis and pregnancy complications, the need for specific treatment, and the potential for non-thrombotic manifestations.

Despite efforts made to identify provoking risk factors for VTE, they are found in less than 50% of cases of deep vein thrombosis (DVT).[1] Thrombophilia is one of the elements that increases the risk of VTE, although it is relatively rare[2] in comparison with more traditional risk factors such as immobility, surgery, neoplastic disease, and obesity. However, the rate of thrombophilia is higher in patients with a first or recurrent episodes of VTE.[3] Testing for inherited thrombophilia (IT) is controversial in the setting of VTE.[4,5] In contrast, testing for acquired thrombophilia in the setting of arterial thromboembolism may be of relevant clinical utility in guiding patient care.[6–9] The patient management in terms of type of anticoagulant, therapy duration, and association of adjunctive antiplatelet therapy may be influenced by the presence of thrombophilia.

Inherited thrombophilia

IT involves abnormalities of genes responsible for the synthesis of coagulation factors. Gene alterations include loss-of-function mutations affecting antithrombin (AT), protein C, and protein S, and gain-of-function mutations known as factor V Leiden (FVL) and the prothrombin variant G20210A (PVG/A)[4] (➔ Table 23.1). Deficiency of AT, protein C, or protein S is associated with a high risk of developing initial VTE (estimated as more than nine times that of the general population), but these conditions are fortunately uncommon (each occurring in <0.5% of the general population).

FVL and PVG/A are associated with a modest risk of developing initial VTE (two to five times that of the general population) and are relatively common (2–5% in Caucasians).[10] Conversely, IT is a poor predictor of recurrent VTE, as the relative risk compared with VTE patients without IT is modest.

Inherited thrombophilia testing

Guidelines on IT testing are lacking, and the role of testing outside specific cases is controversial.[11] Indeed, VTE risk scores (DASH, HERDOO2, Vienna) do not endorse it. Testing is clinically useful in carriers of severe IT, notably those with confirmed deficiency of AT, protein C, or protein S, and those with homozygous FVL or homozygous PVG/A, or heterozygous for the two combined genetic abnormalities. These patients are candidates for indefinite anticoagulant treatment after a first episode of VTE.[12] In contrast, no evidence for a clinical benefit of extended anticoagulant treatment is currently available for carriers of heterozygous FVL or PVG/A. Testing could also help in primary prevention of relatives of IT-positive patients.

Oral anticoagulant therapy and duration of anticoagulation after a first episode of venous thromboembolism

Treatment of acute VTE does not differ from the usual care in patients with IT. Direct-acting oral anticoagulants (DOACs) can be used as a first-line treatment in the acute phase and in the long term. Indeed, in a case–control study, the use of DOACs did not differ in terms of efficacy and safety from the standard heparin/vitamin K antagonist (VKA) regimen.[13] As shown in ➔ Table 23.1, IT (with the exception of very rare FVL homozygosis) does not substantially increase the risk of recurrent VTE. Thus, screening for IT has little role in determining the duration of anticoagulation[4] that should rather be guided by the presence of other risk factors.

Special situations: pregnancy and puerperium

The occurrence of VTE is approximately 1–2 per 1000 pregnant women.[14] The standard treatment of VTE in pregnancy is anticoagulation with therapeutic dose of low-molecular-weight heparins (LMWHs), which do not cross the placenta and thus are not teratogenic.[15] The risk of VTE increases throughout pregnancy and is highest in the puerperium.[16] Among the numerous risk factors for VTE in pregnancy and in the puerperium, a previous VTE episode, positive family history for VTE, and IT are of major importance.[17,18] Known thrombophilia increases the risk of recurrent VTE in pregnant women, and accurate prophylaxis with LMWH during pregnancy and for 6 weeks after delivery is warranted. The optimal dose of LMWH prophylaxis, especially in the antepartum period, is still a matter of debate.[19] In the absence of VTE history or of additional predisposing factors, the presence of a weak thrombophilia, such as heterozygous FVL alone, does not usually require LMWH prophylaxis.[20] In case of severe IT and no previous VTE, a family history of VTE, as well as additional VTE risk factors, should be considered, and the decision for LMWH prophylaxis should be taken on an individual basis.

Table 23.1 Prevalence and thrombosis risk for inherited causes of thrombophilia

	Prevalence (%)	RR of initial VTE	RR of recurrent VTE
Weak			
Factor V Leiden	5–7	3.5–5.5	1.1–1.8
Prothrombin variant (G20210A)	1–2	2.2–3.5	0.7–2.3
Strong			
Antithrombin deficiency	0.02	10–30	2.6
Protein C deficiency	0.2–0.5	10	1.8
Protein S deficiency	0.1–0.7	9.6	1.0
Homozygous for factor V Leiden	0.06–0.25	6.8	19.3
Homozygous for prothrombin variant	Rare	2.2–20.7	Uncertain
Double heterozygosity (Leiden and prothrombin)	0.1	1.1–5.0	2.7

RR, relative risk; VTE, venous thromboembolism.

Source data from Stevens SM, Woller SC, Bauer KA, et al. Guidance for the evaluation and treatment of hereditary and acquired thrombophilia. J Thromb Thrombolysis. 2016;41(1):154–64. doi: 10.1007/s11239-015-1316-1.

Acquired thrombophilia

Acquired thrombophilia encompasses a large group of clinical conditions that are associated with an increased risk of thrombosis. These include classical risk factors for VTE—such as increasing age, immobilization, and recent surgery—and many others. Treatment of these conditions is beyond the scope of this chapter that will focus on selected causes of acquired thrombophilia (➔ Table 23.2).

Antiphospholipid syndrome

Antiphospholipid syndrome (APS) is a condition defined by a clinical event (thrombosis or pregnancy morbidity) and the presence of persistently positive antiphospholipid antibodies (aPL)[25] (➔ Figure 23.1). VTE generally occurs in deep veins of the lower extremities (DVT) or pulmonary veins [pulmonary embolism (PE)], but uncommon sites—such as cerebral, mesenteric, and upper limb veins—may also be affected. The most common arterial involvement is the cerebral circulation (stroke/transient ischaemic attack), but arterial thrombosis can occur in the coronary and peripheral arteries as well. Thrombosis on both native (Libman–Sacks endocarditis) and prosthetic valves are also observed.[9] The estimated prevalence of APS is 50 cases (95% confidence interval 42–58 cases) per 100,000 people.[21] The estimated aPL frequency in DVT is 9.5%,[26] but in patients with a first unprovoked VTE, the presence of aPL could be up to 25%.[27] Out of 100 cases of APS, 80 are thrombotic and 20 are associated with pregnancy morbidity.[26] Patients with chronic thromboembolic pulmonary hypertension (CTEPH) present a positive aPL profile in 12% of cases.[28] All the three tests reported in ➔ Figure 23.1 are mandatory for the diagnosis, and must be confirmed 12 weeks apart. Triple-positive patients (positive for all the three tests) are at high risk of recurrence.[29]

The suspicion of APS increases when unexplained thrombosis occurs in young patients, VTE is unprovoked or provoked by mild risk factors, or VTE occurs in uncommon sites or in patients with associated systemic lupus erythematosus or other autoimmune diseases.[30,31] In patients already on anticoagulant treatment, aPL testing needs particular attention for possible lupus anticoagulant false-positive results[32–37](➔ Figure 23.2).

Table 23.2 Selected causes of acquired thrombophilia

Condition	Prevalence
Antiphospholipid syndrome	42–58 per 100,000 people[21]
Heparin-induced thrombocytopenia	5% patients/year[a]
Paroxysmal nocturnal haemoglobinuria	0.05–0.15 per 100,000 people[22]
Polycythemia vera and essential thrombocythaemia	22–24 per 100,000 people[23]
Sickle cell disease[b]	~25 per 100,000 people[24]

[a] Mainly caused by unfractionated heparin.
[b] Sickle cell disease is an inherited thrombophilia not involving coagulation factors.

Antithrombotic therapy

Type of anticoagulant

Rivaroxaban was tested for efficacy and safety against warfarin in the TRAPS trial. This was a prospective, randomized, phase-III, open-label, non-inferiority trial.[38,39] Patients were stratified for sex and autoimmune diseases and randomized to receive rivaroxaban 20 mg once daily (15 mg if creatinine clearance 30–50 mL/min) or warfarin to maintain an international normalized ratio (INR) between 2 and 3. The trial was prematurely terminated, after the

Current classification criteria for APS

Antiphospholipid syndrome requires the combination of at least one clinical and one laboratory criterion.

Clinical criteria: a. vascular thrombosis or b. pregnancy morbidity

a. Objectively proven venous, arterial, or small vessell thrombosis
b. One or more unexplained deaths of a morphologically normal fetus after10 week of gestation or >3 unexplained consecutive spontaneous abortions before the 10th week of gestation

Laboratory criteria: a. Lupus anticoagulant (LA); b. anticardiolipin antibodies (aCL); c. anti **β2-glycoprotein I antibodies (aβ2GPI) at medium high titre present on 2 occasions at least 12 weeks apart.**

Figure 23.1 Classification criteria for the antiphospholipid syndrome (APS). Note that these are classification and not diagnostic criteria. Multiple positive laboratory tests (e.g. triple positivity) and multiple episodes of both venous and arterial thrombosis and pregnancy morbidity identify patients at higher risk of recurrence. aβ2GPI, anti-beta$_2$ glycoprotein I antibodies; aCL, anticardiolipin antibodies; aPS/PT, antiphosphatidylserine/prothrombin antibodies.

Source data from Miyakis S, Lockshin MD, Atsumi T, et al. International consensus statement on an update of the classification criteria for definite antiphospholipid syndrome (APS). J Thromb Haemost. 2006;4(2):295–306. doi: 10.1111/j.1538-7836.2006.01753.x.

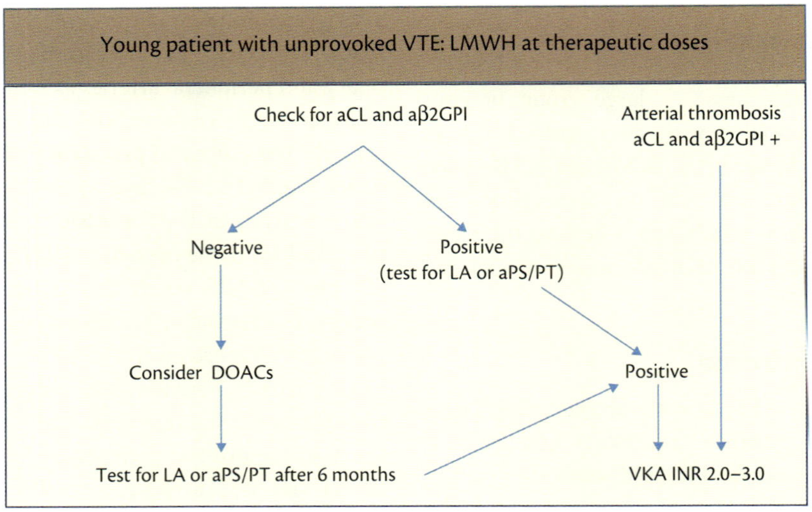

Figure 23.2 How we treat suspected thrombotic APS. In young patients with unprovoked VTE or VTE provoked by mild risk factors, an initial treatment with therapeutic dose of LMWH is recommended taking into consideration renal function and patient bleeding risk. Check for immunological tests [anti-cardiolipin (aCL) and anti-beta$_2$ glycoprotein I (aβ2GPI antibodies)] that are unaffected by the presence of anticoagulants. If negative, direct oral anticoagulants (DOACs) may be considered. If positive and the patient is lupus anticoagulant (LA) positive or a surrogate test for LA [antiphosphatidylserine/prothrombin antibodies (aPS/PT)] is positive, then a vitamin K antagonist (VKA) at standard intensity [international normalized ratio (INR) 2.0–3.0] should be used. After 6 months of DOACs, check for LA: if positive, VKA should be considered. In case of arterial thrombosis and aCL and aβ2GPI antibodies are positive, VKAs are the suggested treatment.

Source data from Pengo V. Additional laboratory tests to improve on the diagnosis of antiphospholipid syndrome: Response from Pengo. J Thromb Haemost. 2020;18(11):3118–3119. doi: 10.1111/jth.15026.

randomization of 120 patients, due to excess arterial thromboembolic events (four ischaemic strokes and three myocardial infarctions in the rivaroxaban arm vs none in the warfarin group). A similar randomized trial gave similar results.[40] Nine patients in the rivaroxaban group had an ischaemic stroke compared to none in the VKA group. A third randomized open-label trial[41] compared apixaban 2.5 mg twice daily versus warfarin (target INR 2–3) for 12 months. Due to an increased incidence of events with apixaban 2.5 mg twice daily, the protocol was first modified to apixaban 5 mg twice daily and then patients with prior arterial thrombosis were excluded for excess risk with apixaban. The study ended prematurely due to an increased risk of stroke in patients receiving apixaban (6 out of 23 in the apixaban arm versus 0 out of 25 in the warfarin arm). Taken together, these data suggest that warfarin is the best treatment option in high-risk APS patients.

Given the up-to-date evidence, high-risk (i.e. those with a triple-positive laboratory profile) APS patients should not be treated with DOACs.[42] Whether this caution can be translated to patients with a single- or double-positive laboratory profile in currently unknown. In high-risk settings, such as pregnancy or around surgery, a LMWH at intermediate/therapeutic dose should be used according to individual patient risk.[43]

Intensity and duration of VKA treatment

High-intensity warfarin (INR >3.0) was a suggested treatment in patients with previous arterial events.[44] However, two randomized controlled trials showed that standard-intensity anticoagulation (INR 2.0–3.0) performed better than high-intensity anticoagulation (INR >3.0)[45,46] in terms of thrombosis recurrence and major and minor bleeding events. Long-term treatment is generally indicated in APS patients with venous or arterial thrombosis. Recurrence after anticoagulation suspension is high among APS patients, even in the absence of aPL persistence.[47]

Recurrence while on treatment

In case of treatment failure,[29] adherence and persistence to therapy should be investigated in the first place. Although EULAR guidelines[48] suggest either increasing INR range to 3–4 or switching to LMWH, we believe the best option is the addition of low-dose aspirin to warfarin. Indeed, the increase of INR target increases both the risk of thrombosis and bleeding[45,46]; in addition, LMWH is unsuitable for long-term treatment.

Chronic thromboembolic pulmonary hypertension

CTEPH is a type of pulmonary hypertension characterized by a mean pulmonary artery pressure of 25 mmHg or higher in the presence of persistent thrombi and vascular remodelling in the pulmonary circulation.[49] Recurrent PE is a major risk factor for CTEPH[50] and might be common in patients with APS. Indeed, among patients with CTEPH the rate of aPL antibody-positivity was as high as 12%,[28] and most patients had a high-risk triple-positive aPL profile.[51]

Heparin-induced thrombocytopenia

Heparin-induced thrombocytopenia (HIT) is a serious immunoglobulin-mediated complication precipitated by the generation of heparin–platelet factor 4 (PF4) antibodies,[52] leading to consumption thrombocytopenia and a high risk of venous and arterial thrombosis,[53] including DVT/PE, myocardial infarction, stroke, and peripheral artery thrombosis.[54] HIT can occur in up to 5% of patients exposed to heparin products, and up to 50% of patients develop thromboembolic complications with a mortality of 30%.[55] HIT usually occurs 5–14 days after the start of heparin therapy and is prevalent with unfractionated heparin rather than with LMWH.[56] Albeit infrequent, HIT may develop either early (after a recent previous exposure to heparin) or late after heparin exposure.[57] The presence of HIT may be estimated using the 4Ts score,—Thrombocytopenia, Timing, Thrombosis, and the absence of other explanations for Thrombosis[53] (➔ Table 23.3). Together with pre-test probability, there are two commercially available assays to help in the diagnosis of HIT.[58]

Thromboembolic complications of HIT comprise the development of large-vessel venous thrombosis (DVT and PE) and, less frequently, arterial thrombosis (myocardial infarction, stroke, peripheral artery thrombosis). Moreover, there are a number of unusual characteristic sequelae of HIT (warfarin-associated venous limb gangrene, bilateral adrenal haemorrhagic infarction, heparin-induced skin lesions), or acute systemic reactions following intravenous heparin bolus, such as chills, fever, dyspnoea, chest pain, and flushing.[54]

HIT treatment

The treatment of HIT should be initiated when a 4Ts score is 4 or more (➔ Table 23.3).[59] Treatment starts with immediate heparin cessation (including heparin flushes, heparin-coated catheters, and heparin used for device patency) and switching to a non-heparin anticoagulant. Non-heparin anticoagulants include argatroban, bivalirudin, danaparoid, fondaparinux, or DOACs.[60]

Argatroban

Argatroban is a rapid synthetic direct thrombin inhibitor that reversibly binds to the thrombin active site. Due to the short duration of action (<1 hour), it is the preferred option for critically ill patients, patients who are at increased risk of bleeding, or patients who might require an urgent procedure.[60] Switching from heparin to argatroban requires baseline activated partial thromboplastin time (aPTT) determination and continuous infusion at 2 micrograms/kg/min. The aPTT should be checked after 2 hours and after every dosage adjustment (not to exceed 10 micrograms/kg/min), until reaching a target aPTT of 1.5–3.0 times the baseline aPTT (not to exceed 100 seconds).[61] Argatroban metabolized by the liver, and thus requires a lower starting rate and more frequent aPTT monitoring in patients with hepatic dysfunction, heart failure, and/or multiorgan failure.[62] Argatroban produces a false INR elevation and a specific protocol must be followed when bridging back to warfarin.[63]

Bivalirudin, fondaparinux, and DOACs

Bivalirudin is another direct thrombin inhibitor that is preferentially used in cardiac catheterization and cardiac surgery, as an alternative to heparin.

Fondaparinux is commonly used for the treatment of HIT. It is safe, effective, and convenient for both in- and out-of-hospital use. Fondaparinux has similar effectiveness and safety as argatroban in patients with suspected HIT even at prophylactic doses in patients with no indication for full anticoagulation[64] or without thrombosis.[65] Fondaparinux is contraindicated in severe renal failure and with a creatinine clearance less than 30 mL/min (➔ Figure 23.3).

There is growing evidence on the use of DOACs in the treatment of HIT. Current guidelines list DOACs as an acceptable treatment option with the same doses and modalities as in the setting of VTE.[55]

Vaccine-induced thrombocytopenia thrombosis

Vaccine-induced thrombocytopenia thrombosis, also known as autoimmune HIT, is a very rare condition similar to HIT but occurring without heparin exposure.[66] The condition became notorious with adenoviral vector-based COVID-19 vaccines, where it manifested with a combination of cerebral venous sinus thrombosis and thrombocytopenia 4–28 days after vaccination.[67] Treatment consists of the use of non-heparin anticoagulants such as argatroban, fondaparinux, or DOACs. Early treatment with intravenous immunoglobulin or plasmapheresis should be strongly considered.[68]

Table 23.3 The 4Ts scoring system

4Ts category	2 points	1 point	0 points
Thrombocytopenia	Platelet count fall > 50% and platelet nadir ≥ 20 × 10^9/L	Platelet count 30–50% or platelet nadir 10–20x10^9/L	Platelet count fall <30% or platelet nadir <10 × 10^9/L
Thrombocytopenia (Timing)	Onset days 5–10 or onset ≤1 day (prior heparin exposure within 30 days)	Probably with days 5–10 fall. Onset after day 10. Fall ≤1 day (prior heparin exposure 30–100 days ago)	Platelet count ≤4 days without recent exposure
Thrombosis	New thrombosis or skin necrosis; acute systemic reaction post-intravenous unfractionated heparin bolus	Progressive or recurrent thrombosis; non-necrotizing skin lesions; suspected thrombosis (not proven)	None
Thrombocytopenia (Other causes)	No	Possible	Definite

1–3 points low probability; 4–5 points intermediate probability; 6–8 points high probability.

Source data from Cuker A, Gimotty PA, Crowther MA, Warkentin TE. Predictive value of the 4Ts scoring system for heparin-induced thrombocytopenia: a systematic review and meta-analysis. Blood. 2012;120(20):4160–7. doi: 10.1182/blood-2012-07-443051.

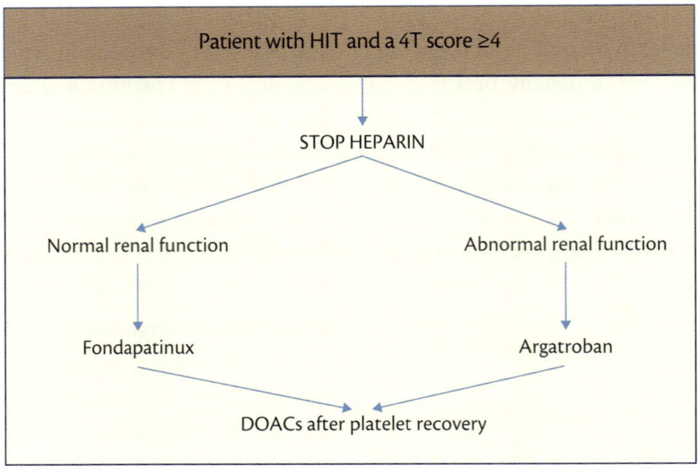

Figure 23.3 How we treat HIT with a 4T score of 4 or more. Immediately stop heparin. Then consider renal function: if normal, use fondaparinux at therapeutic dose. If renal function is impaired (<30 mL/min), use argatroban (bivalirudin in the catheter laboratory or in case of cardiac surgery). When platelet count returns to normal, consider starting treatment with a DOAC, or VKA in case of arterial thrombosis or contraindication to DOACs.

Paroxysmal nocturnal haemoglobinuria

Paroxysmal nocturnal haemoglobinuria (PNH) is a rare (prevalence 0.5–1.5 per million),[22] acquired, life-threatening disease, caused by a somatic mutation of the phosphatidylinositol glycan A gene (*PIGA*) in bone marrow stem cells, creating defective 'PNH' blood cells. In this condition, uncontrolled complement activity leads to systemic complications, principally through intravascular haemolysis and platelet activation.[69] Thrombosis in PNH may occur at any site, but is more common at unusual sites. Visceral (hepatic, spontaneous Budd–Chiari syndrome, mesenteric, portal, splenic, inferior vena cava) or cerebral (superior sagittal sinus) venous thrombosis often precedes the diagnosis of PNH. Thrombosis may involve the myocardium, leading to compromised cardiac function in the long term. Treatment consists of immediate full anticoagulation with heparin therapy (a LMWH with target anti-Xa levels 0.5–1.0 U) in adjunction to eculizumab, a C5 complement inhibitor.

Other than case series and reports, especially with rivaroxaban,[70] there are no reports from ad hoc studies with DOACs. The use of DOACs in this condition is attractive, but should be reserved to carefully selected patients.[71]

Polycythaemia vera and essential thrombocythaemia

Polycythaemia vera (PV) and essential thrombocythaemia (ET) are chronic myeloproliferative neoplasms, with a prevalence in the US of 22 per 100,000 and 24 per 100,000 for PV and ET, respectively.[23] PV and ET are associated with a particularly increased risk for thrombosis, especially in the arterial circulation.[72] Major thrombotic events at the time of diagnosis range from 34–39% for PV and 10–29% for ET, and are somewhat lower during follow-up. Treatment measures include low-dose aspirin, phlebotomy (target haematocrit 45% in case of PV), and, in high-risk patients (with PV or ET), hydroxyurea with a starting dose 500 mg twice daily.[73]

Sickle cell disease

Sickle cell disease is an inherited condition due to mutation of the β-globin gene that generates the sickle haemoglobin (HbS). Abnormal polymerization of Hb tetramers upon deoxygenation causes red blood cell deformation (sickle shape), leading to small vessel occlusion in both the venous and the arterial circulation, resulting in intermittent painful episodes, haemolytic anaemia, and vascular inflammation. Episodes of VTE are frequent in patients with sickle cell disease, and treatment does not differ from that of non-sickle cell disease patients. In a retrospective single-centre study,[74] most VTE was catheter associated or post hospital discharge. DOACs are the recommended treatment option due to their risk/benefit profile.[74,75] Extended anticoagulation beyond 3 months is recommended even in case of provoked VTE. Both haemorrhagic and ischaemic stroke may occur, and prompt blood transfusion to reduce HbS is the recommended treatment.

Combined oral contraceptives

Soon after the introduction of combined oral contraceptives (COCs, combination of progestogens with oestrogens) in 1960, WM Jordan reported a case of PE in a 40-year-old nurse who had taken this drug for endometriosis.[76] Given the diffusion of COC as a method of contraception worldwide, even a small increase in the risk thrombosis translates to a relevant healthcare problem.[77] Over the years, new generations of COC with progressively lower oestrogen content were proposed (third-generation COC). In one meta-analysis,[78] the odds ratio of VTE for third-generation versus second-generation COC was 1.7 (95% confidence interval 1.4–2.0). Activated protein C resistance is the main coagulation alteration in COC users, and could explain both VTE and arterial thrombosis (e.g. ischaemic stroke).[79] The presence of thrombophilic alterations (FVL and prothrombin G20210A mutation) increases the risk of VTE.[80,81] The need for thrombophilia screening before COC prescription has been long debated and is generally not recommended. Before prescribing a COC, VTE risk factors, such as positive family history, age over 35 years, smoking more than 15 cigarettes per day, diabetes with vascular disease, obesity with body mass index greater than 30 kg/m^2, and migraine with aura, should be assessed.[82]

Malignancies

Cancer promotes a hypercoagulable state increasing the risk for VTE by ninefold[83] that in turn significantly reduces survival.[84] Risk factors for VTE are patient related (e.g. age, obesity, and previous VTE), cancer related (e.g. active cancer and cancer type), and treatment related (e.g. major surgery and chemotherapy). The risk of thrombosis can be assessed with the Khorana prediction score (➔ Table 23.4),[85] and studies suggest a benefit of thromboprophylaxis in patients with a score of 2 or higher.[86] In hospitalized medical or surgical oncology patients, heparin or fondaparinux at prophylactic dose are generally used. For ambulatory patients, apixaban 2.5 mg twice daily, rivaroxaban 10 mg once daily, or LMWH are the recommended drugs.[86] In case of contraindication to anticoagulation, mechanical prophylaxis is indicated.

For treatment of cancer-associated thrombosis, LMWH has been the gold standard since the publication of the CLOT trial in 2003,[87] and dalteparin has been the comparator for DOACs in subsequent cancer-associated VTE trials. DOACs have emerged as a valid option.[88–90] A meta-analysis of three studies[91] that utilized edoxaban,[88] rivaroxaban,[92] and apixaban[90] showed that DOACs are more effective than LMWH for prevention of VTE recurrence at the price of an increased risk for non-major bleeding.[93] DOACs are thus considered agents of choice in cancer-associated thrombosis.[94] LMWH (dalteparin, tinzaparin, and enoxaparin) can be used in case of DOAC contraindications, active gastrointestinal or urothelial cancer, thrombocytopenia (<50,000 platelets/μL), renal impairment, or history of major bleeding.[95] Patients should be treated for 6 months and reassessed for risk of recurrence and bleeding every 3 months. Suspension of anticoagulant therapy should be considered in the absence of active cancer and ongoing cancer therapy.

Table 23.4 The risk of thrombosis assessed with the Khorana prediction score. A value of 3 or more indicates the need for VTE prophylaxis

Characteristic	Risk score
Type of cancer: stomach, pancreas	+2
Type of cancer: lung, lymphoma, gynaecological, bladder, testicular	+1
Pre-chemotherapy platelet count ≥350 × 10^9/L	+1
Haemoglobin level <10 g/dL or using red blood cell growth factors	+1
Pre-chemotherapy leucocyte count >11 × 10^9/L	+1
BMI ≥35 kg/m^2	+1

Source data from Khorana AA, DeSancho MT, Liebman H, Rosovsky R, Connors JM, Zwicker J. Prediction and Prevention of Cancer-Associated Thromboembolism. Oncologist. 2021;26(1):e2–7. doi: 10.1002/onco.13569.

Acquired thrombotic microangiopathies

Thrombotic microangiopathies encompass various diseases characterized by microangiopathic haemolytic anaemia, platelet clumping and consequent thrombocytopaenia, and organ failure of variable severity.

Catastrophic antiphospholipid syndrome

Catastrophic antiphospholipid syndrome (CAPS) might complicate the clinical course of APS in 1% of cases.[96] This condition leads to death in 50% of cases as multiple vascular occlusive events, usually affecting small vessels, determine multiple organ failure. Precipitating factors of CAPS include infections, surgery, malignancy, contraceptives, pregnancy/puerperium, withdrawal of warfarin or subtherapeutic (<2.0) INR, systemic lupus erythematosus flares, and trauma.[32] Initial clinical signs of CAPS often include cutaneous necrosis and a decline in platelet count.[97] Treatment consists of a combination of unfractionated heparin at therapeutic doses, glucocorticoids, plasma exchange, and/or intravenous immunoglobulins.[32,98,99]

Other thrombotic microangiopathies

Besides CAPS, a broad range of alternative thrombotic microangiopathies should be considered in the differential diagnosis during clinical workup as shown in ➔ Table 23.5.[100]

Thrombotic thrombocytopenic purpura is attributable in most cases to antibodies against ADAMTS13, a metalloproteinase able to break down large prothrombotic multimers of von Willebrand factor. These patients present a severe neurological involvement, and in 90% of cases the cause of death is a myocardial infarction. ADAMTS13 supplements via plasmapheresis or immunosuppression are treatment options in thrombotic thrombocytopenic purpura.

Haemolytic uraemic syndrome (HUS) secondary to a toxin produced by *Shigella* infection is characterized by a rapid onset of renal involvement associated with episodes of diarrhoea in children. Treatment includes kidney replacement therapy and hydration. Atypical haemolytic uraemic syndrome is a genetic, life-threatening, chronic disease of complement-mediated thrombotic microangiopathy, the prognosis of which has improved after the introduction of C5 complement inhibitors (such as eculizumab).

The haemolysis, elevated liver enzymes, and low platelets (HELLP) syndrome may arise between the 27th and the 37th week of gestation in multiparous women. The clinical presentation is characterized by abdominal pain with nausea and vomiting, elevated liver enzymes, and renal failure. Patients with the HELLP syndrome should be routinely treated with corticosteroids.

Table 23.5 Distinctive features of thrombotic microangiopathies

	Previous history	Fibrinogen	Haemolytic anaemia	Schistocytes	Thrombocytopenia	Antibodies
CAPS	CPAPS/SLE	Normal/high	+/−	+	+	aPL
TTP	Infection (?)	Normal/high	+	++	++	Anti-ADAMTS13
HUS	Infection	Normal/high	+	+	+	−
HELLP	Pregnancy	Normal/high	+	+/−	++	−
DIC	Sepsis	Low	+/−	+/−	++ −	−

aPL, antiphospholipid antibodies; CAPS, catastrophic antiphospholipid syndrome; DIC disseminated intravascular coagulation; HELLP, haemolysis, elevated liver enzymes, and low platelets; HUS, haemolytic uraemic syndrome; SLE, systemic lupus erythematosus; TTP, thrombotic thrombocytopenic purpura.

Source data from Emmi G, Silvestri E, Squatrito D, et al. An approach to differential diagnosis of antiphospholipid antibody syndrome and related conditions. ScientificWorldJournal. 2014;2014:341342. doi: 10.1155/2014/341342.

Disseminated intravascular coagulation usually occurs in patients with sepsis. The treatment of choice are antibiotics against the index infection.

What's new

- In women with IT, there is no need for VTE prophylaxis with LMWH in pregnancy and puerperium in the absence of previous VTE unless severe thrombophilia or other risk factors are present.
- VKA treatment (INR 2.0–3.0) is mandatory for the prevention of recurrent thrombosis in high-risk (triple-positive) patients with APS. Do not use DOACs in this setting.
- In APS patients, in case of treatment failure, possible causes should be investigated, and the addition of low-dose aspirin should be considered.
- In patients with HIT, after stopping heparin, argatroban or fondaparinux are the drugs of choice.
- Heparin therapy in adjunction to monoclonal antibody therapy with eculizumab (a C5 complement inhibitor) is indicated in the treatment of thrombosis in patients with PNH.
- Low-dose aspirin is indicated in PV and ET.
- In sickle cell disease, conventional anticoagulant treatment with DOACs is recommended in case of VTE, while no antithrombotic treatment is advised for ischaemic stroke.
- In the prevention and treatment of cancer-associated thrombosis, DOACs have emerged as the drugs of choice.

Guideline recommendations

- LMWH is the treatment of choice of VTE during pregnancy with no clear dosage indication.[12]
- No evidence for a clinical benefit of extended anticoagulant treatment in patients with VTE and carriers of heterozygous FVL or prothrombin 20210A mutation.[12]
- Patients with VTE and severe thrombophilia are candidates for indefinite anticoagulant treatment.[12]
- DOACs are not an alternative to VKAs for patients with the APS.[12]
- Unfractionated heparin may predispose to HIT.[12]
- Third-generation COCs are associated with a higher VTE risk than the second-generation COC.[12]
- Edoxaban or rivaroxaban should be considered as an alternative to LMWH with caution for patients with gastrointestinal cancer (increased bleeding risk with DOACs).[12]

What's next

- Drug discovery and development in antithrombotic therapy are still a high priority. Indeed, studies with inhibitors of factor XI or factor XIa have shown antithrombotic efficacy with minimal effects on bleeding.
- Studies on primary prevention of VTE with low-dose DOACs for patients with severe IT are highly warranted.
- Studies of DOAC treatment in patients with APS and lower risk profiles (double- and single-positive patients) are necessary.
- Counselling on contraception and contraceptive use may help in reducing VTE in COC users.
- Studies are ongoing on treatment of VTE in cancer patients at increased bleeding risk and in special categories, such as incidental VTE, splanchnic vein thrombosis, or catheter-related thrombosis.

References

1. Heit JA. The epidemiology of venous thromboembolism in the community: implications for prevention and management. J Thromb Thrombolysis. 2006;21:23–9.
2. Khan S, Dickerman JD. Hereditary thrombophilia. Thromb J. 2006;4:15.
3. Roldan V, Lecumberri R, Munoz-Torrero JF, et al. Thrombophilia testing in patients with venous thromboembolism. Findings from the RIETE registry. Thromb Res. 2009;124:174–7.
4. Stevens SM, Woller SC, Bauer KA, et al. Guidance for the evaluation and treatment of hereditary and acquired thrombophilia. J Thromb Thrombolysis. 2016;41:154–64.
5. Carroll BJ, Piazza G. Hypercoagulable states in arterial and venous thrombosis: when, how, and who to test? Vasc Med. 2018;23:388–99.
6. Stoykova J, Dimitrova V, Tasheva I, Dosev L, Zlatareva-Gronkova N, Petrov I. Acute coronary syndrome and thrombophilia in young patients: clinical data, experience. Eur Heart J. 2020;41(Suppl 2):1553.

7. Agewall S, Beltrame JF, Reynolds HR, et al. ESC working group position paper on myocardial infarction with non-obstructive coronary arteries. Eur Heart J. 2016;38:143–53.
8. Cheng C, Cheng GY, Denas G, Pengo V. Arterial thrombosis in antiphospholipid syndrome (APS): clinical approach and treatment. A systematic review. Blood Rev. 2021;48:100788.
9. Denas G, Jose SP, Bracco A, Zoppellaro G, Pengo V. Antiphospholipid syndrome and the heart: a case series and literature review. Autoimmun Rev. 2015;14:214–22.
10. Kearon C. Influence of hereditary or acquired thrombophilias on the treatment of venous thromboembolism. Curr Opin Hematol. 2012;19:363–70.
11. Mazzolai L, Aboyans V, Ageno W, et al. Diagnosis and management of acute deep vein thrombosis: a joint consensus document from the European Society of Cardiology working groups of aorta and peripheral vascular diseases and pulmonary circulation and right ventricular function. Eur Heart J. 2018;39:4208–18.
12. Konstantinides SV, Meyer G. The 2019 ESC Guidelines on the diagnosis and management of acute pulmonary embolism. Eur Heart J. 2019;40:3453–5.
13. Campello E, Spiezia L, Simion C, et al. Direct oral anticoagulants in patients with inherited thrombophilia and venous thromboembolism: a prospective cohort study. J Am Heart Assoc. 2020;9:e018917.
14. Hart C, Bauersachs R, Scholz U, et al. Prevention of venous thromboembolism during pregnancy and the puerperium with a special focus on women with hereditary thrombophilia or prior VTE—position paper of the Working Group in Women's Health of the Society of Thrombosis and Haemostasis (GTH). Hamostaseologie. 2020;40:572–90.
15. Fogerty AE. Management of venous thromboembolism in pregnancy. Curr Treat Options Cardiovasc Med. 2018;20:69.
16. Bates SM, Middeldorp S, Rodger M, James AH, Greer I. Guidance for the treatment and prevention of obstetric-associated venous thromboembolism. J Thromb Thrombolysis. 2016;41:92–128.
17. Middeldorp S, Naue C, Kohler C. Thrombophilia, thrombosis and thromboprophylaxis in pregnancy: for what and in whom? Hamostaseologie. 2022;42:54–64.
18. Robertson L, Wu O, Langhorne P, et al. Thrombophilia in pregnancy: a systematic review. Br J Haematol. 2006;132:171–96.
19. Rodger M. Pregnancy and venous thromboembolism: 'TIPPS' for risk stratification. Hematology Am Soc Hematol Educ Program. 2014;2014:387–92.
20. Bates SM, Rajasekhar A, Middeldorp S, et al. American Society of Hematology 2018 guidelines for management of venous thromboembolism: venous thromboembolism in the context of pregnancy. Blood Adv. 2018;2:3317–59.
21. Duarte-Garcia A, Pham MM, Crowson CS, et al. The epidemiology of antiphospholipid syndrome: a population-based study. Arthritis Rheumatol. 2019;71:1545–52.
22. Parker CJ. Update on the diagnosis and management of paroxysmal nocturnal hemoglobinuria. Hematology Am Soc Hematol Educ Program. 2016;2016:208–16.
23. Ma X, Vanasse G, Cartmel B, Wang Y, Selinger HA. Prevalence of polycythemia vera and essential thrombocythemia. Am J Hematol. 2008;83:359–62.
24. Brousseau DC, Panepinto JA, Nimmer M, Hoffmann RG. The number of people with sickle-cell disease in the United States: national and state estimates. Am J Hematol. 2010;85:77–8.
25. Miyakis S, Lockshin MD, Atsumi T, et al. International consensus statement on an update of the classification criteria for definite antiphospholipid syndrome (APS). J Thromb Haemost. 2006;4:295–306.
26. Andreoli L, Chighizola CB, Banzato A, Pons-Estel GJ, Ramire de Jesus G, Erkan D. Estimated frequency of antiphospholipid antibodies in patients with pregnancy morbidity, stroke, myocardial infarction, and deep vein thrombosis: a critical review of the literature. Arthritis Care Res (Hoboken). 2013;65:1869–73.
27. Kearon C, Parpia S, Spencer FA, et al. Antiphospholipid antibodies and recurrent thrombosis after a first unprovoked venous thromboembolism. Blood. 2018;131:2151–60.
28. Cheng CY, Zhang YX, Denas G, Du Y, Jing ZC, Pengo V. Prevalence of antiphospholipid (aPL) antibodies among patients with chronic thromboembolic pulmonary hypertension: a systematic review and meta-analysis. Intern Emerg Med. 2019;14:521–7.
29. Pengo V, Ruffatti A, Legnani C, et al. Clinical course of high-risk patients diagnosed with antiphospholipid syndrome. J Thromb Haemost. 2010;8:237–42.
30. Devreese KMJ, Ortel TL, Pengo V, de Laat B. Laboratory criteria for antiphospholipid syndrome: reply. J Thromb Haemost. 2018;16:2117–9.
31. Farmer-Boatwright MK, Roubey RA. Venous thrombosis in the antiphospholipid syndrome. Arterioscler Thromb Vasc Biol. 2009;29:321–5.
32. Ruffatti A, De Silvestro G, Marson P, et al. Catastrophic antiphospholipid syndrome: lessons from 14 cases successfully treated in a single center. A narrative report. J Autoimmun. 2018;93:124–30.
33. Anderson M, Belmont HM. Severe thrombotic events associated with pre-procedural interruption of anticoagulation in systemic lupus erythematosus with secondary antiphospholipid syndrome: cases and literature review. Lupus. 2022;31:261–7.
34. Pengo V. Additional laboratory tests to improve on the diagnosis of antiphospholipid syndrome: response from Pengo. J Thromb Haemost. 2020;18:3118–19.
35. Hoxha A, Banzato A, Ruffatti A, Pengo V. Detection of lupus anticoagulant in the era of direct oral anticoagulants. Autoimmun Rev. 2017;16:173–8.
36. Moore GW, Jones PO, Platton S, et al. International multicenter, multiplatform study to validate Taipan snake venom time as a lupus anticoagulant screening test with ecarin time as the confirmatory test: communication from the ISTH SSC Subcommittee on Lupus Anticoagulant/Antiphospholipid Antibodies. J Thromb Haemost. 2021;19:3177–92.
37. Tripodi A, Scalambrino E, Chantarangkul V, et al. Impact of a commercially available DOAC absorbent on two integrated procedures for lupus anticoagulant detection. Thromb Res. 2021;204:32–9.
38. Pengo V, Denas G, Zoppellaro G, et al. Rivaroxaban vs warfarin in high-risk patients with antiphospholipid syndrome. Blood. 2018;132:1365–71.
39. Pengo V, Banzato A, Bison E, Zoppellaro G, Padayattil Jose S, Denas G. Efficacy and safety of rivaroxaban vs warfarin in high-risk patients with antiphospholipid syndrome: rationale and design of the Trial on Rivaroxaban in AntiPhospholipid Syndrome (TRAPS) trial. Lupus. 2016;25:301–6.
40. Ordi-Ros J, Saez-Comet L, Perez-Conesa M, et al. Rivaroxaban versus vitamin K antagonist in antiphospholipid syndrome: a randomized noninferiority trial. Ann Intern Med. 2019;171:685–94.
41. Woller SC, Stevens SM, Kaplan D, et al. Apixaban compared with warfarin to prevent thrombosis in thrombotic antiphospholipid syndrome: a randomized trial. Blood Adv. 2022;6:1661–70.
42. Pharmacovigilance Risk Assessment Committee. PRAC recommendations on signals. May 2019 edition. Amsterdam: European Medicines Agency; 2019.

43. Skeith L. Anticoagulating patients with high-risk acquired thrombophilias. Blood. 2018;132:2219–29.
44. Pengo V, Ruiz-Irastorza G, Denas G, Andreoli L, Khamashta M, Tincani A. High intensity anticoagulation in the prevention of the recurrence of arterial thrombosis in antiphospholipid syndrome: 'PROS' and 'CONS'. Autoimmun Rev. 2012;11:577–80.
45. Crowther MA, Ginsberg JS, Julian J, et al. A comparison of two intensities of warfarin for the prevention of recurrent thrombosis in patients with the antiphospholipid antibody syndrome. N Engl J Med. 2003;349:1133–8.
46. Finazzi G, Marchioli R, Brancaccio V, et al. A randomized clinical trial of high-intensity warfarin vs. conventional antithrombotic therapy for the prevention of recurrent thrombosis in patients with the antiphospholipid syndrome (WAPS). J Thromb Haemost. 2005;3:848–53.
47. Comarmond C, Jego P, Veyssier-Belot C, et al. Cessation of oral anticoagulants in antiphospholipid syndrome. Lupus. 2017;26:1291–6.
48. Tektonidou MG, Andreoli L, Limper M, et al. EULAR recommendations for the management of antiphospholipid syndrome in adults. Ann Rheum Dis. 2019;78:1296–304.
49. Keogh AM, Mayer E, Benza RL, et al. Interventional and surgical modalities of treatment in pulmonary hypertension. J Am Coll Cardiol. 2009;54:S67–77.
50. Pengo V, Lensing AW, Prins MH, et al. Incidence of chronic thromboembolic pulmonary hypertension after pulmonary embolism. N Engl J Med. 2004;350:2257–64.
51. Jiang X, Du Y, Cheng CY, et al. Antiphospholipid syndrome in chronic thromboembolic pulmonary hypertension: a well-defined subgroup of patients. Thromb Haemost. 2019;119:1403–8.
52. Jang IK, Hursting MJ. When heparins promote thrombosis: review of heparin-induced thrombocytopenia. Circulation. 2005;111:2671–83.
53. Warkentin TE. Heparin-induced thrombocytopenia: diagnosis and management. Circulation. 2004;110:e454–8.
54. Warkentin TE. Clinical presentation of heparin-induced thrombocytopenia. Semin Hematol. 1998;35:9–16.
55. Nicolas D, Nicolas S, Hodgens A, Reed M. Heparin Induced Thrombocytopenia. Treasure Island, FL: StatPearls; 2022.
56. Kelton JG, Warkentin TE. Heparin-induced thrombocytopenia: a historical perspective. Blood. 2008;112:2607–16.
57. Baroletti SA, Goldhaber SZ. Heparin-induced thrombocytopenia. Circulation. 2006;114:e355–6.
58. Bakchoul T, Giptner A, Bein G, Santoso S, Sachs UJ. Performance characteristics of two commercially available IgG-specific immunoassays in the assessment of heparin-induced thrombocytopenia (HIT). Thromb Res. 2011;127:345–8.
59. Cuker A, Gimotty PA, Crowther MA, Warkentin TE. Predictive value of the 4Ts scoring system for heparin-induced thrombocytopenia: a systematic review and meta-analysis. Blood. 2012;120:4160–7.
60. Cuker A, Arepally GM, Chong BH, et al. American Society of Hematology 2018 guidelines for management of venous thromboembolism: heparin-induced thrombocytopenia. Blood Adv. 2018;2:3360–92.
61. Babuin L, Pengo V. Argatroban in the management of heparin-induced thrombocytopenia. Vasc Health Risk Manag. 2010;6:813–19.
62. Bambrah RK, Pham DC, Rana F. Argatroban in heparin-induced thrombocytopenia: rationale for use and place in therapy. Ther Adv Chronic Dis. 2013;4:302–4.
63. Grouzi E. Update on argatroban for the prophylaxis and treatment of heparin-induced thrombocytopenia type II. J Blood Med. 2014;5:131–41.
64. Kang M, Alahmadi M, Sawh S, Kovacs MJ, Lazo-Langner A. Fondaparinux for the treatment of suspected heparin-induced thrombocytopenia: a propensity score-matched study. Blood. 2015;125:924–9.
65. Grouzi E, Kyriakou E, Panagou I, Spiliotopoulou I. Fondaparinux for the treatment of acute heparin-induced thrombocytopenia: a single-center experience. Clin Appl Thromb Hemost. 2010;16:663–7.
66. Greinacher A, Selleng K, Warkentin TE. Autoimmune heparin-induced thrombocytopenia. J Thromb Haemost. 2017;15:2099–114.
67. Greinacher A, Thiele T, Warkentin TE, Weisser K, Kyrle PA, Eichinger S. Thrombotic thrombocytopenia after ChAdOx1 nCov-19 vaccination. N Engl J Med. 2021;384:2092–101.
68. Makris M, Pavord S, Lester W, Scully M, Hunt B. Vaccine-induced immune thrombocytopenia and thrombosis (VITT). Res Pract Thromb Haemost. 2021;5:e12529.
69. Hill A, Kelly RJ, Hillmen P. Thrombosis in paroxysmal nocturnal hemoglobinuria. Blood. 2013;121:4985–96.
70. Dragoni F, Chiarotti F, Iori AP, La Rocca U, Cafolla A. Antithrombotic therapy with rivaroxaban in five patients with paroxysmal nocturnal haemoglobinuria and thrombotic events. Thromb J. 2018;16:26.
71. Skeith L. Anticoagulating patients with high-risk acquired thrombophilias. Hematol Am Soc Hematol Educ Program. 2018;2018:439–49.
72. Tefferi A, Elliott M. Thrombosis in myeloproliferative disorders: prevalence, prognostic factors, and the role of leukocytes and JAK2V617F. Semin Thromb Hemost. 2007;33:313–20.
73. Tefferi A, Barbui T. Polycythemia vera and essential thrombocythemia: 2017 update on diagnosis, risk-stratification, and management. Am J Hematol. 2017;92:94–108.
74. Srisuwananukorn A, Raslan R, Zhang X, et al. Clinical, laboratory, and genetic risk factors for thrombosis in sickle cell disease. Blood Adv. 2020;4:1978–86.
75. Shet AS, Wun T. How I diagnose and treat venous thromboembolism in sickle cell disease. Blood. 2018;132:1761–9.
76. Jordan WM AJ. Pulmonary embolism. Lancet. 1961;278:1146.7.
77. Morimont L, Haguet H, Dogne JM, Gaspard U, Douxfils J. Combined oral contraceptives and venous thromboembolism: review and perspective to mitigate the risk. Front Endocrinol (Lausanne). 2021;12:769187.
78. Kemmeren JM, Algra A, Grobbee DE. Third generation oral contraceptives and risk of venous thrombosis: meta-analysis. BMJ. 2001;323:131–4.
79. Lidegaard O, Lokkegaard E, Jensen A, Skovlund CW, Keiding N. Thrombotic stroke and myocardial infarction with hormonal contraception. N Engl J Med. 2012;366:2257–66.
80. Vandenbroucke JP, Koster T, Briet E, Reitsma PH, Bertina RM, Rosendaal FR. Increased risk of venous thrombosis in oral-contraceptive users who are carriers of factor V Leiden mutation. Lancet. 1994;344:1453–7.
81. Legnani C, Palareti G, Guazzaloca G, et al. Venous thromboembolism in young women; role of thrombophilic mutations and oral contraceptive use. Eur Heart J. 2002;23:984–90.
82. Curtis KM, Tepper NK, Jatlaoui TC, et al. U.S. medical eligibility criteria for contraceptive use, 2016. MMWR Recomm Rep. 2016;65:1–103.
83. Mulder FI, Horvath-Puho E, van Es N, et al. Venous thromboembolism in cancer patients: a population-based cohort study. Blood. 2021;137:1959–69.
84. Sorensen HT, Mellemkjaer L, Olsen JH, Baron JA. Prognosis of cancers associated with venous thromboembolism. N Engl J Med. 2000;343:1846–50.
85. Khorana AA, Kuderer NM, Culakova E, Lyman GH, Francis CW. Development and validation of a predictive model for chemotherapy-associated thrombosis. Blood. 2008;111:4902–7.

86. Streiff MB, Holmstrom B, Angelini D, et al. Cancer-associated venous thromboembolic disease, version 2.2021, NCCN Clinical Practice Guidelines in Oncology. J Natl Compr Canc Netw. 2021;19:1181–201.
87. Lee AY, Levine MN, Baker RI, et al. Low-molecular-weight heparin versus a coumarin for the prevention of recurrent venous thromboembolism in patients with cancer. N Engl J Med. 2003;349:146–53.
88. Raskob GE, van Es N, Verhamme P, et al. Edoxaban for the treatment of cancer-associated venous thromboembolism. N Engl J Med. 2018;378:615–24.
89. Khorana AA, Soff GA, Kakkar AK, et al. Rivaroxaban for thromboprophylaxis in high-risk ambulatory patients with cancer. N Engl J Med. 2019;380:720–8.
90. Agnelli G, Becattini C, Meyer G, et al. Apixaban for the treatment of venous thromboembolism associated with cancer. N Engl J Med. 2020;382:1599–607.
91. Mulder FI, Bosch FTM, Young AM, et al. Direct oral anticoagulants for cancer-associated venous thromboembolism: a systematic review and meta-analysis. Blood. 2020;136:1433–41.
92. Young AM, Marshall A, Thirlwall J, et al. Comparison of an oral factor Xa inhibitor with low molecular weight heparin in patients with cancer with venous thromboembolism: results of a randomized trial (SELECT-D). J Clin Oncol. 2018;36:2017–23.
93. Desai R, Koipallil GK, Thomas N, et al. Efficacy and safety of direct oral anticoagulants for secondary prevention of cancer associated thrombosis: a meta-analysis of randomized controlled trials. Sci Rep. 2020;10:18945.
94. Khorana AA, Mackman N, Falanga A, et al. Cancer-associated venous thromboembolism. Nat Rev Dis Primers. 2022;8:11.
95. Carrier M, Blais N, Crowther M, et al. Treatment algorithm in cancer-associated thrombosis: Canadian expert consensus. Curr Oncol. 2018;25:329–37.
96. Cervera R, Piette JC, Font J, et al. Antiphospholipid syndrome: clinical and immunologic manifestations and patterns of disease expression in a cohort of 1,000 patients. Arthritis Rheum. 2002;46:1019–27.
97. Pontara E, Banzato A, Bison E, et al. Thrombocytopenia in high-risk patients with antiphospholipid syndrome. J Thromb Haemost. 2018;16:529–32.
98. Legault K, Schunemann H, Hillis C, et al. McMaster RARE-Bestpractices clinical practice guideline on diagnosis and management of the catastrophic antiphospholipid syndrome. J Thromb Haemost. 2018;16:1656–64.
99. Marson P, Bagatella P, Bortolati M, et al. Plasma exchange for the management of the catastrophic antiphospholipid syndrome: importance of the type of fluid replacement. J Intern Med. 2008;264:201–3.
100. Emmi G, Silvestri E, Squatrito D, et al. An approach to differential diagnosis of antiphospholipid antibody syndrome and related conditions. ScientificWorldJournal. 2014;2014:341342.

CHAPTER 24

Prevention and treatment of bleeding related to antithrombotic drugs

Roxana Mehran, Alessandro Spirito, Davide Cao, and George Dangas

Contents

Summary

Antiplatelet and anticoagulant therapy reduce the occurrence of ischaemic events both in primary and secondary prevention in different cardiovascular conditions. However, these benefits come at the expense of higher bleeding complications, especially when different types of antithrombotic medications are combined. For decades, bleeding was thought to be an unavoidable side effect of antithrombotic therapy and of marginal relevance compared to ischaemic events. Yet, in recent years, major bleeding has been proven to impact mortality to a similar extent as ischaemic events. For these reasons, adoption of bleeding avoidance strategies is pivotal in the management of patients on antithrombotic therapy. These include an upfront bleeding risk assessment, accurate selection of candidates for invasive procedures, prevention of vascular access-related bleeding, modulation of antithrombotic therapy, and regular follow-up visits to reassess the bleeding risk and adjust the treatment. In case of major, life-threatening bleeding, prompt treatment including reversal of antithrombotic treatment is required.

Prevention of bleeding

Introduction

Antiplatelet and anticoagulant therapy have been shown effective in reducing the occurrence of ischaemic events both in primary and secondary prevention in different cardiovascular conditions (➔ Figure 24.1). However, this benefit comes at the expense of higher bleeding complications, especially when a combination of different antithrombotic medications is used (➔ Figure 24.2a). In recent years, major bleeding has been proven to impact mortality to a similar extent as ischaemic events[1–3] (➔ Figure 24.2b). Moreover, bleeding is associated with longer lengths of hospital stay and increased healthcare costs.[4] For these reasons, the attention of clinicians and researchers turned to implementing bleeding avoidance strategies,[1] which are discussed in the following sections.

Bleeding risk assessment

Assessing individual bleeding and ischaemic risk upfront is critical for tailoring antithrombotic therapy and minimizing future complications.[1] For patients undergoing

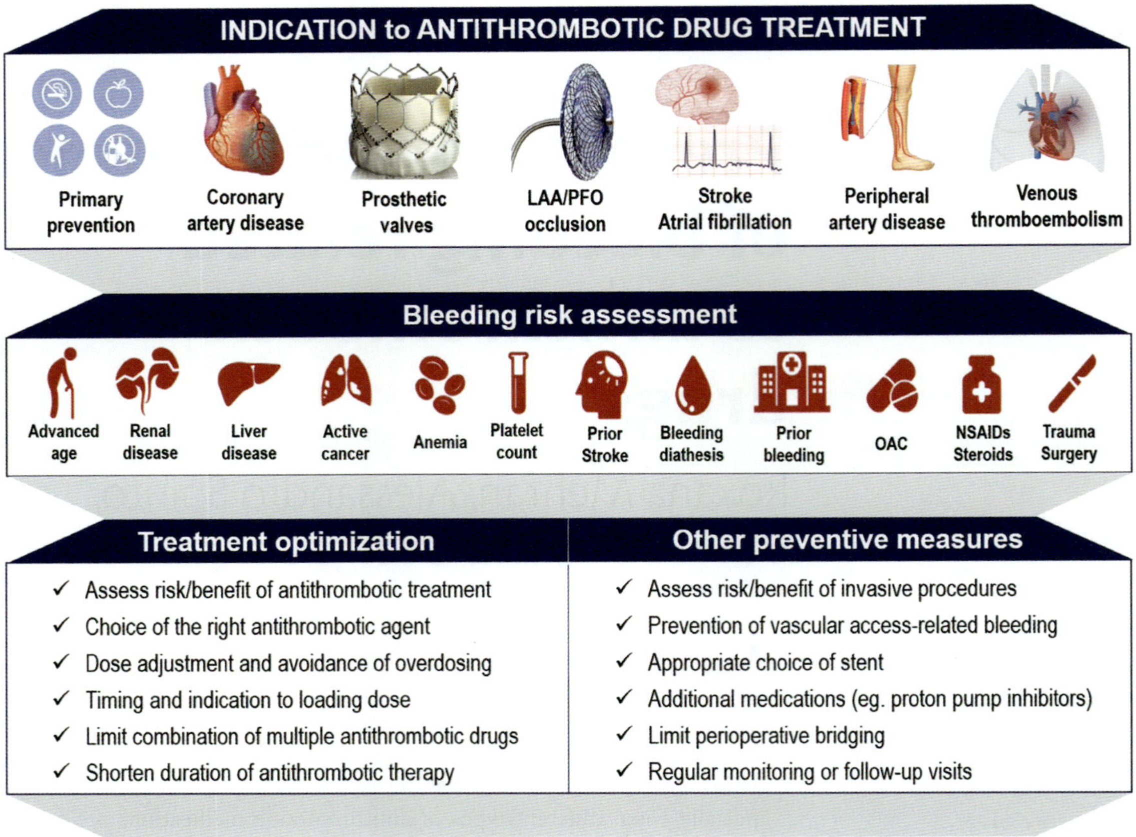

Figure 24.1 General principles of bleeding avoidance strategies in cardiovascular diseases requiring an antithrombotic treatment. In the depicted clinical scenarios, bleeding avoidance strategies include first bleeding risk assessment and thereafter optimization of antithrombotic treatment as well as other preventive measure. LAA, left atrial appendage; NSAIDs, non-steroidal anti-inflammatory drugs; OAC, oral anticoagulation; PFO, patent foramen ovale.

percutaneous coronary intervention (PCI), several tools to estimate bleeding risk at different time points (i.e. in hospital, at 30 days, at 1 year, or at longer follow-up) are available.[2,5,6] However, only some of these have been validated and have shown good predictive value[1,2] (➔ Table 24.1). In 2019, the Academic Research Consortium (ARC) proposed a definition of high bleeding risk (HBR) using 14 major and six minor criteria. The presence of at least one major or two minor criteria is expected to yield a 4% or greater risk of type 3 or 5 bleeding according to Bleeding Academic Research Consortium (BARC) scale or at least a 1% risk of intracranial haemorrhage at 1 year after PCI (➔ Table 24.1).[7] International guidelines for the management of patients undergoing PCI or with acute coronary syndrome (ACS) recommend to assess bleeding risk using validated tools and, in case of HBR, to adjust antithrombotic therapy irrespective of the concomitant ischaemic risk.[1,5,8–10] Of note, the impact of routine bleeding risk assessment on outcomes has not yet been tested in randomized controlled trials and therefore the efficacy of these tools remains unclear.[5]

In patients with atrial fibrillation (AF), anticoagulation is generally recommended if the CHA_2DS_2-VASc score is equal or greater than 1 in men or 2 in women. According to current guidelines, bleeding risk should be assessed using the HAS-BLED score[8] (➔ Table 24.1). Score calculation allows modifiable bleeding risk factors to be identified and estimates the need for closer clinical follow-up but should not affect the decision to begin anticoagulation therapy or its dose.[11] In patient at very high risk for bleeding, left atrial appendage closure (LAAC) can be considered as an alternative to oral anticoagulation (OAC) for stroke prevention (➔ Heparins, heparin derivatives and bivalirudin).

The importance of bleeding risk assessment has become evident even for non-PCI interventions, such as transcatheter aortic valve implantation (TAVI), peripheral percutaneous transluminal angioplasty (PTA), and venous thromboembolism (VTE).

In patients undergoing TAVI, the recently developed PREDICT-TAVR score including six items showed a good predictive ability for the occurrence of bleeding at 30 days (➔ Table 24.1). Nonetheless, it remains unclear how this information would affect the clinical management. Indeed, guidelines recommend to modulate antithrombotic therapy after TAVI solely based on the indication to OAC and/or concomitant coronary stenting, in the absence of which aspirin monotherapy should be preferred.[12]

In patients with peripheral artery disease (PAD) undergoing PTA, assessment of bleeding risk is recommended but there is no consensus on which risk assessment tool should be used. The OAC^3-PAD score was recently developed to predict major bleeding at 1 year from PAD diagnosis (➔ Table 24.1). In HBR patients undergoing PTA without an indication for anticoagulation, aspirin or clopidogrel or vitamin K antagonist (VKA) monotherapy rather than standard 1-month dual antiplatelet therapy (DAPT) is

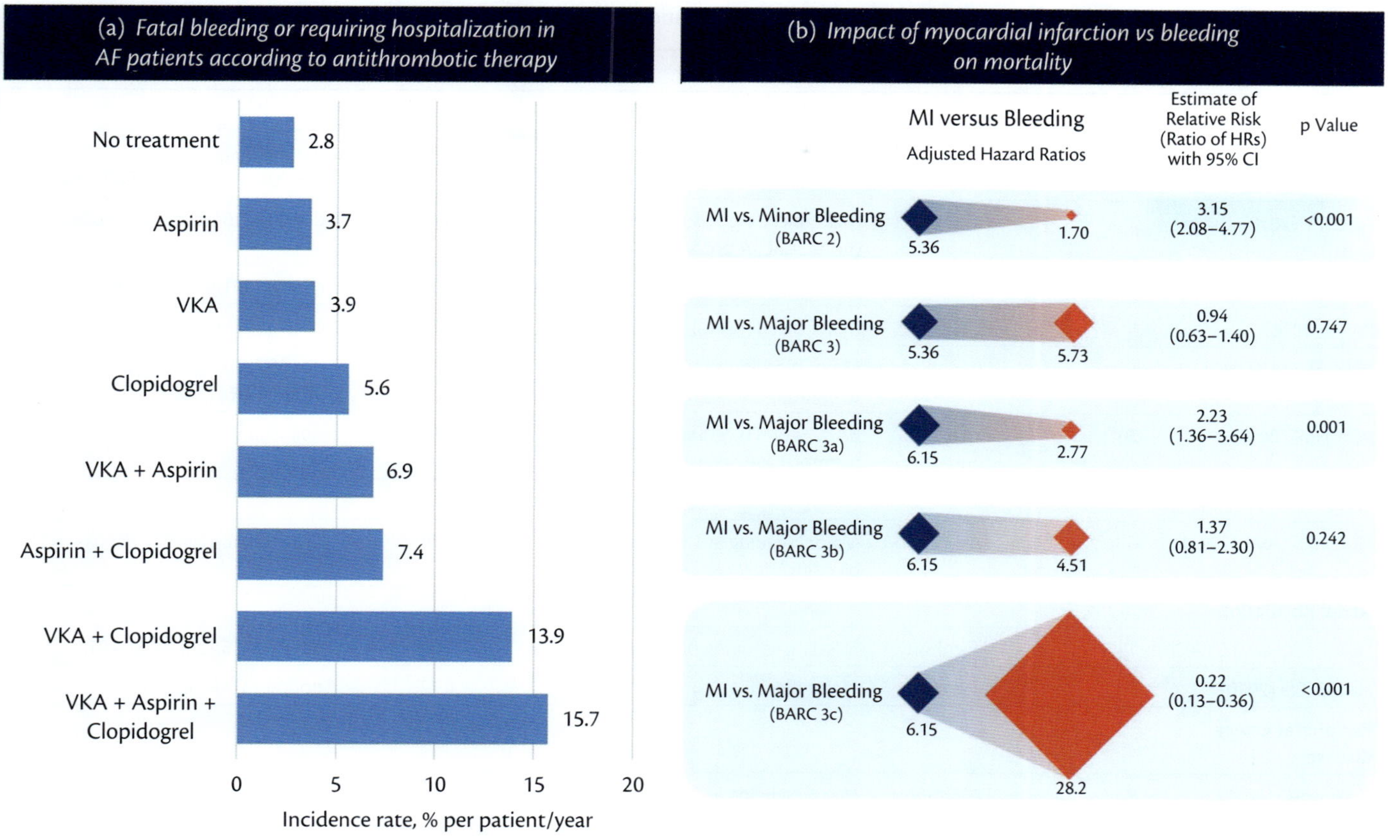

Figure 24.2 Rates and impact on mortality of bleeding events in patients on antithrombotic therapy. (a) Crude rate of fatal bleeding or bleeding requiring hospitalization in 118,606 patients discharged alive from a Danish hospital with a first-time diagnosis of atrial fibrillation (AF) stratified by antithrombotic treatment at discharge. (b) Impact of myocardial infarction (MI) versus bleeding classified according to Bleeding Academic Research Consortium (BARC) scale in 12,702 patients with non-ST-segment elevation acute coronary syndrome treated with vorapaxar or placebo and free from MI at 30 days. BARC 3b bleeding was associated with a risk of mortality similar to MI, BARC 3c with a higher risk. VKA, vitamin K antagonist.

(a) Source data from Hansen ML, Sørensen R, Clausen MT, Fet al. Risk of bleeding with single, dual, or triple therapy with warfarin, aspirin, and clopidogrel in patients with atrial fibrillation. Arch Intern Med. 2010 Sep 13;170(16):1433–41. doi: 10.1001/archinternmed.2010.271.

(b) Reproduced from Valgimigli M, Costa F, Lokhnygina Y, et al. Trade-off of myocardial infarction vs. bleeding types on mortality after acute coronary syndrome: lessons from the Thrombin Receptor Antagonist for Clinical Event Reduction in Acute Coronary Syndrome (TRACER) randomized trial. Eur Heart J. 2017 Mar 14;38(11):804–810. doi: 10.1093/eurheartj/ehw525.

recommended. For HBR patients with an indication for OAC, the addition of an antiplatelet agent should be avoided.[13]

Over the last 20 years, several bleeding risk assessment tools were created for patients with VTE (➔ Table 24.1). However, their use in clinical practice is limited by the modest predictive ability (c-statistic ~0.6).[11,14] Bleeding risk assessment allows modifiable bleeding risk factors to be identified and treated, but it should not impact the anticoagulation regimen in the first 6 months. Beyond this time point, the decision to continue anticoagulant treatment and the dose should take into account the benefits as well as the potential bleeding harm.[15]

Aspirin

For decades, aspirin has been a cornerstone of primary prevention, even in patients at low or moderate risk for coronary heart disease. However, recent evidence demonstrated no or only modest reduction of ischaemic events with aspirin in primary prevention and a consistently higher risk of major bleeding, especially intracranial and gastrointestinal.[16] Hence, in the absence of established atherosclerotic cardiovascular disease, aspirin use should be restricted to patients with diabetes or at high cardiovascular risk and no contraindications, such as HBR or age over 70 years.[17,18]

Aspirin is recommended for secondary prevention in patients with documented atherosclerotic cardiovascular disease (e.g. after myocardial infarction, ACS, arterial revascularization procedures, stroke, etc.). In these patients the benefit of low-dose aspirin on ischaemic event reduction exceeds the bleeding harm irrespective of bleeding risk or age.[17,18]

Given that up to 50% of major bleeds associated with aspirin are gastrointestinal, gastroprotection with proton pump inhibitors (PPIs) should be considered in the presence of some high-risk features (➔ Table 24.2).[17–19]

Oral platelet $P2Y_{12}$ inhibitors

The addition of $P2Y_{12}$ inhibitors to aspirin—a combination named DAPT—for a limited duration immediately after arterial revascularization procedures or acute cardiovascular events has been shown to be superior to aspirin alone in reducing the risk of stent thrombosis but also non-stent-related events, such

Table 24.1 Bleeding risk assessment tools with internal or external validation

Risk assessment tool	No. of items	Derivation	Bleeding outcome	c-statistic	Reference doi
PCI					
CRUSADE (2009)	8	NSTEMI cohort	In-hospital major bleeding[a]	0.72[b], 0.71[c]	doi: 10.1161/CIRCULATIONAHA.108.828541
ACUITY (2010)	7	ACS cohort	Major bleeding at 30 days[a] (non-CABG-related)	0.74[b]	doi: 10.1016/j.jacc.2009.09.076
DAPT (2016)	9	PCI cohort	Major bleeding at 1 year (GUSTO criteria)	0.68[b], 0.64[c]	doi: 10.1001/jama.2016.3775
PARIS (2016)	6	PCI cohort	Major bleeding at 2 years (BARC type 3 or 5)	0.72[b], 0.64[c]	doi: 10.1016/j.jacc.2016.02.064
PRECISE-DAPT (2017)	5	PCI cohort	Major bleeding after discharge (TIMI definition)	0.73[b] 0.66[c], 0.70[c]	doi: 10.1016/S0140-6736(17)30397-5
ARC-HBR (2019)	20	Expert consensus	BARC 3 or 5 bleeding or intracranial haemorrhage risk at 1 year	0.64–0.68[c]	doi: 10.1093/eurheartj/ehz372
TAVI					
PREDICT-TAVR (2021)	6	TAVR cohort	Major bleeding at 1 month (VARC-2 bleeding)	0.78[c]	doi: 10.1016/j.jcin.2021.03.024
Atrial fibrillation					
HEMORR$_2$HAGES (2006)	12	AF cohort	Bleeding requiring hospitalization[a]	0.67[c]	doi: 10.1016/j.ahj.2005.04.017
HAS-BLED (2010)	8	AF cohort	Major bleeding at 1 year[a]	0.72[c]	doi: 10.1378/chest.10-0134
Peripheral artery disease					
OAC^3-PAD (2022)	8	PAD cohort	Major bleeding at 1 year (ISTH adapted definition)	0.69[c]	doi: 10.1016/j.ejvs.2021.12.019
Venous thromboembolism					
Kuijer (1999)	3	VTE cohort	Major bleeding at 3 months[a]	0.55[c]	doi: 10.1001/archinte.159.5.457
RIETE (2008)	6	VTE cohort	Major bleeding at 3 months[a]	0.51–0.61[c]	doi: 10.1160/TH08-03-0193
IMPROVE (2011)	10	Acute VTE	In-hospital major and CRNM bleeding (ISTH definition)	0.63[c]	doi: 10.1378/chest.09-3081
ACCP (2016)	17	VTE cohort	Major bleeding between 3 and 12 months (ISTH definition)	0.55–0.56[c]	doi: 10.1016/j.chest.2015.11.026
VTE-BLEED (2016)	6	VTE cohort	Major bleeding between 1 and 6 months (ISTH definition)	0.66–0.71[c]	doi: 10.1183/13993003.00280-2016
Seiler et al. (2017)	7	VTE cohort	Major bleeding at 3 years[a]	0.68[c]	doi: 10.1160/TH17-03-0162

[a] Study specific definition.

[b] Derivation cohort.

[c] Validation cohort.

ACS, acute coronary syndrome; AF, atrial fibrillation; BARC, Bleeding Academic Research Consortium; CABG, coronary artery bypass graft; GUSTO, Global Use of Strategies to Open Occluded Arteries; ISTH, International Society on Thrombosis and Haemostasis; NSTEMI, non-ST-segment elevation myocardial infarction; PCI, percutaneous coronary intervention; TAVI, transcatheter aortic valve implantation; TIMI, Thrombolysis in Myocardial Infarction; VARC, Valve academic research consortium; VTE, venous thromboembolism.

as recurrent myocardial infarction or stroke.[2,5,6,9,10,13] Several strategies can reduce the bleeding risk associated with DAPT (➔ Table 24.2).

First, the choice of P2Y$_{12}$ inhibitor is crucial. Compared to potent P2Y$_{12}$ inhibitors (i.e. ticagrelor and prasugrel), clopidogrel is less effective in preventing recurrent ischaemic events but is associated with fewer bleeding complications.[20,21] Clopidogrel is preferred for patients on OAC and in case of previous intracranial haemorrhage.[2,5] Prasugrel should be avoided in patients with a body weight less than 60 kg, previous transient ischaemic attack, or ischaemic stroke and in elderly patients a reduced dose (5 mg instead of 10 mg per day) should be considered. The ongoing development of an agent to rapidly reverse the effect of ticagrelor could make this agent an appropriate choice for HBR patients.[1]

P2Y$_{12}$ loading dose before PCI (i.e. pretreatment) should be avoided in patients with chronic coronary syndrome or ACS without ST-elevation. Pretreatment with P2Y$_{12}$ might be considered in the presence of ST-elevation or in ACS patients undergoing delayed coronary angiography.[5,9]

DAPT is generally recommended for at least 6 months after elective procedures and for 12 months after ACS.[5,6,9] Over recent

Table 24.2 Summary of bleeding avoidance strategies

Aspirin	
Primary prevention	Avoid if low or moderate risk of major adverse cardiovascular events Avoid in HBR patients (e.g. >70 years old) without established CVD
Oral P2Y$_{12}$ inhibitors	
PCI or ACS	Clopidogrel if concomitant OAC or prior intracranial haemorrhage Avoid prasugrel if body weight <60 kg, previous TIA, ischaemic stroke, or age ≥75 years (or prasugrel 5 mg in this latter group) No pretreatment except in STEMI or NSTE-ACS with delayed CAG Short DAPT: aspirin or P2Y$_{12}$ inhibitors monotherapy after 1–3 months of DAPT Guided or unguided de-escalation after 1 month ± test for clopidogrel resistance Triple therapy no longer than 1 month
TAVI	P2Y$_{12}$ in addition to aspirin not recommended Clopidogrel-based DAPT for 1–6 months only after coronary stenting
PAD	1-month DAPT after percutaneous revascularization No P2Y$_{12}$ inhibitors in case of surgical revascularization or concomitant OAC
LAAC	Clopidogrel-based DAPT no longer than 3 months after LAAC If bleeding risk very high, 1-month clopidogrel-based DAPT or SAPT
PFO occlusion	Shorten DAPT from 6 up to 1 month after occlusion
Glycoprotein IIb/IIIa inhibitors and cangrelor	
Indications	Only in bailout situations in patients undergoing PCI Bridging before surgery in patients at very high ischaemic risk Use cangrelor if rapid platelet inhibition required in P2Y$_{12}$-naïve patients
Dose adjustment	If GFR<30 mL/min: no eptifibatide, ↓ tirofiban dose by 50% If GFR 30–49 mL/min: ↓ eptifibatide dose by 50%
Monitoring	Interrupt administration if relevant thrombocytopenia or bleeding suspicion
Heparins, heparin derivatives, bivalirudin	
Dose adjustment	Dose calculated based on patient's weight, age, and renal function If GFR <15 mL/min, UFH indicated If GFR 15–30 mL/min, dose adjustment required for all agents except UFH
PCI	Periprocedural anticoagulation preferentially with UFH If UFH: ACT target 250–300; ACT target 200–250 s with GPIIb/IIIa inhibitor Bivalirudin in HBR patients with low ischaemic risk (stent thrombosis); not if active bleeding, malignant hypertension, or subacute bacterial endocarditis In ACS patients with upstream enoxaparin, IV enoxaparin better than UFH
VTE	Initial anticoagulation with LMWH or fondaparinux preferred over UFH If GFR <30 mL/min or primary reperfusion planned, UFH better
Vitamin K antagonist	
	First choice in specific situations such as severe renal dysfunction and mechanical valve prosthesis; otherwise DOACs preferable In case of elective PCI/PTA: avoid interruption; no UFH if INR >2.5
Direct oral anticoagulants (DOACs)	
Dose adjustment	Rivaroxaban: 15 mg OD if GFR 15–49 mL/min or concomitant APT Apixaban; 2.5 mg BD if at least 2 of 3 criteria: age ≥80 years, body weight ≤60 kg, creatinine ≥133 μmol/L (≥1.5 mg/dL) Edoxaban 30 mg OD if GFR 15–50 mL/min, weight ≤60 kg, concomitant drugs[a] Dabigatran: 110 mg BD if age >80 years, HBR, concomitant APT or verapamil
PCI	No interruption in case of elective percutaneous intervention If no interruption, low-dose periprocedural anticoagulation (e.g. enoxaparin 0.5 mg/kg IV or UFH 60 IU/kg)
DPI	Avoid in HBR patients
TAVI	VKA preferred; OAC only if other indication (e.g. AF, VTE)
VTE	Discontinuation or dose reduction (apixaban 2.5 mg BD or rivaroxaban 10 mg OD) 6 months after acute event in HBR patients
Stroke	DOACs initiation between 4 and 14 days after acute cardioembolic stroke

(continued)

Table 24.2 Continued

Fibrinolysis or thrombolytic therapy	
Indications	STEMI if primary PCI not available within 120 minutes from diagnosis Bailout treatment if no-reflow or a thrombotic complication First line treatment for high-risk pulmonary embolism or ischaemic stroke
Contraindications	See Chapter 13
Dose adjustment	If age ≥75 years, 50% tenecteplase dose If concomitant enoxaparin, 75% tenecteplase dose
Other	Avoid clopidogrel or enoxaparin loading with tenecteplase
Other prevention measures	
Invasive procedures	Evaluate benefit/risk for invasive procedures in high-risk patients Opt for non-invasive diagnostic tests (e.g. CCTA)
Vascular access	Radial access and haemostasis with wristband recommended If femoral access, target a 'safe zone' with fluoroscopy or US guidance and use of vascular closure devices
Coronary stent	Use stents suitable for earlier DAPT discontinuation (see text) BMS is no longer the standard of care for HBR patients Achieve optimal stent expansion
PPI and *H. pylori*	PPI recommended if age ≥75 years, concomitant steroid or NSAIDs administration, combined antiplatelet therapy plus OAC therapy, and at high risk of gastrointestinal bleeding (i.e. prior peptic ulcer or gastrointestinal bleed) Routine screening and eradication of *H. pylori*
Bridging	Avoid before non-cardiac surgery except in very high-risk patients (e.g. mechanical valve prosthesis, AF with very high CHA_2DS_2-VASc score, very recent stent implantation)
Follow-up	Regular monitoring or follow-up visits while patients on antithrombotic therapy

[a] Dronedarone, ciclosporin, erythromycin or ketoconazole.

ACS, acute coronary syndrome; ACT, activated clotting time; AF, atrial fibrillation; APT, antiplatelet therapy; BD, twice daily; BMS, bare metal stent; CAG, coronary angiography; CCTA, coronary computed tomography angiography; CVD, cardiovascular disease; DAPT, dual antiplatelet therapy; DOAC, direct oral anticoagulant; GFR, glomerular filtration rate; GP, glycoprotein; HBR, high bleeding risk; INR, international normalized ratio; LAAC, left atrial appendage closure; LMWH, low-molecular-weight heparin (e.g. enoxaparin); NSAIDs, non-steroidal anti-inflammatory drugs; OAC, oral anticoagulation; OD, once daily; PAD, peripheral artery disease; PCI, percutaneous coronary intervention; PFO, patent foramen ovale; PPI, proton pump inhibitor; PTA, percutaneous transluminal angioplasty; PTS, patients; SAPT, single antiplatelet therapy; STEMI, ST-segment elevation myocardial infarction; TAVI, transcatheter aortic valve implantation; TIA, transient ischaemic attack; UFH, unfractionated heparin; US, ultrasound; VKA, vitamin K antagonist; VTE, venous thromboembolism.

years, alternative regimens shortening the duration or modulating the intensity of DAPT to reduce bleeding risk have been investigated. In HBR patients, a 3-month or even 1-month DAPT followed by aspirin or $P2Y_{12}$ inhibitor monotherapy after implantation of drug-eluting stents has shown similar efficacy and safety to standard DAPT.[22–24] Another option is de-escalation; it consists of a DAPT with a potent $P2Y_{12}$ inhibitor, which is switched to clopidogrel or to a lower dose of prasugrel or ticagrelor at the latest 1 month after PCI. De-escalation can be decided after exclusion of clopidogrel resistance using platelet function or genetic testing (guided de-escalation) or routinely without any test (unguided de-escalation). A meta-analysis of randomized controlled trials showed a significant decrease of bleeding and ischaemic events with de-escalation compared to standard DAPT.[25] Further evidence is needed to support a broader application in clinical practice.

In patients undergoing PCI with an indication to OAC, combination with DAPT (i.e. triple therapy) should be as short as possible and clopidogrel represents the $P2Y_{12}$ inhibitor of choice.[8,10,26]

Continuation of DAPT beyond 12 months after PCI has been proven effective in reducing recurrent ischaemic events in the long term at the cost of increased bleeding complications.[27,28] Therefore, this regimen should be restricted to non-HBR patients at high ischaemic risk.[5,10]

In recent years, several studies investigated the optimal antithrombotic regimen for patients undergoing TAVI. Those patients should be treated with aspirin monotherapy, except those with an indication to OAC (e.g. AF or previous VTE) in whom continuation of OAC monotherapy is recommended. The addition of a $P2Y_{12}$ inhibitor (or aspirin) is recommended only in case of recent coronary revascularization but it should not exceed 6 months.[12]

After LAAC, a 1- to 3-month clopidogrel-based DAPT is usually prescribed to avoid the formation of thrombi on the surface of the implanted device before complete endothelization, even though the evidence supporting this practice is limited. Based on expert consensus, in patients at very HBR, DAPT for 1 month or less or a single antiplatelet agent should be considered.[8]

Similarly, after percutaneous patent foramen ovale (PFO) occlusion, the recommended 6-month DAPT duration can be shortened up to 1 month in the presence of HBR features.[29]

In PAD patients undergoing PTA, DAPT should be prescribed for no longer than 1 month; in patients on OAC, the addition of an antiplatelet agent is discouraged.[13]

Intravenous or subcutaneous P2Y$_{12}$ inhibitors

In recent years, intravenous or subcutaneous P2Y$_{12}$ inhibitors with a very rapid onset and offset of action (within minutes) have been developed. The intravenous agent cangrelor can be used in P2Y$_{12}$ inhibitor-naïve patients for which a rapid platelet inhibition is desirable, such as patients with ST-elevation myocardial infarction (STEMI) or cardiogenic shock who are unable to swallow oral antiplatelet agents.[1,30] Compared with glycoprotein (GP)-IIb/IIIa inhibitors, cangrelor is associated with less bleeding complications. The subcutaneous P2Y$_{12}$ inhibitor selatogrel is a novel compound with similar pharmacodynamics properties, that is, rapid onset and offset of action, which showed promising efficacy and safety in small trials.[31]

Glycoprotein IIb/IIIa inhibitors

GPIIb/IIIa inhibitors are potent intravenous inhibitors of platelet aggregation. In the past, these agents were broadly used in ACS patients to inhibit platelet aggregation until the onset of action of clopidogrel or dipyridamole was achieved. Because of the high rate of bleeding complications associated with their use and the availability of rapidly acting P2Y$_{12}$ inhibitors, these agents are now indicated only as a 'bailout' strategy in case of ACS with high thrombotic burden with no-reflow phenomenon or thrombotic complications during PCI, or as a bridge before surgery in patients at very high ischaemic risk (e.g. coronary stenting <1 month before surgery).[5,6,9] Overdosing of GPIIb/IIIa inhibitors should be avoided and their dose should be adjusted to renal function (➔ Table 24.2). New compounds under development and not yet available for clinical use, such as revacept, a competitive antagonist to platelet glycoprotein VI, or conformation-specific GP inhibitors, outside-in signalling GP inhibitors, or platelet-targeted CD39 may provide more consistent platelet inhibition with a limited bleeding risk.[1,32]

Heparins, heparin derivatives, and bivalirudin

Heparins and heparin derivatives are indicated in several clinical situations, such as anticoagulation during PCI, acute treatment of ACS, prevention and treatment of VTE, or as bridging until OAC is fully effective. Bleeding avoidance strategies when using these agents encompass the choice of the right agent, dose, and activity monitoring.

In patients undergoing PCI, unfractionated heparin (UFH) is the agent of choice for periprocedural anticoagulation; enoxaparin, bivalirudin, or argatroban can be alternatively administered. To decrease the bleeding risk associated with UFH, activated clotting time should be regularly assessed during PCI, targeting a therapeutic of range of 250–300 seconds (in case of concomitant administration of GPIIb/IIIa inhibitors between 200 and 250 seconds).[5] Bivalirudin is associated with less bleeding but also with higher rates of stent thrombosis; for these reasons it can be employed in HBR patients if ischaemic risk is low.[5,6] Enoxaparin might reduce death, myocardial infarction, and major bleeding compared to UFH,[33] but adequately powered and dedicated randomized controlled trials are needed to recommend its use over other available agents. In ACS patients treated with upstream subcutaneous enoxaparin, intravenous enoxaparin rather than UFH should be administered during PCI to decrease the bleeding risk (➔ Table 24.2).

In VTE, low-molecular-weight heparin (LMWH) and fondaparinux are preferred over UFH for initial anticoagulation in pulmonary embolism, as they carry a lower risk of inducing major bleeding and heparin-induced thrombocytopenia. However, if primary reperfusion treatment is necessary or in case of serious renal impairment (glomerular filtration rate <30 mL/min), UFH is a safer option.[15]

Dose of heparins and heparin derivatives should be calculated taking into account the patient's weight, age and renal function (➔ Table 24.2).

Vitamin K antagonists

Vitamin K antagonists (VKAs) have been the only OAC available for 50 years. With the advent of direct oral anticoagulants (DOACs) (➔ Oral factor Xa inhibitors, dabigatran, and forthcoming oral factor XIa and factor XII inhibitors), VKAs represent the first-line treatment only in some specific situations, such as patients with severely impaired renal function or a mechanical valve prosthesis. For several other indications (e.g. stroke prevention in patients with AF, and VTE), DOAC should be considered to reduce intracranial bleeding and provide better protection from ischaemic events.[8,34] Moreover, DOACs should be preferred over VKAs when concomitant antiplatelet therapy is indicated.[8,26]

When a VKA is administered, the lower range of the recommended international normalized ratio (INR) range should be targeted and the risk of drug–drug interactions continuously assessed. In case of elective PCI, interruption of a VKA is not advised. Periprocedural UFH should not be administered if INR is greater than 2.5.

The duration of triple therapy (combination of DAPT and OAC) should not exceed 1 month. After 6–12 months, continuation of OAC alone is recommended in patients with concomitant coronary artery disease, unless ischaemic risk is considered very high and bleeding risk low. Routine PPI use is recommended when OAC and antiplatelet therapy are combined.[18]

LAAC is an available alternative to OAC in AF patients at very high risk of bleeding to prevent stroke and decrease bleeding complications.[35] The patient should be able to tolerate 1–3 months of DAPT regimen or at least 2–4 weeks of single antiplatelet therapy (SAPT) after LAAC. Of note, these regimens, which are widely adopted in clinical practice, have not been tested in dedicated randomized controlled trials.[8]

Oral factor Xa inhibitors, dabigatran, and forthcoming oral factor XIa and factor XII inhibitors

DOACs include three direct factor Xa inhibitors—apixaban, edoxaban, and rivaroxaban—and the direct thrombin inhibitor, dabigatran. DOACs have stable plasma concentrations and do not require regular monitoring. DOACs compared to VKAs are more effective in preventing thromboembolism and are associated with lower rates of intracranial haemorrhage, lower or comparable major bleeding, and higher or comparable gastrointestinal bleeding.[34] For these reasons, DOACs became the agents of choice for several cardiovascular diseases for which OAC is indicated. None of these agents can be administered in patients with a glomerular filtration rate less than 15 mL/min.

Strategies for bleeding prevention with these agents include dose adjustment and avoidance of drug interactions. Indications to dose adjustment of DOACs are reported in ➔ Table 24.2. Off-label dose adjustments are not recommended since safety and efficacy data are not available.

In case of elective PCI, interruption of DOACs is not advised. Regardless of the timing of the last administration of DOACs, low-dose parenteral anticoagulation (e.g. enoxaparin 0.5 mg/kg intravenously or UFH 60 IU/kg) can be safely administered.

After an acute cardioembolic stroke, OAC should be initiated between 4 and 14 days after the onset of neurological symptoms.[36]

Dual pathway inhibition, consisting of the combination of very low-dose rivaroxaban (2.5 mg) with an antiplatelet agent in patients without an OAC indication, has been shown to decrease recurrent ischaemic events in patients with recent ACS or known coronary or PAD.[5,13,37,38] However, this strategy should be avoided in HBR patients because of increased bleeding rates compared to standard antiplatelet therapy.

Use of DOACs in patients undergoing TAVI without an OAC indication (e.g. AF) should be avoided, given the risk of bleeding complications and limited benefit in ischaemic event prevention.[12]

In patients with VTE, the risk and benefits of continuation of anticoagulation beyond 6 months after the acute event should be carefully assessed. In HBR patients with a reasonably low risk of VTE recurrence, DOAC discontinuation should be considered or alternatively a reduced dose of apixaban (2.5 mg twice daily) or rivaroxaban (10 mg once daily) (➔ Table 24.2).[11] New OACs under development that inhibit factor XI and factor XII may attenuate the risk of thrombosis with limited effects on haemostasis.[32,39]

Thrombolytic therapy

The use of thrombolytic therapy to treat myocardial infarction significantly declined with the advent of PCI. Thrombolysis is currently indicated only for STEMI patients if primary PCI is not available within 120 minutes from diagnosis or as bailout treatment in case of no-reflow or a thrombotic complication.[6] However, thrombolysis remains a first-line treatment in other acute cardiovascular conditions, such as high-risk pulmonary embolism and ischaemic stroke.[15] Before administration, the presence of absolute and relative contraindications should be assessed (➔ Chapter 13).

The dose of thrombolytic agents is calculated based on the patient's weight and concomitant medications (➔ Table 24.2).[5,6,9]

Other preventive measures

In addition to optimization of antithrombotic medications, other measures have proven to be effective in bleeding risk prevention among patients on antithrombotic therapy (➔ Figure 24.1 and ➔ Table 24.2).

In HBR patients, the risk/benefit of any invasive procedure should be carefully evaluated; non-invasive diagnostic tests (e.g. computed tomography angiography) should be preferred over coronary angiography.

In patients undergoing PCI, radial access should be preferred over a femoral access to reduce major bleeding and mortality[5,6,9] (➔ Figure 24.3). If femoral access is deemed necessary, punctures should be performed under fluoroscopy or ultrasonography guidance to target a 'safe zone' and use of vascular closure devices is advised (➔ Figure 24.3). In case of radial access, haemostasis can be achieved by using wristbands.[1]

Newer stent platforms (e.g. Resolute Onyx™, Synergy™, Xience™, BioFreedom™, Ultimaster™) have been shown to be safe with ultra-short DAPT regimens and should be preferred to reduce the risk of bleeding, whereas use of bare metal stents is no longer recommended.[40]

Since recurrent ischaemic complications may require an intensification of antithrombotic therapy, any measure reducing ischaemic events can be indirectly considered as a bleeding avoidance strategy. Optimization of stent deployment to reduce the stent-related complications (e.g. by means of intravascular imaging) and strict control of cardiovascular risk factors are of paramount importance.

In general, bridging of antithrombotic therapies before non-cardiac surgery should be avoided except in patients at very high-risk for cardiovascular events, such as those with mechanical valve prosthesis, AF with very high CHA_2DS_2-VASc score or very recent stent implantation (➔ Chapter 25).

Routine screening and eradication of *Helicobacter pylori* and therapy with PPI inhibitors are strongly recommended since gastrointestinal bleeding is the most frequent type of bleeding in patients on antithrombotic therapy. Indications for PPI are reported in ➔ Table 24.2. Non-steroidal anti-inflammatory drugs should be avoided.[1] During antithrombotic therapy, regular visits are recommended to address modifiable bleeding risk factors and adjust the therapy if needed.

Treatment of bleeding

Introduction to reversal of antithrombotic drugs

Major bleeding related to oral antithrombotic drugs is a clinical emergency where patients may necessitate rapid restoration of normal haemostatic functions on top of standard supportive measures (e.g. blood transfusions, vasopressors, fluid infusion, mechanical compression, or intervention at the bleeding site).[41] In case of life-threatening bleeding, immediate drug discontinuation is mandatory but generally not sufficient to promptly restore procoagulant pathways since oral antithrombotic drugs exert their effect for days after the last intake. Hence, pharmacological agents allowing immediate reversal of the inhibition of

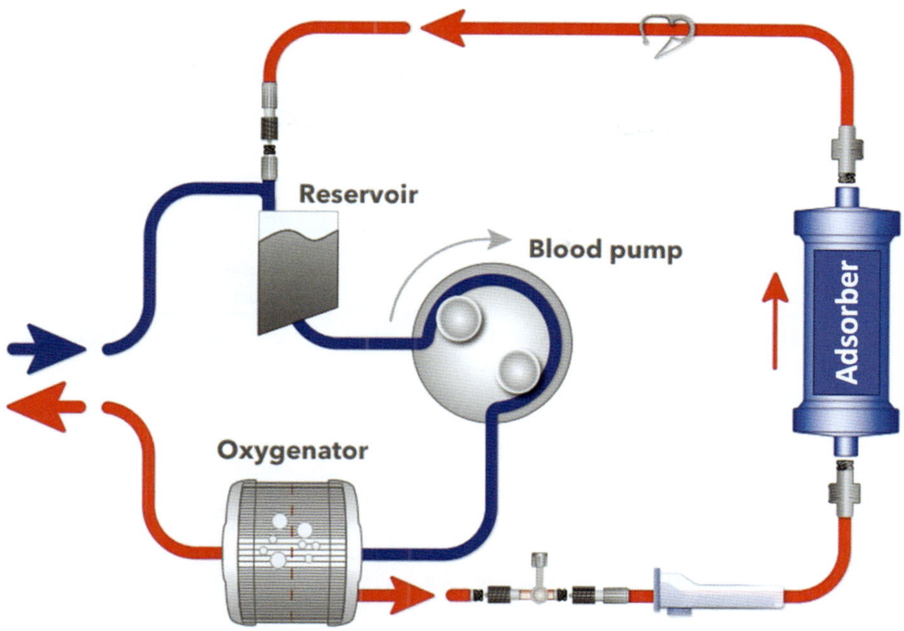

Figure 24.3 Haemoadsorption device for antithrombotic drug removal. The device is integrated as a parallel shunt circuit to the main cardiopulmonary bypass circuit. Blood flow intake to the parallel circuit is after the pump in the main circuit, and blood flow return from the parallel circuit is to the blood reservoir in the main circuit.

Reproduced from Gibson CM, Mack MJ, Lee VT, et al. Rationale and design of the safe and timely antithrombotic removal—ticagrelor (STAR-T) trial: a prospective, multi-center, double-blind, randomized controlled trial evaluating reductions in postoperative bleeding with intraoperative removal of ticagrelor by the drugsorb™-ATR device in patients undergoing cardiothoracic surgery within 48 hours from last ticagrelor dose. Am Heart J. 2022 Mar;245:19–28. doi: 10.1016/j.ahj.2021.10.188 with permission from Elsevier.

platelet or coagulation factors activity represent a key therapeutic option.[42,43] Some reversal strategies may also be considered before proceeding to surgery to mitigate perioperative bleeding complications.

Pooled platelet and coagulation factors supplementation have long been used in this setting despite limited supporting evidence. More recently, newer targeted strategies for antithrombotic drug reversal have emerged and include monoclonal antibodies and recombinant factors that bind to the specific drug (➔ Table 24.3). It must be noted, however, that potential harms related to the prothrombotic effects of reversal agents have been described and their use should only be considered in case of life-threatening bleeding.[44,45]

Reversal of antiplatelet drugs

Platelet transfusion

The effectiveness of platelet transfusion to restore platelet function in patients with an ongoing haemorrhage related to antiplatelet therapy is uncertain and contingent on the specific drug being reversed and the time of last intake. Platelet transfusion seems to adequately reverse the effects of aspirin, clopidogrel, and prasugrel,[46,47] but less so for ticagrelor.[48–53] Moreover, transfusions should be given only after the active metabolites of antiplatelet drugs are no longer present at therapeutic concentrations in the bloodstream: at least 2 hours from the last dose of aspirin or 4–5 hours with enteric-coated preparations, and 4 hours from the last dose of clopidogrel and prasugrel when absorption is not delayed by opiate.

In vitro experiments evaluating functional recovery of platelet reactivity with platelet supplementation in antiplatelet-treated patients have yielded mixed results. Clinical studies in patients with a major bleed have observed a higher risk of adverse events and worse outcomes with platelet transfusion.[54,55] These unfavourable findings may relate to the prothrombotic and proinflammatory effects of transfusions of blood products in general, and platelets in particular.[56,57] Guidelines fail to provide specific recommendations either in favour of or against the use of platelet transfusions in patients undergoing urgent surgical procedures.[58]

Platelet-rich plasma has been suggested to restore platelet function in ticagrelor-treated patients.[59] This effect might be related to the presence of proteins found in human serum. Albumin administration has also been proposed as an option to bind and neutralize circulating ticagrelor.[59] Nevertheless, currently there are no clinical data supporting these strategies *in vivo*.

Reversal of ticagrelor

Bentracimab is a neutralizing recombinant monoclonal antibody fragment that binds to free ticagrelor and its active metabolite with approximately 100-fold greater affinity than the affinity of ticagrelor for the $P2Y_{12}$ receptor.[60] In a phase I randomized, placebo-controlled trial in heathy volunteers, ticagrelor reversal following bentracimab administration

Table 24.3 Reversal agents for antithrombotic drugs

Agent	Drug reversed	Structure	Mechanism of action	Mode of administration	Dosage(s)	Onset of action (minutes)	Offset of action (hours)
Bentracimab	Ticagrelor	Human monoclonal antibody	Antigen-binding fragment	IV bolus followed by prolonged infusion	6 g (bolus) over 10 minutes; 6 g loading infusion over 4 hours; 6 g maintenance infusion over 12 hours	5	24
Idarucizumab	Dabigatran	Humanized monoclonal antibody	Thrombin analogue	IV bolus or infusion (two boluses given no longer than 15 minutes apart)	2×2.5 mg	<5	24–72
Andexanet alfa	Direct and indirect factor Xa inhibitors[a]	Recombinant truncated human factor Xa variant	Decoy receptor	IV bolus followed by 2-hour infusion	400–800 mg bolus; 480–960 mg infusion	2	12
Ciraparantag	All DOACs, heparin and fondaparinux	Small cationic molecule	Hydrogen bonding and charge–charge interactions with DOACs and heparins	IV bolus	100–300 mg	5–10	24
PCC/aPCC	VKA, DOACs, heparin, and fondaparinux	Proteins C and S, factors II, VII, IX, and X	Increase plasma levels of haemostatic factors	IV infusion	04-F PCC: 2000 IU aPCC: 50 IU/kg	Immediate	6–72

[a] Limited action on low-molecular-weight heparin.

4-F, four factor; aPCC, activated prothrombin complex concentrate; DOACs, direct oral anticoagulants; IV, intravenous; PCC, prothrombin complex concentrate; VKA, vitamin K antagonist.

occurred shortly (within 5 minutes) and was sustained for 16–24 hours in patients who received the highest doses, with excellent tolerability and no prothrombotic rebound effect.[61] An interim analysis from the REVERSE-IT study on 150 patients with reported use of ticagrelor within 3 days, of whom 142 required urgent surgery (mainly coronary artery bypass grafting) and eight had major haemorrhage, demonstrated immediate and sustained reversal of ticagrelor's platelet inhibition within 5–10 minutes following infusion, with more than 90% of patients achieving protocol-defined good or excellent haemostasis within 24 hours.[62]

Reversal of anticoagulant drugs

Reversal of heparins

Protamine sulphate rapidly reverses the anticoagulant effect of UFH by preventing its interaction with antithrombin.[63] One milligram of protamine neutralizes approximately 80–100 units of UFH. Beyond 50 mg, however, protamine itself may exert an anticoagulant effect.

Protamine is less effective in reversing LMWH activity as it incompletely reverses factor Xa inhibition despite complete neutralization of the antithrombin effect. This results in only about a 60% reversal of LMWH effects.[63] The risk of allergic reactions associated with the use of protamine should be carefully monitored.

Reversal of vitamin K antagonists

In patients with VKA-associated bleeding, prothrombin complex concentrates (PCCs) and activated PCC can restore haemostasis and normalize the INR within few minutes.[64] PCCs come in both three- and four-factor complexes that include the vitamin K-dependent cofactors II, IX, and X. The four-factor complexes include a higher concentration of factor VII and are generally preferred over three-factor PCCs.[65] In the absence of PCCs, fresh frozen plasma may be considered.[66]

Vitamin K (phytomenadione), either intravenous or oral, reverses the anticoagulant effect of VKA over several hours, so it is generally administered in combination with PCCs or fresh frozen plasma.[67]

Reversal of factor IIa (thrombin) inhibitors

Idarucizumab is a humanized monoclonal antibody that irreversibly binds to free and thrombin-bound dabigatran with a 350-fold greater affinity than thrombin.[68] Indications for treatment include reversal of dabigatran, when needed, for emergency surgery/urgent procedures or life-threatening or uncontrolled bleeding. Among healthy volunteers, idarucizumab infusion immediately reduced circulating unbound dabigatran, reversed dabigatran-induced anticoagulation, and restored normal haemostasis.[69] In the phase III RE-VERSE AD study, idarucizumab rapidly and consistently reversed the anticoagulant effect of dabigatran among patients with uncontrolled gastrointestinal or neurological bleeds, or undergoing urgent surgery.[70] At 90 days, thrombotic events had occurred in 6.3% of the bleeding cohort and 7.4% of the surgical cohort, not deemed to be related to the study drug. However, the product label still carries a warning against thromboembolic risk.

Reversal of factor Xa inhibitors

Andexanet alfa is a specific reversal agent that neutralizes the anticoagulant effects of both direct and indirect factor Xa inhibitors. This enzymatically inactive recombinant modified human factor Xa decoy protein binds with high affinity to the active site of apixaban, rivaroxaban, edoxaban, UFH and LMWH, and fondaparinux.[71] Andexanet alfa was shown to sequester factor Xa inhibitors within the vascular space and rapidly normalize haemostasis.[72] In the phase IIIb/IV ANNEXA-4 study, andexanet alfa reduced anti-factor Xa activity and restored haemostasis in patients with acute major bleeding associated with the use of apixaban or rivaroxaban (as well as edoxaban or enoxaparin in a smaller portion of patients), with 82% of subjects achieving excellent or good haemostasis at 12 hours after the infusion.[73] Nonetheless, concerns have been raised about the 10% rate of thrombotic events reported in the study.

Universal anticoagulant reversal

Ciraparantag is a small molecule that binds non-covalently to heparins and DOACs (both factor Xa and direct thrombin inhibitors).[74] Two recent dose-ranging trials in healthy subjects showed sustained reversal of apixaban and rivaroxaban.[75] Although promising, ciraparantag as a therapeutic agent has not yet been studied in phase III clinical trials. Moreover, when compared to other reversal agents such as andexanet alfa, ciraparantag was shown to have weaker affinity and direct reversal activity for heparins, rivaroxaban, and edoxaban.[76]

PCCs and activated PCCs have been proposed as second-line strategies when the specific DOAC reversal agent is not available, despite debated evidence.[77,78] PCCs can induce a non-specific reversal of DOAC-related coagulopathy by overloading the coagulation cascade with upstream factors. However, some of these coagulation factors could also be in turn inhibited by the circulating unbound DOAC metabolites, which limits their effectiveness and explains the wide variability in haemostasis restoration. In addition, the use of PCCs is also limited by their potential prothrombotic effects.[79]

Other haemostatic agents

Tranexamic acid is a synthetic lysine derivative that inhibits fibrinolysis by blocking the lysine binding sites on plasminogen.[80] It was developed in the 1960s and is increasingly considered a universal haemostatic agent.[81] In randomized controlled trials, tranexamic acid demonstrated a significant reduction in bleeding complications after surgery without increasing thrombotic risk, but at the cost of more postoperative seizure with administration of high doses (>2 g/day) and especially during cardiac surgery.[82–84] Conversely, among healthy volunteers treated with supratherapeutic doses of rivaroxaban, tranexamic acid did not have any effect on either thrombin generation or bleeding in a skin biopsy model.[85]

Desmopressin (DDAVP) improves platelet function by increasing the release of factors VIII and von Willebrand factor.[86] DDAVP has been suggested for patients on antiplatelet agents with active bleeding (intracranial haemorrhage) despite conflicting results from relatively small and low-quality studies.[87,88]

Removal of oral antithrombotic drugs

Removal of antithrombotic drugs from the patient's blood can be achieved by incorporating an adsorber device into an extracorporeal haemoperfusion circuit such as cardiopulmonary bypass or continuous renal replacement therapy (➔ Figure 24.3). Haemoadsorption involves passing the blood directly through a sorbent material for selective removal of specific molecules. Adsorption devices may be useful in patients on antithrombotic drugs requiring urgent/non-deferrable surgery with a significant risk of bleeding complications.

An *in vitro* recirculation model with the CytoSorb™ device (CytoSorbents, NJ, USA) and bovine whole blood demonstrated a removal rate at 30, 60, 120, and 360 minutes of 81.5%, 96.3%, 99.3%, and greater than 99.8% for apixaban; 80.7%, 95.1%, 98.9%, and greater than 99.5% for rivaroxaban; and 62.5%; 75%, 86.6%, and greater than 99% for ticagrelor, respectively.[89] Consistent results were observed in models using dabigatran and edoxaban.[90,91] Two randomized trials of ticagrelor and rivaroxaban or apixaban removal in patients undergoing urgent/emergency cardiac surgery are currently ongoing.[92]

What's new

- Bleeding avoidance strategies include upfront assessment of bleeding risk, careful choice of antithrombotic agents, and other prevention measures, such as reduction of periprocedural bleeding, use of PPIs, and avoidance of bridging of antithrombotic therapies.
- Aspirin in primary prevention should be restricted to patients with diabetes or at high cardiovascular risk without contraindications, such as HBR or age over 70 years.
- $P2Y_{12}$ loading dose before PCI should be limited to STEMI.
- Short-term DAPT or de-escalation to less potent antiplatelet regimens are recommended to reduce bleeding risk.
- Fibrinolysis and GPIIb/IIIa inhibitors should be used only in very specific (bail-out) clinical situations.
- DOACs should be preferred to VKAs in patients with non-valvular AF, VTE, or stroke.
- Measures to reverse antithrombotic drugs include platelet transfusion, PCCs, fresh frozen plasma, and targeted reversal agents.
- Adsorption devices may be useful in patients on antithrombotic drugs requiring urgent/non-deferrable surgery with a significant risk of bleeding complications.

Guideline recommendations

2020 European Society of Cardiology (ESC) Guidelines for the management of acute coronary syndromes in patients presenting without persistent ST-segment elevation

- The use of risk scores designed to evaluate the benefits and risks of different DAPT durations may be considered. (IIb A)
- To estimate bleeding risk, the use of scores may be considered in patients undergoing coronary angiography. (IIb B)
- GPIIb/IIIa antagonists should be considered for bailout if there is evidence of no-reflow or a thrombotic complication. (IIa C)
- Treatment with GPIIb/IIIa antagonists in patients in whom coronary anatomy is not known is not recommended. (III A)
- It is not recommended to administer routine pre-treatment with a $P2Y_{12}$ receptor inhibitor in patients in whom coronary anatomy is not known and an early invasive management is planned. (III A)
- It is recommended to select anticoagulation according to both ischaemic and bleeding risks, and according to the efficacy/safety profile of the chosen agent. (I C)
- Discontinuation of parenteral anticoagulation should be considered immediately after an invasive procedure. (IIa C)
- Crossover of UFH and LMWH is not recommended. (III B)
- After stent implantation with high risk of bleeding (e.g. PRECISE-DAPT ≥25 or ARC-HBR criteria met), discontinuation of $P2Y_{12}$ receptor inhibitor therapy after 3 months should be considered. (IIa B)
- After stent implantation in patients undergoing a strategy of DAPT, stopping aspirin after 3–6 months should be considered, depending on the balance between the ischaemic and bleeding risk. (IIa A)
- De-escalation of $P2Y_{12}$ receptor inhibitor treatment (e.g. with a switch from prasugrel or ticagrelor to clopidogrel) may be considered as an alternative DAPT strategy, especially for ACS patients deemed unsuitable for potent platelet inhibition. De-escalation may be done unguided based on clinical judgement or guided by platelet function testing or cytochrome P450 2C19 genotyping, depending on the patient's risk profile and availability of respective assays. (IIb A)
- In patients with AF and CHA_2DS_2-VASc score of 1 or greater in men and 2 or greater in women, after a short period of triple antithrombotic therapy (up to 1 week from the acute event), dual antithrombotic therapy is recommended as the default strategy using a DOAC at the recommended dose for stroke prevention and a single oral antiplatelet agent (preferably clopidogrel). (I A)
- When rivaroxaban is used and concerns about HBR prevail over stent thrombosis or ischaemic stroke, rivaroxaban 15 mg once daily should be considered in preference to rivaroxaban 20 mg once daily for the duration of concomitant SAPT or DAPT. (IIa B)
- In patients at HBR (HAS-BLED ≥3), dabigatran 110 mg twice daily should be considered in preference to dabigatran 150 mg twice daily for the duration of concomitant SAPT or DAPT to mitigate bleeding risk. (IIa B)
- The use of ticagrelor or prasugrel as part of triple antithrombotic therapy is not recommended. (III C)
- In patients with dabigatran-associated ongoing life-threatening bleeding, the administration of the specific antidote for dabigatran—idarucizumab—should be considered. (IIa B)
- In patients with rivaroxaban-, apixaban-, or edoxaban-associated ongoing life-threatening bleeding, the administration of the specific antidote—andexanet alfa—may be considered. (IIb B)
- In patients with VKA-associated life-threatening bleeding events, rapid reversal of anticoagulation with four-factor PCC rather than with fresh frozen plasma or recombinant activated factor VII should be considered. In addition, repetitive 10 mg intravenous doses of vitamin K should be administered by slow injection. (IIa C)
- In patients with DOAC-associated ongoing life-threatening bleeding, the administration of PCCs or activated PCCs should be considered when the specific antidote is unavailable. (IIa C)
- Radial access is recommended as the standard approach, unless there are overriding procedural considerations. (I A)
- Concomitant use of a PPI is recommended in patients receiving aspirin monotherapy, DAPT, double antithrombotic therapy, triple antithrombotic therapy, or OAC monotherapy who are at high risk of gastrointestinal bleeding in order to reduce the risk of gastric bleeds. (I A)

2021 ESC Guidelines on cardiovascular disease prevention in clinical practice

- Antiplatelet therapy is not recommended in individuals with low/moderate cardiovascular risk due to the increased risk of major bleeding. (III A)
- In patients with diabetes mellitus at high or very high cardiovascular disease risk, low-dose aspirin may be considered for primary prevention in the absence of clear contraindications. (IIb)
- Concomitant use of a PPI is recommended in patients receiving antiplatelet therapy who are at high risk of gastrointestinal bleeding. (I A)
- Adding a second antithrombotic drug (a $P2Y_{12}$ inhibitor or low-dose rivaroxaban) to aspirin for long-term secondary prevention should be considered in patients with a high risk of ischaemic events and without high bleeding risk. (IIa A)
- In patients with chronic coronary syndrome, clopidogrel 75 mg daily is recommended, in addition to aspirin, for 6 months following coronary stenting, irrespective of stent type, unless a shorter duration (1–3 months) is indicated due to risk or the occurrence of life-threatening bleeding. (I A)

2018 ESC/European Association for Cardio-Thoracic Surgery (EACTS) Guidelines on myocardial revascularization
Recommendations for antithrombotic treatment in stable coronary artery disease patients undergoing percutaneous coronary intervention:

- In patients with spontaneous coronary artery dissection considered at high bleeding risk (e.g. PRECISE-DAPT ≥25), DAPT should be considered for 3 months. (IIa)
- In patients with spontaneous coronary artery dissection in whom 3-month DAPT poses safety concerns, DAPT may be considered for 1 month. (IIb C)
- GPIIb/IIIa antagonists should be considered only for bailout. (IIa C)

2017 ESC Guidelines for the management of acute myocardial infarction in patients presenting with ST-segment elevation

- GPIIb/IIIa inhibitors should be considered for bailout if there is evidence of no-reflow or a thrombotic complication. (IIa C)
- A half-dose of tenecteplase should be considered in patients ≥75 years of age. (IIa B)
- Radial access is recommended over femoral access if performed by an experienced radial operator. (I A).
- A PPI in combination with DAPT is recommended in patients at high risk of gastrointestinal bleeding. (I B)
- In patients who are at high risk of severe bleeding complications, discontinuation of $P2Y_{12}$ inhibitor therapy after 6 months should be considered. (IIa B)
- The use of ticagrelor or prasugrel is not recommended as part of triple antithrombotic therapy with aspirin and OAC. (III C)

2017 ESC focused update on dual antiplatelet therapy in coronary artery disease developed in collaboration with EACTS

- It is recommended to reassess the type, dose, and duration of DAPT in patients with actionable bleeding complications while on treatment. (I C)

What's next

- Novel antithrombotic regimens such as complete aspirin-free regimen after PCI or new de-escalation strategies.
- Novel antithrombotic compounds potentially associated with a lower risk of bleeding complications: lipid–aspirin complex, subcutaneous reversible non-thienopyridine $P2Y_{12}$ inhibitor, new inhibitors of platelet glycoproteins, and factor XIa and XIIa inhibitors.
- Specific reversal agents are investigated, such as bentracimab for ticagrelor, and ciraparantag for factor Xa and direct thrombin inhibitors.

Drug dosing

Antithrombotic agents: see Table 24.2.
Reversal agents available for clinical use:

- Protamine sulphate 10 mg intravenously for every 1000–2000 IU of UFH (maximum 50 mg).
- 4-Factor PCC 25–50 U/kg based on INR as a single-dose intravenous infusion.
- Vitamin K up to 10 mg as intravenous infusion.
- Idarucizumab 5 g (two 2.5-g boluses no more than 15 minutes apart), as intravenous bolus (reversal agent for dabigatran).
- Andexanet alfa 400–800 mg intravenous bolus followed by 4–8 mg/min infusion for 120 minutes (reversal agent for factor Xa inhibitors).

References

1. Capodanno D, Bhatt DL, Gibson CM, et al. Bleeding avoidance strategies in percutaneous coronary intervention. Nat Rev Cardiol. 2022;19:117–32.
2. Valgimigli M, Bueno H, Byrne RA, et al. 2017 ESC focused update on dual antiplatelet therapy in coronary artery disease developed in collaboration with EACTS: the Task Force for dual antiplatelet therapy in coronary artery disease of the European Society of Cardiology (ESC) and of the European Association for Cardio-Thoracic Surgery (EACTS). Eur Heart J. 2017;39:213–60.
3. Valgimigli M, Costa F, Lokhnygina Y, et al. Trade-off of myocardial infarction vs. bleeding types on mortality after acute coronary syndrome: lessons from the Thrombin Receptor Antagonist for Clinical Event Reduction in Acute Coronary Syndrome (TRACER) randomized trial. Eur Heart J. 2017;38:804–10.
4. Steg PG, Huber K, Andreotti F, et al. Bleeding in acute coronary syndromes and percutaneous coronary interventions: position paper by the Working Group on Thrombosis of the European Society of Cardiology. Eur Heart J. 2011;32:1854–64.
5. Collet JP, Thiele H, Barbato E, et al. 2020 ESC Guidelines for the management of acute coronary syndromes in patients presenting without persistent ST-segment elevation. Eur Heart J. 2021;42:1289–367.
6. Ibanez B, James S, Agewall S, et al. 2017 ESC Guidelines for the management of acute myocardial infarction in patients presenting with ST-segment elevation: the Task Force for the management of acute myocardial infarction in patients presenting with ST-segment elevation of the European Society of Cardiology (ESC). Eur Heart J. 2018;39:119–77.
7. Urban P, Mehran R, Colleran R, et al. Defining high bleeding risk in patients undergoing percutaneous coronary intervention. Circulation. 2019;140:240–61.
8. Hindricks G, Potpara T, Dagres N, et al. 2020 ESC Guidelines for the diagnosis and management of atrial fibrillation developed in collaboration with the European Association for Cardio-Thoracic Surgery (EACTS): the Task Force for the diagnosis and management of atrial fibrillation of the European Society of Cardiology (ESC). Developed

with the special contribution of the European Heart Rhythm Association (EHRA) of the ESC. Eur Heart J. 2021;42:373–498.
9. Lawton JS, Tamis-Holland JE, Bangalore S, et al. 2021 ACC/AHA/SCAI guideline for coronary artery revascularization: executive summary: a report of the American College of Cardiology/American Heart Association Joint Committee on Clinical Practice Guidelines. Circulation. 2022;145:e4–17.
10. Neumann FJ, Sousa-Uva M, Ahlsson A, et al. 2018 ESC/EACTS Guidelines on myocardial revascularization. Eur Heart J. 2019;40:87–165.
11. Gorog DA, Gue YX, Chao T-F, et al. Assessment and mitigation of bleeding risk in atrial fibrillation and venous thromboembolism: a position paper from the ESC Working Group on Thrombosis, in collaboration with the European Heart Rhythm Association, the Association for Acute CardioVascular Care and the Asia-Pacific Heart Rhythm Society. EP Europace. 2022;24:1844–71.
12. Ten Berg J, Sibbing D, Rocca B, et al. Management of antithrombotic therapy in patients undergoing transcatheter aortic valve implantation: a consensus document of the ESC Working Group on Thrombosis and the European Association of Percutaneous Cardiovascular Interventions (EAPCI), in collaboration with the ESC Council on Valvular Heart Disease. Eur Heart J. 2021;42:2265–9.
13. Aboyans V, Ricco JB, Bartelink MEL, et al. 2017 ESC Guidelines on the diagnosis and treatment of peripheral arterial diseases, in collaboration with the European Society for Vascular Surgery (ESVS): document covering atherosclerotic disease of extracranial carotid and vertebral, mesenteric, renal, upper and lower extremity arteries. Endorsed by: the European Stroke Organization (ESO)The Task Force for the Diagnosis and Treatment of Peripheral Arterial Diseases of the European Society of Cardiology (ESC) and of the European Society for Vascular Surgery (ESVS). Eur Heart J. 2018;39:763–816.
14. de Winter MA, van Es N, Buller HR, Visseren FLJ, Nijkeuter M. Prediction models for recurrence and bleeding in patients with venous thromboembolism: a systematic review and critical appraisal. Thromb Res. 2021;199:85–96.
15. Konstantinides SV, Meyer G, Becattini C, et al. 2019 ESC Guidelines for the diagnosis and management of acute pulmonary embolism developed in collaboration with the European Respiratory Society (ERS): the Task Force for the diagnosis and management of acute pulmonary embolism of the European Society of Cardiology (ESC). Eur Heart J. 2020;41:543–603.
16. Zheng SL, Roddick AJ. Association of aspirin use for primary prevention with cardiovascular events and bleeding events: a systematic review and meta-analysis. JAMA. 2019;321:277–87.
17. Arnett DK, Blumenthal RS, Albert MA, et al. 2019 ACC/AHA guideline on the primary prevention of cardiovascular disease: a report of the American College of Cardiology/American Heart Association Task Force on Clinical Practice Guidelines. Circulation. 2019;140:e596–646.
18. Visseren FLJ, Mach F, Smulders YM, et al. 2021 ESC Guidelines on cardiovascular disease prevention in clinical practice: developed by the Task Force for cardiovascular disease prevention in clinical practice with representatives of the European Society of Cardiology and 12 medical societies with the special contribution of the European Association of Preventive Cardiology (EAPC). Eur Heart J. 2021;42:3227–337.
19. Lai KC, Lam SK, Chu KM, et al. Lansoprazole for the prevention of recurrences of ulcer complications from long-term low-dose aspirin use. N Engl J Med. 2002;346:2033–8.
20. Wallentin L, Becker RC, Budaj A, et al. Ticagrelor versus clopidogrel in patients with acute coronary syndromes. N Engl J Med. 2009;361:1045–57.
21. Wiviott SD, Braunwald E, McCabe CH, et al. Prasugrel versus clopidogrel in patients with acute coronary syndromes. N Engl J Med. 2007;357:2001–15.
22. P2Y12 inhibitor monotherapy or dual antiplatelet therapy after coronary revascularisation: individual patient level meta-analysis of randomised controlled trials. BMJ. 2022;376:o239.
23. Mehran R, Baber U, Sharma SK, et al. Ticagrelor with or without aspirin in high-risk patients after PCI. N Engl J Med. 2019;381:2032–42.
24. Valgimigli M, Frigoli E, Heg D, et al. Dual antiplatelet therapy after PCI in patients at high bleeding risk. N Engl J Med. 2021;385:1643–55.
25. Tavenier AH, Mehran R, Chiarito M, et al. Guided and unguided de-escalation from potent P2Y12 inhibitors among patients with acute coronary syndrome: a meta-analysis. Eur Heart J Cardiovasc Pharmacother. 2022;8:492–502.
26. Angiolillo DJ, Bhatt DL, Cannon CP, et al. Antithrombotic therapy in patients with atrial fibrillation treated with oral anticoagulation undergoing percutaneous coronary intervention: a North American perspective: 2021 update. Circulation 2021;143:583–96.
27. Koo BK, Kang J, Park KW, et al. Aspirin versus clopidogrel for chronic maintenance monotherapy after percutaneous coronary intervention (HOST-EXAM): an investigator-initiated, prospective, randomised, open-label, multicentre trial. Lancet. 2021;397:2487–96.
28. Mauri L, Kereiakes DJ, Yeh RW, et al. Twelve or 30 months of dual antiplatelet therapy after drug-eluting stents. N Engl J Med. 2014;371:2155–66.
29. Pristipino C, Sievert H, D'Ascenzo F, et al. European position paper on the management of patients with patent foramen ovale. General approach and left circulation thromboembolism. EuroIntervention. 2019;14:1389–402.
30. Majmundar M, Kansara T, Jain A, et al. Meta-analysis of the role of cangrelor for patients undergoing percutaneous coronary intervention. Am J Cardiol. 2019;123:1069–75.
31. Milluzzo RP, Franchina GA, Capodanno D, Angiolillo DJ. Selatogrel, a novel P2Y12 inhibitor: a review of the pharmacology and clinical development. Expert Opin Investig Drugs. 2020;29:537–546.
32. Zwart B, Parker WAE, Storey RF. New antithrombotic drugs in acute coronary syndrome. J Clin Med. 2020;9:2059.
33. Silvain J, Beygui F, Barthelemy O, et al. Efficacy and safety of enoxaparin versus unfractionated heparin during percutaneous coronary intervention: systematic review and meta-analysis. BMJ. 2012;344:e553.
34. Ruff CT, Giugliano RP, Braunwald E, et al. Comparison of the efficacy and safety of new oral anticoagulants with warfarin in patients with atrial fibrillation: a meta-analysis of randomised trials. Lancet. 2014;383:955–62.
35. Reddy VY, Doshi SK, Kar S, et al. 5-Year outcomes after left atrial appendage closure: from the PREVAIL and PROTECT AF trials. J Am Coll Cardiol. 2017;70:2964–75.
36. Powers WJ, Rabinstein AA, Ackerson T, et al. Guidelines for the early management of patients with acute ischemic stroke: 2019 update to the 2018 guidelines for the early management of acute ischemic stroke: a guideline for healthcare professionals from the American Heart Association/American Stroke Association. Stroke. 2019;50:e344–418.
37. Mega JL, Braunwald E, Wiviott SD, et al. Rivaroxaban in patients with a recent acute coronary syndrome. N Engl J Med. 2012;366:9–19.
38. Eikelboom JW, Connolly SJ, Bosch J, et al. Rivaroxaban with or without aspirin in stable cardiovascular disease. N Engl J Med. 2017;377:1319–30.

39. Hsu C, Hutt E, Bloomfield DM, Gailani D, Weitz JI. Factor XI inhibition to uncouple thrombosis from hemostasis: JACC review topic of the week. J Am Coll Cardiol. 2021;78:625–31.
40. Capodanno D. Evolving landscapes in coronary stents for patients at high bleeding risk. Circ Cardiovasc Interv. 2021;14:e010591.
41. Spahn DR, Bouillon B, Cerny V, et al. The European guideline on management of major bleeding and coagulopathy following trauma: fifth edition. Crit Care. 2019;23:98.
42. Greenberg SM, Ziai WC, Cordonnier C, et al. 2022 Guideline for the management of patients with spontaneous intracerebral hemorrhage: a guideline from the American Heart Association/American Stroke Association. Stroke. 2022;53:e282–361.
43. Christensen H, Cordonnier C, Kõrv J, et al. European Stroke Organisation guideline on reversal of oral anticoagulants in acute intracerebral haemorrhage. Eur Stroke J. 2019;4:294–306.
44. Cuker A, Burnett A, Triller D, et al. Reversal of direct oral anticoagulants: guidance from the Anticoagulation Forum. Am J Hematol. 2019;94:697–709.
45. Godier A, Albaladejo P, The French Working Group On Perioperative Haemostasis (GIHP) Group. Management of bleeding events associated with antiplatelet therapy: evidence, uncertainties and pitfalls. J Clin Med. 2020;9:2318.
46. Vilahur G, Choi BG, Zafar MU, et al. Normalization of platelet reactivity in clopidogrel-treated subjects. J Thromb Haemost. 2007;5:82–90.
47. Zafar MU, Santos-Gallego C, Vorchheimer DA, et al. Platelet function normalization after a prasugrel loading-dose: time-dependent effect of platelet supplementation. J Thromb Haemost. 2013;11:100–6.
48. Hansson EC, Shams Hakimi C, Åström-Olsson K, et al. Effects of ex vivo platelet supplementation on platelet aggregability in blood samples from patients treated with acetylsalicylic acid, clopidogrel, or ticagrelor. Br J Anaesth. 2014;112:570–5.
49. Godier A, Taylor G, Gaussem P. Inefficacy of platelet transfusion to reverse ticagrelor. N Engl J Med. 2015;372:196–7.
50. Teng R, Carlson GF, Nylander S, Andersson TL. Effects of autologous platelet transfusion on platelet inhibition in ticagrelor-treated and clopidogrel-treated subjects. J Thromb Haemost. 2016;14:2342–52.
51. Bonhomme F, Bonvini R, Reny JL, Poncet A, Fontana P. Impact of non-inhibited platelet supplementation on platelet reactivity in patients treated with prasugrel or ticagrelor for an acute coronary syndrome: an ex vivo study. Platelets. 2015;26:324–30.
52. Martin AC, Berndt C, Calmette L, et al. The effectiveness of platelet supplementation for the reversal of ticagrelor-induced inhibition of platelet aggregation: an in-vitro study. Eur J Anaesthesiol. 2016;33:361–7.
53. Zafar MU, Smith DA, Baber U, et al. Impact of timing on the functional recovery achieved with platelet supplementation after treatment with ticagrelor. Circ Cardiovasc Interv. 2017;10:e005120.
54. Baharoglu MI, Cordonnier C, Al-Shahi Salman R, et al. Platelet transfusion versus standard care after acute stroke due to spontaneous cerebral haemorrhage associated with antiplatelet therapy (PATCH): a randomised, open-label, phase 3 trial. Lancet. 2016;387:2605–13.
55. Zakko L, Rustagi T, Douglas M, Laine L. No benefit from platelet transfusion for gastrointestinal bleeding in patients taking antiplatelet agents. Clin Gastroenterol Hepatol. 2017;15:46–52.
56. Goel R, Ness PM, Takemoto CM, Krishnamurti L, King KE, Tobian AA. Platelet transfusions in platelet consumptive disorders are associated with arterial thrombosis and in-hospital mortality. Blood. 2015;125:1470–6.
57. Ducrocq G, Gonzalez-Juanatey JR, Puymirat E, et al. Effect of a restrictive vs liberal blood transfusion strategy on major cardiovascular events among patients with acute myocardial infarction and anemia: the REALITY randomized clinical trial. JAMA. 2021;325:552–60.
58. Kaufman RM, Djulbegovic B, Gernsheimer T, et al. Platelet transfusion: a clinical practice guideline from the AABB. Ann Intern Med. 2015;162:205–13.
59. Schoener L, Jellinghaus S, Richter B, et al. Reversal of the platelet inhibitory effect of the P2Y(12) inhibitors clopidogrel, prasugrel, and ticagrelor in vitro: a new approach to an old issue. Clin Res Cardiol. 2017;106:868–74.
60. Buchanan A, Newton P, Pehrsson S, et al. Structural and functional characterization of a specific antidote for ticagrelor. Blood. 2015;125:3484–90.
61. Bhatt DL, Pollack CV, Weitz JI, et al. Antibody-based ticagrelor reversal agent in healthy volunteers. N Engl J Med. 2019;380:1825–33.
62. Bhatt DL, Pollack CV, Mazer CD, et al. Bentracimab for ticagrelor reversal in patients undergoing urgent surgery. NEJM Evid. 2021;1:3.
63. Yee J, Kaide CG. Emergency reversal of anticoagulation. West J Emerg Med. 2019;20:770–83.
64. Dentali F, Ageno W, Crowther M. Treatment of coumarin-associated coagulopathy: a systematic review and proposed treatment algorithms. J Thromb Haemost. 2006;4:1853–63.
65. Hellstern P. Production and composition of prothrombin complex concentrates: correlation between composition and therapeutic efficiency. Thromb Res. 1999;95:S7–12.
66. Steiner T, Poli S, Griebe M, et al. Fresh frozen plasma versus prothrombin complex concentrate in patients with intracranial haemorrhage related to vitamin K antagonists (INCH): a randomised trial. Lancet Neurol. 2016;15:566–73.
67. Dezee KJ, Shimeall WT, Douglas KM, Shumway NM, O'Malley P G. Treatment of excessive anticoagulation with phytonadione (vitamin K): a meta-analysis. Arch Intern Med. 2006;166:391–7.
68. Pollack CV Jr, Reilly PA, Eikelboom J, et al. Idarucizumab for dabigatran reversal. N Engl J Med. 2015;373:511–20.
69. Glund S, Stangier J, Schmohl M, et al. Safety, tolerability, and efficacy of idarucizumab for the reversal of the anticoagulant effect of dabigatran in healthy male volunteers: a randomised, placebo-controlled, double-blind phase 1 trial. Lancet. 2015;386:680–90.
70. Pollack CV, Reilly PA, van Ryn J, et al. Idarucizumab for dabigatran reversal—full cohort analysis. N Engl J Med. 2017;377:431–41.
71. Lu G, DeGuzman FR, Hollenbach SJ, et al. A specific antidote for reversal of anticoagulation by direct and indirect inhibitors of coagulation factor Xa. Nat Med. 2013;19:446–51.
72. Siegal DM, Curnutte JT, Connolly SJ, et al. Andexanet alfa for the reversal of factor Xa inhibitor activity. N Engl J Med. 2015;373:2413–24.
73. Connolly SJ, Crowther M, Eikelboom JW, et al. Full study report of andexanet alfa for bleeding associated with factor Xa inhibitors. N Engl J Med. 2019;380:1326–35.
74. Ansell J, Laulicht BE, Bakhru SH, et al. Ciraparantag, an anticoagulant reversal drug: mechanism of action, pharmacokinetics, and reversal of anticoagulants. Blood. 2021;137:115–25.
75. Ansell J, Bakhru S, Laulicht BE, Tracey G, Villano S, Freedman D. Ciraparantag reverses the anticoagulant activity of apixaban and rivaroxaban in healthy elderly subjects. Eur Heart J. 2021;43:985–92.
76. Kalathottukaren MT, Creagh AL, Abbina S, et al. Comparison of reversal activity and mechanism of action of UHRA, andexanet, and PER977 on heparin and oral FXa inhibitors. Blood Adv. 2018;2:2104–14.
77. Kaide CG, Gulseth MP. Current strategies for the management of bleeding associated with direct oral anticoagulants and a review of investigational reversal agents. J Emerg Med. 2020;58:217–33.

78. Gómez-Outes A, Alcubilla P, Calvo-Rojas G, et al. Meta-analysis of reversal agents for severe bleeding associated with direct oral anticoagulants. J Am Coll Cardiol. 2021;77:2987–3001.
79. Rawal A, Ardeshna D, Minhas S, Cave B, Ibeguogu U, Khouzam R. Current status of oral anticoagulant reversal strategies: a review. Ann Transl Med. 2019;7:411.
80. Hunt BJ. The current place of tranexamic acid in the management of bleeding. Anaesthesia. 2015;70(Suppl 1):50–3.
81. Tengborn L, Blombäck M, Berntorp E. Tranexamic acid—an old drug still going strong and making a revival. Thromb Res. 2015;135:231–42.
82. Myles PS, Smith JA, Forbes A, et al. Tranexamic acid in patients undergoing coronary-artery surgery. N Engl J Med. 2017;376:136–48.
83. Devereaux PJ, Marcucci M, Painter TW, et al. Tranexamic acid in patients undergoing noncardiac surgery. N Engl J Med. 2022;386:1986–97.
84. Murao S, Nakata H, Roberts I, Yamakawa K. Effect of tranexamic acid on thrombotic events and seizures in bleeding patients: a systematic review and meta-analysis. Crit Care. 2021;25:380.
85. Levy JH, Moore KT, Neal MD, et al. Rivaroxaban reversal with prothrombin complex concentrate or tranexamic acid in healthy volunteers. J Thromb Haemost. 2018;16:54–64.
86. Kaufmann JE, Vischer UM. Cellular mechanisms of the hemostatic effects of desmopressin (DDAVP). J Thromb Haemost. 2003;1:682–9.
87. Frontera JA, Lewin JJ 3rd, Rabinstein AA, et al. Guideline for reversal of antithrombotics in intracranial hemorrhage: executive summary. a statement for healthcare professionals from the Neurocritical Care Society and the Society of Critical Care Medicine. Crit Care Med. 2016;44:2251–7.
88. Andersen LK, Hvas AM, Hvas CL. Effect of desmopressin on platelet dysfunction during antiplatelet therapy: a systematic review. Neurocrit Care. 2021;34:1026–46.
89. Tripathi R, Morales J, Lee V, et al. Antithrombotic drug removal from whole blood using haemoadsorption with a porous polymer bead sorbent. Eur Heart J Cardiovasc Pharmacother. 2022;8:847–56.
90. Angheloiu AA, Angheloiu GO. Removal of dabigatran using sorbent hemadsorption. Int J Cardiol. 2019;293:73–5.
91. Angheloiu AA, Tan Y, Ruse C, Shaffer SA, Angheloiu GO. In-vitro sorbent-mediated removal of edoxaban from human plasma and albumin solution. Drugs R D. 2020;20:217–23.
92. Gibson CM, Mack MJ, Lee VT, et al. Rationale and design of the safe and timely antithrombotic removal—ticagrelor (STAR-T) trial: a prospective, multi-center, double-blind, randomized controlled trial evaluating reductions in postoperative bleeding with intraoperative removal of ticagrelor by the drugsorb™-ATR device in patients undergoing cardiothoracic surgery within 48 hours from last ticagrelor dose. Am Heart J. 2021;245:19–28.

CHAPTER 25

Management of patients treated with antithrombotic drugs undergoing surgery

Michael Maeng, Steen Dalby Kristensen, and Jolanta M. Siller-Matula

Contents

Summary

Numerous prothrombotic, inflammatory, and haemodynamic factors related to surgery can increase the risk of ischaemia in patients with known or unknown underlying cardiovascular disease. Therefore, a standardized approach and a stepwise evaluation of risk of bleeding and ischaemic events related to surgery is strongly recommended in the decision-making process regarding the perioperative continuation or interruption of antithrombotic drugs. Prior to surgery, the patient's net perioperative outcome should be assessed in a multidisciplinary team involving perioperative care specialists. Based on an individualized risk assessment, the periprocedural antithrombotic strategy including continuing, pausing, or reversal as well as resumption of antithrombotic therapy should be decided. Decisions regarding antithrombotic therapy during surgery must be made with the goal of achieving an optimal balance between the potential benefit of preventing perioperative thrombotic events and avoiding bleeding complications.

Introduction

It was recently shown that the 5-year risk of all-cause mortality in case of a periprocedural myocardial infarction in relation to non-cardiac surgery (NCS) was 68% while being 38% for patients with spontaneous, non-operative myocardial infarctions,[1] underlining the importance of providing a careful evaluation of NCS patients. Approximately 5% of the world's population undergoes major surgery annually and this number is increasing due to the higher morbidity associated with an ageing population.[2] Comorbidities are common in these patients and treatments with antithrombotic drugs have often been initiated. For example, a recently published study indicated that 18% of adults undergoing NCS had a history of coronary artery disease while 5% had a history of stroke.[3] Furthermore, two large registries in patients undergoing percutaneous coronary interventions (PCIs) showed that 11–23% of these patients underwent surgery after PCI within 1 year.[4,5] Patient-related factors (severity of cardiovascular disease, comorbidities, age, and type and combination of antiplatelet or anticoagulant agents) and procedure-related factors (acute vs elective, duration, and type of the procedure) determine the risk of ischaemic and bleeding complications in patients treated with antithrombotic agents.[3,6,7] When patients receiving antithrombotic therapy need surgery, the scenario is like a double-edged sword: continuation increases the risk of bleeding complications, while interruption enhances the risk of ischaemic events. Moreover, surgery itself and bleeding-related transfusion of blood products may induce a prothrombotic state, which significantly increases the risk of myocardial ischaemia and all-cause death.[3,8–10] Therefore, it is of major importance to prevent bleeding complications associated with antithrombotic treatment in patients undergoing surgery.

Aim

The aim of this chapter is to provide a concise overview of the management of patients treated with antithrombotic drugs undergoing surgery. Emphasis is put on a stepwise evaluation of bleeding and ischaemic risks associated with discontinuation or interruption of antithrombotic drugs. Such an individualized risk assessment, which might result in continuation or withholding of antithrombotic therapy, or sometimes postponing the time point of surgery, aims to optimize the patient's net perioperative outcome. A comprehensive review of the literature on NCS was published by the European Society of Cardiology (ESC) in 2022 and we refer to these guidelines when more detailed or specific information is needed.[11] Importantly, the current chapter also includes cardiac surgery.

Perioperative management of antithrombotic agents

The evidence for reducing the risk of cardiovascular events with antithrombotic drugs is solid. Pausing or altering the intensity of treatment may thus increase the risk of thromboembolic complications, especially in the setting of acute treatment of thrombosis but also in secondary prevention.[12–15] In turn, surgical procedures or invasive interventions during continued antithrombotic treatment can increase the risk of bleeding events.[16] The risk of bleeding depends on the type of the surgical procedure, urgency of the operation, type of antithrombotic treatment, and patient-related factors such as a history of previous bleeding, age, renal function, haemorrhagic diathesis (coagulopathy, thrombocytopenia, etc.), concomitant medication, and comorbidity.

Therefore, a meticulous plan for the perioperative management of antithrombotic treatment is crucial to reduce both risk of bleeding and thrombotic events. Management of patients treated with antiplatelet or anticoagulant drugs with need for urgent or elective surgery should focus on patient- and procedure-related factors with an objective to improve the net perioperative clinical benefit. Importantly, the pharmacological properties and characteristics of the antithrombotic drugs should be taken into consideration (see specific chapters in ➔ Section 2) when interruption of therapy is necessary.[15,17] The risk of bleeding associated with the type of procedure (➔ Table 25.1) should be estimated in the decision-making process and a decision on continuation or interruption of the antithrombotic drugs has to be made. If a decision to interrupt antithrombotic treatment is taken, one must also determine the time point for this discontinuation as well as the optimal timing of surgery (if elective or non-urgent) in patients requiring long-term antithrombotic therapy. Interventions with a relatively high risk of bleeding (➔ Table 25.1) in patients with a very high risk of thrombotic events (➔ Figures 25.1 and 25.2) constitute a special challenge, for example, in patients with recurrent cardiovascular events or recent revascularization with coronary stent implantation. In these situations, the invasive procedure is most often performed during continued or modified antithrombotic treatment with careful haemostasis. Patients will benefit from a perioperative risk assessment focusing on

Table 25.1 Perioperative bleeding risk according to the type of intervention/surgery

Low risk	Moderate risk	High risk
◆ Cataract surgery ◆ Dermatological procedures (e.g. biopsy) ◆ Coronary angiography ◆ Permanent pacemaker insertion or internal defibrillator placement (if bridging anticoagulation is not used) ◆ Selected procedures (e.g. thoracentesis, paracentesis, arthrocentesis) ◆ Gastroscopy or colonoscopy without biopsies ◆ Dental extractions (1 or 2 teeth), endodontic (root canal) procedure ◆ Subgingival scaling or other cleaning	◆ Other intrathoracic surgery ◆ Other orthopaedic surgery ◆ Other vascular surgery ◆ Non-cataract ophthalmological surgery ◆ Selected procedures (e.g. bone marrow biopsy, lymph node biopsy) ◆ Complex dental procedure (e.g. multiple tooth extractions) ◆ Other intra-abdominal surgery (e.g. laparoscopic cholecystectomy, hernia repair, colon resection) ◆ Other general surgery (e.g. breast) ◆ Gastroscopy or colonoscopy with biopsies	◆ Neurosurgery (intracranial or spinal) ◆ Any surgery or procedure with neuraxial (spinal or epidural) anaesthesia ◆ Cardiac surgery (e.g. coronary artery bypass graft, heart valve replacement) ◆ Major intra-abdominal surgery (e.g. intestinal anastomosis) ◆ Major vascular surgery (e.g. aortic aneurysm repair, aortofemoral bypass) ◆ Major orthopaedic surgery (e.g. hip or knee replacement) ◆ Lung resection surgery ◆ Extensive cancer surgery (e.g. pancreas, liver) ◆ Reconstructive plastic surgery ◆ Selected procedures (e.g. kidney biopsy, prostate biopsy, cervical cone biopsy, pericardiocentesis, colonic polypectomy) ◆ Urological surgery (e.g. prostatectomy, bladder tumour resection)

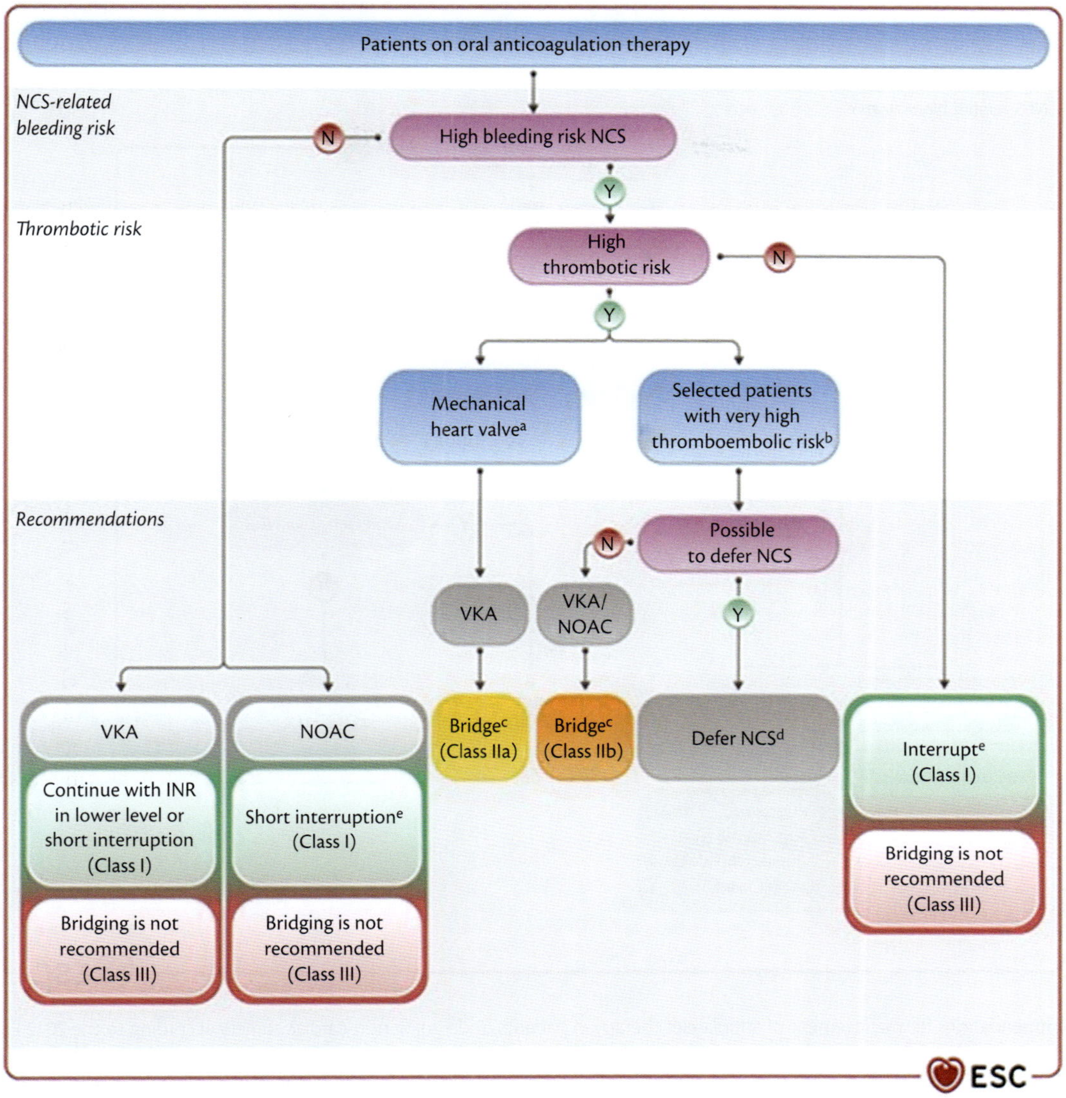

Figure 25.1 Recommendations for management of oral anticoagulation therapy in patients undergoing non-cardiac surgery according to the 2022 ESC Guidelines on cardiovascular assessment and management of patients undergoing non-cardiac surgery.[11] CHA_2DS_2-VASc, congestive heart failure, hypertension, age 75 years or older, diabetes mellitus, stroke, vascular disease, age 65–74 years, sex category (female); N, no; NCS, non-cardiac surgery; NOAC, non-vitamin K antagonist oral anticoagulant; VKA, vitamin K antagonist; VTE, venous thromboembolism. Y, yes. [a] Mechanical aortic valve replacement (AVR) and any thromboembolic risk factor (atrial fibrillation, previous thromboembolism, severe left ventricular dysfunction, hypercoagulable state), or older-generation mechanical AVR, or a mechanical mitral valve replacement. [b] Recent stroke less than 3 months, high risk of VTE recurrences (e.g. antithrombin 3 deficiency or protein C and/or S deficiency), left ventricular apex thrombus, atrial fibrillation with a very high stroke risk. [c] Bridging with unfractionated heparin or LMWH. [d] For example, longer than months after stroke/VTE. [e] For VKA and NOAC management during NCS, see E Tables 25.3 and 25.4.

Halvorsen S, Mehilli J, Cassese S, et al.; ESC Scientific Document Group. 2022 ESC Guidelines on cardiovascular assessment and management of patients undergoing non-cardiac surgery. Eur Heart J. 2022 Oct 14;43(39):3826–3924. doi: 10.1093/eurheartj/ehac270. Copyright European Society of Cardiology. Reproduced with permission from Oxford University Press.

weighting ischaemic versus bleeding risks by a multidisciplinary team including a cardiologist, surgeon, anaesthesiologist, and in some cases also a neurologist, haematologist, or vascular specialist. Patients who experience a perioperative bleeding event and require a reversal drug, need careful haemostatic monitoring and interdisciplinary decision-making to reinforce an early reuptake of the antithrombotic treatment, as a prothrombotic rebound might occur.

➲ Figures 25.1 and 25.2 illustrate the current recommendations for management of antiplatelet and oral anticoagulation therapy, respectively, in patients undergoing NCS according to the 2022 ESC Guidelines on cardiovascular assessment and management of patients undergoing NCS.[11] Most procedures with low-to-moderate bleeding risk can be performed without interruption of antithrombotic treatment, but individualized assessment is important, as some procedures can be associated with low bleeding

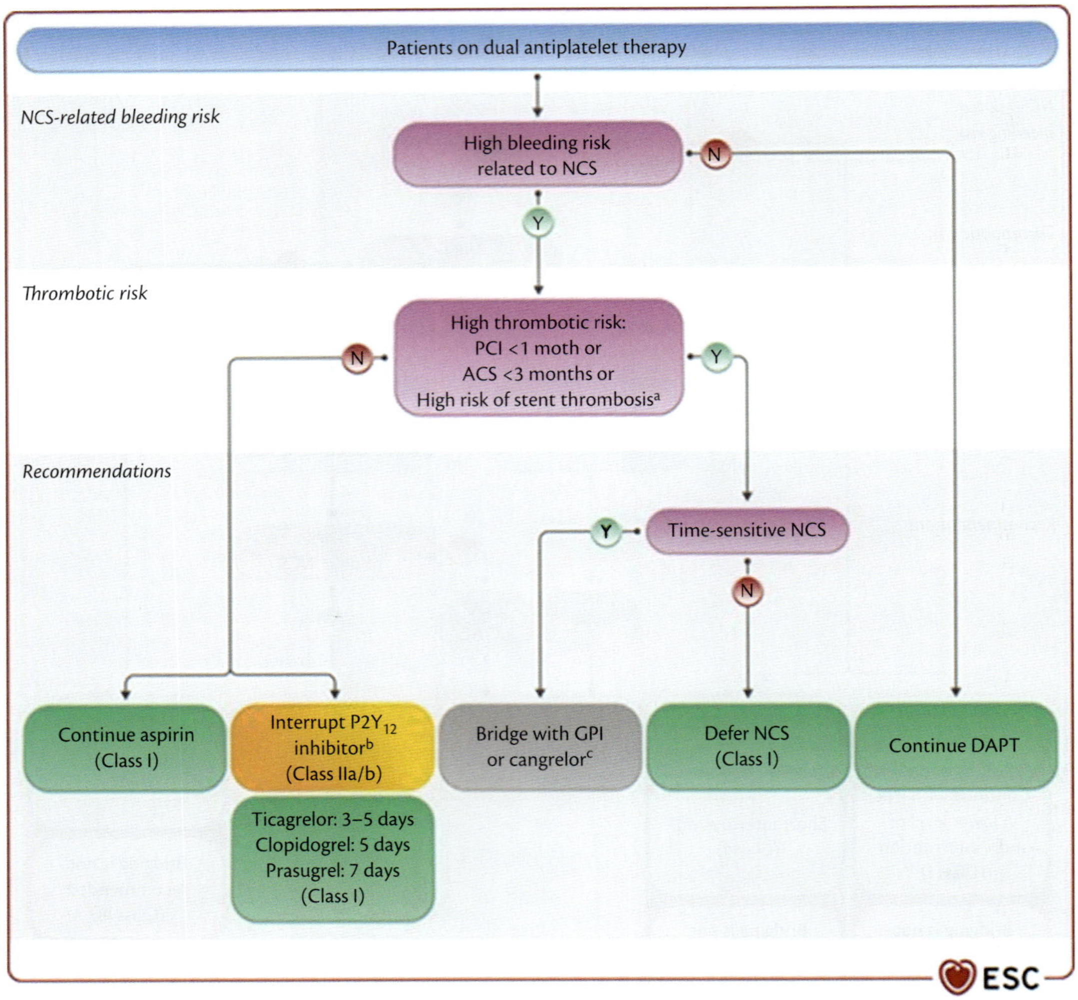

Figure 25.2 Recommendations for management of antiplatelet therapy in patients undergoing non-cardiac surgery according to the 2022 ESC Guidelines on cardiovascular assessment and management of patients undergoing non-cardiac surgery.[11] ACS, acute coronary syndrome; DAPT, dual antiplatelet therapy; GPI, glycoprotein IIb/IIIa inhibitors; PCI, percutaneous coronary intervention; N, no; NCS, non-cardiac surgery. Y, yes. [a] High risk of perioperative stent thrombosis defined by at least one of the following: history of stent thrombosis under antiplatelet therapy, reduced left ventricular ejection fraction (<40%), poorly controlled diabetes, severely impaired renal function/haemodialysis, recent complex PCI (i.e. severely calcified lesion, left main PCI, chronic total occlusion, bifurcational/crush technique, bypass graft PCI), or stent malapposition/residual dissection. [b] Timing of resumption after interdisciplinary risk assessment as soon as possible (within 48 hours) after surgery. [c] For dosing, see Table 25.2.

Halvorsen S, Mehilli J, Cassese S, et al.; ESC Scientific Document Group. 2022 ESC Guidelines on cardiovascular assessment and management of patients undergoing non-cardiac surgery. Eur Heart J. 2022 Oct 14;43(39):3826–3924. doi: 10.1093/eurheartj/ehac270. Copyright European Society of Cardiology. Reproduced with permission from Oxford University Press.

risk, but potentially large consequences of even a small bleed (e.g. intracranial surgery). The management of the antithrombotic treatment will also depend on whether the procedure is elective or acute. The former allows planning and adjustment of treatment, whereas in the case of acute surgery, antithrombotic treatment may need to be reversed.

Antithrombotic drugs: platelet inhibitors

Single antiplatelet therapy with aspirin in patients with cardiovascular disease

Aspirin used for *primary* prevention of cardiovascular disease does not reduce all-cause or cardiovascular mortality and results in an insufficient risk/benefit ratio.[18,19] Thus, in healthy individuals aspirin should be withdrawn prior to NCS and should in general not be resumed.

In contrast to primary prevention, aspirin has an established role for *secondary* or *tertiary* prevention of major adverse cardiovascular events (MACE) in patients with established cardiovascular disease.[19–21] The effect of perioperative aspirin use was investigated in the randomized, placebo-controlled POISE-2 trial[22] including more than 10,000 patients undergoing NCS.[22] Only 33% of patients had a history of vascular disease: 23% coronary artery disease, 5% stroke, and 9% PAD. In the overall study population, aspirin did not reduce the rates of the composite of death or non-fatal myocardial infarction [hazard ratio (HR) 0.99, 95% confidence interval (CI) 0.86–1.15] but increased the risk of major bleeding events (HR 1.23, 95% CI 1.01–1.49) at 30 days.[22]

Thus, in general it should be considered to interrupt aspirin before surgery. However, in the analysis of patients who had undergone prior PCI (n = 470), aspirin significantly reduced MACE (HR 0.50, 95% CI 0.26–0.95) and myocardial infarction (HR 0.44, 95% CI 0.22–0.87) without an increase in major bleeding events,[23] supporting perioperative aspirin use in patients with a history of PCI.

Single antiplatelet therapy with $P2Y_{12}$ inhibitors in patients with coronary artery disease, or stroke

$P2Y_{12}$ inhibitor monotherapy is an emerging approach, especially in patient at high bleeding risk.[24–30] Unfortunately, there is very limited evidence on perioperative management of patients on $P2Y_{12}$ inhibitor monotherapy. One way to circumvent this lack of evidence is to switch from the $P2Y_{12}$ inhibitor to aspirin 75 mg daily 7 days prior to surgery. Moreover, most surgeons are more comfortable with performing surgery in patients on aspirin than on a $P2Y_{12}$ inhibitor.

Dual antiplatelet therapy

Dual antiplatelet therapy (DAPT) with $P2Y_{12}$ inhibitors and aspirin is recommended after PCI or acute coronary syndrome.[14,26,31–34] During the first year after PCI, up to 10% of patients will undergo major NCS.[35–37] Studies reported a twofold higher risk for cardiac events in PCI versus non-PCI patients undergoing NCS.[5,35,36,38–40] The most important predictors for intra-/perioperative ischaemia are timing of NCS in relation to PCI and the urgency of surgery.[37,41–44] A meta-analysis including more than 50,000 patients has shown that preoperative use of clopidogrel on top of aspirin in patients undergoing CABG was associated with a 2.5-fold increased risk of reoperation for bleeding and a 1.47-fold increased risk of death while not diminishing the risk for myocardial infarction or MACE.[16] Further, a randomized study including 2100 CABG patients showed that continuation of aspirin during the operation neither resulted in a lower risk of death or thrombotic complications nor in a higher risk of bleeding than that with placebo.[45] In patients undergoing NCS, preoperative use of clopidogrel on top of aspirin was associated with a twofold increased risk of reoperation for major bleeding but did not reduce the risk of MACE or death.[16] Thus, a single antiplatelet strategy with low-dose aspirin is preferred whenever possible.

Timing of surgery and antiplatelet drug discontinuation

Patients receiving antiplatelet therapy for *primary* prevention can have this treatment paused or stopped at least 7 days prior to surgery. For patients receiving *secondary* or *tertiary* prevention with antiplatelet agents, the two most important messages are (1) postpone surgery for at least 30 days post PCI, and (2) aim for surgery with perioperative single platelet inhibition with low-dose aspirin.[5,35,41,46] This is not always possible but should be pursued.

Platelets have a lifespan of 8–10 days, which is an important indicator for the time point of interruption of irreversible platelet inhibitors such as aspirin and the adenosine diphosphate (ADP) inhibitors clopidogrel and prasugrel. After cessation of the treatment with platelet inhibitors, functional platelets are released daily corresponding to approximately 10% of the normal platelet pool. As the platelet count is usually 150–350 × 10^9/L, and since normal haemostasis is possible with >50 × 10^9/L of functional platelets, normal haemostasis is expected after a 3–4-day aspirin pause.[47] The platelet inhibitory effect of the $P2Y_{12}$ inhibitors decreases more slowly than for acetylsalicylic acid,[46] so normal haemostasis requires a slightly longer treatment pause: at least 3, but usually 5, days for the reversible platelet inhibitor ticagrelor, 5 days for clopidogrel, and 7 days for prasugrel (➔ Table 25.2). In general, $P2Y_{12}$ inhibitors can be resumed when there is sufficient haemostasis, for example, in the evening on the day of surgery or in the morning the day after surgery.

Independently of the timing of surgery, aspirin should be continued in patients with an indication for DAPT. Particular attention is required for certain neurosurgical or ophthalmological operations (➔ Table 25.1), which usually require a 1-week pause of any platelet inhibitor.[46] In patients with a recent PCI who need to undergo a surgical procedure where discontinuation of all platelet inhibitors is needed due to an extensive bleeding risk, we suggest that the operation is performed in hospitals with 24/7 availability of a catheterization laboratory and that bridging with cangrelor (see dose in ➔ Table 25.2) is considered.

Elective surgery

Some guidelines suggest that *elective* surgery in patients on DAPT treated with PCI should be delayed until completion of the recommended DAPT duration, which is on average 6 months for elective PCI and 12 months after acute coronary syndrome.[26,31] Observational studies reflecting daily practical practice, however, report that elective surgery is commonly being performed within the recommended DAPT period. Further, a large Danish observational study showed that NCS appeared equally safe for 1–3, 4–6, and 6–12 months after PCI.[5] As such, the ESC consensus document on DAPT suggests that NCS can be considered at 1 month post PCI whenever relevant.[46]

Time-sensitive surgery

Recent studies and meta-analyses suggest that shortening DAPT duration to 1–3 months after PCI is associated with acceptable rates of MACE and stent thrombosis and a decrease in bleeding risks,[5,24,25,41] indicating that for *time-sensitive* surgery it might be an option to shorten DAPT duration to 1–3 months (depending on the ischaemic risk). Recent evidence from a large Danish registry suggested that patients with either acute coronary syndromes or stable angina pectoris, who underwent surgery between 1 and 12 months after stent implantation, had a risk for myocardial infarction and death that was similar to the risk observed in surgical patients *without* coronary artery disease.[41] If DAPT cannot be interrupted due to a very high risk of stent thrombosis or ischaemia, bridging therapy with the intravenous platelet inhibitors cangrelor, tirofiban, or eptifibatide might be an option[48–50] (➔ Figure 25.1 and ➔ Table 25.2). However, with modern stenting techniques the risk of stent thrombosis is low, especially when surgery is performed more than 30 days after PCI. In a cohort of 458 patients undergoing moderate- to high-risk surgery within 12 months post PCI, only four patients developed stent thrombosis and all of these occurred when surgery was performed within 30 days after PCI.[35] Several studies indicate that platelet function testing can also be

Table 25.2 Key characteristics of currently used antiplatelet agents related to their interruption/discontinuation for surgical procedures

	Aspirin **Low dose (75–100 mg)**	**Clopidogrel** **75 mg**	**Prasugrel** **10 mg**	**Ticagrelor** **90 mg**	**Cangrelor** Bridging dose: 0.75 mcg/kg/min	**Eptifibatide** Bridging dose: 2.0 mcg/kg/min; if GFR <50 mL/min: 1.0 mcg/kg/min	**Tirofiban** Bridging dose: 0.1 mcg/kg/min; if GFR <50 mL/min: 0.05 mcg/kg/min
Target	COX-1	$P2Y_{12}$	$P2Y_{12}$	$P2Y_{12}$	$P2Y_{12}$	GPIIb/IIIa	GPIIb/IIIa
Reversibility	Irreversible	Irreversible	Irreversible	Reversible	Reversible	Reversible	Reversible
Duration of action after the last dose	3–10 days	3–10 days	7–10 days	3–5 days	1 hour	4 hours	8 hours
Periprocedural management	*Primary prevention:* Discontinuation/interruption 7 days before surgery *Secondary prevention:* In patients with prior PCI, acute coronary syndrome, or stroke, aspirin should be continued during the perioperative period. If the peri-operative bleeding risk is high, aspirin might be discontinued 3 days before surgery in patients without a history of PCI. If the perioperative bleeding risk is very high, aspirin might be discontinued 7 days before surgery	*Interruption:* 5 days before surgery	*Interruption:* 7 days before surgery	*Interruption:* 3–5 days before surgery	*Discontinuation:* 1–2 hours before surgery, if used for the bridging to surgery	*Discontinuation:* 4–6 hours before surgery, if used for the bridging to surgery	*Discontinuation:* 8–10 hours before surgery, if used for the bridging to surgery

COX-1, cyclooxygenase-1; GFR, glomerular filtration rate; GPIIb/IIIa, glycoprotein IIb/IIIa; PCI, percutaneous coronary intervention.

used to guide timing of surgery after antiplatelet therapy cessation.[51–55] Moreover, platelet function testing can help to identify patients who are at increased risk for surgery-related bleeding or thrombosis on single antiplatelet therapy or DAPT.[21,56–58]

Urgent surgery and reversal of the antiplatelet effect

If urgent surgery is performed during DAPT and the patient experiences major perioperative bleeding, transfusion of platelets is indicated. In this context, it is important to be aware that ticagrelor also inhibits aggregation of transfused platelets.[59] Some data indicate that additional infusion of albumin can bind ticagrelor and therefore reduce its inhibitory effect.[60] Recently, PB2452, a specific reversal agent for ticagrelor, was shown to provide immediate and sustained reversal of the antiplatelet effects of ticagrelor in animal and human studies[61,62] but the PB2452 antidote is not available at the time of writing this chapter. In case of severe bleeding, desmopressin 0.3 micrograms/kg intravenously and/or tranexamic acid 1 g intravenously can be used.

Antithrombotic drugs: oral anticoagulants

Approximately 25% of patients taking oral anticoagulant therapy will require surgery during a period of 24 months.[63] It is essential, in relation to elective surgical procedures, to decide whether drug discontinuation and bridging should be recommended. This will depend on the type of oral anticoagulant, the indication for use, and the type of surgery.

Vitamin K antagonists

Vitamin K antagonists (VKAs) inhibit the formation of coagulation factors II, VII, IX, and X and include phenprocoumon (half-life 100 hours), warfarin (half-life 36–48 hours), and acenocoumarol (half-life 12 hours) (➔ Table 25.3). As pharmacological properties of VKA differ markedly from direct oral anticoagulants (➔ Tables 25.3 and 25.4), perioperative management of VKA is more challenging. The long half-life of phenprocoumon and warfarin necessitates a longer treatment pause (➔ Table 25.3). Importantly, after the initiation of VKA treatment after surgery, it takes 4–6 days to reach the maximum effect, exposing the patient to a relatively long period in which the anticoagulant treatment is suboptimal and the risk of thrombosis is thus increased. This can be accepted in some patients but if the thromboembolic risk is high, intravenous unfractionated heparin infusion or subcutaneous low-molecular-weight heparin (LMWH; dalteparin, tinzaparin, or enoxaparin) should be used before and after the procedure until the international normalized ratio (INR) is in the therapeutic interval again. Heparin bridging should not be confused with the lower-dose LMWH used in some patients for postoperative thromboembolic prophylaxis.

Table 25.3 Key characteristics of vitamin K antagonists related to their interruption/discontinuation for surgical procedures

	Phenprocoumon	Warfarin	Acenocoumarol
Mechanism of action	Inhibits formation of factor II, VII, IX, and X	Inhibits formation of factor II, VII, IX, and X	Inhibits formation of factor II, VII, IX, and X
Time to maximum therapeutic effect	3–4 days	3–4 days	1–2 days
Half-time	100 hours	36–48 hours	12 hours
Duration of discontinuation before surgery	7 days	5 days	3 days
Start with heparin bridging after VKA discontinuation in high thromboembolic risk patients	Day 5	Day 3	Day 2
Reversal	Vitamin K PCC	Vitamin K PCC	Vitamin K PCC

PCC, prothrombin complex concentrate; VKA, vitamin K antagonist.

Surgery in patients treated with VKAs for atrial fibrillation, venous thromboembolism, or pulmonary embolism

Minor surgery with a low bleeding risk (➔ Table 25.1) can be done without VKA interruption aiming for a slightly lower INR threshold (e.g. 2.0). The BRIDGE trial confirmed the safety of warfarin interruption (3–5 days) without bridging in patients with atrial fibrillation.[64] The Postoperative LMWH bridging for patients at high risk of arterial thromboembolism (PERIOP2) trial showed that LMWH after the procedure was not associated with a significant benefit to prevent major thromboembolism in patients with atrial fibrillation.[65] Nevertheless, bridging with heparins might be an option for patients with very high thrombotic risk (AF with CHA_2DS_2-VASc score >6, embolic stroke <3 months, or high risk of venous thromboembolism or pulmonary embolism recurrence).[65–67] In patients with previous coronary stent implantation, bridging with aspirin should be considered using the same arguments as mentioned previously in the sections on single antiplatelet therapy and DAPT.

Surgery with VKAs in patients with mechanical heart valves

Therapeutic anticoagulation is of crucial importance in patients with mechanical heart valves. Therefore, no VKA interruption with INR at the lower level of the therapeutic range should be considered for minor invasive procedures. The evidence is unclear whether bridging improves outcome and the decision to bridge should be done based on the risk for thromboembolism.[65] In patients with a moderate-to-high risk of thromboembolism such as mechanical mitral or aortic valve plus any additional thromboembolic risk factor or an older-generation mechanical aortic valve, bridging with heparin should be considered. Primarily, only APTT-guided intravenous unfractionated heparin (UFH) was used for bridging in patients with mechanical heart valves. Currently, although off-label, subcutaneous LMWH[68] at a therapeutic dose is administered in the majority of patients with the dose adjusted for renal impairment. In patients with renal impairment or severely obese individuals, anti-factor (F)-Xa activity monitoring may be useful with target levels from 0.5 to 1.0 U/mL.

Reversal of the anticoagulant effect of VKAs

The anticoagulant effect of VKA can be reversed with administration of vitamin K. Nevertheless, the effect occurs slowly: the incipient effect is seen after 6 hours, and the maximum effect occurs after 24–36 hours. Vitamin K can thus be used in patients with increased INR and bleeding risk but has limited effect in the setting of acute bleeding during ongoing VKA treatment. In case of the need for downregulation of INR or in the case of minor bleeding, 1.0–2.5 mg of vitamin K can be given orally (e.g. on a sugar lump) or intravenously. If the bleeding is severe, a higher dose (e.g. 5 or 10 mg) of vitamin K, often supplemented with intravenous fresh frozen plasma (10–30 mL/kg), or a coagulation factor concentrate such as prothrombin complex concentrate, which contains the four coagulation factors (FII, FVII, FIX, and FX). In contrast to vitamin K, the effect of prothrombin complex concentrate occurs within 15–30 minutes.

Direct oral anticoagulants

The newer group of oral anticoagulants directly inhibits some of the blood clotting factors and they are therefore referred to as direct oral anticoagulants (DOACs). DOACs have several advantages related to the perioperative management: lower risk of bleeding, shorter half-lives, no need for bridging, and availability of specific antidotes (➔ Table 25.4). It is essential that DOACs have very short onsets and half-lives. The anticoagulant effect occurs early after the start of treatment and decreases rapidly upon pause. This allows a very short interruption for the surgical procedure. Even if an interruption is needed, no bridging is usually necessary although bridging with aspirin should be considered in patients with previous coronary stent implantation as argued above.

Most frequently a shorter interruption of 1–2 days is sufficient. As DOACs are excreted renally, the anticoagulant effect decreases more slowly when renal function is impaired, and in patients with renal impairment a pause of up to 4 days is required (➔ Table 25.5). Treatment with DOACS can be resumed when there is regular haemostasis (usually 6–8 hours after surgery).

Surgery with direct oral anticoagulants

Elective surgical intervention

In patients undergoing elective surgical interventions, the perioperative management is dependent on the inhibitor type (FIIa vs FXa), periprocedural risk of bleeding, and renal function (➔ Table 25.5). It is important to emphasize that no bridging with heparins is recommended.[69–71]

Table 25.4 Key characteristics of direct oral anticoagulants (dabigatran etexilate, rivaroxaban, apixaban, and edoxaban) related to their interruption/discontinuation for surgical procedures

	Dabigatran	Rivaroxaban	Apixaban	Edoxaban
Mechanism of action	Thrombin (factor II) inhibitor	Factor Xa inhibitor	Factor Xa inhibitor	Factor Xa inhibitor
Time to onset of the effect	2–3 hours	1–3 hours	1–2 hours	1–2 hours
Half-time	7–17 hours	5–13 hours	8–15 hours	10–14 hours
Duration of action after last dose	24 hours	24 hours	24 hours	24 hours
Last dose intake before discontinuation for surgery	24–96 hours, dependent on renal function and perioperative bleeding risk	24–48 hours, dependent on renal function and perioperative bleeding risk	24–48 hours, dependent on renal function and perioperative bleeding risk	24–48 hours, dependent on renal function and perioperative bleeding risk
Restart	6–8 hours after surgery For high postoperative bleeding risk: 48–72 hours after surgery; postoperative bridging with thromboprophylaxis dose	6–8 hours after surgery For high postoperative bleeding risk: 48–72 hours after surgery; postoperative bridging with thromboprophylaxis dose	6–8 hours after surgery For high postoperative bleeding risk: 48–72 hours after surgery; postoperative bridging with thromboprophylaxis dose	6–8 hours after surgery For high postoperative bleeding risk: 48–72 hours after surgery; postoperative bridging with thromboprophylaxis dose
Reversal	Idarucizumab	PCC Andexanet alfa	PCC Andexanet alfa	PCC

PCC, prothrombin complex concentrate.

Urgent surgical intervention

For urgent surgery, DOACs should be immediately discontinued and a panel of coagulation tests should be performed. In additional to the classical tests, ecarin clotting assay for dabigatran and anti-FXa chromogenic assays for FXa inhibitors, as well as the DOAC plasma levels should be assessed to guide the decision about use of the reversal agents.[71] Importantly, the clinical presentation and the indication for surgery should also guide the management of bleeding.

Reversal of the anticoagulant effect of DOACs

A specific antidote, idarucizumab, has been developed for the thrombin inhibitor dabigatran, which binds with very high affinity to the metabolites of dabigatran. Idarucizumab was tested in an open-label prospective trial in patients on dabigatran experiencing acute major bleeding or requiring urgent surgical intervention.[72] The antidote quickly (within a few minutes) and effectively abolished the anticoagulant effect of dabigatran.[72] It can be used for life-threatening or uncontrolled bleeding and in some cases also prior to acute surgery in a non-bleeding patient treated with dabigatran. The effect of rivaroxaban and apixaban, FXa inhibitors, can be reversed with the antidote andexanet alfa. The effect of andexanet alfa has not been tested for use in edoxaban-treated patients. Importantly, andexanet alfa was only tested in patients with acute major bleeding under therapy, but not in those requiring urgent surgery.[73] Andexanet alfa non-specifically binds all FXa inhibitors (as unfractionated heparin or LMWH) [71] and its effect is short-lasting. Both antidotes are expensive, and andexanet alfa is not widely available. In a recent meta-analysis of DOAC-related bleedings, the haemostasis rate was around 80% for idarucizumab, andexanet alfa, and prothrombin complex concentrates.[74] Thus, if the specific antidotes are not available, reversal with prothrombin complex concentrates should be strongly considered.

The ➔ Drug dosing box provides the dosing of drugs that will assist in reversal of antithrombotic therapy.

Table 25.5 Timing of last direct oral anticoagulant dose before a surgical procedure and perioperative bleeding risk

GFR (ml/min)	Perioperative bleeding risk			
	Factor Xa inhibitors: apixaban, rivaroxaban, edoxaban		Factor IIa inhibitor: dabigatran	
	Low risk	High risk	Low risk	High risk
≥80	24 h	48 h	24 h	48 h
50–79	24 h	48 h	36 h	72 h
30–49	24 h	48 h	48 h	96 h
15–29	36 h	48 h	Not indicated	Not indicated

What's next

- There is a lack of evidence regarding bridging strategies before emergent or time-sensitive NCS in patients considered to be at high risk of thromboembolic events.
- Studies on patients undergoing NCS regarding optimal INR among mechanical valve carriers and use of DOAC antidotes are needed.
- More evidence is needed in patients undergoing NCS on $P2Y_{12}$-inhibitor monotherapy.
- Novel anticoagulant drugs may include inhibitors of FXI or FXII, which are promising alternatives based on epidemiological and preclinical evidence.

Drug dosing

Drug dosing specific for perioperative bleeding and thrombosis management

- Vitamin K: 2–10 mg depending on the INR value.
- Prothrombin complex concentrate: INR 2–4, 25 U/kg; INR 4–6, 35 U/kg; INR greater than 6, 50 U/kg; maximum dose of 5000 U at 100 kg of body weight.
- Cangrelor bridging dose: 0.75 micrograms/kg/min.
- Tirofiban bridging dose: 0.1 micrograms/kg/min; if creatinine clearance less than 50 mL/min, adjust to 0.05 micrograms/kg/min.
- Eptifibatide bridging dose: 2.0 micrograms/kg/min; if creatinine clearance is less than 50 mL/min, adjust to 1.0 micrograms/kg/min.
- Idarucizumab: 5 g intravenously divided into two 2.5 g doses administered 15 minutes apart.
- Andexanet alfa: a high dose is used when the last dose of apixaban was greater than 5 mg or the last dose of rivaroxaban greater than 10 mg plus this last dose of apixaban/rivaroxaban was taken within 8 hours prior to start of andexanet alfa. Otherwise the low dose is recommended.
  - Low dose: 400 mg intravenous bolus over 15 minutes followed by 480 mg infusion over 2 hours.
  - High dose: 800 mg intravenous bolus over 15 minutes followed by 960 mg infusion over 2 hours.
- LMWH for bridging in patients treated with oral anticoagulants: a therapeutic dose twice a day adjusted for renal impairment. Anti-FXa activity monitoring with target levels from 0.5 to 1.0 U/mL may be considered.

References

1. Korsgaard S, Schmidt M, Maeng M, et al. Long-term outcomes of perioperative versus nonoperative myocardial infarction: a Danish population-based cohort study (2000–2016). Circ Cardiovasc Qual Outcomes. 2022;15:e008212.
2. Weiser TG, Haynes AB, Molina G, et al. Estimate of the global volume of surgery in 2012: an assessment supporting improved health outcomes. Lancet. 2015;385(Suppl 2):S11.
3. Vascular Events in Noncardiac Surgery Patients Cohort Evaluation Study Investigators, Spence J, LeManach Y, et al. Association between complications and death within 30 days after noncardiac surgery. CMAJ. 2019;191:E830–7.
4. Lee OH, Hong SJ, Ahn CM, et al. The incidence of non-cardiac surgery in patients treated with drug-eluting stents according to age. J Invasive Cardiol. 2019;31:E9–14.
5. Egholm G, Kristensen SD, Thim T, et al. Risk associated with surgery within 12 months after coronary drug-eluting stent implantation. J Am Coll Cardiol. 2016;68:2622–32.
6. Norderud K, Egholm G, Thim T, et al. Validation of the European Society of Cardiology and European Society of Anaesthesiology non-cardiac surgery risk score in patients treated with coronary drug-eluting stent implantation. Eur Heart J Qual Care Clin Outcomes. 2019;5:22–7.
7. Smilowitz NR, Gupta N, Guo Y, Beckman JA, Bangalore S, Berger JS. Trends in cardiovascular risk factor and disease prevalence in patients undergoing non-cardiac surgery. Heart. 2018;104:1180–6.
8. Kamel H, Johnston SC, Kirkham JC, et al. Association between major perioperative hemorrhage and stroke or Q-wave myocardial infarction. Circulation. 2012;126:207–12.
9. CRASH-2 Trial Collaborators, Shakur H, Roberts I, et al. Effects of tranexamic acid on death, vascular occlusive events, and blood transfusion in trauma patients with significant haemorrhage (CRASH-2): a randomised, placebo-controlled trial. Lancet. 2010;376:23–32.
10. Kougias P, Sharath S, Barshes NR, Chen M, Mills JL, Sr. Effect of postoperative anemia and baseline cardiac risk on serious adverse outcomes after major vascular interventions. J Vasc Surg. 2017;66:1836–43.
11. Halvorsen S, Mehilli J, Cassese S, et al. 2022 ESC Guidelines on cardiovascular assessment and management of patients undergoing non-cardiac surgery. Eur Heart J. 2022;43:3826–924.
12. Komosa A, Perek B, Rzymski P, et al. Platelet function in patients undergoing surgical and transcatheter aortic valve replacement: a comparative study. Kardiol Pol. 2021;79:554–61.
13. Kozinski M, Rejszel-Baranowska J, Mlodawska E, Siller-Matula JM, Tomaszuk-Kazberuk A. Updated overview of evidence on optimal antithrombotic therapy in patients with atrial fibrillation undergoing percutanous coronary intervention. Postepy Kardiol Interwencyjnej. 2020;16:127–37.
14. Kubica J, Adamski P, Niezgoda P, et al. Prolonged antithrombotic therapy in patients after acute coronary syndrome: a critical appraisal of current European Society of Cardiology guidelines. Cardiol J. 2020;27:661–76.
15. Siller-Matula JM, Krumphuber J, Jilma B. Pharmacokinetic, pharmacodynamic and clinical profile of novel antiplatelet drugs targeting vascular diseases. Br J Pharmacol. 2010;159:502–17.
16. Siller-Matula JM, Petre A, Delle-Karth G, et al. Impact of preoperative use of P2Y12 receptor inhibitors on clinical outcomes in cardiac and non-cardiac surgery: a systematic review and meta-analysis. Eur Heart J Acute Cardiovasc Care. 2017;6:753–70.
17. Siller-Matula JM, Jilma B. Ticagrelor: from discovery to phase III clinical trial. Future Cardiol. 2010;6:753–64.
18. Gelbenegger G, Postula M, Pecen L, et al. Aspirin for primary prevention of cardiovascular disease: a meta-analysis with a particular focus on subgroups. BMC Med. 2019;17:198.
19. Siller-Matula JM. Hemorrhagic complications associated with aspirin: an underestimated hazard in clinical practice? JAMA. 2012;307:2318–20.
20. Piepoli MF, Hoes AW, Agewall S, et al. 2016 European Guidelines on cardiovascular disease prevention in clinical practice: the Sixth Joint Task Force of the European Society of Cardiology and Other Societies on Cardiovascular Disease Prevention in Clinical Practice (constituted by representatives of 10 societies and by invited experts) developed with the special contribution of the European Association for Cardiovascular Prevention & Rehabilitation (EACPR). Eur Heart J. 2016;37:2315–81.

21. Siller-Matula JM, Delle-Karth G, Christ G, et al. Dual non-responsiveness to antiplatelet treatment is a stronger predictor of cardiac adverse events than isolated non-responsiveness to clopidogrel or aspirin. Int J Cardiol. 2013;167:430–5.
22. Devereaux PJ, Mrkobrada M, Sessler DI, et al. Aspirin in patients undergoing noncardiac surgery. N Engl J Med. 2014;370:1494–503.
23. Graham MM, Sessler DI, Parlow JL, et al. Aspirin in patients with previous percutaneous coronary intervention undergoing noncardiac surgery. Ann Intern Med. 2018;168:237–44.
24. Gelbenegger G, Erari-Canyurt U, Grafeneder J, et al. Optimal duration and combination of antiplatelet therapies following percutaneous coronary intervention: a meta-analysis. Vascul Pharmacol. 2021;138:106858.
25. Gelbenegger G, Schoergenhofer C, Jilma B, et al. Efficacy and safety of ticagrelor monotherapy in patients undergoing percutaneous coronary intervention: a meta-analysis. Clin Pharmacol Ther. 2021;110:424–31.
26. Collet JP, Thiele H, Barbato E, et al. 2020 ESC Guidelines for the management of acute coronary syndromes in patients presenting without persistent ST-segment elevation. Eur Heart J. 2021;42:1289–367.
27. Mehran R, Baber U, Sharma SK, et al. Ticagrelor with or without aspirin in high-risk patients after PCI. N Engl J Med. 2019;381:2032–2042.
28. Vranckx P, Valgimigli M, Juni P, et al. Ticagrelor plus aspirin for 1 month, followed by ticagrelor monotherapy for 23 months vs aspirin plus clopidogrel or ticagrelor for 12 months, followed by aspirin monotherapy for 12 months after implantation of a drug-eluting stent: a multicentre, open-label, randomised superiority trial. Lancet. 2018;392:940–9.
29. Watanabe H, Domei T, Morimoto T, et al. Effect of 1-month dual antiplatelet therapy followed by clopidogrel vs 12-month dual antiplatelet therapy on cardiovascular and bleeding events in patients receiving pci: the STOPDAPT-2 randomized clinical trial. JAMA. 2019;321:2414–27.
30. Siller-Matula J, Schror K, Wojta J, Huber K. Thienopyridines in cardiovascular disease: focus on clopidogrel resistance. Thromb Haemost. 2007;97:385–93.
31. Knuuti J, Wijns W, Saraste A, et al. 2019 ESC Guidelines for the diagnosis and management of chronic coronary syndromes. Eur Heart J. 2020;41:407–77.
32. Kubica J, Adamski P, Ladny JR, et al. Pre-hospital treatment of patients with acute coronary syndrome: recommendations for medical emergency teams. Expert position update 2022. Cardiol J. 2022;29:540–2.
33. Komosa A, Lesiak M, Krasinski Z, et al. Optimal timing of P2Y12 inhibitor loading in patients undergoing PCI: a meta-analysis. Thromb Haemost. 2019;119:1000–20.
34. Siller-Matula JM, Gruber C, Francesconi M, et al. The net clinical benefit of personalized antiplatelet therapy in patients undergoing percutaneous coronary intervention. Clin Sci (Lond). 2015;128:121–30.
35. Egholm G, Thim T, Olesen KK, et al. Dual anti-platelet therapy after coronary drug-eluting stent implantation and surgery-associated major adverse events. Thromb Haemost. 2016;116:172–80.
36. Berger PB, Kleiman NS, Pencina MJ, et al. Frequency of major noncardiac surgery and subsequent adverse events in the year after drug-eluting stent placement results from the EVENT (Evaluation of Drug-Eluting Stents and Ischemic Events) Registry. JACC Cardiovasc Interv. 2010;3:920–7.
37. Saia F, Belotti LMB, Guastaroba P, et al. Risk of adverse cardiac and bleeding events following cardiac and noncardiac surgery in patients with coronary stent: how important is the interplay between stent type and time from stenting to surgery? Circ Cardiovasc Qual Outcomes. 2016;9:39–47.
38. Huber KC, Evans MA, Bresnahan JF, Gibbons RJ, Holmes DR Jr. Outcome of noncardiac operations in patients with severe coronary artery disease successfully treated preoperatively with coronary angioplasty. Mayo Clin Proc. 1992;67:15–21.
39. Holcomb CN, Graham LA, Richman JS, Itani KMF, Maddox TM, Hawn MT. The incremental risk of coronary stents on postoperative adverse events: a matched cohort study. Ann Surg. 2016;263:924–30.
40. Mahmoud KD, Sanon S, Habermann EB, et al. Perioperative cardiovascular risk of prior coronary stent implantation among patients undergoing noncardiac surgery. J Am Coll Cardiol. 2016;67:1038–49.
41. Thim T, Egholm G, Kristensen SD, et al. Risk of myocardial infarction and death after noncardiac surgery performed within the first year after coronary drug-eluting stent implantation for acute coronary syndrome or stable angina pectoris. Am J Cardiol. 2021;160:14–20.
42. Holcomb CN, Hollis RH, Graham LA, et al. Association of coronary stent indication with postoperative outcomes following noncardiac surgery. JAMA Surg. 2016;151:462.
43. Rodriguez A, Guilera N, Mases A, et al. Management of antiplatelet therapy in patients with coronary stents undergoing noncardiac surgery: association with adverse events. Br J Anaesth. 2018;120:67–76.
44. Armstrong EJ, Graham L, Waldo SW, Valle JA, Maddox TM, Hawn MT. Patient and lesion-specific characteristics predict risk of major adverse cardiovascular events among patients with previous percutaneous coronary intervention undergoing noncardiac surgery. Catheter Cardiovasc Interv. 2017;89:617–27.
45. Myles PS, Smith JA, Forbes A, et al. Stopping vs. continuing aspirin before coronary artery surgery. N Engl J Med. 2016;374:728–37.
46. Valgimigli M, Bueno H, Byrne RA, et al. 2017 ESC focused update on dual antiplatelet therapy in coronary artery disease developed in collaboration with EACTS: the Task Force for dual antiplatelet therapy in coronary artery disease of the European Society of Cardiology (ESC) and of the European Association for Cardio-Thoracic Surgery (EACTS). Eur Heart J. 2018;39:213–60.
47. Patrono C, Andreotti F, Arnesen H, et al. Antiplatelet agents for the treatment and prevention of atherothrombosis. Eur Heart J. 2011;32:2922–32.
48. Angiolillo DJ, Firstenberg MS, Price MJ, et al. Bridging antiplatelet therapy with cangrelor in patients undergoing cardiac surgery: a randomized controlled trial. JAMA. 2012;307:265–74.
49. Walker EA, Dager WE. Bridging with tirofiban during oral antiplatelet interruption: a single-center case series analysis including patients on hemodialysis. Pharmacotherapy. 2017;37:888–92.
50. Wu F, Ma K, Xiang R, et al. Efficacy and safety of a bridging strategy that uses intravenous platelet glycoprotein receptor inhibitors for patients undergoing surgery after coronary stent implantation: a meta-analysis. BMC Cardiovasc Disord. 2022;22:125.
51. Mahla E, Tantry US, Schoerghuber M, Gurbel PA. Platelet function testing in patients on antiplatelet therapy before cardiac surgery. Anesthesiology. 2020;133:1263–76.
52. Mahla E, Metzler H, Bornemann-Cimenti H, et al. Platelet inhibition and bleeding in patients undergoing non-cardiac surgery—the BIANCA observational study. Thromb Haemost. 2018;118:864–72.
53. Siller-Matula JM, Trenk D, Schror K, et al. How to improve the concept of individualised antiplatelet therapy with P2Y12 receptor inhibitors—is an algorithm the answer? Thromb Haemost. 2015;113:37–52.
54. Siller-Matula JM, Trenk D, Schror K, et al. Response variability to P2Y12 receptor inhibitors: expectations and reality. JACC Cardiovasc Interv. 2013;6:1111–28.

55. Siller-Matula JM, Akca B, Neunteufl T, et al. Inter-patient variability of platelet reactivity in patients treated with prasugrel and ticagrelor. Platelets. 2016;27:373–7.
56. Mahla E, Metzler H, Bornemann-Cimenti H, et al. Platelet inhibition and bleeding in patients undergoing non-cardiac surgery—the BIANCA Observational Study. Thromb Haemost. 2018;118: 864–72.
57. Mahla E, Tantry US, Pruller F, Gurbel PA. Is there a role for preoperative platelet function testing in patients undergoing cardiac surgery during antiplatelet therapy? Circulation. 2018;138:2145–59.
58. Mahla E, Suarez TA, Bliden KP, et al. Platelet function measurement-based strategy to reduce bleeding and waiting time in clopidogrel-treated patients undergoing coronary artery bypass graft surgery: the timing based on platelet function strategy to reduce clopidogrel-associated bleeding related to CABG (TARGET-CABG) study. Circ Cardiovasc Interv. 2012;5:261–9.
59. Hobl EL, Derhaschnig U, Firbas C, Schoergenhofer C, Schwameis M, Jilma B. Reversal strategy in antagonizing the P2Y12 -inhibitor ticagrelor. Eur J Clin Invest. 2013;43:1258–61.
60. Angheloiu GO, Gugiu GB, Ruse C, Pandey R, Dasari RR, Whatling C. Ticagrelor removal from human blood. JACC Basic Transl Sci. 2017;2:135–45.
61. Pehrsson S, Johansson KJ, Janefeldt A, et al. Hemostatic effects of the ticagrelor antidote MEDI2452 in pigs treated with ticagrelor on a background of aspirin. J Thromb Haemost. 2017;15: 1213–22.
62. Bhatt DL, Pollack CV, Weitz JI, et al. Antibody-based ticagrelor reversal agent in healthy volunteers. N Engl J Med. 2019;380:1825–33.
63. Beyer-Westendorf J, Gelbricht V, Forster K, et al. Peri-interventional management of novel oral anticoagulants in daily care: results from the prospective Dresden NOAC registry. Eur Heart J. 2014;35:1888–96.
64. Douketis JD, Spyropoulos AC, Kaatz S, et al. Perioperative bridging anticoagulation in patients with atrial fibrillation. N Engl J Med. 2015;373:823–33.
65. Kovacs MJ, Wells PS, Anderson DR, et al. Postoperative low molecular weight heparin bridging treatment for patients at high risk of arterial thromboembolism (PERIOP2): double blind randomised controlled trial. BMJ. 2021;373:n1205.
66. Doherty JU, Gluckman TJ, Hucker WJ, et al. 2017 ACC expert consensus decision pathway for periprocedural management of anticoagulation in patients with nonvalvular atrial fibrillation: a report of the American College of Cardiology Clinical Expert Consensus Document Task Force. J Am Coll Cardiol. 2017;69:871–98.
67. Otto CM, Nishimura RA, Bonow RO, et al. 2020 ACC/AHA Guideline for the management of patients with valvular heart disease: executive summary: a report of the American College of Cardiology/American Heart Association Joint Committee on Clinical Practice Guidelines. Circulation. 2021;143:e35–71.
68. Caldeira D, David C, Santos AT, Costa J, Pinto FJ, Ferreira JJ. Efficacy and safety of low molecular weight heparin in patients with mechanical heart valves: systematic review and meta-analysis. J Thromb Haemost. 2014;12:650–9.
69. Hindricks G, Potpara T, Dagres N, et al. 2020 ESC Guidelines for the diagnosis and management of atrial fibrillation developed in collaboration with the European Association for Cardio-Thoracic Surgery (EACTS). Eur Heart J. 2021;42:373–498.
70. Levy JH, Ageno W, Chan NC, et al. When and how to use antidotes for the reversal of direct oral anticoagulants: guidance from the SSC of the ISTH. J Thromb Haemost. 2016;14:623–7.
71. Steffel J, Collins R, Antz M, et al. 2021 European Heart Rhythm Association practical guide on the use of non-vitamin k antagonist oral anticoagulants in patients with atrial fibrillation. Europace. 2021;23:1612–76.
72. Pollack CV Jr, Reilly PA, van Ryn J, et al. Idarucizumab for dabigatran reversal—full cohort analysis. N Engl J Med. 2017;377:431–41.
73. Connolly SJ, Crowther M, Eikelboom JW, et al. Full study report of andexanet alfa for bleeding associated with factor Xa inhibitors. N Engl J Med. 2019;380:1326–35.
74. Gomez-Outes A, Alcubilla P, Calvo-Rojas G, et al. Meta-analysis of reversal agents for severe bleeding associated with direct oral anticoagulants. J Am Coll Cardiol. 2021;77:2987–3001.

CHAPTER 26

Antithrombotic therapy in patients with atrial fibrillation and recent coronary stenting, with or without an acute coronary syndrome

Alexander C. Fanaroff, Renato D. Lopes, and John H. Alexander

Contents

Summary

Many patients with atrial fibrillation (AF) will ultimately undergo percutaneous coronary intervention (PCI) at some point in their lifetime. Though antithrombotic therapy is indicated for both conditions, anticoagulation is most effective for stroke prophylaxis in AF and dual antiplatelet therapy is most effective for prevention of stent thrombosis and myocardial infarction after PCI. However, the use of so-called triple therapy (oral anticoagulation + P2Y12 inhibitor + aspirin) in patients with AF who undergo PCI is associated with unacceptably high rates of bleeding. Over the past decade, multiple clinical trials have tested alternate antithrombotic regimens in this patient population. Overall, these trials have indicated that the combination of a non-vitamin K antagonist oral anticoagulant plus clopidogrel, with only a short (7–30 days) course of aspirin, hits the sweet spot of limiting bleeding while still providing acceptable protection from stroke, stent thrombosis, and myocardial infarction.

Introduction

Coronary artery disease (CAD) and atrial fibrillation (AF) are very common and increase sharply in prevalence with age. CAD affects 7% of US adults overall, but 16% of those aged between 60 and 79 years and 28% of those over 80 years.[1] Similarly, AF affects 1% of US adults overall, but 3% of those aged between 60 and 79 years and 9% of those over 80 years.[2] CAD and AF share other risk factors, including hypertension, obesity, diabetes mellitus, smoking, and a sedentary lifestyle.[3] Given this overlap in risk factors, it is unsurprising that AF and CAD frequently co-occur. Among all patients with atherosclerotic vascular disease, approximately 10% have AF, including 10% of those undergoing percutaneous coronary intervention (PCI) and 20% of patients aged over 65 years presenting with myocardial infarction (MI).[4–6] Other studies have estimated that up to 15% of patients with AF will undergo PCI at some point during their lifetime.[7]

The most serious complications of both disease processes are mediated by thrombosis; however, the nature of the thrombotic substrate differs substantially. Thrombosis in CAD develops at the site of a ruptured or eroded atherosclerotic plaque within the coronary arteries (or associated with non-endothelialized coronary stent struts), acutely interrupting coronary blood flow and leading to subendocardial or transmural MI. By contrast, thrombosis in AF is not mediated by endothelial injury, but by stasis within the left atrium and left atrial appendage. Embolization of left atrial thrombus causes stroke or systemic embolism. These differences in mechanism and location of thrombus formation in AF and CAD have important implications for the antithrombotic management of these conditions: anticoagulants most effectively reduce stroke and systemic embolism in patients with AF, whereas antiplatelet agents most effectively reduce recurrent MI and stent thrombosis in patients with CAD undergoing PCI.

In this chapter, we will describe historical challenges in determining optimal antithrombotic therapy for patients with AF undergoing PCI, discuss randomized controlled trials conducted in the last decade that established the combination of a non-vitamin K antagonist oral anticoagulant (NOAC) and $P2Y_{12}$ inhibitor as the optimal regimen in these patients, and summarize best practices for management of these patients.

A historical perspective

In the 1980s, six randomized controlled trials compared warfarin versus placebo and/or antiplatelet therapy for the prevention of stroke and systemic embolism in patients with AF.[8–13] In a systematic review and meta-analysis of these trials, warfarin reduced stroke or systemic embolism by 64% versus placebo and 39% versus antiplatelet therapy.[14] For this reason, consensus guidelines published in the 1990s included a class I recommendation for the use of anticoagulation with warfarin to prevent stroke in patients with AF. Concomitantly, other randomized controlled trials established best practices for prevention of thrombosis in patients undergoing PCI with newly developed coronary stents. The first of these trials, the Stent Anticoagulation Restenosis Study (STARS), evaluated three antithrombotic regimens—aspirin alone, aspirin plus warfarin, and aspirin plus the first-generation $P2Y_{12}$ inhibitor ticlopidine [dual antiplatelet therapy (DAPT)]—for the prevention of the composite of death, target vessel revascularization, stent thrombosis, or MI within 30 days after PCI.[15] Patients randomized to DAPT had the lowest incidence of the composite outcome (0.5% vs 3.6% with aspirin alone and 2.7% with aspirin plus warfarin), and lower incidence of haemorrhagic complications than patients randomized to aspirin plus warfarin (5.5 vs 6.2%). This trial established DAPT as superior to anticoagulation for the prevention of thrombotic events in patients undergoing PCI. Thus, by the end of the 1990s, these parallel streams of research led to recommendations for oral anticoagulation (OAC) to prevent stroke in patients with AF and DAPT to prevent arterial thrombotic events in patients undergoing PCI. Triple antithrombotic therapy with aspirin, clopidogrel, and warfarin was thus recommended for patients with AF who underwent PCI.

However, population-based studies showed that the rate of bleeding requiring hospitalization exceeded 10% per year among patients with AF treated with triple therapy.[16–18] Other data showed strong associations between bleeding, quality of life, and clinical outcomes.[19–21] Together, these data made clear that alternative antithrombotic combinations were needed in patients with AF undergoing PCI. At the same time, development of new antithrombotic agents—the more potent $P2Y_{12}$ inhibitors prasugrel and ticagrelor, and the NOACs dabigatran, rivaroxaban, apixaban, and edoxaban—increased the number of agents available to be included in these combinations. The stage was set for a series of pivotal clinical trials that established best practices for antithrombotic therapy among patients with AF who undergo PCI.

Trials of antithrombotic therapy in patients with atrial fibrillation who undergo percutaneous coronary intervention

For a number of reasons, pivotal clinical trials of alternative antithrombotic therapies in patients with AF undergoing PCI focused on bleeding avoidance rather than prevention of ischaemic events. Since these patients had an indication for three antithrombotic agents, the obvious strategy for reducing bleeding was to drop one of the agents. However, it was not obvious which agent should be dropped or how long it should be continued prior to stopping, and there were thousands of potential combinations that could be tested (➔ Figure 26.1). Eight major clinical trials have been conducted in this patient population, evaluating six broad antithrombotic strategies (➔ Table 26.1): (1) warfarin + $P2Y_{12}$ inhibitor + aspirin for 6–12 months (warfarin-based triple antithrombotic therapy); (2) NOAC + $P2Y_{12}$ inhibitor + aspirin for 6–12 months (NOAC-based triple antithrombotic therapy); (3) low-dose NOAC + $P2Y_{12}$ inhibitor + aspirin for 6–12 months; (4) warfarin + $P2Y_{12}$ inhibitor for 6–12 months + aspirin for 7–30 days (warfarin-based double antithrombotic therapy); (5) NOAC + $P2Y_{12}$ inhibitor + aspirin for 7–30 days (NOAC-based double antithrombotic therapy); and (6) oral anticoagulant (OAC; warfarin or NOAC) + aspirin for 6–12 months + $P2Y_{12}$ inhibitor for 4–6 weeks. In all of these trials, more than 90% of patients were treated with clopidogrel, and few were treated with the more potent $P2Y_{12}$ inhibitors ticagrelor or prasugrel. Of these eight clinical trials, five focused on comparing a strategy of double antithrombotic therapy versus triple antithrombotic therapy.

The WOEST (What is the Optimal antiplatElet and anticoagulant therapy in patients with oral anticoagulation and coronary stenTing) trial randomized 573 patients who were undergoing

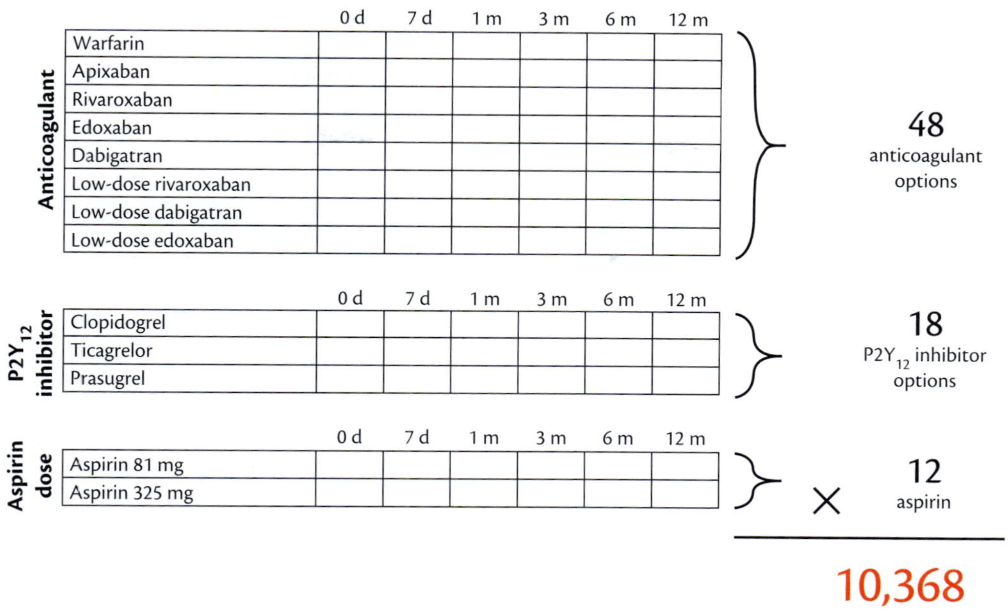

Figure 26.1 Options for antithrombotic regimens in patients with atrial fibrillation undergoing percutaneous coronary intervention. With eight anticoagulant options/doses approved, three $P2Y_{12}$ inhibitors, and two aspirin doses, each of which can be continued for 0 days, 7 days, 1 month, 3 months, 6 months, or 12 months, there are 10,368 ways to combine antithrombotic agents to manage patients with AF undergoing PCI.

PCI and had an indication for OAC (AF in 69%, mechanical heart valve in 10%) to either warfarin-based triple antithrombotic therapy or warfarin-based double antithrombotic therapy.[22] Over 1-year follow up, 19.4% of patients in the double therapy arm had any bleeding event (n = 54) compared with 44.4% patients in the triple therapy arm (n = 126) [hazard ratio (HR) 0.36, 95% confidence interval (CI) 0.26–0.50]. The trial's primary ischaemic endpoint—a composite of death, MI, stroke, target vessel revascularization, and stent thrombosis—occurred in 11.1% of patients randomized to double therapy and 17.6% of those randomized to triple therapy (HR 0.60, 95% CI 0.38–0.94). Though WOEST demonstrated the superiority of double antithrombotic therapy compared with triple antithrombotic therapy for the prevention of both bleeding and ischaemic endpoints, the trial was small with an implausibly large effect size (especially with respect to ischaemic events), and guideline recommendations did not change.[23]

However, by the time WOEST was published in 2012, several clinical trials demonstrating the superiority of the NOACs compared with warfarin with respect to major bleeding and non-inferiority for the prevention of stroke were completed,[24–27] and dabigatran, rivaroxaban, apixaban, and edoxaban were subsequently approved by regulatory authorities. These new OACs had a favourable safety profile compared with warfarin, and their potential utility in patients with AF at high risk of bleeding on warfarin—including those with an indication for DAPT—was clear. However, the pivotal trials evaluating NOACs in patients with AF largely excluded patients with an indication for DAPT. A series of trials enrolling patients with AF undergoing PCI were designed to close this gap in the literature. Unlike WOEST, the indication for anticoagulation in all of these patients was non-valvular AF, as the NOACs were not approved for patients with mechanical valves or rheumatic mitral stenosis, and used different dosing regimens for patients with venous thromboembolism.

PIONEER AF-PCI (Open-Label, Randomized, Controlled, Multicenter Study Exploring Two Treatment Strategies of Rivaroxaban and a Dose-Adjusted Oral Vitamin K Antagonist Treatment Strategy in Subjects with Atrial Fibrillation who Undergo Percutaneous Coronary Intervention) enrolled 2124 patients with AF who had undergone PCI within 72 hours.[28] Patients were randomized to one of three regimens: (1) warfarin-based triple therapy; (2) rivaroxaban 15 mg daily + $P2Y_{12}$ inhibitor; or (3) very-low-dose rivaroxaban (2.5 mg twice daily) + $P2Y_{12}$ inhibitor + aspirin. The trial's primary bleeding outcome—a composite of Thrombolysis in Myocardial Infarction (TIMI) major bleeding, TIMI minor bleeding, and bleeding requiring medical attention over 12-month follow-up—occurred in 26.7% of patients in the warfarin-based triple therapy arm, 16.8% of those in the rivaroxaban-based double therapy arm (HR 0.59, 95% CI 0.47–0.76), and 18.0% of those in the very-low-dose rivaroxaban triple therapy arm (HR 0.63, 95% CI 0.50–0.80). The composite of death from cardiovascular causes, MI, or stroke—a key secondary outcome for which the trial was not powered—occurred in 6.0% of the warfarin-based triple therapy arm, 6.5% of the rivaroxaban-based double therapy arm (HR 1.08, 95% CI 0.69–1.68), and 6.0% of the very-low-dose rivaroxaban triple therapy arm (HR 0.93, 95% CI 0.59–1.48). Neither of the rivaroxaban arms used the dose of rivaroxaban approved for prevention of stroke in non-valvular AF (20 mg daily), and the trial had no prespecified hypothesis with respect to the effect of the treatments on the incidence of ischaemic events.

RE-DUAL PCI (Evaluation of Dual Therapy With Dabigatran vs. Triple Therapy With Warfarin in Patients With AF That Undergo a PCI With Stenting) enrolled 2725 patients with non-valvular AF who

Table 26.1 Major clinical trials of antithrombotic regimens in patients with atrial fibrillation undergoing percutaneous coronary intervention

Trial	Patient population	Regimens evaluated (n)	Major findings
WOEST	Patients with an indication for anticoagulation (67% AF) undergoing PCI (27% for ACS)	◆ Warfarin + clopidogrel + aspirin (284) ◆ Warfarin + clopidogrel (279)	◆ Double therapy reduced the risk of any bleeding versus triple therapy (HR 0.36, 95% CI 0.26–0.50)
RE-DUAL PCI	Patients with non-valvular AF who underwent PCI (51% for ACS) within 120 hours of randomization	◆ Warfarin + clopidogrel + aspirin (981) ◆ Dabigatran 110 mg BD + clopidogrel (981) ◆ Dabigatran 150 mg BD + clopidogrel (763)	◆ Compared with warfarin-based triple therapy, double antithrombotic therapy with 150 mg BD dabigatran reduced the incidence of ISTH major or clinically relevant non-major bleeding (HR 0.72, 95% CI 0.58–0.88), as did double antithrombotic therapy with 110 mg dabigatran (HR 0.52, 95% CI 0.42–0.63)
PIONEER AF-PCI	Patients with non-valvular AF who underwent PCI (52% for ACS) within 72 hours of randomization	◆ Warfarin + clopidogrel + aspirin (706) ◆ Rivaroxaban 15 mg daily + clopidogrel (709) ◆ Rivaroxaban 2.5 mg BD + clopidogrel + aspirin (709)	◆ Compared with warfarin-based triple therapy, rivaroxaban-based double antithrombotic therapy reduced the risk of TIMI major bleeding, TIMI minor bleeding, or bleeding requiring medical attention (HR 0.59, 95% CI 0.47–0.76), as did very low-dose rivaroxaban-based triple therapy (HR 0.63, 95% CI 0.50–0.80) ◆ There were no significant differences between groups in the incidence of the composite of CV death, MI, and stroke
AUGUSTUS	Patients with non-valvular AF who underwent PCI for ACS (37%), PCI for CCS (39%), or had a medically managed ACS (24%) within 14 days of randomization	◆ OAC + clopidogrel + aspirin (2307) ◆ OAC + clopidogrel + placebo (2307) ◆ Apixaban 5 mg daily + clopidogrel + ASA/placebo (2306) ◆ Warfarin + clopidogrel + ASA/placebo (2308)	◆ Aspirin (vs placebo) increased the risk of ISTH major or clinically relevant non-major bleeding (HR 1.89, 95% CI 1.59–2.24) ◆ There was no difference between aspirin and placebo in the incidence of the composite of death and hospitalization ◆ Apixaban (vs warfarin) reduced the risk of ISTH major or clinically relevant non-major bleeding (HR 0.69, 95% CI 0.58–0.81) ◆ Apixaban (vs warfarin) reduced the risk of death and hospitalization (HR 0.83, 95% CI 0.74–0.93) ◆ There was no difference between groups (apixaban vs warfarin and aspirin vs placebo) in the incidence of the composite of death and ischaemic events
ENTRUST AF-PCI	Patients with non-valvular AF who underwent PCI (52% for ACS) within 5 days of randomization	◆ Warfarin + clopidogrel + aspirin (755) ◆ Edoxaban 60 mg daily + clopidogrel (751)	◆ Edoxaban-based double therapy was non-inferior to warfarin-based triple therapy for the composite of ISTH major and clinically relevant non-major bleeding (HR 0.83, 95% CI 0.65–1.05)
ISAR-TRIPLE	Patients with an indication for anticoagulation (83% AF) undergoing PCI (33% for ACS)	◆ Warfarin + aspirin + 6 weeks clopidogrel (307) ◆ Warfarin + + aspirin + 6 months clopidogrel (307)	◆ There was no difference between treatment arms in the composite of death, MI, stent thrombosis, stroke, and major bleeding (HR 1.14, 95% CI 0.68–1.41)
SAFE-A	Patients with non-valvular AF who underwent PCI within 72 hours of randomization	◆ Apixaban 5 mg BD + aspirin + 6 months clopidogrel (106) ◆ Apixaban 5 mg BD + aspirin + 1 month clopidogrel (102)	◆ The trial was stopped early prior to completing enrolment; there was no difference between groups in the primary endpoint of any bleeding (HR 0.70, 95% CI 0.33–1.47)
MASTER DAPT (OAC stratum)	Patients with an indication for anticoagulation (AF in 84%) who underwent PCI (42% for ACS) 30–44 days prior	◆ OAC + clopidogrel + aspirin (818) ◆ OAC + clopidogrel (848)	◆ There was no difference between arms in net adverse clinical events (composite of death, MI, stroke, and BARC 3 or 5 bleeding) (HR 0.83, 95% CI 0.60–1.15)

ACS, acute coronary syndrome; AF, atrial fibrillation; BARC, Bleeding Academic Research Consortium; BD, twice daily; CCS, chronic coronary syndrome; CI, confidence interval; HR, hazard ratio; ISTH, International Society of Thrombosis and Hemostasis; MI, myocardial infarction; TIMI, Thrombolysis in Myocardial Infarction.

had undergone PCI within the previous 120 hours, and randomly assigned them to warfarin-based triple therapy, full-dose dabigatran-based (150 mg twice daily) double therapy, or low-dose dabigatran-based (110 mg twice daily) double therapy.[29] Over 12-month follow-up, International Society for Thrombosis and Hemostasis (ISTH) major or clinically relevant non-major bleeding occurred in 26.9% of patients in the warfarin-based triple therapy arm compared with 15.4% of patients in the dabigatran 110 mg double therapy group (HR 0.52, 95% CI 0.42–0.63) and 20.2% of patients in the dabigatran 150 mg double therapy group (HR 0.72, 95% CI 0.58–0.88). The primary ischaemic event endpoint—a composite of MI, stroke, systemic embolism, death, and unplanned revascularization—occurred in 13.4% of patients in the triple therapy arm compared with 15.2% in the 110 mg double therapy group (HR 1.13, 95% CI 0.90–1.43) and 11.8% in the 150 mg double therapy group (HR 0.89, 95% CI 0.67–1.19). Definite stent thrombosis was rare, occurring in less than 1% of patients in each arm. When considering the results of this trial, it is important to note that the 110 mg dose of dabigatran is not approved in the US; the 150 mg dose is approved for stroke prevention in patients with non-valvular AF.

ENTRUST-AF PCI (Edoxaban-based versus vitamin K antagonist-based antithrombotic regimen after successful coronary stenting in patients with atrial fibrillation) compared warfarin-based triple therapy to full-dose edoxaban-based double therapy (60 mg daily) in 1506 patients with AF undergoing PCI.[30] The trial's primary outcome, ISTH major or clinically relevant non-major bleeding, occurred in 20.1% of patients in the warfarin-based triple therapy arm compared with 17.0% of patients in the edoxaban-based double therapy arm (HR 0.83, 95% CI 0.65–1.05). The primary ischaemic event endpoint—the composite of cardiovascular death, stroke, systemic embolism, MI, and definite stent thrombosis—occurred in 6.0% of patients in the warfarin triple therapy arm compared with 6.5% in the edoxaban double therapy arm (HR 1.06, 95% CI 0.71–1.69). ENTRUST-AF was designed as a non-inferiority trial, and though edoxaban-based double therapy was non-inferior to warfarin-based triple therapy in terms of ISTH major or clinically relevant non-major bleeding, it was not superior.

Unlike prior trials of NOACs in patients with AF undergoing PCI, which compared NOAC-based double therapy versus warfarin-based triple therapy, AUGUSTUS (The Open-Label, 2 × 2 Factorial, Randomized, Controlled Clinical Trial to Evaluate the Safety of Apixaban vs Vitamin K Antagonist and Aspirin vs Aspirin Placebo in Patients with Atrial Fibrillation and Acute Coronary Syndrome and/or Percutaneous Coronary Intervention) was designed as a 2 × 2 factorial trial, in which 4614 patients were randomly assigned to either aspirin 81 mg or matching placebo, and to either full-dose apixaban (5 mg twice daily, or 2.5 mg twice daily in patients meeting two of three dose-reduction criteria) or warfarin (dose adjusted to achieve a target INR 2.0–3.0).[31] This design allowed a direct comparison between double and triple antithrombotic therapy and between NOACs and warfarin. AUGUSTUS enrolled patients undergoing PCI or with a medically managed acute coronary syndrome (ACS), and 37.3% had ACS with PCI, 38.8% elective PCI, and 23.9% medically managed ACS. The primary bleeding outcome, ISTH major or clinically relevant non-major bleeding, occurred in 10.5% of patients randomized to warfarin and 14.7% of patients randomized to warfarin (HR 0.69, 95% CI 0.58–0.81) over 6-month follow-up; the primary bleeding outcome occurred in 16.1% of patients randomized to aspirin and 9.0% of patients randomized to placebo. The composite of all-cause death, MI, definite or probable stent thrombosis, stroke, and urgent revascularization—the trial's primary ischaemic endpoint—occurred in 6.7% of patients randomized to apixaban compared with 7.1% randomized to warfarin (HR 0.93, 95% CI 0.75–1.16), and 6.5% of patients randomized to aspirin compared with 7.3% randomized to placebo (HR 0.89, 95% CI 0.71–1.11). The composite of all-cause death and hospitalization, the trial's other key secondary outcome, occurred in 23.5% of patients randomized to apixaban compared with 27.4% randomized to warfarin (HR 0.83, 95% CI 0.74–0.93), and 26.2% of patients randomized to aspirin compared with 24.7% randomized to placebo (HR 1.08, 95% CI 0.96–1.21). Though not formally evaluated in this way, the design of AUGUSTUS effectively created four treatment regimens: warfarin-based triple therapy, apixaban-based triple therapy, warfarin-based double therapy, and apixaban-based double therapy. The primary bleeding outcome occurred in 18.7% of patients randomized to warfarin-based triple therapy, 13.8% randomized to apixaban-based triple therapy, 10.9% randomized to warfarin-based double therapy, and 7.3% randomized to apixaban-based double therapy.

Broadly, these five trials all had arms comparing long-term triple antithrombotic therapy versus short-term (~7 days) triple therapy followed by long-term double antithrombotic therapy with an OAC plus clopidogrel, but three other trials have evaluated alternative antithrombotic regimens in this population. MASTER DAPT (Management of High Bleeding Risk Patients Post Bioresorbable Polymer Coated Stent Implantation with an Abbreviated versus Standard DAPT Regimen) evaluated standard versus abbreviated duration DAPT in 5204 patients at high bleeding risk undergoing PCI,[32] including 1666 patients on OAC. In the OAC stratum of MASTER DAPT, patients were enrolled 30–44 days after their index PCI and randomized to immediately stopping DAPT (and continuing single antiplatelet therapy alone) or continuing DAPT for at least 2 additional months. Functionally MASTER DAPT tested a strategy of 30 days of triple antithrombotic therapy followed by double antithrombotic therapy versus triple antithrombotic therapy. Among patients in the OAC stratum, the trial's primary bleeding outcome (BARC 2, 3, or 5 bleeding) occurred in 9.9% of patients randomized to 1 month of triple antithrombotic therapy versus 11.7% of those randomized to 3 months (HR 0.83, 95% CI 0.62–1.12); the composite of all-cause death, MI, and stroke occurred in 5.9% of those randomized to 1 month of triple therapy and 6.7% of those randomized to 3 months (HR 0.88, 95% CI 0.60–1.30).

Two small prior trials have evaluated regimens that eliminated a $P2Y_{12}$ inhibitor. ISAR-TRIPLE (Triple Therapy in Patients on Oral Anticoagulation After Drug Eluting Stent Implantation) randomized 605 patients on OAC who underwent drug-eluting stent implantation to OAC and aspirin plus either 6 weeks or 6 months of clopidogrel.[33] There were no significant between-group differences in either TIMI major bleeding or the composite of death, MI, definite stent thrombosis, and ischaemic stroke. Similarly, SAFE-A randomized patients with AF undergoing PCI to apixaban 5 mg twice daily plus aspirin plus either 1 month or 6 months of $P2Y_{12}$ inhibitor therapy.[34] Due to slow accrual, SAFE-A was stopped early after enrolling 210 of a planned 600 patients. There was no significant difference in the rate of the trial's primary bleeding or ischaemic events.

Integrating evidence from major randomized controlled trials to develop treatment recommendations—meta-analyses and subgroup analyses

Summary HRs for trial-defined primary bleeding and ischaemic events for experimental regimens compared with triple antithrombotic therapy are shown in ➔ Figure 25.2. Broadly, the

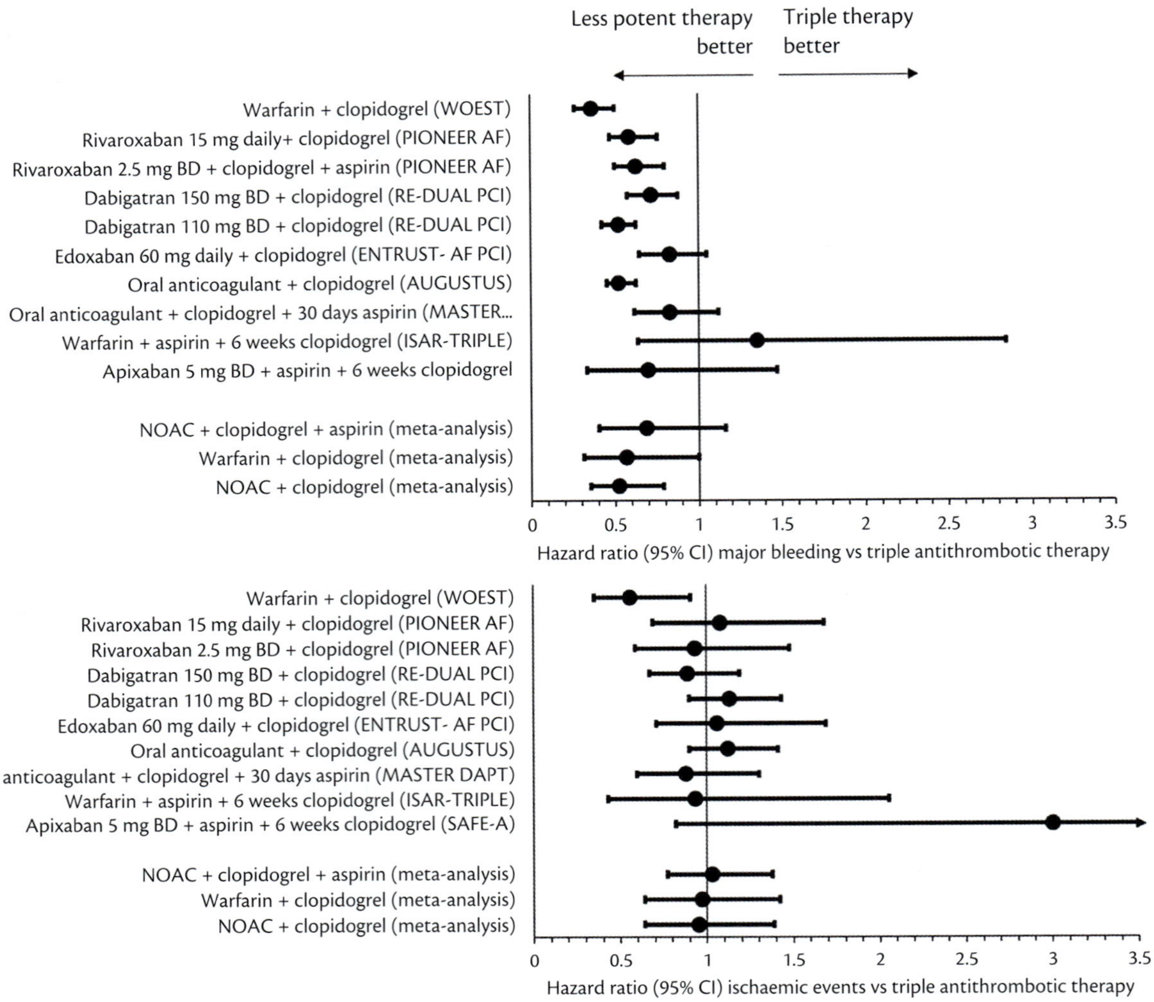

Figure 26.2 Hazard ratios for major bleeding and ischaemic events for less potent antithrombotic therapies compared with triple antithrombotic therapy. Shown are hazard ratios for trial-defined bleeding (top panel) and trial-defined ischaemic events for the experimental arms compared with vitamin K antagonist-based triple antithrombotic therapy in all major trials of antithrombotic therapy in patients with atrial fibrillation with acute coronary syndromes and/or undergoing percutaneous coronary intervention. Trial-defined primary bleeding outcomes were any bleeding (WOEST, SAFE-A), TIMI minor, major bleeding or any bleeding requiring clinical attention (PIONEER AF PCI), ISTH major or clinically relevant non-major bleeding (RE-DUAL PCI, ENTRUST AF-PCI, AUGUSTUS), TIMI major bleeding (ISAR-TRIPLE), BARC 2–5 bleeding (MASTER DAPT). Trial-defined primary ischaemic outcomes were the composite of death, MI, stroke, target vessel revascularization, and stent thrombosis (WOEST); the composite of cardiovascular death, MI, and stroke (PIONEER AF PCI); the composite of death, MI, stroke, systemic embolism, and unplanned revascularization (RE-DUAL PCI); the composite of cardiovascular death, stroke, systemic embolism, MI, and definite stent thrombosis (ENTRUST AF-PCI); the composite of death, MI, definite or probable stent thrombosis, stroke, and urgent revascularization (AUGUSTUS); the composite of death, MI, and stroke (MASTER DAPT); the composite of death, MI, stent thrombosis, and ischaemic stroke (ISAR-TRIPLE); and the composite of death, MI, stroke, and systemic embolism (SAFE-A). BD, twice daily.

strategy studied in WOEST, RE-DUAL PCI, PIONEER AF PCI, ENTRUST-AF PCI, and AUGUSTUS of stopping aspirin within approximately 7 days after PCI or ACS has shown the greatest reduction in bleeding without any difference in ischaemic events compared with triple antithrombotic therapy. These trials have also been combined in several meta-analyses. In a network meta-analysis that used warfarin-based triple therapy as the reference, the odds ratio (95% CI) for TIMI major bleeding was 0.69 (0.40–1.16) for NOAC plus DAPT, 0.57 (0.31–1.00) for warfarin plus $P2Y_{12}$ inhibitor, and 0.52 (0.35–0.79) for NOAC plus $P2Y_{12}$ inhibitor.[35] For trial-defined primary ischaemic outcomes, the odds ratios were 1.03 (0.77–1.38) for NOAC plus $P2Y_{12}$ inhibitor, 0.97 (0.64–1.42) for warfarin plus $P2Y_{12}$ inhibitor, and 0.95 (0.64–1.39) for NOAC plus DAPT. There were no significant differences in all-cause death, stroke, MI, or stent thrombosis. A trial sequential analysis of RE-DUAL PCI, PIONEER AF PCI, AUGUSTUS, and ENTRUST-AF PCI showed that with the data gathered from these four trials, it is possible to exclude the potential that triple therapy reduces the relative risk of ischaemic outcomes by 20% or more compared with double therapy.[36] When comparing individual NOAC-containing regimens, apixaban-based double therapy was associated with the greatest reduction in clinically significant bleeding compared with warfarin-based triple therapy; all NOAC-based double therapy regimens had similar risks of ischaemic events.

Other meta-analyses, recognizing the heterogeneity in study endpoints and the challenges in weighting ischaemic and bleeding events, have explored the effect of antithrombotic regimen on clearly serious events like death, stent thrombosis, and intracranial bleeding. Across the five major trials, there is no effect of antithrombotic treatment strategy on all-cause death.[35,36] Stent thrombosis and intracranial haemorrhage are rare: among 11,542 patients enrolled in WOEST, PIONEER AF PCI, RE-DUAL PCI, ENTRUST-AF PCI, and AUGUSTUS, there were 108 definite or probable stent thrombosis events and 62 intracranial haemorrhages. Despite the low numbers of events, double antithrombotic therapy reduces the risk of intracranial haemorrhage and increases the risk of definite or probable stent thrombosis compared with triple antithrombotic therapy.[35–37] However, due to the rarity of stent thrombosis, the absolute risk increase of stent thrombosis with double antithrombotic therapy was 0.4%, and one would need to treat 274 patients with triple antithrombotic therapy to prevent one stent thrombosis event. Among those 274 patients, there would be eight excess major or clinically relevant non-major bleeding events, including one intracranial haemorrhage.[38]

Though the combined results of major clinical trials indicate that double antithrombotic therapy with NOAC and clopidogrel represents the population-level sweet spot for limiting bleeding events while still providing protection against MI, stent thrombosis, and stroke, investigators have sought to identify subgroups of patients who might benefit from triple antithrombotic therapy. Recognizing that subgroup analyses are inherently underpowered, in secondary analyses of PIONEER AF-PCI, RE-DUAL PCI, ENTRUST-AF PCI, and AUGUSTUS investigators have found no interaction between indication for DAPT (medically managed ACS vs invasively managed ACS vs PCI for chronic coronary syndrome vs STEMI), urgency of revascularization, location of culprit artery, severity of angiographic stenosis, presence of bifurcation, presence of thrombus, type of stent, length of stent, number of stents, baseline DAPT score, PRECISE-DAPT score, CHA_2DS_2 score, HAS-BLED score, renal function, diabetes, heart failure, or use of proton pump inhibitor and the risk/benefit trade-off of double versus triple antithrombotic therapy.[28–31,39–49] The risk/benefit trade-off of double versus triple antithrombotic therapy does, however, change over time. In a landmark analysis of AUGUSTUS, aspirin (versus placebo) increased the absolute risk of severe bleeding by 1% over the first 30 days, while reducing ischaemic events by 1% over the same time period.[50] From 30 days to 6 months, however, aspirin increased the absolute risk of severe bleeding by 1% while reducing ischaemic events by 0.2%. These data suggest that for the first 30 days after PCI or ACS, triple therapy offers an equal trade-off between increased bleeding and reduced ischaemic events, but after that time frame, aspirin continues to increase bleeding with diminishing effects on ischaemic events.

Because less potent antithrombotic strategies necessarily reduce bleeding risk while increasing ischaemic risk,[51] determining the best strategy for antithrombotic therapy in patients with AF who suffer ACS or undergo PCI requires integrating the increased risk of ischaemic events and lower risk of bleeding with less potent antithrombotic therapy versus the lower risk of ischaemic events and greater risk of bleeding with more potent antithrombotic therapy. This requires making an apples-to-oranges comparison that is essentially impossible on the individual patient level. Bleeding events are much more common, but ischaemic events may be more severe (➔ Figure 26.3).[52] In patients undergoing PCI, the severity of future ischaemic events may be partially mediated by the location of the stent, but most post-PCI ischaemic events are not in the previously stented vessel.[53]

The best approximation of the evidence therefore requires several assumptions about the relative effect of bleeding and ischaemic events on clearly patient-centred outcomes like all-cause death and quality of life. Because major bleeding and recurrent MI have similar effects on quality of life and prognosis,[19–21,54] and because bleeding occurs with greater frequency, double antithrombotic therapy with NOAC plus a $P2Y_{12}$ inhibitor is the optimal strategy for prevention of ischaemic events while limiting excess bleeding at the population level.[52] However, for individual patients, the relative importance of bleeding and ischaemic events may differ based on patient preferences, details of anatomy, and other factors, highlighting the importance of shared decision-making in this patient population.

Best practices for percutaneous coronary intervention in patients with atrial fibrillation—guideline recommendations and beyond

Consistent with the results of WOEST, PIONEER AF PCI, RE-DUAL PCI, ENTRUST AF-PCI, AUGUSTUS, and MASTER DAPT, the 2021 American College of Cardiology (ACC)/American Heart Association (AHA) guideline for coronary artery revascularization recommends treating patients with AF who undergo PCI with triple therapy (OAC, $P2Y_{12}$ inhibitor, and aspirin) for 1–4 weeks followed by OAC plus $P2Y_{12}$ inhibitor (without aspirin) for 6–12 months [class I, level of evidence (LOE) B].[55] The guideline gives a weaker recommendation, based on AUGUSTUS, in favour of a NOAC over warfarin (class 2A, LOE B). Similarly, the 2020 European Society (ESC) Guideline for the diagnosis and management of AF recommends early cessation of aspirin (≤1 week) after PCI in patients with AF followed by 6 months of OAC plus $P2Y_{12}$ inhibitor in patients undergoing PCI for chronic coronary syndromes and 12 months of anticoagulation plus $P2Y_{12}$ inhibitor in patients with ACS (class I, LOE A).[56] Longer-term triple antithrombotic therapy can be considered when the risk of stent thrombosis outweighs the risk of bleeding (class IIA, LOE C). The ESC Guideline gives a strong recommendation in favour of NOACs in preference to warfarin in patients with AF who undergo PCI and do not have a mechanical valve or severe mitral stenosis (class I, LOE A). The 2021 North American Consensus on the management of antithrombotic therapy in patients with AF undergoing PCI largely mirrors the ESC guideline: it recommends stopping aspirin at the time of hospital discharge or up to 1 week after PCI, choosing a NOAC in preference to warfarin in the absence of contraindications, and continuing a NOAC plus $P2Y_{12}$ inhibitor for 1 year after PCI.[57] It allows that triple antithrombotic therapy may be continued for up to 30 days in patients at particularly high thrombotic risk and acceptably low bleeding risk. It also recommends clopidogrel in preference to other $P2Y_{12}$ inhibitors in this cohort of patients, while allowing that ticagrelor may be used in patients at low bleeding risk.

We agree with these data-driven recommendations, and offer several other best practices (➔ Table 26.2).

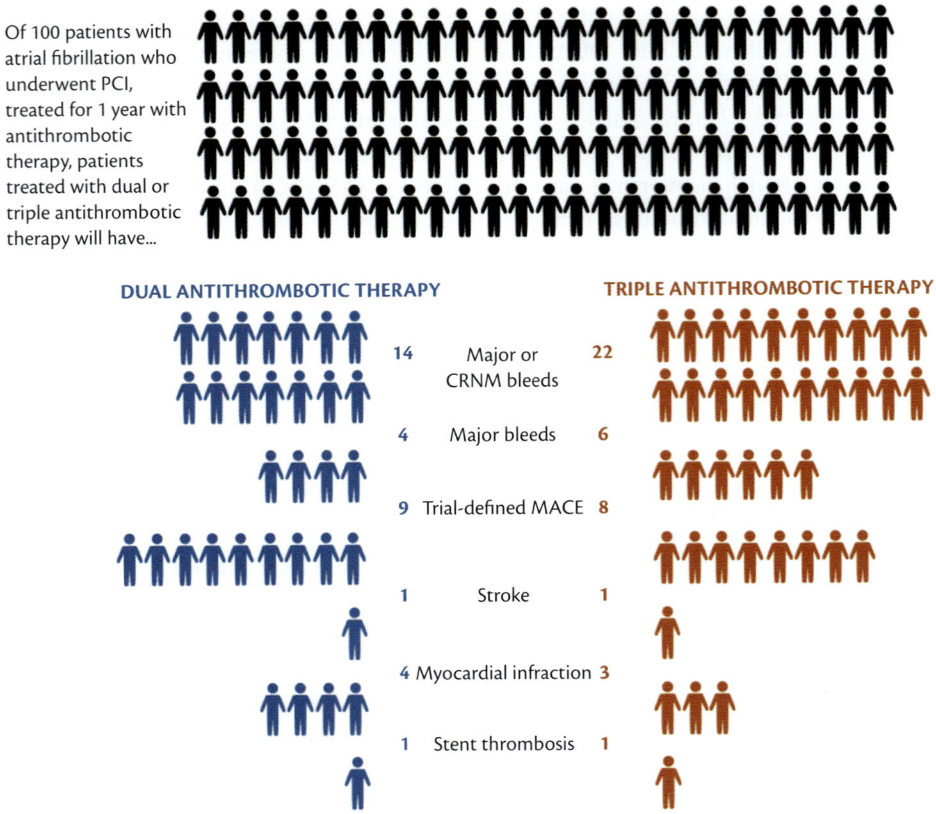

Figure 26.3 Absolute risks of bleeding and ischaemic events with double and triple antithrombotic therapy in patients with atrial fibrillation (AF) undergoing percutaneous coronary intervention (PCI). Across major trials of triple versus double antithrombotic therapy in patients with AF undergoing PCI, double therapy is associated with a 6% absolute reduction in major or clinically relevant non-major bleeding (CRNMB) and a 2% reduction in major bleeding compared with triple therapy, with a smaller (1%) absolute increase in trial-defined major adverse cardiovascular events (MACE) and myocardial infarction.

Reproduced from De Caterina R, Agewall S, Andreotti F, et al. Great debate: triple antithrombotic therapy in patients with atrial fibrillation undergoing coronary stenting should be limited to 1 week. Eur Heart J. 2022 Oct 7;43(37):3512–3527. doi: 10.1093/eurheartj/ehac294 with permission from Oxford University Press.

First, especially among patients whose indication for PCI is chronic coronary syndrome, it is reasonable to consider not performing PCI at all. Performing PCI in patients with AF necessitates temporary escalation of antithrombotic therapy with attendant increased risks of bleeding,[25,31] and coronary revascularization performed in patients with chronic coronary syndromes does not reduce the incidence of death or MI compared with medical therapy.[58,59] These facts should be considered when deciding whether to perform PCI at all in patients with AF, and incorporated in a shared decision-making process. Second, in patients with AF who ultimately do undergo PCI, operators should use drug-eluting stents, and not bare metal stents. Though early-generation drug-eluting stents had long delays to endothelialization requiring longer-term antiplatelet treatment, 70% of contemporary drug-eluting stent struts were covered within 2 weeks of PCI and up to 93% were covered within 1 month.[60–62] In clinical trials, contemporary drug-eluting stents reduced the risk of stent thrombosis and target vessel revascularization compared with

Table 26.2 Best practices for performing percutaneous coronary intervention in patients with atrial fibrillation

Pre-procedure	◆ Maximize medical therapy, especially antianginal therapy, prior to performing PCI in patients with chronic coronary syndrome
Intra-procedure	◆ Use latest generation drug-eluting stents ◆ Use intravascular imaging to optimize stent size, expansion, and apposition, and to identify rare stent-related complications ◆ Manage intraprocedural antithrombotic therapy per usual with loading doses of aspirin and $P2Y_{12}$ inhibitor, and anticoagulation with heparin, low-molecular-weight heparin, or bivalirudin
Post-procedure	◆ Continue triple antithrombotic therapy with aspirin, $P2Y_{12}$ inhibitor, and oral anticoagulation for ≤7 days after PCI ◆ Clopidogrel should be used preferentially to other $P2Y_{12}$ inhibitors ◆ NOACs should be used preferentially to warfarin in patients for whom these agents are indicated ◆ Stop aspirin ≤7 days after PCI and continue antithrombotic therapy with a NOAC (in appropriate patients) plus clopidogrel for 6–12 months ◆ After 6–12 months, stop clopidogrel and continue NOAC alone for long-term thromboprophylaxis

NOAC, non-vitamin K antagonist oral anticoagulant; PCI, percutaneous coronary intervention.

bare metal stents.[63,64] Lastly, PCI operators should seek to optimize stent sizing and placement through the use of intravascular imaging. In a meta-analysis of nine randomized controlled trials, intravenous ultrasound guidance, compared with angiography alone, reduced major adverse cardiac events by 40% and definite/probable stent thrombosis by 55%.[65] For patients with AF undergoing PCI, optimizing stent placement is critical, since underexpanded or mal-apposed stents are more likely to thrombose,[66] perhaps especially in patients receiving guideline-directed single antiplatelet therapy.

Unanswered questions

Despite multiple randomized controlled trials that have established double antithrombotic therapy with a NOAC plus $P2Y_{12}$ inhibitor as the standard of care for patients with AF undergoing PCI, multiple questions remain.

- Nearly all patients in major clinical trials enrolling patients with AF undergoing PCI were treated with clopidogrel. Is there a role for the more potent $P2Y_{12}$ inhibitors in this population?
- Though clinical trials have evaluated many potential antithrombotic strategies, there are literally thousands of combinations that have not been tested. Some of the more promising ones include stopping OAC for 1 month after PCI and treating with DAPT (including a high-potency $P2Y_{12}$ inhibitor) alone, and not starting antiplatelet therapy at all after PCI and managing patients with OAC alone. Are one of these strategies superior to double antithrombotic therapy with OAC and a $P2Y_{12}$ inhibitor?
- A subset of patients will have multiple recurrent ischaemic events over long-term follow-up, necessitating multiple rounds of escalated antithrombotic therapy with the attendant increased risk of bleeding.[66] Is it possible to identify these patients early and consider non-pharmacological methods of stroke prophylaxis, like percutaneous or surgical left atrial appendage occlusion?
- Lastly, advances in both PCI and stroke prophylaxis in AF (both pharmacological and non-pharmacological) will need to be evaluated in this special population. How should next-generation stents and bioresorbable scaffolds, novel antithrombotic agents (including factor XIa inhibitors), and novel techniques for surgical and percutaneous left atrial appendage exclusion be used in patients with AF undergoing PCI?

Conclusion

Patients with AF undergoing PCI represent a subgroup at high risk for bleeding events because they have strong, evidence-based indications for OAC as well as DAPT with aspirin and a $P2Y_{12}$ inhibitor, but the combination of these three agents is associated with unacceptably high rates of bleeding. Randomized controlled trials have established double antithrombotic therapy with a NOAC plus clopidogrel, with aspirin continued for 7–30 days following PCI, as the 'sweet spot' strategy which prevents recurrent ischaemic events to a similar extent as triple antithrombotic therapy with a dramatically lower incidence of major bleeding. For that reason, consensus guidelines recommend this antithrombotic strategy. However, when faced with patients with AF and a potential indication for PCI, it is important to consider the indication for PCI carefully, as even double antithrombotic therapy carries a greater risk of major and clinically relevant bleeding than OAC alone, and to ensure that PCI is performed optimally with latest-generation drug-eluting stents and image guidance to reduce the risk of stent failure.

What's new

- Though so-called triple antithrombotic therapy with OAC, aspirin, and a $P2Y_{12}$ inhibitor is indicated for patients with AF who undergo PCI, rates of hospitalization for major bleeding approach 10% in patients treated with this combination.
- Five major clinical trials conducted in patients with AF who underwent PCI have demonstrated that the combination of a NOAC plus $P2Y_{12}$ inhibitor represents the 'sweet spot' for limiting major bleeding while preventing stroke, stent thrombosis, and MI.
- Together, these trials indicate that the combination of NOAC plus $P2Y_{12}$ inhibitor reduces the risk of major bleeding by 48% compared with warfarin-based triple therapy, with no significant effect on ischaemic events; with more than 16,000 patients enrolled across the five major clinical trials, it is possible to exclude the possibility that triple therapy reduces the relative risk of ischaemic events by more than 20% compared with double therapy.
- Secondary analyses of these trials have failed to identify a subgroup of patients who benefits from longer-term triple therapy, and consensus guidelines recommend a short (<30 days) period of triple therapy followed by 6–12 months of double therapy in most patients with AF who undergo PCI.

Guideline recommendations

- In AF patients with ACS undergoing an uncomplicated PCI, early cessation (≤1 week) of aspirin and continuation of dual therapy with an OAC and a $P2Y_{12}$ inhibitor (preferably clopidogrel) for up to 12 months is recommended if the risk of stent thrombosis is low or if concerns about bleeding risk prevail over concerns about stent thrombosis, irrespective of the type of stent used (class I, LOE A).[56]
- Triple therapy with aspirin, clopidogrel, and an OAC for longer than 1 week after an ACS should be considered when risk of stent thrombosis outweighs the bleeding risk, with the total duration (≤1 month) decided according to assessment of these risks, and the treatment plan should be clearly specified at hospital discharge (class IIa, LOE C).[56]

- After uncomplicated PCI, early cessation (≤1 week) of aspirin and continuation of dual therapy with OAC and clopidogrel for up to 6 months is recommended if the risk of stent thrombosis is low or if concerns about bleeding risk prevail over concerns about stent thrombosis, irrespective of the type of stent used (class I, LOE A).[56]
- Triple therapy with aspirin, clopidogrel, and an OAC for longer than 1 week should be considered when risk of stent thrombosis outweighs the bleeding risk, with the total duration (≤1 month) decided according to assessment of these risks, and the treatment plan should be clearly specified at hospital discharge (class IIa, LOE C).[56]
- In AF patients eligible for NOACs, it is recommended to use a NOAC in preference to a warfarin in combination with antiplatelet therapy (class I, LOE A).[56]
- In patients at high bleeding risk (HAS-BLED ≥3), rivaroxaban 15 mg daily should be considered in preference to rivaroxaban 20 mg daily for the duration of concomitant single or DAPT, to mitigate bleeding risk (class IIa, LOE B).[56]
- In patients at high bleeding risk (HAS-BLED ≥3), dabigatran 110 mg twice daily should be considered in preference to dabigatran 150 mg twice daily for the duration of concomitant single or DAPT, to mitigate bleeding risk (class IIa, LOE B).[56]
- In AF patients with an indication for warfarin in combination with antiplatelet therapy, the warfarin dosing should be carefully regulated with a target INR of 2.0–2.5 and time in therapeutic range of 70% or more.[56]

What's next

- How will the role of device-based therapies for stroke prophylaxis evolve as successive iterations of these devices become safer and more effective?
- Factor XIa inhibitors have demonstrated a favourable safety profile compared with Xa inhibitors for stroke prophylaxis in patients with AF. What will their role be in patients with AF who undergo PCI, and which antiplatelet agents should they be combined with?
- Is there a role for more potent $P2Y_{12}$ inhibitors in patients with AF who undergo PCI, either in combination with OACs or during a short post-PCI anticoagulation holiday?
- Is it possible to further personalize antithrombotic therapy after PCI in patients with AF, such that intensity of antithrombotic therapy can be tailored to an individual's risk of bleeding and ischaemic events? Might strategies not yet tested in major clinical trials (continuation of anticoagulation without antiplatelet therapy, potent DAPT without anticoagulation, non-pharmacological stroke prophylaxis plus DAPT) be optimal in certain patient populations?

References

1. Virani SS, Alonso A, Benjamin EJ, et al. Heart disease and stroke statistics—2020 update: a report from the American Heart Association. Circulation. 2020;141(9):e139–596.
2. Go AS, Hylek EM, Phillips KA, et al. Prevalence of diagnosed atrial fibrillation in adults: national implications for rhythm management and stroke prevention: the AnTicoagulation and Risk Factors In Atrial Fibrillation (ATRIA) Study. JAMA. 2001;285(18):2370.
3. Kornej J, Börschel CS, Benjamin EJ, Schnabel RB. Epidemiology of atrial fibrillation in the 21st century: novel methods and new insights. Circ Res. 2020;127(1):4–20.
4. Fosbol EL, Wang TY, Li S, et al. Safety and effectiveness of antithrombotic strategies in older adult patients with atrial fibrillation and non–ST elevation myocardial infarction. Am Heart J. 2012;163(4):720–8.
5. Ruff CT, Bhatt DL, Steg PHG, et al. Long-term cardiovascular outcomes in patients with atrial fibrillation and atherothrombosis in the REACH Registry. Int J Cardiol. 2014;170(3):413–18.
6. Morita Y, Hamaguchi T, Yamaji Y, et al. Temporal trends in prevalence and outcomes of atrial fibrillation in patients undergoing percutaneous coronary intervention. Clin Cardiol. 2019;43(1):33–42.
7. Capodanno D, Huber K, Mehran R, et al. Management of antithrombotic therapy in atrial fibrillation patients undergoing PCI: JACC state-of-the-art review. J Am Coll Cardiol. 2019;74(1):83–99.
8. Boston Area Anticoagulation Trial for Atrial Fibrillation Investigators, Singer DE, Hughes RA, et al. The effect of low-dose warfarin on the risk of stroke in patients with nonrheumatic atrial fibrillation. N Engl J Med. 1990;323(22):1505–11.
9. Stroke Prevention in Atrial Fibrillation Study. Final results. Circulation. 1991;84(2):527–39.
10. Connolly SJ, Laupacis A, Gent M, Roberts RS, Cairns JA, Joyner C. Canadian Atrial Fibrillation Anticoagulation (CAFA) study. J Am Coll Cardiol. 1991;18(2):349–55.
11. Ezekowitz MD, Bridgers SL, James KE, et al. Warfarin in the prevention of stroke associated with nonrheumatic atrial fibrillation. Veterans Affairs Stroke Prevention in Nonrheumatic Atrial Fibrillation Investigators. N Engl J Med. 1992;327(20):1406–12.
12. Petersen P, Godtfredsen J, Boysen G, Andersen E, Andersen B. Placebo-controlled, randomised trial of warfarin and aspirin for prevention of thromboembolic complications in chronic atrial fibrillation: the Copenhagen AFASAK study. Lancet. 1989;333(8631):175–9.
13. EAFT (European Atrial Fibrillation Trial) Study Group. Secondary prevention in non-rheumatic atrial fibrillation after transient ischaemic attack or minor stroke. Lancet. 1993;342(8882):1255–62.
14. Hart RG, Pearce LA, Aguilar MI. Meta-analysis: antithrombotic therapy to prevent stroke in patients who have nonvalvular atrial fibrillation. Ann Intern Med. 2007;146(12):857–67.
15. Leon MB, Baim DS, Popma JJ, et al. A clinical trial comparing three antithrombotic-drug regimens after coronary-artery stenting. N Engl J Med. 1998;339(23):1665–71.
16. Lamberts M, Gislason GH, Olesen JB, et al. Oral anticoagulation and antiplatelets in atrial fibrillation patients after myocardial infarction and coronary intervention. J Am Coll Cardiol. 2013;62(11):981–9.

17. van Rein N, Heide-Jørgensen U, Lijfering Willem M, et al. Major bleeding rates in atrial fibrillation patients on single, dual, or triple antithrombotic therapy. Circulation. 2019;139(6):775–86.
18. Lamberts M, Gislason GH, Lip GYH, et al. Antiplatelet therapy for stable coronary artery disease in atrial fibrillation patients taking an oral anticoagulant: a nationwide cohort study. Circulation. 2014;129(15):1577–85.
19. Lewis EF, Li Y, Pfeffer MA, et al. Impact of cardiovascular events on change in quality of life and utilities in patients after myocardial infarction: a VALIANT study (valsartan in acute myocardial infarction). JACC Heart Fail. 2014;2(2):159–65.
20. Amin AP, Wang TY, McCoy L, et al. Impact of bleeding on quality of life in patients on DAPT: insights from TRANSLATE-ACS. J Am Coll Cardiol. 2016;67(1):59–65.
21. Mehran R, Pocock SJ, Stone GW, et al. Associations of major bleeding and myocardial infarction with the incidence and timing of mortality in patients presenting with non-ST-elevation acute coronary syndromes: a risk model from the ACUITY trial. Eur Heart J. 2009;30(12):1457–66.
22. Dewilde WJM, Oirbans T, Verheugt FWA, et al. Use of clopidogrel with or without aspirin in patients taking oral anticoagulant therapy and undergoing percutaneous coronary intervention: an open-label, randomised, controlled trial. Lancet. 2013;381(9872):1107–15.
23. Gibson CM, Mehran R, Bode C, et al. An open-label, randomized, controlled, multicenter study exploring two treatment strategies of rivaroxaban and a dose-adjusted oral vitamin k antagonist treatment strategy in subjects with atrial fibrillation who undergo percutaneous coronary intervention (PIONEER AF-PCI). Am Heart J. 2015;169(4):472–8.
24. Connolly SJ, Ezekowitz MD, Yusuf S, et al. Dabigatran versus warfarin in patients with atrial fibrillation. N Engl J Med. 2009;361(12):1139–51.
25. Granger CB, Alexander JH, McMurray JJ, et al. Apixaban versus warfarin in patients with atrial fibrillation. N Engl J Med. 2011;365(11):981–92.
26. Patel MR, Mahaffey KW, Garg J, et al. Rivaroxaban versus warfarin in nonvalvular atrial fibrillation. N Engl J Med. 2011;365(10):883–91.
27. Giugliano RP, Ruff CT, Braunwald E, et al. Edoxaban versus warfarin in patients with atrial fibrillation. N Engl J Med. 2013;369(22):2093–104.
28. Gibson CM, Mehran R, Bode C, et al. Prevention of bleeding in patients with atrial fibrillation undergoing PCI. N Engl J Med. 2016;375(25):2423–34.
29. Cannon CP, Bhatt DL, Oldgren J, et al. Dual antithrombotic therapy with dabigatran after PCI in atrial fibrillation. N Engl J Med. 2017 19;377(16):1513–24.
30. Vranckx P, Valgimigli M, Eckardt L, et al. Edoxaban-based versus vitamin K antagonist-based antithrombotic regimen after successful coronary stenting in patients with atrial fibrillation (ENTRUST-AF PCI): a randomised, open-label, phase 3b trial. Lancet. 2019;394(10206):1335–43.
31. Lopes RD, Heizer G, Aronson R, et al. Antithrombotic therapy after acute coronary syndrome or PCI in atrial fibrillation. N Engl J Med. 2019;380(16):1509–24.
32. Valgimigli M, Frigoli E, Heg D, et al. Dual antiplatelet therapy after PCI in patients at high bleeding risk. N Engl J Med. 2021;385(18):1643–55.
33. Fiedler KA, Maeng M, Mehilli J, et al. Duration of triple therapy in patients requiring oral anticoagulation after drug-eluting stent implantation: the ISAR-TRIPLE trial. J Am Coll Cardiol. 2015;65(16):1619–29.
34. Hoshi T, Sato A, Hiraya D, et al. Short-duration triple antithrombotic therapy for atrial fibrillation patients who require coronary stenting: results of the SAFE-A study. EuroIntervention. 2020;16(2):e164–72.
35. Lopes RD, Hong H, Harskamp RE, et al. Optimal antithrombotic regimens for patients with atrial fibrillation undergoing percutaneous coronary intervention: an updated network meta-analysis. JAMA Cardiol. 2020;5(5):1–8.
36. Capodanno D, Di Maio M, Greco A, et al. Safety and efficacy of double antithrombotic therapy with non-vitamin K antagonist oral anticoagulants in patients with atrial fibrillation undergoing percutaneous coronary intervention: a systematic review and meta-analysis. J Am Heart Assoc. 2020;9(16):e017212.
37. Galli M, Andreotti F, D'Amario D, Porto I, Crea F. Stent thrombosis with dual antithrombotic therapy in atrial fibrillation—ACS/PCI trials. J Am Coll Cardiol. 2020;75(14):1727–8.
38. Galli M, Andreotti F, Porto I, Crea F. Intracranial haemorrhages vs. stent thromboses with direct oral anticoagulant plus single antiplatelet agent or triple antithrombotic therapy: a meta-analysis of randomized trials in atrial fibrillation and percutaneous coronary intervention/acute coronary syndrome patients. EP Europace. 2020;22(4):538–46.
39. Vranckx P, Valgimigli M, Eckardt L, et al. Edoxaban in atrial fibrillation patients with percutaneous coronary intervention by acute or chronic coronary syndrome presentation: a pre-specified analysis of the ENTRUST-AF PCI trial. Eur Heart J. 2020;41(47):4497–504.
40. Zeymer U, Leiva O, Hohnloser SH, et al. Dual antithrombotic therapy with dabigatran in patients with atrial fibrillation after percutaneous coronary intervention for ST elevation myocardial infarction: results from the randomised RE-DUAL PCI trial. EuroIntervention. 2021;17(6):474–80.
41. Kerneis M, Gibson CM, Chi G, et al. Effect of procedure and coronary lesion characteristics on clinical outcomes among atrial fibrillation patients undergoing percutaneous coronary intervention: insights from the PIONEER AF-PCI trial. JACC Cardiovasc Interv. 2018;11(7):626–34.
42. Berry NC, Mauri L, Steg PG, et al. Effect of lesion complexity and clinical risk factors on the efficacy and safety of dabigatran dual therapy versus warfarin triple therapy in atrial fibrillation after percutaneous coronary intervention: a subgroup analysis from the REDUAL PCI trial. Circ Cardiovasc Interv. 2020;13(4):e008349.
43. Lip GYH, Mauri L, Montalescot G, et al. Relationship of stroke and bleeding risk profiles to efficacy and safety of dabigatran dual therapy versus warfarin triple therapy in atrial fibrillation after percutaneous coronary intervention: an ancillary analysis from the RE-DUAL PCI trial. Am Heart J. 2019;212:13–22.
44. Hohnloser SH, Steg PG, Oldgren J, et al. Renal function and outcomes with dabigatran dual antithrombotic therapy in atrial fibrillation patients after PCI. JACC Cardiovasc Interv. 2019;12(16):1553–61.
45. Maeng M, Steg PG, Bhatt DL, et al. Dabigatran dual therapy versus warfarin triple therapy post-PCI in patients with atrial fibrillation and diabetes. JACC Cardiovasc Interv. 2019;12(23):2346–55.
46. Nicolau JC, Bhatt DL, Hohnloser SH, et al. Dabigatran dual therapy vs warfarin triple therapy post-percutaneous coronary intervention in patients with atrial fibrillation with/without a proton pump inhibitor: a pre-specified analysis of the RE-DUAL PCI trial. Drugs. 2020;80(10):995–1005.
47. Costa F, Valgimigli M, Steg PG, et al. Antithrombotic therapy according to baseline bleeding risk in patients with atrial fibrillation undergoing percutaneous coronary intervention: applying the PRECISE-DAPT score in RE-DUAL PCI. Eur Heart J Cardiovasc Pharmacother. 2020;8(3):216–26.

48. Harskamp RE, Fanaroff AC, Lopes RD, et al. Antithrombotic therapy in patients with atrial fibrillation after acute coronary syndromes or percutaneous intervention. J Am Coll Cardiol. 2022;79(5):417–27.
49. Fudim M, Wojdyla DM, Alexander JH, et al. Efficacy and safety of antithrombotic therapy in patients with atrial fibrillation, recent acute coronary syndrome, or percutaneous coronary intervention and a history of heart failure: insights from the AUGUSTUS trial. J Am Heart Assoc. 2021;10(24):e023143.
50. Alexander JH, Wojdyla D, Vora AN, et al. Risk/benefit tradeoff of antithrombotic therapy in patients with atrial fibrillation early and late after an acute coronary syndrome or percutaneous coronary intervention: insights from AUGUSTUS. Circulation. 2020;141(20):1618–27.
51. Fanaroff AC, Hasselblad V, Roe MT, et al. Antithrombotic agents for secondary prevention after acute coronary syndromes: a systematic review and network meta-analysis. Int J Cardiol. 2017;214:87–96.
52. De Caterina R, Agewall S, Andreotti F, et al. Great debate: triple antithrombotic therapy in patients with atrial fibrillation undergoing coronary stenting should be limited to 1 week. Eur Heart J. 2022;43(37):3512–27.
53. Mauri L, Kereiakes DJ, Yeh RW, et al. Twelve or 30 months of dual antiplatelet therapy after drug-eluting stents. N Engl J Med. 2014;371(23):2155–66.
54. Mehran R, Pocock S, Nikolsky E, et al. Impact of bleeding on mortality after percutaneous coronary intervention results from a patient-level pooled analysis of the REPLACE-2 (randomized evaluation of PCI linking angiomax to reduced clinical events), ACUITY (acute catheterization and urgent intervention triage strategy), and HORIZONS-AMI (harmonizing outcomes with revascularization and stents in acute myocardial infarction) trials. JACC Cardiovasc Interv. 2011;4(6):654–64.
55. Lawton JS, Tamis-Holland JE, Bangalore S, et al. 2021 ACC/AHA/SCAI guideline for coronary artery revascularization. J Am Coll Cardiol. 2022;79(2):e21–129.
56. Hindricks G, Potpara T, Dagres N, et al. 2020 ESC Guidelines for the diagnosis and management of atrial fibrillation developed in collaboration with the European Association for Cardio-Thoracic Surgery (EACTS): the Task Force for the diagnosis and management of atrial fibrillation of the European Society of Cardiology (ESC) Developed with the special contribution of the European Heart Rhythm Association (EHRA) of the ESC. Eur Heart J. 2021;42(5):373–498.
57. Angiolillo DJ, Bhatt DL, Cannon CP, et al. Antithrombotic therapy in patients with atrial fibrillation treated with oral anticoagulation undergoing percutaneous coronary intervention: a North American perspective: 2021 update. Circulation. 2021;143(6):583–96.
58. Boden WE, O'Rourke RA, Teo KK, et al. Optimal medical therapy with or without PCI for stable coronary disease. N Engl J Med. 2007;356(15):1503–16.
59. Maron DJ, Hochman JS, Reynolds HR, et al. Initial invasive or conservative strategy for stable coronary disease. N Engl J Med. 2020;382(15):1395–407.
60. Oishi Y, Tsujita H, Ogura K, et al. Early vascular response to ultrathin biodegradable polymer sirolimus-eluting stents for the treatment of ST-elevation myocardial infarction after plaque rupture. Int Heart J. 2021;62(1):42–9.
61. Ogura K, Tsujita H, Oishi Y, et al. Early vascular healing following bioresorbable-polymer sirolimus-eluting stent placement compared to that with durable-polymer everolimus-eluting stent. Int Heart J. 2021;62(3):510–19.
62. Miura T, Ueki Y, Senda K, et al. Early vascular response of ultra-thin bioresorbable polymer sirolimus-eluting stents assessed by optical frequency domain imaging: the EVALUATION study. Cardiovasc Interv Ther. 2021;36(3):281–8.
63. Shah R, Rao SV, Latham SB, Kandzari DE. Efficacy and safety of drug-eluting stents optimized for biocompatibility vs bare-metal stents with a single month of dual antiplatelet therapy: a meta-analysis. JAMA Cardiol. 2018;3(11):1050–9.
64. Piccolo R, Bonaa KH, Efthimiou O, et al. Drug-eluting or bare-metal stents for percutaneous coronary intervention: a systematic review and individual patient data meta-analysis of randomised clinical trials. Lancet. 2019;393(10190):2503–10.
65. Gao XF, Wang ZM, Wang F, et al. Intravascular ultrasound guidance reduces cardiac death and coronary revascularization in patients undergoing drug-eluting stent implantation: results from a meta-analysis of 9 randomized trials and 4724 patients. Int J Cardiovasc Imaging. 2019;35(2):239–47.
66. Nissen SE, Yock P. Intravascular ultrasound: novel pathophysiological insights and current clinical applications. Circulation. 2001;103(4):604–16.
67. Fanaroff AC, Li S, Marquis-Gravel G, et al. Atrial fibrillation and coronary artery disease: a long-term perspective on the need for combined antithrombotic therapy. Circ Cardiovasc Interv. 2021;14(12):e011232.

CHAPTER 27

Prevention and treatment of venous and arterial thrombosis in patients with specific conditions: diabetes, renal insufficiency, thrombophilia, and pregnancy

Stefan Agewall, Vanessa Roldán, and Francisco Marín

Contents

Summary

There are special populations that require specific preventive and therapeutic measures, either because of increased thrombotic risk, like diabetes mellitus or thrombophilia, or because they need an adaptation of the treatment to their characteristics, such as renal impairment or pregnancy. The dosing of some antithrombotic drugs is highly dependent on renal function so dosages should be adjusted. Several antithrombotics are contraindicated in pregnancy. The relationships between antithrombotic therapy and these clinical conditions are developed in this chapter.

Introduction

Cardiovascular disease is a major cause of morbidity and mortality worldwide, with the lifetime risk exceeding 60%. Thrombosis is a major complication of cardiovascular disease, leading to myocardial infarction (MI), acute ischaemic stroke, or venous thromboembolism (VTE). Rates differ among age groups and sex, and different clinical conditions. Management of cardiovascular disease varies based on this heterogeneity.

Diabetes mellitus

Epidemiology

Patients with diabetes mellitus (DM) have a greater average atherosclerotic plaque burden than patients without DM, and the onset of thromboembolic complications occurs at an earlier age. The prevalence of type 1 and type 2 DM and the frequency of impaired glucose tolerance continues to increase worldwide, mainly associated with the expansion of Western lifestyles.[1] Importantly, this increased prevalence of DM in a population of advancing age and higher comorbidities will confer a complex scenario and is a major health issue. The Emerging Risk Factor Collaboration, a meta-analysis of more than 100 prospective studies, showed that DM (data on DM type were unavailable) confers a double increased risk of cardiovascular events, independent of other risk factors.[2] The Swedish National Diabetes Register has demonstrated the deteriorated cardiovascular prognosis in both types of DM. Age at onset of type 1 DM is an important determinant of survival, as well as all cardiovascular outcomes, with highest excess risk in women.[3] In type 2 DM, the excess risks of death from any cause and cardiovascular death increased with younger age (<55 years), worse glycaemic control, and greater severity of renal complications.[4]

The haemostatic response has an important physiological role in the response to trauma but, if it becomes activated inappropriately, thrombosis can be triggered. The clinical effects of thrombosis arise primarily from its location, such as in the coronary arteries leading to acute coronary syndrome (ACS, including MI and unstable angina), cerebral arteries leading to thrombotic stroke, peripheral arteries leading to acute limb ischaemia or deep limb veins leading to deep vein thrombosis (DVT).

As the European Society of Cardiology (ESC) Guidelines on cardiovascular prevention in clinical practice recognized, the presence of prediabetes, in addition to both types of DM, are independent risk factors for cardiovascular disease.[5] While difficult to completely exclude the effects of confounders such as obesity and hypertension, epidemiological data suggest a causal association between DM and atrial fibrillation (AF), including that poor glycaemic control and longer DM duration increase AF risk.[6] Interestingly, patients with DM presenting with an ACS, more frequently present with non-typical symptoms, more frequently have multifocal coronary stenoses, less frequently receive guideline-indicated care, are treated with significant delay, and have worse clinical outcomes than non-diabetic patients.[7]

The duration of DM and glycaemic control were also associated with AF (each year with DM conferred a 3% increase in the risk of AF), while a haemoglobin A1c (HbA1c) level of greater than 9% was associated with a nearly twofold increase in AF risk.[8] A meta-analysis of 11 studies with more than 100,000 AF cases in 168,6097 subjects showed a 40% greater risk of AF in the presence of DM, but the effect was attenuated after adjustment for multiple risk factors [relative risk (RR) 1.24, 95% confidence interval (CI) 1.06–1.44], while the population-attributable estimate for AF owing to DM was 2.5% (95% CI 0.1–3.9).[9] DM is a recognized risk factor for embolism,[10] and accordingly this variable is included in the CHA_2DS_2-VASc score, the established scheme for embolism stratification in patients with AF. Diabetic patients with a stroke have higher mortality rates than non-diabetic patients[11] and DM was also observed to be associated with an increased risk for major bleeding, although not with intracranial haemorrhage.[10]

While DM is regarded as a weak risk factor for VTE, there are no considerations relating to DM and the usual clinical guidelines for non-DM individuals should generally be followed.

Mechanisms and risk factors

There are clear links between pathological processes associated with DM and those responsible for atherogenesis and thrombosis, including inflammation, platelet activation, and coagulation, that are summarized in ➔ Figure 27.1. Alongside control of glucose levels and optimization of other risk factors, such as dyslipidaemia, hypertension, and smoking cessation, antithrombotic therapy, including antiplatelet therapy and oral anticoagulation, has become a key component of the treatment and prevention of atherothrombotic and cardioembolic events.

Insulin resistance and hyperglycaemia are associated with a cluster of risk factors that result in endothelial dysfunction. Endothelial dysfunction causes endothelial cells to express adhesion molecules, thus attracting inflammatory cells, and increases intercellular permeability, resulting in accumulation of lipoproteins and inflammatory cells within the vessel wall. Increased inflammatory cytokines, including tumour necrosis factor α and interleukin 6, impairs production of the vasodilatory molecule nitric oxide (NO) and modulates activation of PI3K/Akt pathways, further accelerating atherothrombosis in DM. Increased production of advanced glycation end product and formation of reactive oxygen species diminishes endothelial-derived NO and leads to enhanced synthesis of vasoconstrictory prostanoids and endothelin.[12]

DM is associated with increased tissue factor (TF) expression which activates thrombin,[13] converting fibrinogen into fibrin. Increased cellular synthesis of plasminogen activator inhibitor-1 (PAI-1) and fibrinogen, and reduced production of tissue plasminogen activator (tPA), will augment the developing fibrin structure. It has become evident that the fat-laden insulin-resistant adipocyte generates PAI-1, strengthening the link between DM and suppression of fibrinolysis. An upregulation of glycoproteins Ib and IIb/IIIa was observed in patients with DM, and this may trigger thrombus formation via interaction with von Willebrand factor and fibrin molecules.[14] The result is that thrombin generation is increased in individuals with type 1 or type 2 DM.[15]

Preventive measures

As ESC Guidelines on cardiovascular prevention in clinical practice recommend, lifestyle management is a priority for cardiovascular disease prevention and management of DM.[5] Smoking cessation, weight control, and adoption of a healthy lifestyle are recommended for all patients with type 2 DM, and risk factor treatment should be considered in all people with DM, at least those above the age of 40 years. Cardiovascular disease stratification in persons with type 1 DM may be based on the same risk

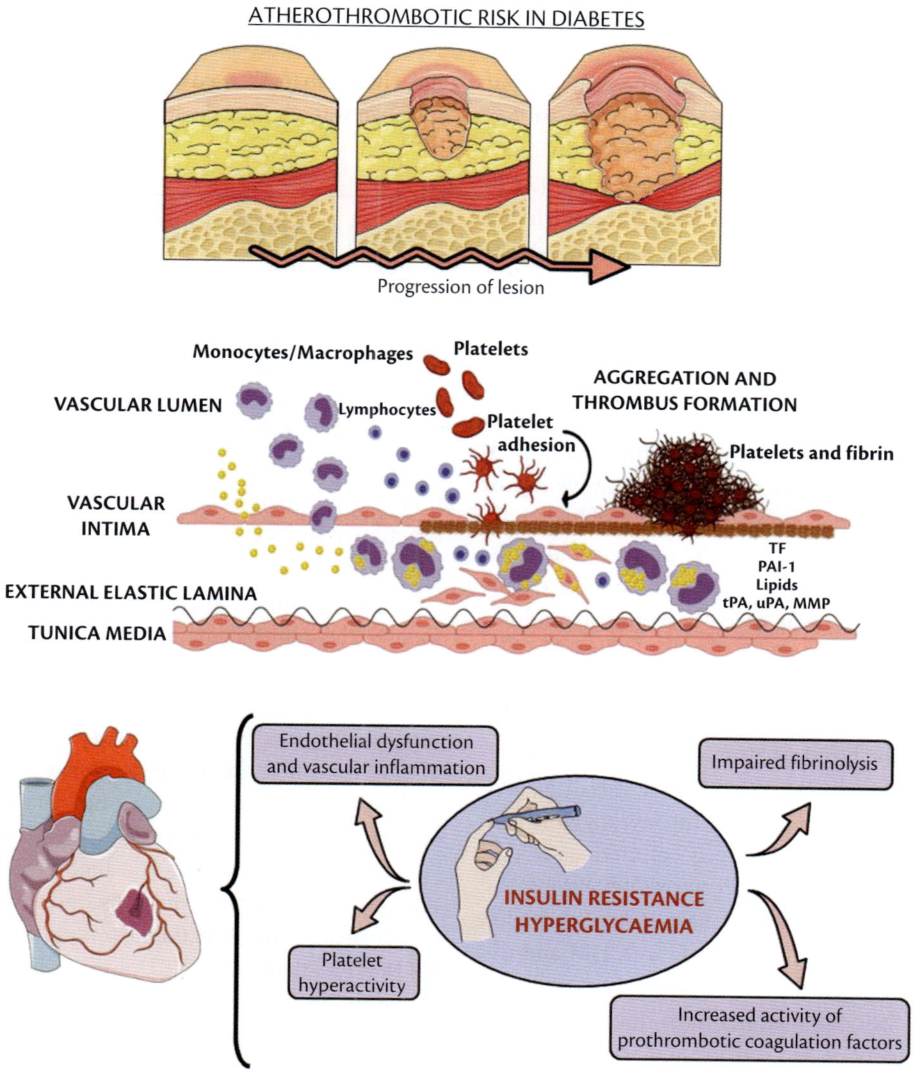

Figure 27.1 Mechanisms of atherothrombosis in diabetic patients. The underlying mechanisms for the high risk of atherothrombotic events in diabetic patients are multifactorial and mainly promoted by insulin resistance and hyperglycaemia, which enable and directly contribute to a proinflammatory and prothrombotic environment. Endothelial dysfunction and damage due to chronic inflammatory response lead to platelet hyperactivity. In addition, enhanced activity or raised plasma levels of prothrombotic coagulation factors (including tissue factor (TF), factor VII, von Willebrand factor, factor VIII, and fibrinogen), increases the risk of thrombosis. This results in very compact fibrin networks with stronger resistance to fibrinolysis, which is the cornerstone of the blood clot in these patients. MMP, matrix metalloproteinase; PAI, plasminogen activator inhibitor; tPA, tissue plasminogen activator; uPA, urokinase plasminogen activator.

classification as for type 2 DM, although the level of evidence for type 1 DM is weaker. A Mediterranean-type diet, where fat sources are derived primarily from monounsaturated oils, may be protective against cardiovascular disease.[5] A combination of aerobic and resistance exercise training is effective in preventing the progression of type 2 DM and for the control of glycaemia.

In the most recent ESC Guidelines, the use of a sodium–glucose co-transporter 2 (SGLT2) inhibitor is recommended in those patients with cardiovascular disease, chronic kidney disease, or heart failure with reduced ejection fraction.[5] These drugs have been demonstrated to improve cardiovascular or cardiorenal outcomes, or even heart failure hospitalizations and cardiovascular events.[5]

In several observational studies, the age-adjusted association of DM with incident AF was no longer significant after multiple adjustments for hypertension, cardiovascular comorbidity, body mass index, or obesity,[9,16] thus suggesting that strategies for AF prevention in DM patients should focus on the control of DM-associated comorbidities (especially the weight and blood pressure control). Intensive glucose lowering (target HbA1c <6.0%) has been associated with similar incident AF rates as less stringent approaches (HbA1c <8.0%), but with increased risk of death and other cardiovascular events.[17] Since silent AF is not uncommon in diabetic patients, some screening attitudes for AF detection might be proposed.[8]

Treatment

When considering the need for antithrombotic therapy, including in patients with DM, it is helpful first to make a distinction between those with an indication for therapeutic anticoagulation and those without. The most common indication is prevention of cardioembolic stroke in those with current or previous AF. The benefit/risk ratio associated with aspirin use in primary prevention is highly debated, as no trial has shown a clear prognostic benefit, particularly in the post-statin era.[18]

Antithrombotic therapy in several distinct groups with DM but without symptomatic atherosclerotic cardiovascular disease has been investigated in a number of trials. The largest individual-level meta-analysis was performed in 2009 and included 95,000 participants from six trials.[19] In individuals with DM, aspirin led to a 12% proportional reduction in the rate of serious vascular events, but this did not reach statistical significance. However, the point estimate was consistent with the statistically significant benefit of aspirin in the non-DM population and the DM population showed an identical trend. Three further trials have been added to the literature since this meta-analysis was performed. Two, JPAD (n = 2539) and POPADAD (n = 1276), were not adequately powered to draw firm conclusions.[20,21] However, most recently ASCEND provided data from 15,480 individuals with DM but without symptomatic atherosclerotic cardiovascular disease who were randomized to receive aspirin 100 mg once daily or placebo.[22] After a mean follow up of 7.4 years, those randomized to aspirin had a significantly reduced rate of serious vascular events (MI, stroke or transient ischaemic attack, or vascular death excluding intracranial haemorrhage) (RR 0.88, 95% CI 0.79–0.97; P = 0.01). However, major bleeding was significantly more frequent when receiving aspirin (RR 1.24, 95% CI 1.09–1.52; P = 0.003), the majority being gastrointestinal. The investigators concluded that the absolute benefits were largely counterbalanced by the risks, despite a favourable, albeit modest, risk/benefit ratio.

Antiplatelet drugs other than aspirin have not been widely studied for primary prevention in individuals with DM and this remains an area for future research.

In high-risk patients, the combination of low-dose rivaroxaban and aspirin may be beneficial for cardiovascular disease. Two trials, ATLAS-ACS TIMI 51 and COMPASS, explore this potential benefit, with more than 30% of the included patients having DM.[23,24] A similar benefit/risk profile of the aspirin/rivaroxaban arm was observed over aspirin alone in both populations (diabetic vs non-diabetic patients). An aspect of potential interest was the finding that in patients with lower extremity artery disease, adverse limb events plus major amputations were reduced by 46%.

Aspirin plus reduced-dose ticagrelor 60 mg twice daily may be considered for high-risk patients and less than 3 years post MI.[25] The relative risk reduction of major adverse cardiovascular events with ticagrelor was similar in the DM and non-DM cohorts.

Oral anticoagulation has demonstrated its efficacy in the reduction of embolism and mortality in those patients with AF and moderate or high risk of thromboembolism.[26] A meta-analysis of the four large non-vitamin K oral anticoagulant (NOAC) trials found no significant interaction between treatment (NOACs vs warfarin) and DM for systemic embolism or major bleeding.[27] However, there are publications that suggest the benefit of some NOACs compared with warfarin. Indeed, a substudy of the RE-LY trial with dabigatran showed a greater absolute risk reduction in embolic events with dabigatran in diabetic compared with non-diabetic patients,[28] whereas a substudy of ARISTOTLE with apixaban observed a consistent reduction of stroke, mortality, and intracranial bleeding in diabetic patients.[29] In a large observational study exploring oral anticoagulation in diabetic patients with AF, apixaban and rivaroxaban showed a lower risk of thromboembolism and apixaban was associated with a lower risk of major bleeding.[30]

Renal insufficiency

Epidemiology

The current recommended staging of chronic kidney disease (CKD) is based on a classification encompassing cause and severity, as expressed by the level of glomerular filtration rate (GFR) and the level of albuminuria,[31] present for longer than 3 months. The GFR explores only one of the components of excretory function, but is widely accepted as the best overall index of kidney function.[32] The prevalence of CKD is increasing.[33] CKD is an independent risk factor for cardiovascular morbidity and mortality.[34] CKD patients often have other comorbid conditions predisposing them to thrombus formation, such as AF, congestive heart failure, left atrial enlargement, hypertension, and DM. Nevertheless, after adjustment for known cardiovascular risk factors, mortality risk progressively increases with worsening CKD.[35] The phenotype of cardiovascular disease associated with CKD is multifactorial, with arterial stiffening causing heart failure, stroke, arrhythmic sudden death, and premature atherosclerosis.[36]

Patients with CKD are at a high risk of developing incident AF.[37] The presence of AF is also associated with a higher risk of advanced renal functional progression among patients with CKD. AF patients with CKD are at higher risk for embolization. However, this may be related to the higher prevalence of different comorbidities. The presence of impaired renal function was closely related to thrombotic/vascular events, bleeding, and mortality in patients with AF.[38,39] However, in 'real-world' cohorts including a broad range of renal (dys)function and stroke risk, CKD does not independently add to the risk of stroke, beyond established stroke risk prediction rules, such as the CHA_2DS_2-VASc score.[40] Renal impairment (defined as creatinine clearance <50 mL/min) also increases the risk of bleeding, and scores 1 point in the HAS-BLED score for predicting major haemorrhage in patients with AF.[26]

Mechanisms and risk factors

Several mechanisms have been proposed to account for why AF is more common in CKD patients. Activation of the renin–angiotensin–aldosterone system, inflammation, myocardial fibrosis, left atrial enlargement, and diastolic dysfunction are more common in patients with CKD.[41] Patients with CKD have abnormalities in haemostasis, which may contribute to their risk for thrombotic and bleeding complications.[42]

Preventive measures

The presence of CKD should be monitored over time: renal function and albuminuria should be measured at least once a year but more frequently if the patient has a high risk of progression and/or where measurement will impact therapeutic decisions.[32]

During a median of 875 days of follow-up, one-fifth of the patients had significant impairment in renal function. Importantly, normal, or mild renal dysfunction at baseline did not exclude the subsequent development of severe renal dysfunction during the follow-up period.[43]

Treatment

CKD is a frequent comorbidity in patients with ACS and is associated with worse short- and long-term clinical outcomes. Despite this high risk, patients are less frequently selected for an invasive treatment strategy and are less commonly treated with guideline-based medications.[44] The patients with CKD appear to be less likely to be admitted to a coronary care unit and had lower rates of coronary angiography and of revascularization.[44] It has also been suggested that patients with CKD may have an impaired response to clopidogrel, which could not be improved by an increase in the clopidogrel dosage.[45] Indeed, in the Clopidogrel in Unstable Angina to Prevent Recurrent Events (CURE) study,[46] and the Clopidogrel for Reduction of Events During Observation (CREDO) trial,[47] clopidogrel compared with placebo reduced the composite endpoint in the global cohorts, and also in those patients with normal renal function, but these benefits of clopidogrel were not observed in patients with mild or moderate renal dysfunction. Importantly, in a substudy of the PLATO trial, patients with CKD showed a remarkable benefit from ticagrelor compared to clopidogrel with a 23% relative risk reduction of the primary ischaemic endpoint and an even more relevant 4.0% absolute and 28% relative risk reduction of all-cause mortality.[48] These findings may suggest an antiplatelet therapy with ticagrelor in ACS patients with CKD in order to reduce mortality and ischaemic events at the price of a slight excess of bleeding.[49]

In patients with mild/moderate CKD (GFR 30–59 mL/min), present evidence on oral anticoagulation suggests that it can be used safely and confers benefit. In this category of patients, both vitamin K antagonists (VKAs) and NOACs have shown similar efficacy. In most studies on NOACs, their safety profile seems to be at least non-inferior or even superior to VKAs.[41] In a recent systematic review and meta-analysis of five trials, including 13,878 AF patients with moderate CKD, NOAC use was associated with reduced risk of thromboembolism [odds ratio (OR) 0.79, 95% CI 0.67–0.94] and lower incidence of major bleeding (OR 0.74, 95% CI 0.65–0.86)[50] compared with warfarin. In individuals with CKD stage 4 (GFR 15–29 mL/min), all guidelines allow the use of warfarin, although the net benefit of oral anticoagulation has never been prospectively assessed in a randomized trial in this patient population. The evidence on NOACs in patients under dialysis is scarce. A recent meta-analysis showed that oral anticoagulation was not associated with a reduced risk of thromboembolism in patients with AF on long-term dialysis, whereas it was associated with significantly higher bleeding risk.[51] So, given the lack of strong evidence, the decision to anticoagulate and (if so) whether to use a NOAC or VKA in patients with end-stage renal failure or on dialysis requires a high degree of individualization.[52]

It has been observed that a progressive deterioration of renal function is common in anticoagulated patients with VKAs[53] and it has been suggested that dabigatran or rivaroxaban may have a preventive effect in this renal deterioration.[53,54]

Thrombophilia

Definitions

Thrombophilia or hypercoagulable state is defined as the set of situations that generate a predisposition to develop thrombotic phenomena. This propensity may be due to enhancement of elements of the haemostatic system and/or weakening of the anticoagulation systems secondary to acquired and inherited risk factors. The term hereditary thrombophilia is applied when the tendency to suffer from thromboembolic episodes is determined by genetic causes. Today, thrombophilia is considered a multigenic disorder in which the clinical expression depends on interactions between multiple genes. In addition, genetic alterations in one or more genes are often not sufficient by themselves to cause a thrombotic event, and the appearance of thrombosis is linked to a concomitant environmental thrombogenic stimulus.[55]

Routine evaluation of inherited thrombophilia in unselected patients is not justified. Patients with hereditary thrombophilia can be initially identified based on a personal and family history of VTE. The clinical characteristics that define inherited thrombophilia are thrombosis at young age (<50 years) with weak provoked risk factors (minor surgery, oral contraceptives, or immobility) or unprovoked VTE, a strong family history of VTE (especially if there are members affected at a young age), recurrent episodes, or unusual localizations, like splanchnic or cerebral veins.[56] However, it is important to note that the hypothetical identification of a hypercoagulable state infrequently would alter the duration of anticoagulation or prevents VTE-related death. So, any benefit of diagnosis should be weighed against the harms of testing including a lack of improved survival, or inappropriate anticoagulation and undue anxiety in the patient (and/or asymptomatic relatives).[57] In recent years, most clinical practice guidelines have made a great effort to minimize the usefulness of hereditary thrombophilia testing for the management of patients with VTE, since the data on its clinical utility are limited, especially in deciding long-term anticoagulation.[58,59]

Mechanisms and epidemiology

Inherited thrombophilia can be caused by two main mechanisms: the first is the loss of function of endogenous anticoagulants, which include deficiency or dysfunction of antithrombin, protein C, or protein S. The second mechanism is gain of function of procoagulant factors which can be caused by increased synthesis of a normal protein [such as the prothrombin 20210A (PT20210A) mutation] or impaired downregulation of a normal protein [such as the factor V Leiden (FVL) mutation]. The latter mechanism includes the most frequent causes of inherited thrombophilia which are considered as mild or low-risk thrombophilia, whereas deficiencies of endogenous anticoagulants are severe or high-risk thrombophilias.[60] In addition, a familial history of VTE constitutes an important risk factor independently of the presence or not of a genetic thrombophilia. Finally, VTE is a multifactorial disease so the interaction with acquired factors is of huge importance. In addition to ageing, the main acquired thromboembolic risk factors are summarized in ➔ Table 27.1.[61,62]

Special mention should be made of the antiphospholipid syndrome which predisposes to both arterial thrombosis and VTE, as well as obstetric morbidity. The diagnosis is based on the presence of at least one clinical criterion (vascular thrombosis or pregnancy complications) and laboratory criteria (presence of lupus anticoagulant, anticardiolipin or anti-beta 2-glycoprotein antibodies, or immunoglobulin (Ig)-G or IgM).[63] Regarding arterial thrombosis, inherited thrombophilia does not play a major role.[64] Here the control of clinical risk factors, which are summarized in ➔ Box 27.1, is more important.[5]

The infection caused by the SARS-CoV-2 virus[65] generates a dysregulated host response to infection, leading in severe cases to a multisystem disease with marked hyperactivity of the immune, endothelial, and coagulation systems.[66] The precise mechanism is not fully understood but a pathogen-induced interplay between the endothelium, the immune system, and the coagulation system is at least in part responsible.[67] Activation of host defence systems results in activation of coagulation and generation of thrombin, a term called thromboinflammation or immunothrombosis. Finally, the proinflammatory environment also results in activated vascular endothelial cells and endothelial injury with resultant prothrombotic properties.[68] Consequently, rates of VTE

Box 27.1 Clinical risk factors for arterial thrombosis

- Cholesterol.
- Blood pressure.
- Cigarette smoking.
- DM.
- Adiposity.
- Age.
- Sex.

Source data from Collet JP, Thiele H, Barbato E, et al.; ESC Scientific Document Group. 2020 ESC Guidelines for the management of acute coronary syndromes in patients presenting without persistent ST-segment elevation. Eur Heart J. 2021;42(14):1289–1367. doi: 10.1093/eurheartj/ehaa575.

Table 27.1 Risk factors for venous thromboembolism

Strong risk factors (OR ≥10)	Major surgery (orthopaedic and neurological)/major trauma Recent (<3 months) hospitalization for acute heart disease or atrial fibrillation/flutter Prior venous thromboembolism Antiphospholipid syndrome Active cancer (depends on type and stage)/chemotherapy Myocardial infarction (within previous 3 months) Spinal cord injury
Moderate risk factors (OR 2–9)	Arthroscopic knee surgery Venous catheters Oral contraception/hormone replacement therapy/*in vitro* fertilization (depends on dose and type of hormone) Pregnancy or postpartum period Inflammatory and autoimmune diseases Infections Active cancer (depends on type and stage)/chemotherapy Congestive heart or respiratory failure Genetic thrombophilia Superficial vein thrombosis (>3 cm from saphenofemoral or saphenopopliteal junctions and >5 cm length) Stroke with residual hemiparesis/hemiplegia Blood transfusion Erythropoiesis-stimulating agents Postpartum period
Weak risk factors (OR <2)	Bed rest (>3 days)/immobility (prolonged sitting position, i.e. travel) Age Obesity Superficial vein thrombosis Varicose veins/chronic vein insufficiency Laparoscopic surgery Diabetes mellitus Arterial hypertension Pregnancy

Source data from Mazzolai L, Ageno W, Alatri A, et al. Second consensus document on diagnosis and management of acute deep vein thrombosis: updated document elaborated by the ESC Working Group on aorta and peripheral vascular diseases and the ESC Working Group on pulmonary circulation and right ventricular function. Eur J Prev Cardiol. 2022;29(8):1248–1263. doi: 10.1093/eurjpc/zwab088; and Konstantinides SV, Meyer G, Becattini C, et al; ESC Scientific Document Group. 2019 ESC Guidelines for the diagnosis and management of acute pulmonary embolism developed in collaboration with the European Respiratory Society (ERS). Eur Heart J. 2020;41(4):543–603. doi: 10.1093/eurheartj/ehz405.

ranging from 2.6% in non-critical patients to 35.3% in critically ill patients have been reported.[69] Thus, the American Society of Hematology and International Society of Thrombosis and Haemostasis guidelines recommend prophylactic anticoagulation with low-molecular-weight heparin (LMWH) in all hospitalized patients with COVID-19.[70] The use of therapeutic doses deserves further investigation, as well as its use in the ambulatory setting.[71]

Management

Once the diagnosis of a VTE is established, full-intensity anticoagulant therapy should be started for at least 3 months. The therapeutic options are a full-dose of LMWH followed by VKA with an international normalized ratio target between 2.0 and 3.0, or NOACs. The latter option is now the first recommended option following the last American College of Chest Physician update. Rivaroxaban and apixaban can be initiated without prior LMWH treatment. Three months of therapy is usually enough for provoked events due to strong and transient risk factors like surgery, trauma, immobility, or acute illness causing hospitalization.[72,73] The risk of recurrence is very low regardless of the presence of thrombophilia[74,75] and thus thrombophilia testing should not be performed in these cases.[76]

In contrast, the risk for recurrence after an unprovoked event is about 10% in the first year and approximately 30% at 5 years, and testing for thrombophilia does not reduce the risk of recurrence.[77] Therefore, several guidelines recommend extended anticoagulation for patients with an unprovoked VTE and a low-to-moderate risk of bleeding.[22,58] If it is planned to stop anticoagulation (either due to haemorrhagic risk or patient value), it could be useful to know if there is an underlying severe thrombophilia which may point in the direction of continued anticoagulation. This is especially important if an antiphospholipid syndrome is suspected. In any case, the risk of recurrence based on other non-modifiable or persistent risk factors such as age, sex, obesity, or D-dimer levels should also be counterweighed especially in those cases with a familial history of VTE.[78] In the case of antiphospholipid syndrome, NOACs should not be used, especially in patients with triple positive tests (presence of lupus anticoagulant, anticardiolipin and anti-beta 2-glycoprotein antibodies, and IgG or IgM) or if the patient has arterial thrombosis.[79]

Prophylaxis in family members

Another goal of thrombophilia testing could be to aid decision-making regarding future VTE prophylaxis after testing of family members; however, evidence for such an approach is limited. As we have mentioned before, a family history of VTE constitutes by itself an important risk factor for the rest of the family, regardless of the presence or not of thrombophilic defects. But it is also important to point out that thrombophilia is included in most risk assessment models for predicting VTE in patients admitted to hospital.[80] In addition, the identification of an inherited thrombophilia in first-degree relatives may result in the avoidance of hormonal contraception in women of childbearing age or the administration of thromboprophylaxis to some patients during pregnancy.

Pregnancy

Epidemiology

Pregnancy confers a four- to fivefold higher risk in women of experiencing a VTE event compared to non-pregnant women. Approximately 75–80% of the patients have DVT and the rest pulmonary embolism (PE). The risk starts at the beginning of the first trimester but with the highest risk in the immediate postpartum period. Six weeks after delivery the risk decreases, and the return to baseline is 12 weeks after.[81] The case fatality rate is overall 3.5%.[82]

Regarding arterial thrombosis, pregnancy is associated with a three- to fourfold increase in acute MI risk compared with age-matched non-pregnant women.[82] Some of these patients have spontaneous coronary artery dissection.

Mechanisms and risk factors

To prevent bleeding, a hypercoagulable state is present during pregnancy. Plasma levels of coagulation factors are elevated whereas natural anticoagulants decrease. At the third trimester, decreased venous flow velocity, venous distension, and obstruction of venous return produced by the growing uterus occur. Finally, delivery constitutes a vascular trauma fulfilling Virchow's triad.[83]

The risk of VTE could be aggravated by the presence of the classical risk factors for VTE (summarized in ➔ Table 27.1) and specifically pregnancy risk factors (➔ Box 27.2).

Box 27.2 Specific pregnancy-related risk factors for venous thromboembolism

- Age over 35 years.
- Nulliparity.
- Multiple gestation.
- Gestational DM.
- Pre(eclampsia).
- Caesarean section.
- Antepartum haemorrhage.
- Postpartum infection.
- Sickle cell disease.
- Systemic lupus erythematosus.
- Smoking.

Source data from Nichols KM, Henkin S, Creager MA. Venous thromboembolism associated with pregnancy: JACC focus seminar. J Am Coll Cardiol. 2020;76(18):2128–2141. doi: 10.1016/j.jacc.2020.06.090.

The strongest risk factor for VTE is a personal history of DVT and/or PE, especially if they occurred during hormone therapy or in a previous pregnancy, with an estimated absolute risk of recurrence between 6% and 10% if no heparin thromboprophylaxis is applied.[84,85]

Inherited thrombophilia carries up to a 15-fold increased risk for VTE during pregnancy, whereas a familial history of VTE, irrespective of the presence of thrombophilia, confers a fourfold higher risk. The highest risk corresponds to the presence of gene mutations such as FVL and PT20210A, especially if they are homozygous or double heterozygous. Unlike non-pregnant patients, deficiency of endogenous anticoagulants (considered as high-risk thrombophilias) conferred a lower thromboembolic risk in pregnancy than FVL or PT20210A, even in heterozygous traits.[86]

In the case of ischaemic heart disease, most of the risk factors are shared with VTE: smoking, age, hypertension, DM, obesity, and dyslipidaemia. More specific pregnancy risk factors are (pre-) eclampsia, thrombophilia, transfusion, postpartum infection, cocaine use, multiparity, and postpartum haemorrhage.[82]

Preventive measures

LMWH has become the drug of choice for the prevention of VTE in pregnant patients. The recommended doses are standard prophylactic dose or half-therapeutic dose schemes. The ESC Guidelines on pregnancy and cardiovascular diseases recommended that patients at high risk for VTE should receive prophylactic enoxaparin at 0.5 IU/kg of body weight once daily or another LMWH at equivalent doses from early pregnancy to 4 weeks after delivery.[82] LMWH is in general well tolerated but not without risks. The use of LMWH could complicate delivery due to unpredicted onset of labour, epidural catheterization, and need for emergent caesarean section.[83] American Society of Hematology guidelines recommend antepartum and postpartum anticoagulant prophylaxis for women not already receiving long-term anticoagulant therapy who have a history of VTE that was unprovoked or was associated with a hormonal risk factor or previous pregnancy.[87]

In the presence of thrombophilia, the recommendation is antepartum antithrombotic prophylaxis to prevent a first venous thromboembolic event for women with antithrombin deficiency who have a family history of VTE and in those who are homozygous for the FVL mutation or who have combined thrombophilia, regardless of family history. This recommendation is in agreement with the American College of Chest Physician guidelines.[87,88] In the postpartum period, the recommendation is for women with combined thrombophilia or who are homozygous for the FVL or PT20210A gene mutation, regardless of family history, or in women with a family history of VTE who have antithrombin, protein C, or protein S deficiency.[87]

Women undergoing assisted reproductive technologies have a twofold higher risk of VTE. However, the absolute risk is low, and most events occur in those who develop an ovarian hyperstimulation syndrome.[89] Only in the latter group is pharmacological prophylaxis recommended.

Treatment

LMWH is the preferred treatment for VTE in pregnant women as it does not cross the placenta and has no teratogenic effects. A once-daily injection is preferred, and the dose is adjusted to the body weight. In ESC Guidelines, a twice-daily dosage is recommended in the case of PE and acute DVT.[82] There is no evidence that monitoring would improve clinical outcomes.[90] Unfractionated heparin (UFH) does not cross the placenta either, but UFH therapy may be associated with thrombocytopenia, osteoporosis, and need for monitoring and frequent dose adjustments. It should only be used in case of massive PE.[82] Delivery poses the greatest risk for bleeding and LMWH should be stopped 12–24 hours before. UFH can also be used prior to labour if the maintenance of anticoagulation is critical, as it can be stopped 4–6 hours before delivery and restarted 4 hours after.[82]

Oral anticoagulation is not recommended in pregnant women with VTE. NOACs cross the placenta and there are no studies about their effects on the fetus. VKAs are teratogenic during the period between the 6th and 12th weeks. Women who are taking oral anticoagulation due to a VTE and become pregnant should change to a LWWH during the pregnancy. For women who are taking a low dose of warfarin (<5 mg/day) the ESC Guidelines recommended the maintenance of warfarin in the first trimester.[91]

In the case of an ACS, low-dose aspirin appears to be safe, but there is little information regarding $P2Y_{12}$ inhibitors. Clopidogrel should be used only when strictly necessary and for the shortest possible duration.[82]

Antithrombotic drugs that can be used in pregnancy are summarized in ➔ Table 27.2, with special consideration of the dosages of LMWH in ➔ Table 27.3. The risk of using thrombolytics in pregnancy seems reasonable taking into account the risk of death in a life-threatening event.[92] Percutaneous and surgical embolectomy may represent alternatives to thrombolysis, if local expertise is available in a timely fashion, which may be preferable due to the high risk of bleeding of thrombolysis.[93]

Conclusion

There are special populations that deserve specific preventive and therapeutic measures, either because of increased thrombotic risk, like DM, or because they need an adaptation of the treatment to their characteristics, such as renal impairment or pregnancy. The dosing of some antithrombotic drugs is highly dependent on renal function so dosages should be adjusted. Several antithrombotics are contraindicated in pregnancy.

Table 27.2 Antithrombotic drugs and pregnancy

	Drug	Dosage	Monitoring	Safe during pregnancy	Safe during breastfeeding
Oral anticoagulants	Warfarin	Variable	INR	No Can be used in second and third trimester in patients with valvular heart disease. Should be stopped 1 month before delivery	Yes
	DOACS	Following SmPC	No	No Cross the placenta	Not known
Heparins	UFH	Variable	aPTT	Yes	Yes
	LMWH (E Table 27.3)	Following SmPC	Not necessary If needed: anti-Xa level	Yes	Yes
Antiplatelet therapy	Aspirin	100 mg	No	Yes	Yes
	Clopidogrel	75 mg	No	Not known Avoid unless necessary	Not known Not recommended

aPTT, activated partial thromboplastin time; DOACS: direct oral anticoagulants; INR, international normalized ratio; LMWH: low-molecular-weight heparin; SmPC: summary of product characteristics; UFH, unfractionated heparin.

Table 27.3 Low-molecular-weight heparin dosing

Drug	Prophylactic dose (every 24 hours)	Therapeutic dose
Dalteparin	5000 U	200 U SC every 24 hours or 100 U every 12 hours
Enoxaparin	40 mg	1 mg/kg every 12 hours
Nadroparin	2850 U	86 U/kg every 12 hours
Tinzaparin	4500 U	175 U/kg every 24 hours
Bemiparin	3500 U	115 U/kg every 24 hours

SC, subcutaneous.

What's new

- DM is considered a main risk factor for cardiovascular disease, in particular atherosclerosis disease. The duration of DM and glycaemic control are associated with AF.
- Antiplatelet therapy in primary prevention of cardiovascular disease in diabetic patients is not recommended, as absolute benefits were largely counterbalanced by the risks of major bleeding.
- CKD is an independent risk factor for cardiovascular morbidity and mortality, and increases the risk of incident AF.
- Clinical utility of hereditary thrombophilia testing for the management of patients with VTE is limited, especially regarding the decision for long-term anticoagulation.
- In provoked VTE anticoagulation can be stopped at 3 months whereas unprovoked episodes in general should maintain anticoagulation indefinitely as long as the patient has an acceptable bleeding risk.
- LMWH has become the drug of choice for both prevention and treatment of VTE in pregnant patients.

Guideline recommendations

- 2021 ESC Guidelines on cardiovascular disease prevention in clinical practice.[5] Excellent review about DM as a cardiovascular risk factor, and the recommendations about the antithrombotic treatment in diabetic patients.
- 2020 ESC Guidelines for the management of acute coronary syndromes in patients presenting without persistent ST-segment elevation.[7] Antithrombotic therapy in different comorbidities in patients with ACS.
- 2020 ESC Guidelines for the diagnosis and management of atrial fibrillation developed in collaboration with the European Association for Cardio-Thoracic Surgery (EACTS).[26] Risk stratification in AF. Antithrombotic recommendation.
- 2019 ESC Guidelines for the diagnosis and management of acute pulmonary embolism developed in collaboration with the European Respiratory Society (ERS): the Task Force for the diagnosis and management of acute pulmonary embolism of the European Society of Cardiology (ESC).[61] Recommendations about prophylaxis and treatment of VTE and performance of inherited thrombophilia testing.
- 2019 ESC Guidelines on diabetes, pre-diabetes, and cardiovascular diseases developed in collaboration with the EASD.[1] Wide review about risk stratification of diabetic patients and the recommended antithrombotic therapy.
- 2018 ESC Guidelines for the management of cardiovascular diseases during pregnancy.[82] Prevention and treatment of antithrombotic therapy in cardiovascular diseases during pregnancy, puerperium, and breastfeeding.

What's next

- More data are expected about potential cardiovascular benefits of the new diabetic drugs.
- Data about antithrombotic therapy in AF patients under haemodialysis—current trials are ongoing.

Drug dosing

See ➔ Tables 27.2 and 27.3.

References

1. Cosentino F, Grant PJ, Aboyans V, et al. 2019 ESC Guidelines on diabetes, pre-diabetes, and cardiovascular diseases developed in collaboration with the EASD. Eur Heart J. 2020;41(2):255–323.
2. Sarwar N, Gao P, Seshasai SR, et al. Diabetes mellitus, fasting blood glucose concentration, and risk of vascular disease: a collaborative meta-analysis of 102 prospective studies. Lancet. 2010;375(9733):2215–22.
3. Rawshani A, Sattar N, Franzén S, et al. Excess mortality and cardiovascular disease in young adults with type 1 diabetes in relation to age at onset: a nationwide, register-based cohort study. Lancet. 2018;392(10146):477–86.
4. Tancredi M, Rosengren A, Svensson AM, et al. Excess mortality among persons with type 2 diabetes. N Engl J Med. 2015;373(18):1720–32.
5. Visseren FLJ, Mach F, Smulders YM, et al. 2021 ESC Guidelines on cardiovascular disease prevention in clinical practice. Eur Heart J. 2021;42(34):3227–337.
6. Kannel WB, Wolf PA, Benjamin EJ, Levy D. Prevalence, incidence, prognosis, and predisposing conditions for atrial fibrillation: population-based estimates. Am J Cardiol. 1998;82(8A):2N–9N.
7. Collet JP, Thiele H, Barbato E, et al. 2020 ESC Guidelines for the management of acute coronary syndromes in patients presenting without persistent ST-segment elevation. Eur Heart J. 2021;42(14):1289–367.
8. Gorenek B, Boriani G, Dan GA, et al. European Heart Rhythm Association (EHRA) position paper on arrhythmia management and device therapies in endocrine disorders, endorsed by Asia Pacific Heart Rhythm Society (APHRS) and Latin American Heart Rhythm Society (LAHRS). Europace. 2018;20(6):895–6.
9. Huxley RR, Filion KB, Konety S, Alonso A. Meta-analysis of cohort and case-control studies of type 2 diabetes mellitus and risk of atrial fibrillation. Am J Cardiol. 2011;108(1):56–62.
10. Friberg L, Rosenqvist M, Lip GY. Evaluation of risk stratification schemes for ischaemic stroke and bleeding in 182 678 patients with atrial fibrillation: the Swedish Atrial Fibrillation cohort study. Eur Heart J. 2012;33(12):1500–10.
11. Stegmayr B, Asplund K. Diabetes as a risk factor for stroke. A population perspective. Diabetologia. 1995;38(9):1061–8.
12. Otamas A, Grant PJ, Ajjan RA. Diabetes and atherothrombosis: the circadian rhythm and role of melatonin in vascular protection. Diab Vasc Dis Res. 2020;17(3):1479164120920582.
13. Soma P, Swanepoel AC, Bester J, Pretorius E. Tissue factor levels in type 2 diabetes mellitus. Inflamm Res. 2017;66(5):365–8.
14. Paneni F, Beckman JA, Creager MA, Cosentino F. Diabetes and vascular disease: pathophysiology, clinical consequences, and medical therapy: part I. Eur Heart J. 2013;34(31):2436–43.
15. Grant PJ. Diabetes mellitus as a prothrombotic condition. J Intern Med. 2007;262(2):157–72.
16. Krahn AD, Manfreda J, Tate RB, Mathewson FA, Cuddy TE. The natural history of atrial fibrillation: incidence, risk factors, and prognosis in the Manitoba Follow-Up Study. Am J Med. 1995;98(5):476–84.
17. Fatemi O, Yuriditsky E, Tsioufis C, et al. Impact of intensive glycemic control on the incidence of atrial fibrillation and associated cardiovascular outcomes in patients with type 2 diabetes mellitus (from the Action to Control Cardiovascular Risk in Diabetes Study). Am J Cardiol. 2014;114(8):1217–22.
18. Ridker PM. Should aspirin be used for primary prevention in the post-statin era? N Engl J Med. 2018;379(16):1572–4.
19. Baigent C, Blackwell L, Collins R, et al. Aspirin in the primary and secondary prevention of vascular disease: collaborative meta-analysis of individual participant data from randomised trials. Lancet. 2009;373(9678):1849–60.
20. Belch J, MacCuish A, Campbell I, et al. The prevention of progression of arterial disease and diabetes (POPADAD) trial: factorial randomised placebo controlled trial of aspirin and antioxidants in patients with diabetes and asymptomatic peripheral arterial disease. BMJ. 2008;337:a1840.
21. Ogawa H, Nakayama M, Morimoto T, et al. Low-dose aspirin for primary prevention of atherosclerotic events in patients with type 2 diabetes: a randomized controlled trial. JAMA. 2008;300(18):2134–41.
22. Bowman L, Mafham M, Wallendszus K, et al. Effects of aspirin for primary prevention in persons with diabetes mellitus. N Engl J Med. 2018;379(16):1529–39.
23. Mega JL, Braunwald E, Wiviott SD, et al. Rivaroxaban in patients with a recent acute coronary syndrome. N Engl J Med. 2012;366(1):9–19.
24. Connolly SJ, Eikelboom JW, Bosch J, et al. Rivaroxaban with or without aspirin in patients with stable coronary artery disease: an international, randomised, double-blind, placebo-controlled trial. Lancet. 2018;391(10117):205–18.
25. Bonaca MP, Bhatt DL, Cohen M, et al. Long-term use of ticagrelor in patients with prior myocardial infarction. N Engl J Med. 2015;372(19):1791–800.
26. Hindricks G, Potpara T, Dagres N, et al. 2020 ESC Guidelines for the diagnosis and management of atrial fibrillation developed in collaboration with the European Association for Cardio-Thoracic Surgery (EACTS). Eur Heart J. 2021;42(5):373–498.
27. Plitt A, McGuire DK, Giugliano RP. Atrial fibrillation, type 2 diabetes, and non-vitamin K antagonist oral anticoagulants: a review. JAMA Cardiol. 2017;2(4):442–8.
28. Brambatti M, Darius H, Oldgren J, et al. Comparison of dabigatran versus warfarin in diabetic patients with atrial fibrillation: results from the RE-LY trial. Int J Cardiol. 2015;196: 127–31.
29. Ezekowitz JA, Lewis BS, Lopes RD, et al. Clinical outcomes of patients with diabetes and atrial fibrillation treated with apixaban: results from the ARISTOTLE trial. Eur Heart J Cardiovasc Pharmacother. 2015;1(2):86–94.
30. Lip GYH, Keshishian AV, Kang AL, et al. Effectiveness and safety of oral anticoagulants in patients with nonvalvular atrial fibrillation and diabetes mellitus. Mayo Clin Proc. 2020;95(5):929–43.
31. Boriani G, Savelieva I, Dan GA, et al. Chronic kidney disease in patients with cardiac rhythm disturbances or implantable electrical devices: clinical significance and implications for decision making—a position paper of the European Heart Rhythm Association endorsed by the Heart Rhythm Society and the Asia Pacific Heart Rhythm Society. Europace. 2015;17(8):1169–96.
32. Stevens PE, Levin A, Kidney Disease: Improving Global Outcomes Chronic Kidney Disease Guideline Development Work Group Members. Evaluation and management of chronic kidney disease: synopsis of the kidney disease: improving global outcomes 2012 clinical practice guideline. Ann Intern Med. 2013;158(11):825–30.
33. Coresh J, Selvin E, Stevens LA, et al. Prevalence of chronic kidney disease in the United States. JAMA. 2007;298(17):2038–47.
34. Mafham M, Emberson J, Landray MJ, Wen CP, Baigent C. Estimated glomerular filtration rate and the risk of major vascular events and all-cause mortality: a meta-analysis. PLoS One. 2011;6(10):e25920.
35. Matsushita K, van der Velde M, Astor BC, et al. Association of estimated glomerular filtration rate and albuminuria with all-cause and cardiovascular mortality in general population cohorts: a collaborative meta-analysis. Lancet. 2010;375(9731):2073–81.
36. Moody WE, Edwards NC, Chue CD, Ferro CJ, Townend JN. Arterial disease in chronic kidney disease. Heart. 2013;99(6):365–72.

37. Bansal N, Fan D, Hsu CY, Ordonez JD, Marcus GM, Go AS. Incident atrial fibrillation and risk of end-stage renal disease in adults with chronic kidney disease. Circulation. 2013;127(5):569–74.
38. Esteve-Pastor MA, Rivera-Caravaca JM, Roldan V, et al. Long-term bleeding risk prediction in 'real world' patients with atrial fibrillation: comparison of the HAS-BLED and ABC-Bleeding risk scores. The Murcia Atrial Fibrillation Project. Thromb Haemost. 2017;117(10):1848–58.
39. Ding WY, Potpara TS, Blomström-Lundqvist C, et al. Impact of renal impairment on atrial fibrillation: ESC-EHRA EORP-AF Long-Term General Registry. Eur J Clin Invest. 2022;52(6):e13745.
40. Roldán V, Marín F, Manzano-Fernandez S, et al. Does chronic kidney disease improve the predictive value of the CHADS2 and CHA2DS2-VASc stroke stratification risk scores for atrial fibrillation? Thromb Haemost. 2013;109(5):956–60.
41. Kumar S, Lim E, Covic A, et al. Anticoagulation in concomitant chronic kidney disease and atrial fibrillation: JACC review topic of the week. J Am Coll Cardiol. 2019;74(17):2204–15.
42. Darlington A, Ferreiro JL, Ueno M, et al. Haemostatic profiles assessed by thromboelastography in patients with end-stage renal disease. Thromb Haemost. 2011;106(1):67–74.
43. Roldán V, Marín F, Fernández H, et al. Renal impairment in a 'real-life' cohort of anticoagulated patients with atrial fibrillation (implications for thromboembolism and bleeding). Am J Cardiol. 2013;111(8):1159–64.
44. Rozenbaum Z, Benchetrit S, Minha S, et al. The effect of admission renal function on the treatment and outcome of patients with acute coronary syndrome. Cardiorenal Med. 2017;7(3):169–78.
45. Park SH, Kim W, Park CS, Kang WY, Hwang SH. A comparison of clopidogrel responsiveness in patients with versus without chronic renal failure. Am J Cardiol. 2009;104(9):1292–5.
46. Best PJ, Steinhubl SR, Berger PB, et al. The efficacy and safety of short- and long-term dual antiplatelet therapy in patients with mild or moderate chronic kidney disease: results from the Clopidogrel for the Reduction of Events During Observation (CREDO) trial. Am Heart J. 2008;155(4):687–93.
47. Keltai M, Tonelli M, Mann JF, et al. Renal function and outcomes in acute coronary syndrome: impact of clopidogrel. Eur J Cardiovasc Prev Rehabil. 2007;14(2):312–8.
48. James S, Budaj A, Aylward P, et al. Ticagrelor versus clopidogrel in acute coronary syndromes in relation to renal function: results from the Platelet Inhibition and Patient Outcomes (PLATO) trial. Circulation. 2010;122(11):1056–67.
49. Montalescot G, Silvain J. Ticagrelor in the renal dysfunction subgroup: subjugated or substantiated? Circulation. 2010;122(11):1049–52.
50. Andò G, Capranzano P. Non-vitamin K antagonist oral anticoagulants in atrial fibrillation patients with chronic kidney disease: a systematic review and network meta-analysis. Int J Cardiol. 2017;231:162–9.
51. Kuno T, Takagi H, Ando T, et al. Oral anticoagulation for patients with atrial fibrillation on long-term hemodialysis. J Am Coll Cardiol. 2020;75(3):273–85.
52. Steffel J, Collins R, Antz M, et al. 2021 European Heart Rhythm Association practical guide on the use of non-vitamin K antagonist oral anticoagulants in patients with atrial fibrillation. Europace. 2021;23(10):1612–76.
53. Yao X, Tangri N, Gersh BJ, et al. Renal outcomes in anticoagulated patients with atrial fibrillation. J Am Coll Cardiol. 2017;70(21):2621–32.
54. López-Gálvez R, Rivera-Caravaca JM, Anguita Sánchez M, et al. Use of rivaroxaban attenuates renal function impairment in patients with atrial fibrillation: insights of the EMIR study. Eur J Clin Invest. 2022;52(9):e13788.
55. Martinelli I, De Stefano V, Mannucci PM. Inherited risk factors for venous thromboembolism. Nat Rev Cardiol. 2014;11(3):140–56.
56. Connors JM. Thrombophilia testing and venous thrombosis. N Engl J Med. 2017;377(12):1177–87.
57. Baglin T, Gray E, Greaves M, et al. Clinical guidelines for testing for heritable thrombophilia. Br J Haematol. 2010;149(2):209–20.
58. Ortel TL, Neumann I, Ageno W, et al. American Society of Hematology 2020 guidelines for management of venous thromboembolism: treatment of deep vein thrombosis and pulmonary embolism. Blood Adv. 2020;4(19):4693–738.
59. Arachchillage DJ, Mackillop L, Chandratheva A, Motawani J, MacCallum P, Laffan M. Guidelines for thrombophilia testing: a British Society for Haematology guideline. Br J Haematol. 2022;198(3):443–58.
60. Middeldorp S. Inherited thrombophilia: a double-edged sword. Hematology Am Soc Hematol Educ Program. 2016;2016(1):1–9.
61. Konstantinides SV, Meyer G, Becattini C, et al. 2019 ESC Guidelines for the diagnosis and management of acute pulmonary embolism developed in collaboration with the European Respiratory Society (ERS): the Task Force for the diagnosis and management of acute pulmonary embolism of the European Society of Cardiology (ESC). Eur Heart J. 2019;40(42):3453–5.
62. Mazzolai L, Ageno W, Alatri A, et al. Second consensus document on diagnosis and management of acute deep vein thrombosis: updated document elaborated by the ESC Working Group on aorta and peripheral vascular diseases and the ESC Working Group on pulmonary circulation and right ventricular function. Eur J Prev Cardiol. 2022;29(8):1248–63.
63. Miyakis S, Lockshin MD, Atsumi T, et al. International consensus statement on an update of the classification criteria for definite antiphospholipid syndrome (APS). J Thromb Haemost. 2006;4(2):295–306.
64. May JE, Moll S. Unexplained arterial thrombosis: approach to diagnosis and treatment. Hematology Am Soc Hematol Educ Program. 2021;2021(1):76–84.
65. Ortega-Paz L, Galli M, Capodanno D, et al. Safety and efficacy of different prophylactic anticoagulation dosing regimens in critically and non-critically ill patients with COVID-19: a systematic review and meta-analysis of randomized controlled trials. Eur Heart J Cardiovasc Pharmacother. 2022;29(8):677–86.
66. Osuchowski MF, Winkler MS, Skirecki T, et al. The COVID-19 puzzle: deciphering pathophysiology and phenotypes of a new disease entity. Lancet Respir Med. 2021;9(6):622–42.
67. Alnima T, Mulder MMG, van Bussel BCT, Ten Cate H. COVID-19 coagulopathy: from pathogenesis to treatment. Acta Haematol. 2022;145(3):282–96.
68. Connors JM, Levy JH. COVID-19 and its implications for thrombosis and anticoagulation. Blood. 2020;135(23):2033–40.
69. Piazza G, Morrow DA. Diagnosis, management, and pathophysiology of arterial and venous thrombosis in COVID-19. JAMA. 2020;324(24):2548–9.
70. Leentjens J, van Haaps TF, Wessels PF, Schutgens REG, Middeldorp S. COVID-19-associated coagulopathy and antithrombotic agents-lessons after 1 year. Lancet Haematol. 2021;8(7):e524–33.
71. Ortega-Paz L, Galli M, Angiolillo DJ. Updated meta-analysis of randomized controlled trials on the safety and efficacy of different prophylactic anticoagulation dosing regimens in non-critically ill hospitalized patients with COVID-19. Eur Heart J Cardiovasc Pharmacother. 2022;8(3):E15–17.
72. Stevens SM, Woller SC, Kreuziger LB, et al. Antithrombotic Therapy for VTE Disease: second update of the CHEST Guideline and Expert Panel Report. Chest. 2021;160(6):e545–608.

73. Witt DM, Nieuwlaat R, Clark NP, et al. American Society of Hematology 2018 guidelines for management of venous thromboembolism: optimal management of anticoagulation therapy. Blood Adv. 2018;2(22):3257–91.
74. Baglin T, Luddington R, Brown K, Baglin C. Incidence of recurrent venous thromboembolism in relation to clinical and thrombophilic risk factors: prospective cohort study. Lancet. 2003;362(9383):523–6.
75. Iorio A, Kearon C, Filippucci E, et al. Risk of recurrence after a first episode of symptomatic venous thromboembolism provoked by a transient risk factor: a systematic review. Arch Intern Med. 2010;170(19):1710–16.
76. Hicks LK, Bering H, Carson KR, et al. The ASH Choosing Wisely® campaign: five hematologic tests and treatments to question. Blood. 2013;122(24):3879–83.
77. Coppens M, Reijnders JH, Middeldorp S, Doggen CJ, Rosendaal FR. Testing for inherited thrombophilia does not reduce the recurrence of venous thrombosis. J Thromb Haemost. 2008;6(9):1474–7.
78. Gaddh M, Rosovsky RP. Venous thromboembolism: genetics and thrombophilias. Semin Respir Crit Care Med. 2021;42(2):271–83.
79. Tektonidou MG, Andreoli L, Limper M, et al. EULAR recommendations for the management of antiphospholipid syndrome in adults. Ann Rheum Dis. 2019;78(10):1296–304.
80. Pandor A, Tonkins M, Goodacre S, et al. Risk assessment models for venous thromboembolism in hospitalised adult patients: a systematic review. BMJ Open. 2021;11(7):e045672.
81. Middeldorp S, Naue C, Köhler C. Thrombophilia, thrombosis and thromboprophylaxis in pregnancy: for what and in whom? Hamostaseologie. 2022;42(1):54–64.
82. Regitz-Zagrosek V, Roos-Hesselink JW, Bauersachs J, et al. 2018 ESC Guidelines for the management of cardiovascular diseases during pregnancy. Eur Heart J. 2018;39(34):3165–241.
83. Nichols KM, Henkin S, Creager MA. Venous thromboembolism associated with pregnancy: JACC focus seminar. J Am Coll Cardiol. 2020;76(18):2128–41.
84. Pabinger I, Grafenhofer H, Kyrle PA, et al. Temporary increase in the risk for recurrence during pregnancy in women with a history of venous thromboembolism. Blood. 2002;100(3):1060–2.
85. De Stefano V, Martinelli I, Rossi E, et al. The risk of recurrent venous thromboembolism in pregnancy and puerperium without antithrombotic prophylaxis. Br J Haematol. 2006;135(3):386–91.
86. Robertson L, Wu O, Langhorne P, et al. Thrombophilia in pregnancy: a systematic review. Br J Haematol. 2006;132(2):171–96.
87. Bates SM, Rajasekhar A, Middeldorp S, et al. American Society of Hematology 2018 guidelines for management of venous thromboembolism: venous thromboembolism in the context of pregnancy. Blood Adv. 2018;2(22):3317–59.
88. Bates SM, Greer IA, Middeldorp S, Veenstra DL, Prabulos AM, Vandvik PO. VTE, thrombophilia, antithrombotic therapy, and pregnancy: Antithrombotic Therapy and Prevention of Thrombosis, 9th ed: American College of Chest Physicians Evidence-Based Clinical Practice Guidelines. Chest. 2012;141(2 Suppl):e691S–736S.
89. Hart C, Bauersachs R, Scholz U, et al. Prevention of venous thromboembolism during pregnancy and the puerperium with a special focus on women with hereditary thrombophilia or prior VTE—position paper of the Working Group in Women's Health of the Society of Thrombosis and Haemostasis (GTH). Hamostaseologie. 2020;40(5):572–90.
90. Middeldorp S, Ganzevoort W. How I treat venous thromboembolism in pregnancy. Blood. 2020;136(19):2133–42.
91. Alshawabkeh L, Economy KE, Valente AM. Anticoagulation during pregnancy: evolving strategies with a focus on mechanical valves. J Am Coll Cardiol. 2016;68(16):1804–13.
92. Sousa Gomes M, Guimarães M, Montenegro N. Thrombolysis in pregnancy: a literature review. J Matern Fetal Neonatal Med. 2019;32(14):2418–28.
93. Martillotti G, Boehlen F, Robert-Ebadi H, Jastrow N, Righini M, Blondon M. Treatment options for severe pulmonary embolism during pregnancy and the postpartum period: a systematic review. J Thromb Haemost. 2017;15(10):1942–50.

CHAPTER 28

Antithrombotic agents and drug–drug interactions

Steven P. Dunn, Craig J. Beavers, and David J. Moliterno

Contents

Summary

Drug–drug interactions affecting antiplatelet and anticoagulant medications are not uncommon, and among patients with cardiovascular disease, many receive polypharmacy thereby increasing the risk for important drug interactions. Such interactions may impact the efficacy or safety, or both, of antithrombotic medications. Since vitamin K antagonists have been widely used in clinical medicine for many years, drug interactions with agents such as warfarin are well known. Over recent years, newer and more potent antiplatelet and anticoagulant agents have been developed, and each of these has an identified potential to be impacted by other medications, primarily by affecting hepatic cytochromes involved with drug metabolism. While many interactions have been identified and alterations of plasma concentrations of drugs have been found, limited meaningful impacts on clinical outcomes have been discerned from large-scale trials. Drugs which importantly alter renal function may also pose a drug clearance issue for agents with a high proportion of the active compound being renally excreted. Lastly, the combination of anticoagulant agents poses the highest risk to patients as the antithrombotic impact is greatest as well as the risk for drug-related interactions among the antithrombotic agents and with other drugs. Recognition of these risks has led to increased scrutiny of anticoagulant safety by clinical care providers, pharmaceutical companies, health agencies, as well as accrediting bodies.

Introduction

Antithrombotic therapy with antiplatelet and anticoagulant agents provides a critical role in the treatment and prevention of cardiovascular disease (CVD). Altogether, CVD remains a leading cause of death with over 17 million deaths each year attributable to CVD, comprising almost one-third of all deaths worldwide.[1] As a result, antiplatelet medications and anticoagulants are some of the most prescribed drug classes in the world. While the goal of effective antithrombotic therapy is to reduce morbidity and mortality due to thrombotic events, avoidance of harm, particularly from haemorrhage, is also a critical factor.

Drug–drug interactions (DDIs) involving either pharmacokinetic or pharmacodynamic alterations of one medication caused by another are routinely encountered.

The reported prevalence varies from less than 10% to as high as 80–90% depending on the population studied and the extent of polypharmacy.[2] Many DDIs do not result in significant patient impact either due to lower levels of alteration and/or a wide therapeutic index of the impacted medication. However, clinically manifested DDIs comprise approximately 10% of all DDIs and contribute to preventable harm.[3] As medication classes with a comparably narrow balance between efficacy and safety, DDIs impacting antiplatelet and anticoagulant therapy are more likely to significantly impact patient care and require a variety of strategies to ameliorate. This chapter focuses on the most encountered DDIs with antithrombotic therapy and the currently recommended management strategies.

Antiplatelet drug–drug interactions

Antiplatelet therapy is broadly prescribed and indicated in the secondary prevention of ischaemic heart disease and the primary and secondary prevention of stroke.

Aspirin

(See also Chapter 5.) Aspirin is commonly utilized as a chronic level of preventative therapy and is minimally impacted by alterations in pharmacokinetic processes. Specifically, the pharmacokinetics of aspirin are not complex as no metabolic activation is required. Drugs affecting liver cytochromes, therefore, do not impact the antiplatelet effect of aspirin. The pharmacodynamic effects of aspirin include heightened bleeding risks, particularly in the presence of other antithrombotic agents. This is discussed in greater detail in circumstances where aspirin is used with oral anticoagulation (OAC) (Chapter 26). Much of the focus of DDIs with antiplatelet therapy therefore focuses on the $P2Y_{12}$ inhibitors both with the thienopyridine class and non-thienopyridines. A summary of these interactions can be found in Table 28.1.

Thienopyridines

(See also Chapter 6.) Thienopyridines (primarily clopidogrel and prasugrel) are prodrugs and require bioactivation by the cytochrome P450 (CYP) system in the liver to an active metabolite which irreversibly binds to the platelet $P2Y_{12}$ receptor to inhibit platelet activation.

- Clopidogrel undergoes a two-step metabolism with an intermediate metabolite primarily via the isoenzymes CYP2C19 and CYP3A4 with CYP2B6, CYP1A2, CYP3A5, and CYP2C9 less involved.[4]
- Prasugrel undergoes a more simplified one-step metabolism to the active metabolite primarily via CYP3A4 and CYP2B6 with CYP2C19, CYP2C9, and CYP2D6 less involved.[5]
- CYP3A4 and CYP2C19 inhibitors:
  - For clopidogrel, CYP2C19 and CYP3A4 are the principal isoenzymes which bioactivate both the parent compound and the intermediate metabolite.
  - Proton pump inhibitors (PPIs) are the best studied DDI with CYP2C19 inhibitors and clopidogrel.
  - Co-administration of PPIs which are moderate inhibitors of CYP2C19 (omeprazole, esomeprazole) reduce active metabolite generation and decrease platelet inhibition as measured by a variety of methods.[6]
  - Retrospective analyses studying the clinical impact of co-administration of PPIs and clopidogrel are mixed but generally associate co-administration of clopidogrel with PPIs with increased rates of CVD events.[7]
  - Prospective trials and assessments of randomized clinical trials are less indicative of a significant clinical impact with co-administration of clopidogrel and PPIs.[8,9]
  - Co-administration of clopidogrel with PPIs that are not CYP2C19 inhibitors or are weak inhibitors (lansoprazole, pantoprazole, rabeprazole) is generally recommended for patients who have an indication for both therapies.[6]
  - Strong CYP3A4 inhibitors (e.g. ketoconazole) have demonstrated pharmacokinetic (decreased active metabolite generation) and pharmacodynamic (reduced platelet inhibition) interactions with clopidogrel with a generally unknown clinical impact.[10]
  - Strong CYP3A4 inhibitors do not appear to significantly impact prasugrel metabolism or its pharmacodynamic effect.[10]
  - Ritonavir (a strong CYP3A4 and CYP2B6 inhibitor) has been shown to significantly decrease prasugrel active metabolite generation and may be clinically relevant.[11]
- CYP inducers:
  - In contrast to inhibitors, CYP inducers may increase active metabolite generation and the platelet-inhibiting effects of thienopyridines.
  - Strong CYP3A4 inducers, such as rifampin, have shown increases in active metabolite generation and increased platelet inhibition with clopidogrel.[12]
  - CYP3A4 inducers do not appear to significantly impact prasugrel metabolism.[13]
- Opioid receptor agonists:
  - Opioid therapy, especially morphine, continues to be recommended and utilized to relieve pain and anxiety in the setting of suspected acute coronary syndromes and is therefore frequently co-administered with dual antiplatelet therapy.
  - Opioid agonists slow gut motility and may impede absorption of antiplatelet therapies.
  - Morphine has been demonstrated to have a negative impact on the pharmacokinetics and pharmacodynamics of clopidogrel, including reduced Cmax, total drug exposure, and reduced platelet inhibition.[14]
  - Morphine use also blunts the effect of prasugrel, resulting in delayed and submaximal absorption and platelet inhibition.[15]
  - Other opiate agonists such as fentanyl appear to result in similar pharmacokinetic and pharmacodynamic alterations with ticagrelor and, presumably, thienopyridines.[16]

Table 28.1 Summary of drug–drug interactions with antiplatelet therapy

Agent	Interacting drug	Interaction mechanism	Management recommendation
Major clinical significance			
Clopidogrel	Anticoagulant agents	Potentiation of bleeding	Minimize overlap to shortest duration indicated (➔ Guideline recommendations) and consider starting proton pump inhibitor
	Opioid agents	Delayed absorption	Avoid if rapid antiplatelet effect needed; consider intravenous antiplatelet therapies
	Proton pump inhibitors (esomeprazole, omeprazole)	CYP2C19 inhibition reducing active metabolite formation	Avoid esomeprazole and omeprazole; use other proton pump inhibitors if indicated
Prasugrel	Anticoagulant agents	Potentiation of bleeding	Avoid in triple therapy regimen
	Opioid agents	Delayed absorption	Avoid if rapid antiplatelet effect needed; consider intravenous antiplatelet therapies
	Ritonavir	Strong CYP3A4 and CYP2B6 inhibitor; reduces active metabolite formation	Avoid combination
Ticagrelor	Anticoagulant agents	Potentiation of bleeding	Avoid in triple therapy regimen
	Opioid agents	Delayed absorption	Avoid if rapid antiplatelet effect needed; consider intravenous antiplatelet therapies
	Strong CYPA4 inhibitors (e.g. clarithromycin, ciclosporin, grapefruit juice, ketoconazole, protease inhibitors, verapamil, voriconazole, etc.)	Reduced metabolism leading to increased toxicities	Avoid combination
	Strong CYPA4 inducers (e.g. rifampin, dexamethasone, phenytoin, carbamazepine, phenobarbital, etc.)	Increased metabolism decreasing therapeutic effect	Avoid combination
Minor clinical significance			
Clopidogrel	Strong CYP3A4 inhibitors (e.g. clarithromycin, ciclosporin, grapefruit juice, ketoconazole, protease inhibitors, verapamil, voriconazole, etc.)	Reduced active metabolite generation	Unknown; may reduce effect
	Strong CYPA4 inducers (e.g. rifampin, dexamethasone, phenytoin, carbamazepine, phenobarbital, etc.)	Increased active metabolite generation	None known; may increase risk of bleeding
Ticagrelor	Aspirin (doses >100 mg)	Efficacy interaction in PLATO trial; no pharmacokinetic or pharmacodynamic effect	Consider lower doses of aspirin which also likely reduce gastrointestinal bleeding

CYP, cytochrome P450.

- The impact on clinical events has been difficult to ascertain though morphine use has been associated with worsened survival and other negative clinical outcomes in a large-scale observational analysis.[17]

Ticagrelor

In contrast to thienopyridines, ticagrelor (a non-thienopyridine) is not a prodrug and is a reversible inhibitor of the $P2Y_{12}$ receptor once absorbed. Ticagrelor is metabolized primarily via CYP3A4 and is a substrate of permeability-glycoprotein (P-gp). Therefore, inhibitors of metabolism will increase the serum concentration and exposure to toxicities and induction of metabolism will decrease the serum concentration and associated platelet inhibition, potentially worsening efficacy outcomes.

- CYP3A4 inhibitors:
  - Co-administration of ticagrelor with strong CYP3A4 inhibitors will significantly increase serum concentration (2.4-fold increase in Cmax with ketoconazole) and are contraindicated.[18] Clinical trials generally excluded patients receiving strong CYP3A4 inhibitors but increases in bleeding and non-platelet-mediated adverse effects (e.g. dyspnoea, bradyarrhythmias) would be expected to increase with co-administration.
  - Moderate CYP3A4 inhibitors (e.g. diltiazem) increase serum concentrations of ticagrelor (69% increase in Cmax with diltiazem) but did not impact clinical outcomes in the PLATO trial.[18,19]
- CYP3A4 inducers:
  - Strong CYP3A4 inducers (e.g. rifampin, dexamethasone, phenytoin, and carbamazepine) significantly increase

ticagrelor metabolism (73% decrease with rifampin in Cmax). Patients receiving strong inducers were excluded from major clinical trials but use is generally not recommended.

- Aspirin:
  - In the PLATO trial, an efficacy interaction was detected whereby aspirin doses of 300 mg or greater co-administered with ticagrelor resulted in decreased clinical efficacy compared to patients receiving less than 300 mg.[20] This interaction was not identified with clopidogrel.
  - Higher aspirin doses do not impact the pharmacokinetics or pharmacodynamics of ticagrelor.[21]
  - Higher doses of aspirin (>100 mg) with ticagrelor are contraindicated in US product labelling despite the lack of any identified mechanism for this interaction.[22] However, higher aspirin doses also generally do not produce greater efficacy for CVD reduction and may increase adverse events.

Anticoagulant drug/food/supplement interactions

The cornerstone in the maintenance management for thromboembolic disease, which includes venous thromboembolism and atrial fibrillation-related stroke, is the use of the OACs. There are three pharmacological categories of OACs, classified based on mechanistic target(s) within the clotting cascade: direct thrombin inhibitors, direct factor Xa inhibitors, and vitamin K antagonists (VKAs). Collectively, the oral direct thrombin inhibitors and factor Xa inhibitors are known as direct oral anticoagulants (DOACs). It is estimated that in the US alone, 6 million patients are treated with anticoagulants.[23] While venous thromboembolism can afflict any patient population, these conditions occur more frequently in patients with advancing age or with multiple comorbidities. Thus, these patients are more likely OAC which could place the patient at increased risk of thrombosis or bleeding event. For example, it is estimated that up to 80% of patients with atrial fibrillation will receive a medication that interacts with their OAC over their lifetime.[24] Given this reality, it is critical for clinicians to have a knowledge of pharmacokinetic and pharmacodynamic interactions associated with OACs as well as common interacting agents and management recommendations.

Direct thrombin inhibitors

(See also ➔ Chapter 10.) Direct thrombin inhibitors work to reduce thrombus formation and thrombin-induced platelet aggregation by inhibiting the conversation of factor II to factor IIa. Currently, there is only one oral direct thrombin inhibitor available which is dabigatran.

- Dabigatran etexilate is a pro-drug undergoing rapid ester hydrolysis to the active form dabigatran with no CYP metabolism.[25]
- Despite its limited CYP metabolism, dabigatran is impacted by P-gp as well as impaired kidney function given its 80% dependence on renal clearance.
- As expected, most of the interactions involve P-gp inhibitors or inducers.

In terms of recommendations for management, the following general guidance statements can be provided as a framework[26]:

- The use of strong inducers of P-gp, defined as an agent that decreases the area under the curve (AUC) of dabigatran by 50%, should be avoided due to the increased risk of therapeutic failure.
- Alternatively, the use of a strong P-gp inhibitor increases exposure dabigatran and the risk of bleeding.
- Thus, given dabigatran is primarily eliminated renally, the use of a strong P-gp inhibitor in conjunction with a creatinine clearance (CrCl) less than 50 mL/min should be avoided.[25]
- The most common major and minor interactions are presented in ➔ Table 28.2.

Direct factor Xa inhibitors

(See also ➔ Chapter 11.) As indicated by their pharmacological class name, the factor Xa inhibitors work on their namesake clotting factor which downstream prevents the conversion of prothrombin to thrombin. There are three oral direct factor Xa inhibitors currently in use: apixaban, edoxaban, and rivaroxaban. While these agents collectively belong to the same class, each has its own unique pharmacokinetic profile which impacts their interactions:

- Apixaban is metabolized 25% hepatically, mainly through CYP3A4 but also with minor contributions from CYP1A2, CYP2C8, CYP2C9, CYP2C19, and CYP2J2.[27]
- In addition, apixaban is a substrate of P-gp and has a 27% dependence on renal clearance.
- Given these factors, it is recommended to avoid apixaban with both strong CYP3A4 inhibitors and P-gp inhibitors.
- However, if a strong CYP3A4 inhibitor cannot be avoided, the dose of apixaban should be reduced by 50% if on a regimen of 5 mg or 10 mg twice daily.
- No dose adjustments should be done with moderate CYP3A4 inhibitors; however, increased monitoring for bleeding should be performed.
- Alternatively, the use of strong CYP3A4 and P-gp inducers should be avoided given the decreased AUC of apixaban and increased thrombotic risk.
- Specific interactions and management are presented in ➔ Table 28.2.
- Unlike apixaban, edoxaban has minimal dependence on CYP3A4; however, like apixaban, edoxaban is a substrate of P-gp and has an approximately 50% dependence on renal clearance.[28]
- Data suggest a significant change in AUC with P-gp inhibitors with or without a CYP3A4 inhibitor.[29]
- ➔ Table 28.2 outlines potential interactions with edoxaban and management recommendations.
- Rivaroxaban has more extensive liver and renal metabolism (51%) compared to the aforementioned oral factor Xa inhibitors.[30]

Table 28.2 Summary of drug/food/supplement–drug interactions with direct acting oral anticoagulants

DOAC	Interacting drug	Interaction mechanism	Management recommendation
Major clinical significance			
All DOACs	Antiplatelet agents	Potentiation of bleeding	Minimize overlap to shortest duration indicated and consider starting proton pump inhibitor
	Apalutamide	Strong CYP3A4 induction	Avoid combination
	Carbamazepine	Strong CYP3A4 induction	Avoid combination
	Enzalutamide	Strong CYP3A4 induction	Avoid combination
	Non-steroidal anti-inflammatory drugs	Cyclooxygenase inhibition	Avoid use unless benefits clearly outweigh risk
	Phenytoin	Strong CYP3A4 induction	Avoid combination
	Rifampin	Strong CYP3A4 induction	Avoid combination
	Ritonavir	Strong CYP3A4 induction	Avoid combination
Apixaban	Itraconazole	Strong P-gp inhibition and moderate CYP3A4 inhibition	Consider alternative, decrease dose by 50% if unavoidable
	Ketoconazole	Strong P-gp inhibition and moderate CYP3A4 inhibition	Consider alternative, decrease dose by 50% if unavoidable
Dabigatran	Ciclosporin	Strong P-gp inhibition	Avoid use
	Dronedarone	P-gp inhibition	Administer dronedarone 2 hours after dabigatran if CrCl is ≥50 mL/min, decrease dose to 75 mg twice daily in patients CrCL <50 mL/min if unavoidable, avoid if CrCl <30 mL/min
	Ketoconazole	Strong P-gp inhibition	Consider alternative, decrease doses to 75 mg twice daily in patients with CrCl <50 mL/min if unavoidable, avoid if <30 mL/min
	Lapatinib	Strong P-gp inhibition	Not studied, avoid combination
Edoxaban	Ciclosporin	Strong P-gp inhibition	Use appropriate unless another P-gp inhibitor is present. Reduce dose of edoxaban by 50% if anticoagulation is for venous thromboembolism or CrCl if <50 mL/min
	Dronedarone	Strong P-gp inhibition	Administer dronedarone 2 hours after edoxaban. Reduce dose of edoxaban by 50% if anticoagulation is for venous thromboembolism or CrCl <50 mL/min
	Itraconazole	Strong P-gp inhibition	Use appropriate unless another P-gp inhibitor is present. Reduce dose of edoxaban by 50% if anticoagulation is for venous thromboembolism or CrCl if <50 mL/min
	Ketoconazole	Strong P-gp inhibition	Use appropriate unless another P-gp inhibitor is present. Reduce dose of edoxaban by 50% if anticoagulation is for venous thromboembolism or CrCl if <50 mL/min
	Lapatinib	Strong P-gp inhibiton	Use appropriate unless another P-gp inhibitor is present. Reduce dose of edoxaban by 50% if anticoagulation is for venous thromboembolism or CrCl if <50 mL/min
	Quinidine	Strong P-gp inhibition	Reduce dose of edoxaban by 50% if anticoagulation is for venous thromboembolism or CrCl if <50 mL/min

(continued)

Table 28.2 Continued

DOAC	Interacting drug	Interaction mechanism	Management recommendation
Rivaroxaban	Dronedarone	Strong P-gp inhibition and moderate CYP3A4 inhibition	Use appropriate unless CrCl is <80 mL/min, otherwise consider alternatives
	Itraconazole	Strong P-gp inhibition and moderate CYP3A4 inhibition	Avoid combination
	Ketoconazole	Strong P-gp inhibition and moderate CYP3A4 inhibition	Avoid combination
	Lapatinib	Strong P-gp inhibition	Not studied, avoid combination
	Protease inhibitors; cobicistat, indinavir, nelfinavir, saquinavir	Strong CYP3A4 inhibition	Appropriate unless if no other pharmacokinetic inhibitor present, otherwise avoid
	Tyrosine kinase inhibitors	Strong CYP3A4 inhibition	Appropriate unless if no other pharmacokinetic inhibitor present, otherwise avoid
Minor clinical significance			
All DOACs	St John's wort	Strong CYP3A4 induction	Limit St John's wort to <4 g/daily
	Grapefruit juice	Strong CYP3A4 induction	Minimize grapefruit juice intake to <200 mL
Apixaban	Dronedarone	Strong P-gp inhibition and moderate CYP3A4 inhibition	Monitor for bleeding
	Ciclosporin	Strong P-gp inhibition and CYP3A4 inhibition	Combination is appropriate, monitor for bleeding
	Nefazodone	Strong CYP3A inhibition	Appropriate if no other pharmacokinetic inhibitor present, otherwise, requires 50% dose reduction
	Posaconazole	Strong CYP3A4 inhibition	Appropriate if no other pharmacokinetic inhibitor present, otherwise, requires 50% dose reduction
	Protease inhibitors; cobicistat, indinavir, nelfinavir, saquinavir	Strong CYP3A4 inhibition	Appropriate if no other pharmacokinetic inhibitor present, otherwise, requires 50% dose reduction
	Tyrosine kinase inhibitors	Strong CYP3A4 inhibition	Appropriate if no other pharmacokinetic inhibitor present, otherwise, requires 50% dose reduction
	Verapamil	Strong P-gp inhibition and moderate CYP3A4 inhibition	Appropriate if no other pharmacokinetic inhibitor present, otherwise, monitor
Dabigatran	Ticagrelor	P-gp inhibition	Administer ticagrelor 2 hours after dabigatran
	Verapamil	P-gp inhibition	Administer verapamil 2 hours after dabigatran
Edoxaban	Verapamil	Strong P-gp inhibition	Reduce dose of edoxaban by 50% if anticoagulation is for venous thromboembolism or CrCl if <50 mL/min
Rivaroxaban	Amiodarone	Weak CYP3A4 and P-gp inhibition	Monitor for bleeding
	Ciclosporin	Strong P-gp inhibition and CYP3A4 inhibition	Appropriate unless CrCl <50 mL/min, then monitor for bleeding
	Nefazodone	Strong CYP3A4 inhibition	Appropriate if no other pharmacokinetic inhibitor present, otherwise, avoid
	Posaconazole	Strong CYP3A4 inhibition	Appropriate if no other pharmacokinetic inhibitor present, otherwise, avoid
	Verapamil	Strong P-gp inhibition and moderate CYP3A4 inhibition	Appropriate unless CrCl is <80 mL/min, otherwise, use diltiazem
	Voriconazole	Strong P-gp inhibition and moderate CYP3A4 inhibition	Appropriate if no other pharmacokinetic inhibitor present, otherwise, avoid

CrCl, creatine clearance; CYP, cytochrome P450; P-gp, P-glycoprotein.

Source data from Mar PL, Gopinathannair R, Gengler BE, et al.; from the American Heart Association Electrocardiography & Arrhythmias Committee of the Council of Clinical Cardiology. Drug interactions affecting oral anticoagulant use. Circ Arrhythm Electrophysiol. 2022;15(6):e007956. doi: 10.1161/CIRCEP.121.007956.

- Liver metabolism primarily occurs via CYP3A4, CYP3A5, and CYP2J2 and, like the other factor Xa inhibitors, rivaroxaban is a substrate for P-gp.
- Given rivaroxaban's greater dependence on liver metabolism, many studies have demonstrated that administration of combined strong CYP3A4 and P-gp inhibitors led to increased major and minor bleeding events.[31]
- Likewise, the use of strong inducers of CYP3A4 or P-gp is likely to lead to therapeutic failure and thrombosis.
- Thus, strong inhibitors and inducers of CYP3A4 and P-gp should be avoided.
- Use of moderate CYP3A4 and P-gp inhibitors is reasonable with monitoring if renal function is normal; however, consideration of avoidance or closer monitoring should occur if CrCl is less than 50 mL/min.
- ➔ Table 28.2 includes recommendations for interactions with rivaroxaban.

Vitamin K antagonists

(See also ➔ Chapter 9.) The VKAs, such as warfarin and acenocoumarol, are vitamin K epoxide reductase inhibitors which impacts the activation of four key components of the clotting cascade: factors II, VII, IX, and X. These agents are dependent on metabolization via CYP2C9 and CYP3A4 as well as some contribution via CYP1A2, CYP2C8, CYP2C18, and CYP2C19. Historically, VKAs were the only means of providing OAC. Thus, they have a rich historical context with literature indicating over 500 distinct described interactions with VKAs.[32] For the majority of these interactions, there is a lack of consensus on clinical significance. Unlike the DOACs, the VKAs can be monitored via the prothrombin time international normalized ratio (INR). Thus, when some interactions may pose a risk, that risk can be limited or mitigated via closer monitoring. Furthermore, certain warfarin drug interactions may be more significant in patients with a genetic polymorphism of CYP2C9.[31] ➔ Table 28.3 provides a list of common VKA interactions and their management recommendations.

Combination antiplatelet and anticoagulant therapy

Combination antiplatelet and anticoagulant therapy is indicated frequently in patients for separate, although sometimes related, conditions. The most common clinical scenario is a patient with atrial fibrillation requiring lifelong anticoagulant therapy to lower the risk of ischaemic stroke while also utilizing antiplatelet therapy for primary or secondary prevention of ischaemic coronary artery disease events, creating a so-called triple therapy regimen. Unfortunately, the pharmacodynamic drug interaction based on multiple antithrombotic pathways being inhibited creates additive bleeding risk, resulting in excess or potentially net harm to the patient while offering comparably little improvement in efficacy. Recent insights into the management of this DDI have indicated the following:

- Co-administration of aspirin with chronic OAC increases gastrointestinal bleeding risk by approximately 40%.[33] The net benefit of aspirin use in a primary prevention population should be re-evaluated in patients who also have indications for anticoagulation.
- Co-administration of dual antiplatelet therapy with chronic OAC increases major bleeding risk over twofold compared to dual antiplatelet therapy alone.[34]
- Multiple randomized clinical trials with DOACs in the setting of percutaneous coronary intervention indicate improved safety outcomes and similar effectiveness with the use of $P2Y_{12}$ inhibitor monotherapy (compared to dual antiplatelet therapy) in combination with DOAC therapy for the interval in which intensive antiplatelet therapy is indicated.[35–37]
- Randomized data with warfarin and $P2Y_{12}$ inhibitor monotherapy compared to continued triple therapy also demonstrate reduced bleeding risk and similar overall efficacy with this combination.[38]
- In general, the overall duration of triple therapy exposure to patients should be limited as much as possible (➔ Guideline recommendations).

Conclusion

Antiplatelet and anticoagulant DDIs are commonly encountered in clinical practice and have potential to significantly impact both the safety and efficacy of medications that already have comparably lower therapeutic indices relative to other medications. Recognition of this risk has led to increased scrutiny of anticoagulant safety by health agencies as well as accrediting bodies. Current systems in place to identify and ameliorate DDIs are largely reliant upon database-centric warning systems in electronic health records or knowledge by the provider or pharmacist, inevitably leading to a detectable prevalence of serious DDIs that are present in population research. Centralized management of antithrombotic therapy through specialized treatment clinics may help to circumvent avoidable DDIs or limit their exposure.[39,40] Similarly, developments in artificial intelligence may provide more timely clinical context to healthcare practitioners. However, the current system depends on some working knowledge in evaluating these scenarios by practitioners with potentially significant consequences for patient efficacy and safety in the management of CVD.

What's new

- DDIs with antithrombotic therapy can significantly impact both efficacy and safety of these critical agents in the prevention and treatment of CVD.
- Opioid co-administration is increasingly recognized to delay absorption and the therapeutic effect of oral antiplatelet drugs given in the setting of acute coronary syndromes though the exact clinical significance and management is still being investigated.
- Aspirin doses greater than 100 mg are still recognized as contraindicated with ticagrelor by some regulatory agencies though no mechanism or pharmacodynamic impact has been described.

Table 28.3 Summary of drug/food/supplement–drug interactions with vitamin K antagonists

Interacting drug	Interaction mechanism	Management recommendation
Acetaminophen	CYP enzyme inhibition	When doses of acetaminophen exceed 2 g/day, closer monitoring of INR levels is warranted
All antibiotics	Alteration in gut flora production of vitamin K	Close monitoring of INR levels
Amiodarone	CYP2C9 and CYP3A4 inhibition	Decrease warfarin dose by 25%
Antiplatelet therapies	Potentiation of bleeding	Minimize overlap to shortest duration indicated and consider starting a proton pump inhibitor
Aprepitant	CYP enzyme induction	Close monitoring of INR levels
Atorvastatin	CYP3A4 inhibition	Close monitoring of INR levels
Azithromycin	CYP inhibition	Closer monitoring of INR levels
Capecitabine	Possible enzyme induction	Closer monitoring of INR levels
Carbamazepine	CYP enzyme induction	Increase warfarin dose by 50% with close follow-up
Ciprofloxacin	CYP1A2 inhibition	Closer monitoring of INR
Clarithromycin	CYP3A4 inhibition	Closer monitoring of INR
Cloxacillin	CYP3A4 induction	Closer monitoring of INR
Cranberry juice	CYP enzyme inhibition	Consume no more than 700 mL per day
Danazol	Inhibition of metabolism	Closer monitoring of INR
Dronedarone	CYP3A4 inhibition	Closer monitoring of INR
Ethanol	CYP2C9 inhibition	Avoid excessive alcoholic consumption (<60 g/day)
Enzalutamide	CYP induction	Closer monitoring of INR
Erythromycin	CYP3A4 inhibition	Closer monitoring of INR
Flucloxacillin	CYP3A4 induction	Closer monitoring of INR
Fluconazole	CYP2C9 inhibition	Use alternative, if possible, otherwise closer monitoring is warranted
Fluorouracil	Multiple mechanisms	Decrease warfarin dose by 20%
Fluoxetine	CYP2C9 and CYP3A4 inhibition	Consider alternatives such as sertraline, citalopram, or escitalopram; otherwise, closer monitoring of INR levels is warranted
Fluvastatin	CYP2C9 inhibition	Decrease warfarin dose by 25%
Fluvoxamine	CYP2C9 and CYP3A4 inhibition	Consider alternatives such as sertraline, citalopram, or escitalopram; otherwise, closer monitoring of INR levels is warranted
Gemfibrozil	CYP2C9 inhibition	Decrease warfarin dose by 20%
Grapefruit juice	CYP3A4 inhibition	Consume no more than 200 mL per day
Metronidazole	CYP2C9 inhibition	Reduce warfarin dose by 33%
Miconazole	CYP2C9 inhibition	Consider alternative such as nystatin, otherwise consider closer monitoring
Nafcillin	CYP3A4 inhibition	Close monitoring of INR levels; full induction of CYP enzymes occurs in 2–4 weeks after initiation and persists up to 2–4 weeks after discontinuation of nafcillin
Non-steroidal anti-inflammatory drugs	Cyclooxygenase inhibition	Avoid unless benefits clearly outweigh risk
Paclitaxel	Displacement from protein binding or CYP3A4 inhibition	Closer monitoring of INR
Phenytoin	Biphasic interaction with initial displacement from protein binding and then enzyme induction	Closer monitoring of INR
Rifampin	CYP3A4 induction	Closer monitoring of INR
Ritonavir	CYP3A4 inhibition	Closer monitoring of INR
Rosuvastatin	CYP3A4 inhibition	Closer monitoring of INR
Simvastatin	CYP3A4 inhibition	Closer monitoring of INR
St John's wort	CYP induction	Closer monitoring of INR
Sulfonamides	CYP2C9 inhibition	Reduce warfarin dose by 25%
Voriconazole	CYP2C9 inhibition	Use alternative, if possible, otherwise closer monitoring is warranted

CYP, cytochrome P450; INR, international normalized ratio.

Source data from Mar PL, Gopinathannair R, Gengler BE, et al; from the American Heart Association Electrocardiography & Arrhythmias Committee of the Council of Clinical Cardiology. Drug Interactions Affecting Oral Anticoagulant Use. Circ Arrhythm Electrophysiol. 2022;15(6):e007956. doi: 10.1161/CIRCEP.121.007956.

- Strong CYP3A4, P-gp, and combination CYP3A4/P-gp inhibitors and inducers create significant DDIs with most DOACs. While the list of contraindicated therapies is relatively clear, more precision with lesser interactions and management strategies are gradually being defined.

- Combination dual antiplatelet and anticoagulant therapy should not be prescribed for significant lengths of time when there are indications for both. The recommended management strategy is $P2Y_{12}$ inhibitor monotherapy plus anticoagulation when indicated for longer durations.

Guideline recommendations

Guideline recommendations for management of combination anticoagulation and antiplatelet therapy

	2017 ESC focused update on dual antiplatelet therapy[a]	2020 ESC atrial fibrillation guidelines[b]	2021 North American consensus recommendations[c]
Aspirin discontinuation in triple therapy regimen peri-PCI	1 month (IIa, B); up to 6 months in high ischaemic risk and low bleeding risk (IIa, B)	Low stent thrombosis risk or concerns about bleeding risk: 1 week (I, A) Stent thrombosis risk outweighs bleeding risk: 1 month (IIa, C)	Up until time of discharge or a few days longer, generally 1 week; up to 1 month in patients at high thrombotic risk with an acceptable risk of bleeding
Anticoagulant preference	No specific recommendation	NOAC preferred over VKA (I, A)	NOAC preferred over VKA
Antiplatelet preference	The use of ticagrelor or prasugrel is not recommended (III, C)	Clopidogrel is preferred (I, A)	Clopidogrel is preferred; ticagrelor should be reserved for patients at the highest risk of stent thrombosis with acceptable bleeding risk; prasugrel is not recommended
NOAC dosing recommendations	The lowest approved dose effective for stroke prevention tested in AF trials should be considered (IIa, C) Recommend rivaroxaban 15 mg/day when used with antiplatelet therapy (IIb, B)	In patients at high bleeding risk (HAS-BLED ≥3), recommend: ◆ Dabigatran 110 mg twice daily instead of 150 mg twice daily (IIa, B) ◆ Rivaroxaban 15 mg/day instead of 20 mg/day (IIa, B)	Avoid doses lower than those proven effective for stroke prevention in clinical trials Recommend rivaroxaban 15 mg/day with antiplatelet therapy Recommend dabigatran 150 mg twice daily in patients at high thrombotic risk and 110 mg twice daily in patients at high bleeding risk
$P2Y_{12}$ inhibitor discontinuation	Consider at 12 months (IIa, B)	ACS patient: up to 12 months (I, A) Stable PCI: up to 6 months (I, A)	1 year for most patients; consider earlier discontinuation (e.g. 6 months) in patients at low ischaemic risk or high bleeding risk
VKA management	Carefully regulate in the lower part of the INR range and a TTR >65–70%	Carefully regulate with target INR 2.0–2.5 and TTR >70%	INR should be targeted to the lower end of the therapeutic range (e.g. 2.0–2.5)

ACS, acute coronary syndrome; AF, atrial fibrillation; INR, international normalized ratio; NOAC, non-vitamin K antagonist oral anticoagulant; PCI, percutaneous coronary intervention; TTR, time in therapeutic range; VKA, vitamin K antagonist.

[a] Valgimigli M, Bueno H, Byrne RA, et al. 2017 ESC focused update on dual antiplatelet therapy in coronary artery disease developed in collaboration with EACTS. Eur J Cardiothorac Surg. 2018;53(1):34–78. doi: 10.1093/ejcts/ezx334.

[b] Hindricks G, Potpara T, Dagres N, et al. 2020 ESC Guidelines for the diagnosis and management of atrial fibrillation developed in collaboration with the European Association for Cardio-Thoracic Surgery (EACTS). Eur Heart J. 2021;42(5):373–498. doi: 10.1093/eurheartj/ehaa612.

[c] Angiolillo DJ, Bhatt DL, Cannon CP, et al. Antithrombotic therapy in patients with atrial fibrillation treated with oral anticoagulation undergoing percutaneous coronary intervention: a North American perspective: 2021 Update. Circulation. 2021;143(6):583–596. doi: 10.1161/CIRCULATIONAHA.120.050438.

What's next

- More outcomes-based research for lesser but potentially still clinically significant DDIs with antithrombotic therapy will likely occur as utilization over time increases.
- Definitive research and guideline recommendations regarding oral antiplatelet and opioid pharmacotherapy in the setting of acute coronary syndromes are warranted.
- VKAs will continue to be utilized for the foreseeable future but some of the infrastructure dedicated to the safe and effective use of these therapies may decrease. Unique strategies to manage and mitigate spontaneous changes such as DDIs may be useful.
- Increased utilization and research into providing clinicians with timely and useful information about DDIs at the time of prescribing would be valuable.

References

1. World Health Organization. Cardiovascular diseases (CVDs). 2021. Available at: https://www.who.int/news-room/fact-sheets/detail/cardiovascular-diseases-(cvds)
2. de Oliveira LM, Diel JDAC, Nunes A, da Silva Dal Pizzol T. Prevalence of drug interactions in hospitalised elderly patients: a systematic review. Eur J Hosp Pharm. 2021;28:4–9.
3. Gonzaga de Andrade Santos TN, Mendonça da Cruz Macieira G, Cardoso Sodré Alves BM, et al. Prevalence of clinically manifested drug interactions in hospitalized patients: a systematic review and meta-analysis. PLoS One. 2020;15:e0235353.
4. Huber K. Genetic variability in response to clopidogrel therapy: clinical implications. Eur Heart J. 2010;31:2974–6.
5. Schrör K, Siller-Matula JM, Huber K. Pharmacokinetic basis of the antiplatelet action of prasugrel. Fundam Clin Pharmacol. 2012;26:39–46.
6. Frelinger AL 3rd, Lee RD, Mulford DJ, et al. A randomized, 2-period, crossover design study to assess the effects of dexlansoprazole, lansoprazole, esomeprazole, and omeprazole on the steady-state pharmacokinetics and pharmacodynamics of clopidogrel in healthy volunteers. J Am Coll Cardiol. 2012;59:1304–11.
7. Serbin MA, Guzauskas GF, Veenstra DL. Clopidogrel-proton pump inhibitor drug-drug interaction and risk of adverse clinical outcomes among PCI-treated ACS patients: a meta-analysis. J Manag Care Spec Pharm. 2016;22:939–47.
8. Dunn SP, Steinhubl SR, Bauer D, Charnigo RJ, Berger PB, Topol EJ. Impact of proton pump inhibitor therapy on the efficacy of clopidogrel in the CAPRIE and CREDO trials. JAmHeart Assoc. 2013;2:e004564.
9. Bhatt DL, Cryer BL, Contant CF, et al. Clopidogrel with or without omeprazole in coronary artery disease. N Engl J Med. 2010;363:1909–17.
10. Farid NA, Payne CD, Small DS, et al. Cytochrome P450 3A inhibition by ketoconazole affects prasugrel and clopidogrel pharmacokinetics and pharmacodynamics differently. Clin Pharmacol Ther. 2007;81:735–41.
11. Daali Y, Ancrenaz V, Bosilkovska M, Dayer P, Desmeules J. Ritonavir inhibits the two main prasugrel bioactivation pathways in vitro: a potential drug-drug interaction in HIV patients. Metabolism. 2011;60:1584–9.
12. Judge HM, Patil SB, Buckland RJ, Jakubowski JA, Storey RF. Potentiation of clopidogrel active metabolite formation by rifampicin leads to greater P2Y12 receptor blockade and inhibition of platelet aggregation after clopidogrel. J Thromb Haemost. 2010;8:1820–7.
13. Farid NA, Jakubowski JA, Payne CD, et al. Effect of rifampin on the pharmacokinetics and pharmacodynamics of prasugrel in healthy male subjects. Curr Med Res Opin. 2009;25:1821–9.
14. Hobl E-L, Stimpfl T, Ebner J, et al. Morphine decreases clopidogrel concentrations and effects: a randomized, double-blind, placebo-controlled trial. J Am Coll Cardiol. 2014;63:630–5.
15. Hobl E-L, Reiter B, Schoergenhofer C, et al. Morphine interaction with prasugrel: a double-blind, cross-over trial in healthy volunteers. Clin Res Cardiol. 2016;105:349–55.
16. Ibrahim K, Shah R, Goli RR, et al. Fentanyl delays the platelet inhibition effects of oral ticagrelor: full report of the PACIFY randomized clinical trial. Thromb Haemost. 2018;118:1409–18.
17. Meine TJ, Roe MT, Chen AY, et al. Association of intravenous morphine use and outcomes in acute coronary syndromes: results from the CRUSADE Quality Improvement Initiative. Am Heart J. 2005;149:1043–9.
18. Teng R, Butler K. Effect of the CYP3A inhibitors, diltiazem and ketoconazole, on ticagrelor pharmacokinetics in healthy volunteers. J Drug Assess. 2013;2:30–9.
19. Wallentin L, Becker RC, Budaj A, et al. Ticagrelor versus clopidogrel in patients with acute coronary syndromes. N Engl J Med. 2009;361:1045–57.
20. Mahaffey KW, Wojdyla DM, Carroll K, et al. Ticagrelor compared with clopidogrel by geographic region in the Platelet Inhibition and Patient Outcomes (PLATO) trial. Circulation. 2011;124:544–54.
21. Teng R, Maya J, Butler K. Evaluation of the pharmacokinetics and pharmacodynamics of ticagrelor co-administered with aspirin in healthy volunteers. Platelets. 2013;24:615–24.
22. AstraZeneca. Brilinta [package insert]. Sept 2016. Available at: https://www.accessdata.fda.gov/drugsatfda_docs/label/2016/022433s020lbl.pdf
23. Barnes GD, Lucas E, Alexander GC, Goldberger ZD. National trends in ambulatory oral anticoagulant use. Am J Med. 2015;128:1300–5.
24. Suh D-C, Nelson WW, Choi JC, Choi I. Risk of hemorrhage and treatment costs associated with warfarin drug interactions in patients with atrial fibrillation. Clin Ther. 2012;34:1569–82.
25. Boehringer Ingelheim Pharmaceuticals, Inc. Pradaxa [package insert]. Nov 2011. Available at: https://www.accessdata.fda.gov/drugsatfda_docs/label/2011/022512s007lbl.pdf
26. US Food and Drug Administration. Drug development and drug interactions. Table of substrates, inhibitors and inducers. Aug 2022. Available at: https://www.fda.gov/drugs/drug-interactions-labeling/drug-development-and-drug-interactions-table-substrates-inhibitors-and-inducers
27. Bristol-Myers Squibb Company. Eliquis [package insert]. Dec 2012. Available at: https://www.accessdata.fda.gov/drugsatfda_docs/label/2012/202155s000lbl.pdf
28. Daiichi Sankyo, Inc. Savaysa [package insert]. Jan 2015. Available at: https://www.accessdata.fda.gov/drugsatfda_docs/label/2015/206316lbl.pdf
29. Parasrampuria DA, Mendell J, Shi M, Matsushima N, Zahir H, Truitt K. Edoxaban drug-drug interactions with ketoconazole, erythromycin, and cyclosporine. Br J Clin Pharmacol. 2016;82:1591–600.
30. Janssen Pharmaceuticals, Inc. Xarelto [package insert]. May 2016. Available at: https://www.accessdata.fda.gov/drugsatfda_docs/label/2016/202439s017lbl.pdf
31. Mar PL, Gopinathannair R, Gengler BE, et al. Drug interactions affecting oral anticoagulant use. Circ Arrhythm Electrophysiol. 2022;15:e007956.
32. Martins MAP, Carlos PPS, Ribeiro DD, et al. Warfarin drug interactions: a comparative evaluation of the lists provided by five information sources. Eur J Clin Pharmacol. 2011;67:1301–8.
33. García Rodríguez LA, Martín-Pérez M, Hennekens CH, Rothwell PM, Lanas A. Bleeding risk with long-term low-dose aspirin: a systematic review of observational studies. PLoS One. 2016;11:e0160046.

34. Oldgren J, Wallentin L, Alexander JH, et al. New oral anticoagulants in addition to single or dual antiplatelet therapy after an acute coronary syndrome: a systematic review and meta-analysis. Eur Heart J. 2013;34:1670–80.
35. Gibson CM, Mehran R, Bode C, et al. Prevention of bleeding in patients with atrial fibrillation undergoing PCI. N Engl J Med. 2016;375:2423–34.
36. Lopes RD, Heizer G, Aronson R, et al. Antithrombotic therapy after acute coronary syndrome or PCI in atrial fibrillation. N Engl J Med. 2019;380:1509–24.
37. Cannon CP, Bhatt DL, Oldgren J, et al. Dual antithrombotic therapy with dabigatran after PCI in atrial fibrillation. N Engl J Med. 2017;377:1513–24.
38. Dewilde WJM, Oirbans T, Verheugt FWA, et al. Use of clopidogrel with or without aspirin in patients taking oral anticoagulant therapy and undergoing percutaneous coronary intervention: an open-label, randomised, controlled trial. Lancet. 2013;381:1107–15.
39. Haché J, Bonsu KO, Chitsike R, Nguyen H, Young S. Assessment of a pharmacist-led direct oral anticoagulant monitoring clinic. Can J Hosp Pharm. 2021;74:7–14.
40. Uppuluri EM, McComb MN, Shapiro NL. Implementation of a direct oral anticoagulation screening service at a large academic medical center provided by a pharmacist-managed antithrombosis clinic as a method to expand antithrombotic stewardship efforts. J Pharm Pract. 2020;33:271–5.

CHAPTER 29

Personalized antithrombotic therapy: measuring individual variation and monitoring

Wout W.A. van den Broek, Jur M. ten Berg, Dirk Sibbing, and Konstantinos D. Rizas

Contents

Summary

Antithrombotic drugs are frequently prescribed in patients with coronary artery disease, embolic stroke, or atrial fibrillation to prevent thrombosis. However, patients vary widely in their response to these drugs. This interindividual variability can be a result of genetic variation in enzymes that play a role in drug metabolism, though it can also be a consequence of other patient characteristics. A personalized antithrombotic treatment accounts for this interindividual variability with the aim of optimizing the balance between the risk of bleeding and thrombosis. Personalization of antithrombotic therapy might be done by testing for genetic polymorphisms or measuring the patient's response on treatment, both of which have their advantages and disadvantages. This chapter describes the different ways that antithrombotic therapy can be personalized, provides the latest evidence for these strategies, and focuses on the treatment strategies with the most clinical impact.

Introduction: personalized antithrombotic therapy

Patients vary widely in their response to drugs. To a great extent this can be explained by genetic variation, though different patient characteristics, such as age, body weight, kidney disease, and diabetes mellitus, also play a part in this.[1] As this variable response can influence the efficacy or safety of antithrombotic treatment, a personalized antithrombotic therapy could in theory optimize patient outcomes. Personalizing antithrombotic therapy can be done by testing for genetic polymorphisms or measuring the patient's response on treatment. With vitamin K antagonists, this is already standard of care, as the daily dose is based on the international normalized ratio (INR). Regarding antiplatelet therapy, personalizing treatment can be based on specific genetic polymorphisms or by platelet function testing (PFT) (➔ Figure 29.1). Although there is a growing body of evidence suggesting that a personalized antiplatelet therapy can optimize patient outcomes, it is not (yet) routinely used in clinical care. In this chapter we provide the latest evidence, guideline recommendations, and promising developments regarding the personalization of anticoagulants and antiplatelet therapy in patients with cardiovascular disease.

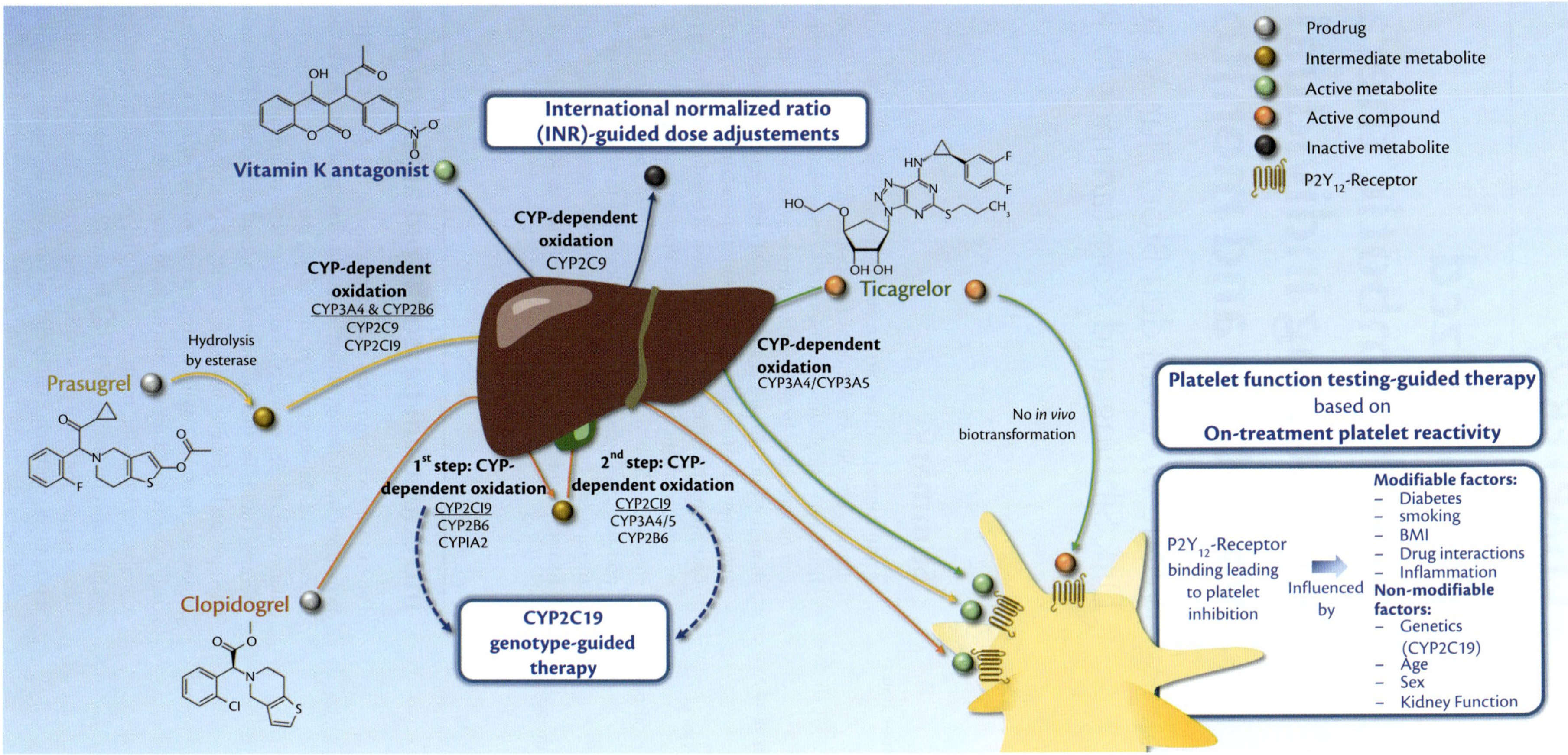

Figure 29.1 Biotransformation and metabolism of the different antithrombotic agents. Antithrombotic therapy can be personalized by (1) using cytochrome P450 (CYP)-2C19 genotype-guided therapy, which is the only genetic polymorphism for which a genotype-guided therapy has been assessed in randomized controlled trials regarding clinical outcomes; or (2) assessing the actual responsiveness to antithrombotic therapy by measuring the international normalized ratio (INR) or on-treatment platelet reactivity, which are influenced by various modifiable and non-modifiable factors.

Pharmacogenetics

Pharmacogenetics is a field of research studying how variation in genes can affect a person's response to drugs. Genetic polymorphisms are nucleotide changes in the reference sequence of a gene that occur in more than 1% of the population.[2] These polymorphisms can influence the action of a drug by altering its pharmacokinetics or pharmacodynamics, often caused by genetic variation in the drug-metabolizing cytochrome P450 (CYP) enzymes. CYP enzymes play a major role in the phase I reactions (oxidation, reduction, and hydrolysis) of drug metabolism, by either converting a drug to its active metabolite or deactivating an active metabolite. In pharmacogenetics, different polymorphisms are indicated with different labels, consisting of an asterisk (*) followed by an Arabic numeral, in which *1 corresponds to a genotype with two standard copies of the normally functional allele, corresponding to the phenotype of extensive metabolizers (EMs). Patients who carry one (heterozygous) or two (homozygous) loss-of-function (LoF) alleles leading to a reduced function of the enzyme are known as intermediate (IMs) or poor metabolizers (PMs), respectively (➔ Table 29.1).[3]

Anticoagulants

The different oral anticoagulants can be divided into two groups, the vitamin K antagonists (VKAs) and the direct oral anticoagulants (DOACs), both primarily used to prevent thrombus formation in low shear stress environments (e.g. fibrillating atria, veins). VKAs (such as acenocoumarol, phenprocoumon, and warfarin) have both a high interindividual and a high intraindividual variability, due to multiple significant food and drug interactions, but their effectivity is also affected by different genetic polymorphisms.[4] Consequently, VKAs have a very narrow therapeutic window, which complicates dosing and necessitates frequent measurements of the international normalized ratio (INR).

The first month of VKA treatment is especially problematic as the therapeutic dose is empirically assessed, with further adjustments made on the basis of trial and error, leading to possible over- or under-anticoagulation with associated potential bleeding or thrombotic events. There are many studies that have assessed the impact of genetic variations on VKA treatment.[5] The genes with the strongest literature support are *CYP2C9* and vitamin K epoxide reductase complex 1 (*VKORC1*), both associated with lower VKA dose requirements and even a higher risk of bleeding.[6] CYP2C9 converts the active drug into inactive metabolites (➔ Figure 29.1). Polymorphisms in *CYP2C9* can lead to high variations in dose response.[7,8] Polymorphisms in the gene encoding VKORC1, which converts vitamin K into its active form and is inhibited by VKAs, also affects the inter-individual variability in warfarin dosing.[9] In 2005 the first warfarin dosing algorithm was published, which included age, height, and *CYP2C9* and *VKORC1* genotype.[10] This led the US Food and Drug Administration (FDA) to modify the warfarin label to include the impact of *CYP2C9* or *VKORC1* gene polymorphisms on dosing in 2007, followed by an additional modification including a pharmacogenetic-guided dosing scheme in 2010. Since then, multiple randomized controlled trials (RCTs) have evaluated the clinical benefit of a personalized VKA strategy using pharmacogenetic algorithm-guided dosing compared with standard dosing strategies.[11–15] A number of meta-analyses have been published showing that genotype-guided dosing improves the time within the therapeutic INR range.[16–18] Moreover, the use of pharmacogenetics in VKA dosing may also reduce bleeding complications; however, not all study results are unequivocal on this.[19–21] Altogether, a personalized pharmacogenetic algorithm can facilitate and improve daily dosing of VKAs, especially when initiating treatment. Hence, the Clinical Pharmacogenetics Implementation Consortium (CPIC) recommends to use these pharmacogenetic algorithms to calculate warfarin dosing,[5] although this is very rarely implemented in clinical practice at the moment.

The newer DOACs (dabigatran, rivaroxaban, apixaban, and edoxaban) have a more convenient therapeutic window and do

Table 29.1 CYP2C19 phenotypes, clopidogrel response, and therapeutic recommendations

Metabolizer phenotype	Examples of CYP2C19 diplotypes	Response to clopidogrel	Therapeutic recommendation[54]	Classification of recommendation (CPIC)[54]
Ultra-rapid metabolizer (UM)	*17/*17	Normal or increased antiplatelet response to clopidogrel	If considering clopidogrel, use at standard dose	Strong
Rapid metabolizer (RM)	*1/*17	Normal or increased antiplatelet response to clopidogrel	If considering clopidogrel, use at standard dose	Strong
Extensive metabolizer (EM)	*1/*1	Normal antiplatelet response to clopidogrel	If considering clopidogrel, use at standard dose	Strong
Intermediate metabolizer (IM)	*1/*2, *1/*3, *2/*17, or *3/*17	Reduced antiplatelet response to clopidogrel	Avoid standard dose clopidogrel. Use prasugrel or ticagrelor at standard dose if no contraindication	Strong
Poor metabolizer (PM)	*2/*2, *2/*3, or *3/*3	Significantly reduced antiplatelet response to clopidogrel	Avoid clopidogrel. Use prasugrel or ticagrelor at standard dose if no contraindication	Strong

not necessitate routine coagulation monitoring, as opposed to VKAs.[22] Despite this, DOACs also have a notable interindividual variability, which may be caused by genetic polymorphisms. Pharmacogenetic testing may help physicians in choosing the most appropriate DOAC treatment. However, currently the evidence is too scarce to recommend routinely genetic testing in patients treated with DOACs.[23]

Antiplatelet therapy

In patients with coronary artery disease (CAD), dual antiplatelet therapy (DAPT) with aspirin and a $P2Y_{12}$ inhibitor (ticagrelor, prasugrel, or clopidogrel) is the cornerstone of medical therapy to prevent the recurrence of thrombotic events.[24–27] Both ticagrelor and prasugrel have a more potent inhibitory effect on platelets, reducing thrombotic events when compared to clopidogrel in large RCTs.[28,29] Accordingly, in patients with an acute coronary syndrome (ACS), ticagrelor or prasugrel are recommended over clopidogrel in the guidelines.[24,25] However, this benefit regarding thrombotic events is counterbalanced by an increased bleeding risk.[28,29] As the prognostic impact of a major bleeding event is comparable to a recurrent thrombotic event, reducing the bleeding risk without affecting efficacy is an extremely important and valuable goal when prescribing DAPT.[30–32]

Aspirin (acetylsalicylic acid) is metabolized by different enzymes [e.g. uridine diphosphate (UDP)-glucuronosyltransferase 1A6, CYP2C9, and N-acetyl transferase 2], but so far no association between genetic polymorphisms and platelet reactivity or clinical outcomes has been demonstrated.[33,34] Ticagrelor is a direct-acting drug, whereas clopidogrel and prasugrel (both thienopyridines) are prodrugs that require cytochrome P450-based *in vivo* conversion to an active metabolite to irreversibly inhibit the $P2Y_{12}$ receptor.[35] The enzyme CYP3A4/5 plays a role in the metabolism of ticagrelor, but no clinically relevant interactions between ticagrelor and genetic polymorphisms are currently known.[36,37] Prasugrel is metabolized to its active metabolite primarily by CYP3A4 and CYP2B6, and to a lesser extent by CYP2C9 and CYP2C19.[38] Common polymorphisms in CYP3A4, CYP2B6, CYP2C9, and CYP2C19 have not been related to relevant pharmacokinetic or pharmacodynamic changes, and carriers of these polymorphisms, treated with prasugrel, did not have an elevated risk of cardiovascular events.[38–40] With clopidogrel it is a different story, as there is a large interindividual variability in pharmacokinetic and pharmacodynamic effects between patients treated with clopidogrel.[41] As a consequence, 30% of patients do not adequately respond to treatment with clopidogrel.[42]

Multiple CYP enzymes play a part (CYP2C19, CYP3A4/5, CYP1A2, CYP2B6, CYP2C9) in the two-step conversion of clopidogrel to its active metabolite; however, CYP2C19 is the main contributor in both steps (➔ Figure 29.1).[43] Carriers of CYP2C19 LoF alleles have a dysfunctional CYP2C19 enzyme, resulting in impaired metabolism of clopidogrel and, as a consequence, in lower levels of the active metabolite.[40] The prevalence of the CYP2C19 polymorphisms (*2 and *3) is estimated to be approximately 25%, 33%, and 55% in the Caucasian, African American, and Asian populations, respectively.[35,44,45] Multiple studies have confirmed that carriers of CYP2C19 LoF alleles have a decreased antiplatelet response and an increased prevalence of high platelet reactivity (HPR).[46–51] Consequently, these patients are at higher risk for thrombotic events, including stent thrombosis.[46,52] This prompted the US FDA to add a 'boxed warning' on the clopidogrel label in 2010, alerting patients and healthcare professionals that clopidogrel treatment is less effective in PMs.[53]

Clinical evidence for a genotype-guided antithrombotic therapy

The US FDA boxed warning on clopidogrel was followed by multiple studies assessing the efficacy and safety of a CYP2C19 genotype-guided strategy in patients with CAD.[42,55–61] The various strategies can be distinguished into 'de-escalation' or 'escalation' of the $P2Y_{12}$ inhibitor therapy. A de-escalation strategy involves switching from the more potent drugs ticagrelor or prasugrel to the less potent clopidogrel in EMs, while escalation involves switching from clopidogrel to ticagrelor or prasugrel in IMs or PMs. De-escalation can be applied in patients with ACS, where current standard treatment is ticagrelor or prasugrel. Escalation of $P2Y_{12}$ inhibitor therapy can be done in patients with a chronic coronary syndrome undergoing percutaneous coronary intervention (PCI), stroke, or peripheral artery disease, where clopidogrel is standard care.

In patients with CAD, multiple randomized trials and non-randomized studies have provided evidence in support for genotyping. The largest randomized trials until now are the Popular Genetics and the TAILOR-PCI studies.[62,63] In the Popular Genetics trial, a genotype-guided de-escalation strategy was assessed in 2488 patients undergoing primary PCI for ST-segment elevation myocardial infarction. In both groups, all patients were treated with aspirin; however, in the genotype-guided group, IMs and PMs were treated with ticagrelor or prasugrel (39%), whereas EMs received clopidogrel (61%). Patients in the control group were treated with ticagrelor according to current guidelines. Genotype-guided $P2Y_{12}$ inhibitor treatment was initiated within 24 hours after randomization and resulted in a lower bleeding incidence compared with standard care with prasugrel or ticagrelor [9.8 vs 12.5%, hazard ratio (HR) 0.78, 95% confidence interval (CI) 0.61–0.98; P = 0.04]. There was no evidence for an increase in thrombotic events in the genotype-guided group.

The TAILOR-PCI study randomized 5302 patients undergoing PCI for ACS or stable CAD between a genotype-guided escalation strategy or conventional therapy.[63] In the genotype-guided group, those identified as CYP2C19 LoF carriers (IMs or PMs) were prescribed ticagrelor (31%), and non-carriers were prescribed clopidogrel (68%). This strategy was compared with clopidogrel treatment in the conventional therapy group. The primary analysis was undertaken in only those patients who were CYP2C19 LoF carriers. There was no statistical difference in primary outcomes regarding cardiovascular death, myocardial infarction, stroke, stent thrombosis, and severe recurrent ischaemia at 12 months (HR 0.66, 95% CI 0.43–1.02; P = 0.06), though the reduced event rates suggest a clinical benefit with the genotype-guided therapy regarding thrombotic outcomes. There was no significant difference in bleeding [Thrombolysis In Myocardial Infarction (TIMI) major or minor bleeding] in the primary analysis cohort. Although the trial was underpowered to detect an effect size less than the prespecified expected 50% relative risk reduction, it showed promising results that offer support for the benefit of a genetically guided therapy. This was also supported by a post hoc analysis for the first 3 months post PCI, which demonstrated a HR of 0.21 (95% CI 0.08–0.54), indicating that the genotype-guided therapy significantly reduced thrombotic risk in the first months, generally the most vulnerable period, after PCI. Furthermore, when allowing for multiple events instead of a time-to-first-event analysis, the genotype-guided therapy was superior to the conventional therapy (HR 0.60, 95% CI 0.41–0.89).

These results are also backed-up by a meta-analysis including 15,949 patients with CAD, showing that carriers of a CYP2C219 LoF allele (*2 or *3) had improved thrombotic outcomes when treated with ticagrelor or prasugrel as compared with those treated with clopidogrel.[64] When ticagrelor or prasugrel was compared with clopidogrel in only wild-type patients (EMs, *1/*1), clopidogrel had comparable efficacy in the prevention of thrombotic events. These results are also consistent with previous large meta-analyses, which demonstrated that clopidogrel-treated patients undergoing PCI who are CYP2C19 IMs or PMs have a higher risk for major adverse cardiovascular events (MACEs) and stent thrombosis compared with CYP2C19 EMs (*1/*1).[65–69] Based on all this evidence, the CPIC recommends to avoid clopidogrel in CYP2C19 IMs and PMs and use an alternative antiplatelet agent, such as prasugrel or ticagrelor, if there are no contraindications.[54] Despite this, a genotype-guided antiplatelet therapy is not yet recommended as standard care in patients with CAD: a genotype-guided de-escalation of $P2Y_{12}$ inhibition currently has a class IIb recommendation, and can be considered for ACS patients deemed unsuitable for potent platelet inhibition.[25]

Nevertheless, based on the growing base of evidence for a genotype-guided DAPT, some centres have implemented a genotype-guided strategy into their clinical practice.[70] Their results are in line with previous meta-analyses, showing that CYP2C19 LoF carriers treated with alternative therapy (ticagrelor or prasugrel) have a lower thrombotic risk when compared with clopidogrel, though the thrombotic risk is similar in those without a LoF allele treated with clopidogrel compared to alternative therapy.

Although most evidence for a genotype-guided antiplatelet treatment comes from trials conducted in patients with CAD, vascular disease is a universal pathophysiological phenomenon that does not adhere to the boundaries of a particular organ. Coherently, a meta-analysis has shown that also in patients with ischaemic stroke or transient ischaemic attack, carriers of a CYP2C19 LoF allele are at greater risk of stroke and of a composite of vascular events than non-carriers.[71] These results are supported by clinical data from the CHANCE-2 trial, which was a RCT in 6412 patients with acute ischaemic stroke or transient ischaemic attack.[72] The trial exclusively enrolled carriers of CYP2C19 LoF alleles, and compared the effects of ticagrelor plus aspirin to standard-dose clopidogrel (75 mg/day) plus aspirin over 90 days. Compared with clopidogrel, ticagrelor-treated IMs and PMs experienced significantly lower rates of stroke and major vascular events, without an increase in moderate or severe bleeding. However, ticagrelor was associated with higher rates of mild bleeding events.

Genetic testing can thus be a valuable tool to aid clinical decision-making, allowing the optimal choice of $P2Y_{12}$ inhibiting therapy. It also has the following advantages: there is no inter-assay variability, no variability of results over time, results are not influenced by extra-patient factors (e.g. timing of the test), and there is no need for the patient to be on treatment. However, genetic testing cannot account for other factors (both modifiable and non-modifiable) affecting the response on antithrombotic drugs (➔ Figure 29.1), and might thus be less accurate in identifying patients with HPR. This can be overcome by the use of PFT, which provides a direct measure of an individual's response to $P2Y_{12}$ inhibitors and automatically accounts for the influence on platelet reactivity of factors like comorbidities, age, sex, and genetics.

Platelet function testing

PFT refers to different *ex vivo* methods aiming to test the ability of platelets to aggregate with each other in response to external aggregating agents. The assessment of PFT has found application in various clinical conditions, including transfusion medicine, identification of patients with bleeding disorders, and monitoring the response to antiplatelet treatment. In particular, monitoring the response of platelets to treatment with $P2Y_{12}$ inhibitors has been evaluated by means of the reactivity of platelet aggregation in response to stimulation with adenosine diphosphate (ADP). The different assays used for the *ex vivo* assessment of platelet reactivity to ADP are classified as point-of-care (VerifyNow, Multiplate, thromboelastography) and laboratory-based methods, such as measurement of vasodilator-stimulated phosphoprotein (VASP) phosphorylation using flow cytometry[73] and light transmission aggregometry (LTA). LTA is considered the gold standard method to investigate patients with suspected abnormalities of primary haemostasis, due to inherited or acquired defects of platelet function. This technique determines platelet aggregation percentage in platelet-rich plasma by measuring the increase in light transmittance in response to the addition of a platelet agonist to the platelet suspension. However, several aspects of the LTA methodology have not been adequately standardized[74] and this method is not routinely used for monitoring subjects on antiplatelet therapy.[75] Regardless of the assay used, the response of platelet aggregation to ADP stimulation has been classified as HPR, low platelet reactivity (LPR), and optimal platelet reactivity (OPR)[76], which is defined as the therapeutic window between LPR and HPR. HPR is associated with increased risk for thrombosis,

Table 29.2 Definition of low and high platelet reactivity for different *ex vivo* assessment methods (point of care: VerifyNow™, Multiplate Analyzer®, and thromboelastography) and laboratory-based methods [using flow-cytometry (measurement of VASP phosphorylation) and LTA]

Assay	LPR	HPR
VerifyNow™ $P2Y_{12}$	85 PRU	208 PRU
Multiplate® Analyzer	18 U	46 U
Thromboelastography (TEG)	31 mm	47 mm
Measurement of VASP phosphorylation	16% PRI	50% PRI
Light transmission aggregometry (LTA)	NA	≥70%

HPR, high platelet reactivity; LPR, low-platelet reactivity; PRI, platelet reactivity index; PRU, platelet reactivity units; VASP, vasodilator-stimulated phosphoprotein.

while LPR is linked to higher risk for bleeding complications.[77] Consequently, patients within the therapeutic window of platelet reactivity have the lowest risk for adverse events.[73] The cut-off values for this categorization are highly dependent on the assay used. Cut-off values for HPR and LPR for the different assays are summarized in ➔ Table 29.2.[73]

Platelet function testing as predictor of events

Current guidelines for antithrombotic therapy in patients undergoing PCI recommend the implementation of DAPT consisting of aspirin and a $P2Y_{12}$ inhibitor for 1–12 months.[25,78,79] However, treatment with all currently available $P2Y_{12}$ inhibitors has been associated with an increased risk for bleeding complications.[28,29,80–82] Moreover, both ischaemic and bleeding events are key counterparts determining the overall patient survival.[83] Therefore, an effort to minimize both complications in PCI-treated patients is an important goal in modern cardiology.[24,84] Monitoring platelet reactivity during treatment with $P2Y_{12}$ inhibitors has been shown to be an important predictor of both bleeding and ischaemic complications, as HPR has been linked to a greater risk for ischaemic complications, while LPR has been associated with a higher incidence of bleeding events.[77] In a meta-analysis combining the results of 17 observational and randomized studies with inclusion of more than 20,000 patients, Aradi et al. demonstrated that, compared with OPR, HPR was associated with a 2.7-fold higher risk for definite or probable stent thromboses [weighted relative risk (RR) 2.73; 95% CI 2.03–3.69; P <0.001].[76] There was no significant advantage of LPR compared to OPR with respect to stent-thromboses (RR 1.06, 95% CI 0.68–1.65; P = 0.78). However, LPR was associated with a 1.7-fold increased risk for clinically relevant major bleeding complications, defined as TIMI major or Bleeding Academic Research Consortium (BARC) type 2 or greater bleeding events (RR 1.74, 95% CI 1.47–2.05; P <0.001).[76] HPR compared to OPR further decreased bleeding events by 16% (RR 0.84, 95% CI 0.71–0.99; P = 0.04). However, it is important to note that, compared with OPR, HPR was associated with higher mortality (RR 1.54, 95% CI 1.22–1.94; P <0.001), while there was no significant difference between LPR and OPR (RR 1.03, 95% CI 0.76–1.40) with respect to all-cause mortality. Based on these results, it can be concluded that a platelet reactivity within the therapeutic window warrants the lowest rate of ischaemic events and bleeding complications.

Platelet function testing-guided escalation in clinical trials

Current guidelines recommend treatment with DAPT based on a potent $P2Y_{12}$ inhibitor (prasugrel or ticagrelor) in patients with ACS undergoing PCI[25,78] and a DAPT therapy with clopidogrel in patients undergoing elective PCI because of stable CAD.[26] Based on the results of previous studies and meta-analyses, the reasonable hypothesis was formulated that PFT-guided DAPT escalation from clopidogrel to a potent $P2Y_{12}$ inhibitor (prasugrel or ticagrelor) or de-escalation from a potent $P2Y_{12}$ inhibitor to clopidogrel could improve outcomes by reducing both ischaemic and bleeding complications. The concept of PFT-guided escalation of DAPT refers to upgrading a $P2Y_{12}$ inhibitor from clopidogrel to prasugrel or ticagrelor in patients with stable CAD undergoing elective PCI exhibiting HPR on clopidogrel. Although this assumption sounds reasonable, none of the major trials testing this hypothesis succeeded in meeting their primary endpoints. The GRAVITAS trial (Gauging Responsiveness With a VerifyNow Assay—Impact on Thrombosis and Safety) [85] was the first major randomized trial in the field of PFT-guided treatment. In this trial, high-dose clopidogrel, instead of a potent $P2Y_{12}$ inhibitor, was used as an escalated regimen. The trial failed to show a benefit of this specific strategy over standard-dosed clopidogrel. The TRIGGER-PCI trial (Testing Platelet Reactivity in Patients Undergoing Elective Stent Placement on Clopidogrel to Guide Alternative Therapy With Prasugrel),[86] which tested prasugrel for PFT-guided treatment escalation in patients undergoing elective PCI, was stopped prematurely because of futility. Finally, the ARCTIC trial (Assessment by a Double Randomization of a Conventional Antiplatelet Strategy Versus a Monitoring-Guided Strategy for Drug-Eluting Stent Implantation and of Treatment Interruption Versus Continuation One Year After Stenting), which used high-dose clopidogrel or short-acting intravenous glycoprotein IIb/IIIa inhibitors or prasugrel (in <10% of patients) as escalated antiplatelet regimens, also failed to show a benefit of escalated DAPT versus clopidogrel. [87] The current European Society of Cardiology (ESC) Guidelines recommend a non-guided escalation strategy (class of recommendation IIb, level of evidence C; ➔ Figure 29.2) from clopidogrel to prasugrel or ticagrelor in specific high-risk situations of elective PCI, such as suboptimal stent deployment or a complex PCI procedure. A PFT-guided approach, although not tested in large randomized trials, might be beneficial in this setting. In a recently published registry-based analysis of long-term outcomes in patients undergoing elective chronic total occlusion PCI, HPR (defined as LTA

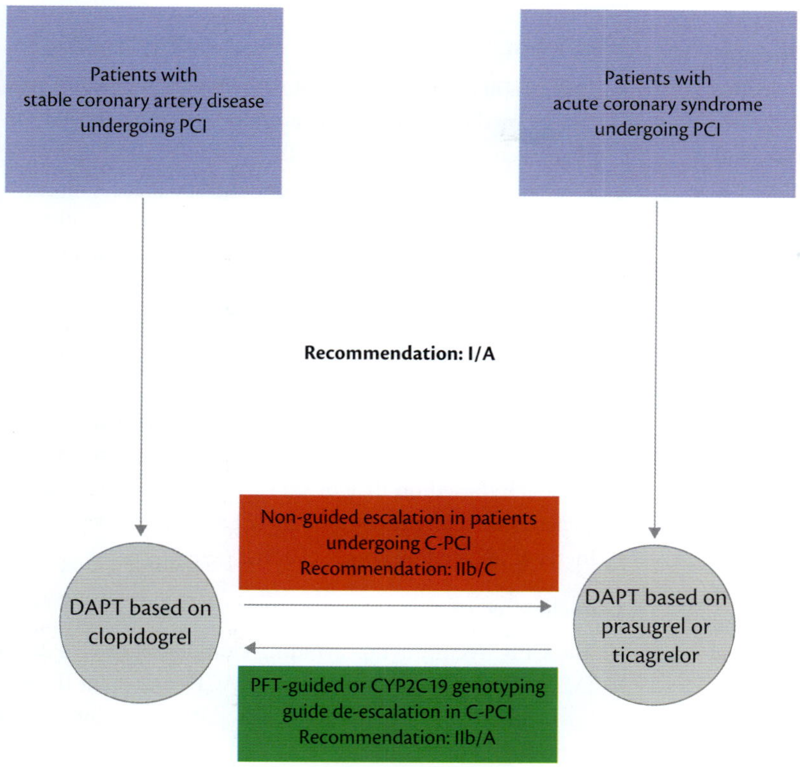

Figure 29.2 Guideline-based recommendations for therapy with $P2Y_{12}$ inhibitors in patients with stable coronary artery disease undergoing elective percutaneous coronary intervention (PCI)[26] and patients undergoing PCI because of an acute coronary syndrome.[25,78] The bottom panel illustrates the recommendations for non-guided escalation in patients undergoing complex PCI (C-PCI) procedures and guided de-escalation based on the results of platelet function testing (PFT) or cytochrome P450 (CYP)-2C19 genotyping.

≥70%) on clopidogrel not being escalated to a potent $P2Y_{12}$ inhibitor was associated with a higher 3-year cardiac mortality rate compared to patients with OPR on clopidogrel (16.8 ± 3.8% vs 4.7 ± 0.8%; P <0.001). Whether patients undergoing elective complex PCI can benefit from a PFT-guided escalation from clopidogrel to a potent $P2Y_{12}$ inhibitor should be further evaluated in future randomized controlled trials.

Platelet function testing-guided de-escalation in clinical trials

De-escalation of antiplatelet therapy from potent $P2Y_{12}$ inhibitors to clopidogrel in patients with ACS undergoing PCI is common in everyday clinical practice and is mainly attributed to bleeding and non-bleeding complications, as well as to socioeconomic factors.[88] It is estimated that the prevalence of unplanned in-hospital de-escalation ranges from 5% to 14%, with an additional 5-8% of unplanned de-escalation taking place after hospital discharge.[84] Moreover, the clinical utility of planned de-escalation of potent $P2Y_{12}$ inhibitors to clopidogrel in patients with ACS undergoing PCI has been tested in three randomized clinical trials. In the Popular Genetics trial a genotype-guided de-escalation strategy was assessed (➔ Clinical evidence for a genotype-guided antithrombotic therapy).[62] The randomized TOPIC (Timing of Optimal Platelet Inhibition After Acute Coronary Syndrome) trial showed that, in patients who have been event free for the first month after an ACS on a combination of aspirin plus a potent $P2Y_{12}$ inhibitor, de-escalation to aspirin plus clopidogrel was associated with reduced bleeding complications.[89] This study did not show any differences in thrombotic events between treatment groups. However, given the limited size of the trial (n = 646) this result should be interpreted cautiously. The TROPICAL-ACS (Testing Responsiveness to Platelet Inhibition on Chronic Antiplatelet Treatment for ACS) trial was a larger trial, which randomized 2610 patients with ACS undergoing PCI to either standard treatment with prasugrel for 12 months or a de-escalation regimen (1 week of prasugrel followed by 1 week of clopidogrel and PFT-guided maintenance therapy with clopidogrel or re-escalation to prasugrel from day 14 after hospital discharge to month 12).[90] Taking into consideration the results of the above-mentioned trials, recent practice guidelines have been updated with a class IIb (level of evidence A) recommendation for a guided (based on PFT or CYP2C19 genotyping) DAPT de-escalation strategy, which may be considered as an alternative DAPT strategy, especially for patients with ACS deemed unsuitable for 12-month potent platelet inhibition[8] (➔ Figure 29.2).

Guided selection of antiplatelet therapy: an appraisal

As discussed above, multiple trials have tried to optimize clinical outcomes by tailoring the $P2Y_{12}$ inhibitor through a genotype- or PFT-guided strategy. However, most of these studies were not powered for hard efficacy outcomes and did not provide unequivocal results. To overcome the limitation of a lack of power, a meta-analysis by Galli et al. assessed the safety and efficacy of guided versus standard selection of antiplatelet therapy in patients, both with chronic coronary syndrome and ACS, undergoing PCI.[91] In this analysis, including 11 RCTs and more than

20,000 patients, guided selection of antiplatelet therapy was associated with a reduction of MACEs compared with standard therapy. In addition, guided antiplatelet therapy also resulted in a reduction of individual efficacy and safety outcomes, like cardiovascular death, myocardial infarction, stent thrombosis, stroke, and minor bleeding. The results were consistent, independent of the test used for guided selection of therapy (PFT vs genetic testing). Outcomes differed according to the strategy used. An escalation strategy was associated with a reduction in ischaemic events without an increase in bleeding, and a de-escalation strategy with a reduction in bleeding without an increase in ischaemic events. Nevertheless, in the specific setting of ACS, physicians may still favour potent $P2Y_{12}$ inhibition, on the one hand due to evidence in support of their use by the large-scale pivotal RCTs,[28,29] and on the other hand since guided selection requires implementation of additional (costly) testing at their local site. However, in a more recent network meta-analysis by Galli et al., the safety and efficacy of guided versus standard selection of antiplatelet therapy was assessed in patients with ACS only, which included 15 RCTs and more than 60,000 patients with ACS.[92] In this analysis clopidogrel was used as the reference treatment. Compared with ticagrelor and prasugrel, a guided antiplatelet approach was the only strategy associated with a reduction in MACE without any significant trade-off in any bleeding, demonstrating that a guided selection of $P2Y_{12}$ inhibition is the strategy with the most favourable balance between safety and efficacy. A guided strategy may also be preferred to standard therapy from an economic perspective. Multiple cost-effectiveness analyses have demonstrated that, by improving outcomes and reducing costs due to the more frequent use of clopidogrel (especially in the setting of ACS), guided selection of antiplatelet therapy can be a cost-effective strategy.[93–95]

Perspective

Currently, a personalized antithrombotic therapy is not (yet) recommended as standard care in the guidelines; however, it can definitely be of great value in selective scenarios. For escalation of $P2Y_{12}$ inhibition, these could be scenarios in which thrombotic risk outweighs bleeding risk. Examples include left main coronary artery stenting, complex lesions, bifurcation PCI, and prior stent thrombosis. For de-escalation strategies, these would include scenarios where patients are at increased risk of bleeding or have experienced bleeding complications. Thus, when personalizing antithrombotic therapy, the patient should be central, taking various clinical, angiographic, procedural, and socioeconomic variables into consideration before opting for a specific strategy. If a guided antiplatelet strategy is implemented, the choice between PFT and genetic testing may depend on the availability of tests and local experience. In general, it is recommended to use point-of-care assays instead of laboratory-based assays. Ultimately, as evidence on PFT- and genotype guided therapy is increasing over the years, with ongoing trials probably further refining the existing evidence, a personalized antithrombotic therapy could become the standard of care in patients undergoing PCI in the future.

What's new

- This chapter provides the latest evidence regarding precision medicine in antithrombotic therapy, based on pharmacogenetics or/and PFT.
- A genotype-guided antithrombotic therapy focuses on identifying common genetic polymorphisms that might influence the antithrombotic effect exerted by oral anticoagulants and antiplatelet medication. So far, CYP2C19 polymorphisms are the only genetic variations for which a genotype-guided therapy has been tested in clinical trials with respect to clinical outcomes in patients with ACS.
- A recent network meta-analysis demonstrated that, compared with ticagrelor and prasugrel, a guided antiplatelet approach (based on PFT or CYP2C19 genotyping) was associated with a reduction in MACEs without a significant increase in bleeding complications.

Guideline recommendations

- The CPIC recommends avoiding clopidogrel in CYP2C19 IMs or PMs in order to prevent MACEs and stent thrombosis, and here rather use an escalated $P2Y_{12}$ inhibitor, such as prasugrel or ticagrelor.
- A platelet reactivity within the therapeutic window warrants the lowest rate of ischaemic events and bleeding complications.
- The current ESC Guidelines recommend a non-guided escalation strategy (class of recommendation IIb, level of evidence C) from clopidogrel to prasugrel or ticagrelor in specific high-risk situations of elective PCI.
- A guided de-escalation of $P2Y_{12}$ inhibition from prasugrel or ticagrelor to clopidogrel, based on PFT or CYP2C19 genotyping, can be considered in patients with ACS deemed unsuitable for treatment with potent platelet inhibitors (class IIb recommendation, level of evidence A).

What's next

- Currently, a personalized antithrombotic therapy is not recommended as standard care in the guidelines; however, it can be of great value as an escalation strategy in patients with high thrombotic risk, or as a de-escalation strategy in patients in whom bleeding risk overweighs thrombotic risk.
- As evidence on PFT- and genotype-guided therapy is increasing over time, a personalized antithrombotic therapy could become the standard of care in patients undergoing a PCI in the future.

Drug dosing

- Aspirin: loading dose of 150–300 mg orally or 75–250 mg intravenously if oral ingestion is not possible, followed by oral maintenance dose of 75–100 mg once daily.
- Clopidogrel: loading dose of 300–600 mg orally, followed by a maintenance dose of 75 mg once daily, no specific dose adjustment in chronic kidney disease patients.

- Prasugrel: loading dose of 60 mg orally, followed by a maintenance dose of 10 mg once daily. In patients with body weight less than 60 kg, a maintenance dose of 5 mg once daily is recommended. In patients aged 75 years and older, prasugrel should be used with caution, but a dose of 5 mg once daily should be used if treatment is deemed necessary. No specific dose adjustment in chronic kidney disease patients. Prior stroke is a contraindication for prasugrel.
- Ticagrelor: loading dose of 180 mg orally, followed by a maintenance dose of 90 mg twice daily, no specific dose adjustment in chronic kidney disease patients.

References

1. Angiolillo DJ, Capodanno D, Danchin N, et al. Derivation, validation, and prognostic utility of a prediction rule for nonresponse to clopidogrel: the ABCD-GENE score. JACC Cardiovasc Interv. 2020;13(5):606–17.
2. Belle DJ, Singh H. Genetic factors in drug metabolism. Am Fam Physician. 2008;77(11):1553–60.
3. Pinto N, Dolan ME. Clinically relevant genetic variations in drug metabolizing enzymes. Curr Drug Metab. 2011;12(5):487–97.
4. Marín F, González-Conejero R, Capranzano P, Bass TA, Roldán V, Angiolillo DJ. Pharmacogenetics in cardiovascular antithrombotic therapy. J Am Coll Cardiol. 2009;54(12):1041–57.
5. Johnson J, Caudle K, Gong L, et al. Clinical Pharmacogenetics Implementation Consortium (CPIC) guideline for pharmacogenetics-guided warfarin dosing: 2017 update. Clin Pharmacol Ther. 2017;102(3):397–404.
6. Verhoef TI, Redekop WK, Daly AK, van Schie RMF, de Boer A, Maitland-van der Zee A-H. Pharmacogenetic-guided dosing of coumarin anticoagulants: algorithms for warfarin, acenocoumarol and phenprocoumon. Br J Clin Pharmacol. 2014;77(4):626–41.
7. Rettie AE, Korzekwa KR, Kunze KL, et al. Hydroxylation of warfarin by human cDNA-expressed cytochrome P-450: a role for P-4502C9 in the etiology of (S)-warfarin-drug interactions. Chem Res Toxicol. 1992;5(1):54–9.
8. Aithal GP, Day CP, Kesteven PJ, Daly AK. Association of polymorphisms in the cytochrome P450 CYP2C9 with warfarin dose requirement and risk of bleeding complications. Lancet. 1999;353(9154):717–9.
9. Rieder MJ, Reiner AP, Gage BF, et al. Effect of VKORC1 haplotypes on transcriptional regulation and warfarin dose. N Engl J Med. 2005;352(22):2285–93.
10. Sconce EA, Khan TI, Wynne HA, et al. The impact of CYP2C9 and VKORC1 genetic polymorphism and patient characteristics upon warfarin dose requirements: proposal for a new dosing regimen. Blood. 2005;106(7):2329–33.
11. Verhoef TI, Ragia G, de Boer A, et al. A randomized trial of genotype-guided dosing of acenocoumarol and phenprocoumon. N Engl J Med. 2013;369(24):2304–12.
12. Pirmohamed M, Burnside G, Eriksson N, et al. A randomized trial of genotype-guided dosing of warfarin. N Engl J Med. 2013;369(24):2294–303.
13. Kimmel SE, French B, Kasner SE, et al. A pharmacogenetic versus a clinical algorithm for warfarin dosing. N Engl J Med. 2013;369(24):2283–93.
14. Cerezo-Manchado JJ, Roldán V, Corral J, et al. Genotype-guided therapy improves initial acenocoumarol dosing. Thromb Haemost. 2016;115(01):117–25.
15. Tong H, Borobia A, Quintana-Díaz M, et al. Acenocoumarol pharmacogenetic dosing algorithm versus usual care in patients with venous thromboembolism: a randomised clinical trial. J Clin Med. 2021;10(13):2949.
16. Tang T, Liu J, Zuo K, et al. Genotype-guided dosing of coumarin anticoagulants. J Cardiovasc Pharmacol Ther. 2015;20(4):387–94.
17. Belley-Cote E, Hanif H, D'Aragon F, et al. Genotype-guided versus standard vitamin K antagonist dosing algorithms in patients initiating anticoagulation. Thromb Haemost. 2015;114(10):768–77.
18. Danese E, Raimondi S, Montagnana M, et al. Effect of CYP 4F2, VKORC 1, and CYP 2C9 in influencing coumarin dose: a single-patient data meta-analysis in more than 15,000 individuals. Clin Pharmacol Ther. 2019;105(6):1477–91.
19. Tse G, Gong M, Li G, et al. Genotype-guided warfarin dosing vs. conventional dosing strategies: a systematic review and meta-analysis of randomized controlled trials. Br J Clin Pharmacol. 2018;84(9):1868–82.
20. Franchini M, Mengoli C, Cruciani M, Bonfanti C, Mannucci PM. Effects on bleeding complications of pharmacogenetic testing for initial dosing of vitamin K antagonists: a systematic review and meta-analysis. J Thromb Haemost. 2014;12(9):1480–7.
21. Stergiopoulos K, Brown DL. Genotype-guided vs clinical dosing of warfarin and its analogues. JAMA Intern Med. 2014;174(8):1330.
22. Maier CL, Duncan A, Hill CE. Pharmacogenetics in oral antithrombotic therapy. Clin Lab Med. 2016;36(3):461–72.
23. Raymond J, Imbert L, Cousin T, et al. Pharmacogenetics of direct oral anticoagulants: a systematic review. J Pers Med. 2021;11(1):37.
24. Valgimigli M, Bueno H, Byrne RA, et al. 2017 ESC focused update on dual antiplatelet therapy in coronary artery disease developed in collaboration with EACTS. Eur J Cardiothoracic Surg. 2017;53(1):34–78.
25. Collet J-P, Thiele H, Barbato E, et al. 2020 ESC Guidelines for the management of acute coronary syndromes in patients presenting without persistent ST-segment elevation. Eur Heart J. 2020;42(14):1289–367.
26. Knuuti J, Wijns W, Flachskampf FA, et al. 2019 ESC Guidelines for the diagnosis and management of chronic coronary syndromes. Eur Heart J. 2020;41(3):407–77.
27. Amsterdam EA, Wenger NK, Brindis RG, et al. 2014 AHA/ACC guideline for the management of patients with non-ST-elevation acute coronary syndromes: a report of the American College of Cardiology/American Heart Association Task Force on Practice Guidelines. J Am Coll Cardiol. 2014;64(24):139–228.
28. Wiviott SD, Braunwald E, McCabe CH, et al. Prasugrel versus clopidogrel in patients with acute coronary syndromes. N Engl J Med. 2007;357(20):2001–15.
29. Wallentin L, Becker RC, Budaj A, et al. Ticagrelor versus clopidogrel in patients with acute coronary syndromes. N Engl J Med. 2009;361(11):1045–57.
30. Vranckx P, Leonardi S, Tebaldi M, et al. Prospective validation of the bleeding academic research consortium classification in the all-comer PRODIGY trial. Eur Heart J. 2014;35(37):2524–9.
31. Vranckx P, White HD, Huang Z, et al. Validation of BARC bleeding criteria in patients with acute coronary syndromes: the TRACER trial. J Am Coll Cardiol. 2016;67(18):2135–44.

32. Généreux P, Giustino G, Witzenbichler B, et al. Incidence, predictors, and impact of post-discharge bleeding after percutaneous coronary intervention. J Am Coll Cardiol. 2015;66(9):1036–45.
33. Agundez J, Martinez C, Perez-Sala D, Carballo M, Torres M, Garcia-Martin E. Pharmacogenomics in aspirin intolerance. Curr Drug Metab. 2009;10(9):998–1008.
34. Postula M, Janicki PK, Rosiak M, et al. Effect of common single-nucleotide polymorphisms in acetylsalicylic acid metabolic pathway genes on platelet reactivity in patients with diabetes. Med Sci Monit. 2013;19(1):394–408.
35. Gurbel PA, Rout A, Tantry US. Pharmacogenetic considerations in antiplatelet therapy. Expert Rev Precis Med Drug Dev. 2020;5(4):235–8.
36. Teng R, Oliver S, Hayes MA, Butler K. Absorption, distribution, metabolism, and excretion of ticagrelor in healthy subjects. Drug Metab Dispos. 2010;38(9):1514–21.
37. Teng R, Butler K. Pharmacokinetics, pharmacodynamics, tolerability and safety of single ascending doses of ticagrelor, a reversibly binding oral P2Y12 receptor antagonist, in healthy subjects. Eur J Clin Pharmacol. 2010;66(5):487–96.
38. European Medicines Agency. Efient: EPAR—product information. Feb 2016. Available at: https://www.ema.europa.eu/en/medicines/human/EPAR/efient
39. Mega JL, Close SL, Wiviott SD, et al. Cytochrome P450 genetic polymorphisms and the response to prasugrel: relationship to pharmacokinetic, pharmacodynamic, and clinical outcomes. Circulation. 2009;119(19):2553–60.
40. Giorgi MA, Cohen Arazi H, Gonzalez CD, Di Girolamo G. Beyond efficacy: pharmacokinetic differences between clopidogrel, prasugrel and ticagrelor. Expert Opin. Pharmacother. 2011;12(8):1285–95.
41. Ancrenaz V, Daali Y, Fontana P, et al. Impact of genetic polymorphisms and drug-drug interactions on clopidogrel and prasugrel response variability. Curr Drug Metab. 2010;11(8):667–77.
42. Roberts JD, Wells GA, Le May MR, et al. Point-of-care genetic testing for personalisation of antiplatelet treatment (RAPID GENE): a prospective, randomised, proof-of-concept trial. Lancet. 2012;379(9827):1705–11.
43. Kazui M, Nishiya Y, Ishizuka T, et al. Identification of the human cytochrome P450 enzymes involved in the two oxidative steps in the bioactivation of clopidogrel to its pharmacologically active metabolite. Drug Metab Dispos. 2010;38(1):92–9.
44. Stouffer GA, Klein MD, Williams AK, Lee CR. Clinical utility of CYP2C19 genotyping to guide antiplatelet therapy in patients with an acute coronary syndrome or undergoing percutaneous coronary intervention brief review. Arter Thromb Vasc Biol. 2019;39:647–52.
45. Fricke-Galindo I, Céspedes-Garro C, Rodrigues-Soares F, et al. Interethnic variation of CYP2C19 alleles, 'predicted' phenotypes and 'measured' metabolic phenotypes across world populations. Pharmacogenomics J. 2016;16(2):113–23.
46. Mega JL, Close SL, Wiviott SD, et al. Cytochrome P-450 polymorphisms and response to clopidogrel. N Engl J Med. 2009;360(4):354–62.
47. Breet NJ, Van Werkum JW, Bouman HJ, et al. Comparison of platelet function tests in predicting clinical outcome in patients undergoing coronary stent implantation. JAMA. 2010;303(8):754–62.
48. Harmsze A, Van Werkum JW, Bouman HJ, et al. Besides CYP2C19*2, the variant allele CYP2C9*3 is associated with higher on-clopidogrel platelet reactivity in patients on dual antiplatelet therapy undergoing elective coronary stent implantation. Pharmacogenet Genomics. 2010;20(1):18–25.
49. Hulot J-S, Bura A, Villard E, et al. Cytochrome P450 2C19 loss-of-function polymorphism is a major determinant of clopidogrel responsiveness in healthy subjects. Blood. 2006;108(7):2244–7.
50. Hochholzer W, Trenk D, Fromm MF, et al. Impact of cytochrome P450 2C19 loss-of-function polymorphism and of major demographic characteristics on residual platelet function after loading and maintenance treatment with clopidogrel in patients undergoing elective coronary stent placement. J Am Coll Cardiol. 2010;55(22):2427–34.
51. Shuldiner AR, O'Connell JR, Bliden KP, et al. Association of cytochrome P450 2C19 genotype with the antiplatelet effect and clinical efficacy of clopidogrel therapy. JAMA. 2009;302(8):849–58.
52. Harmsze AM, Van Werkum JW, Ten Berg JM, et al. CYP2C19*2 and CYP2C9*3 alleles are associated with stent thrombosis: a case-control study. Eur Heart J. 2010;31(24):3046–53.
53. US Food and Drug Administration. FDA Drug Safety Communication: reduced effectiveness of Plavix (clopidogrel) in patients who are poor metabolizers of the drug. March 2017. Available at: https://www.fda.gov/drugs/postmarket-drug-safety-information-patients-and-providers/fda-drug-safety-communication-reduced-effectiveness-plavix-clopidogrel-patients-who-are-poor#ds
54. Lee CR, Luzum JA, Sangkuhl K, et al. Clinical Pharmacogenetics Implementation Consortium guideline for CYP2C19 genotype and clopidogrel therapy: 2022 update. Clin Pharmacol Ther. 2022;112(5):959–67.
55. Deiman BALM, Tonino PAL, Kouhestani K, et al. Reduced number of cardiovascular events and increased cost-effectiveness by genotype-guided antiplatelet therapy in patients undergoing percutaneous coronary interventions in the Netherlands. Netherlands Hear J. 2016;24(10):589–99.
56. Sánchez-Ramos J, Dávila-Fajardo CL, Toledo Frías P, et al. Results of genotype-guided antiplatelet therapy in patients who undergone percutaneous coronary intervention with stent. Int J Cardiol. 2016;225:289–95.
57. Cavallari LH, Lee CR, Beitelshees AL, et al. Multisite investigation of outcomes with implementation of CYP2C19 genotype-guided antiplatelet therapy after percutaneous coronary intervention. JACC Cardiovasc Interv. 2018;11(2):181–91.
58. Xie X, Ma Y-T, Yang Y-N, et al. Personalized antiplatelet therapy according to CYP2C19 genotype after percutaneous coronary intervention: a randomized control trial. Int J Cardiol. 2013;168(4):3736–40.
59. Shen D-L, Wang B, Bai J, et al. Clinical value of CYP2C19 genetic testing for guiding the antiplatelet therapy in a Chinese population. J Cardiovasc Pharmacol. 2016;67(3):232–6.
60. Notarangelo FM, Maglietta G, Bevilacqua P, et al. Pharmacogenomic approach to selecting antiplatelet therapy in patients with acute coronary syndromes: the PHARMCLO trial. J Am Coll Cardiol. 2018;71(17):1869–77.
61. Tuteja S, Glick H, Matthai W, et al. Prospective CYP2C19 genotyping to guide antiplatelet therapy following percutaneous coronary intervention: a pragmatic randomized clinical trial. Circ Genomic Precis Med. 2020;13(1):e002640.
62. Claassens DMF, Vos GJA, Bergmeijer TO, et al. A genotype-guided strategy for oral P2Y12 inhibitors in primary PCI. N Engl J Med. 2019;381(17):1621–31.
63. Pereira NL, Farkouh ME, So D, et al. Effect of genotype-guided oral P2Y12 inhibitor selection vs conventional clopidogrel therapy on ischemic outcomes after percutaneous coronary intervention: the TAILOR-PCI randomized clinical trial. JAMA. 2020;324(8):761–71.
64. Pereira NL, Rihal C, Lennon R, et al. Effect of CYP2C19 genotype on ischemic outcomes during oral P2Y12 inhibitor therapy: a meta-analysis. JACC Cardiovasc Interv. 2021;14(7):739–50.
65. Biswas M, Kali MSK, Biswas TK, Ibrahim B. Risk of major adverse cardiovascular events of CYP2C19 loss-of-function genotype guided prasugrel/ticagrelor vs clopidogrel therapy for acute coronary

syndrome patients undergoing percutaneous coronary intervention: a meta-analysis. Platelets. 2020;32(5):591–600.

66. Lyu SQ, Yang YM, Zhu J, et al. The efficacy and safety of CYP2C19 genotype-guided antiplatelet therapy compared with conventional antiplatelet therapy in patients with acute coronary syndrome or undergoing percutaneous coronary intervention: a meta-analysis of randomized controlled trial. Platelets. 2020;31(8):971–80.
67. Yoon HY, Lee N, Seong JM, Gwak HS. Efficacy and safety of clopidogrel versus prasugrel and ticagrelor for coronary artery disease treatment in patients with CYP2C19 LoF alleles: a systemic review and meta-analysis. Br J Clin Pharmacol. 2020;86(8):1489–98.
68. Kheiri B, Abdalla A, Osman M, et al. Personalized antiplatelet therapy in patients with coronary artery disease undergoing percutaneous coronary intervention: a network meta-analysis of randomized clinical trials. Catheter Cardiovasc Interv. 2019;94(2):181–6.
69. Kheiri B, Osman M, Abdalla A, et al. CYP2C19 pharmacogenetics versus standard of care dosing for selecting antiplatelet therapy in patients with coronary artery disease: a meta-analysis of randomized clinical trials. Catheter Cardiovasc Interv. 2019;93(7):1246–52.
70. Beitelshees AL, Thomas CD, Empey PE, et al. CYP2C19 genotype-guided antiplatelet therapy after percutaneous coronary intervention in diverse clinical settings. J Am Heart Assoc. 2022;11(4):e024159.
71. Pan Y, Chen W, Xu Y, et al. Genetic polymorphisms and clopidogrel efficacy for acute ischemic stroke or transient ischemic attack. Circulation. 2017;135(1):21–33.
72. Wang Y, Meng X, Wang A, et al. Ticagrelor versus clopidogrel in CYP2C19 loss-of-function carriers with stroke or TIA. N Engl J Med. 2021;385(27):2520–30.
73. Sibbing D, Aradi D, Alexopoulos D, et al. Updated expert consensus statement on platelet function and genetic testing for guiding P2Y12 receptor inhibitor treatment in percutaneous coronary intervention. JACC Cardiovasc Interv. 2019;12(16):1521–37.
74. Breddin HK. Can platelet aggregometry be standardized? Platelets. 2005;16(3–4):151–8.
75. Cattaneo M, Cerletti C, Harrison P, et al. Recommendations for the standardization of light transmission aggregometry: a consensus of the working party from the platelet physiology subcommittee of SSC/ISTH. J Thromb Haemost. 2013;11(6):1183–9.
76. Aradi D, Kirtane A, Bonello L, et al. Bleeding and stent thrombosis on P2Y12-inhibitors: collaborative analysis on the role of platelet reactivity for risk stratification after percutaneous coronary intervention. Eur Heart J. 2015;36(27):1762–71.
77. Aradi D, Gross L, Trenk D, et al. Platelet reactivity and clinical outcomes in acute coronary syndrome patients treated with prasugrel and clopidogrel: a pre-specified exploratory analysis from the TROPICAL-ACS trial. Eur Heart J. 2019;40(24):1942–51.
78. Ibanez B, James S, Agewall S, et al. 2017 ESC Guidelines for the management of acute myocardial infarction in patients presenting with ST-segment elevation. Eur Heart J. 2018;39(2):119–77.
79. Neumann F-J, Sousa-Uva M, Ahlsson A, et al. 2018 ESC/EACTS Guidelines on myocardial revascularization. Eur Heart J. 2019;40(2):87–165.
80. Mehta SR, Yusuf S, Peters RJ, et al. Effects of pretreatment with clopidogrel and aspirin followed by long-term therapy in patients undergoing percutaneous coronary intervention: the PCI-CURE study. Lancet. 2001;358(9281):527–33.
81. Antman EM, Wiviott SD, Murphy SA, et al. Early and late benefits of prasugrel in patients with acute coronary syndromes undergoing percutaneous coronary intervention. J Am Coll Cardiol. 2008;51(21):2028–33.
82. Steg PG, Huber K, Andreotti F, et al. Bleeding in acute coronary syndromes and percutaneous coronary interventions: position paper by the Working Group on Thrombosis of the European Society of Cardiology. Eur Heart J. 2011;32(15):1854–64.
83. Valgimigli M, Costa F, Lokhnygina Y, et al. Trade-off of myocardial infarction vs. bleeding types on mortality after acute coronary syndrome: lessons from the thrombin receptor antagonist for clinical event reduction in acute coronary syndrome (TRACER) randomized trial. Eur Heart J. 2017;38(11):804–10.
84. Angiolillo DJ, Rollini F, Storey RF, et al. International expert consensus on switching platelet P2Y 12 receptor-inhibiting therapies. Circulation. 2017;136(20):1955–75.
85. Price MJ, Berger PB, Teirstein PS, et al. Standard- vs high-dose clopidogrel based on platelet function testing after percutaneous coronary intervention: the GRAVITAS randomized trial. JAMA. 2011;305(11):1097–105.
86. Trenk D, Stone GW, Gawaz M, et al. A randomized trial of prasugrel versus clopidogrel in patients with high platelet reactivity on clopidogrel after elective percutaneous coronary intervention with implantation of drug-eluting stents. J Am Coll Cardiol. 2012;59(24):2159–64.
87. Collet J-P, Cuisset T, Rangé G, et al. Bedside monitoring to adjust antiplatelet therapy for coronary stenting. N Engl J Med. 2012;367(22):2100–9.
88. Zettler ME, Peterson ED, McCoy LA, et al. Switching of adenosine diphosphate receptor inhibitor after hospital discharge among myocardial infarction patients: insights from the treatment with adenosine diphosphate receptor inhibitors: longitudinal assessment of treatment patterns and events after. Am Heart J. 2017;183:62–8.
89. Cuisset T, Deharo P, Quilici J, et al. Benefit of switching dual antiplatelet therapy after acute coronary syndrome: the TOPIC (timing of platelet inhibition after acute coronary syndrome) randomized study. Eur Heart J. 2017;38(41):3070–8.
90. Sibbing D, Aradi D, Jacobshagen C, et al. Guided de-escalation of antiplatelet treatment in patients with acute coronary syndrome undergoing percutaneous coronary intervention (TROPICAL-ACS): a randomised, open-label, multicentre trial. Lancet. 2017;390(10104):1747–57.
91. Galli M, Benenati S, Capodanno D, et al. Guided versus standard antiplatelet therapy in patients undergoing percutaneous coronary intervention: a systematic review and meta-analysis. Lancet. 2021;397(10283):1470–83.
92. Galli M, Benenati S, Franchi F, et al. Comparative effects of guided vs. potent P2Y12 inhibitor therapy in acute coronary syndrome: a network meta-analysis of 61 898 patients from 15 randomized trials. Eur Heart J. 2022;43(10):959–67.
93. Limdi NA, Cavallari LH, Lee CR, et al. Cost-effectiveness of CYP2C19-guided antiplatelet therapy in patients with acute coronary syndrome and percutaneous coronary intervention informed by real-world data. Pharmacogenomics J. 2020;20(5):724–35.
94. AlMukdad S, Elewa H, Al-Badriyeh D. Economic evaluations of CYP2C19 genotype-guided antiplatelet therapy compared to the universal use of antiplatelets in patients with acute coronary syndrome: a systematic review. J Cardiovasc Pharmacol Ther. 2020;25(3):201–11.
95. Lomakin N, Rudakova A, Buryachkovskaya L, Serebruany V. Cost-effectiveness of platelet function-guided strategy with clopidogrel or ticagrelor. Eur Cardiol Rev. 2019;14(3):175–8.

CHAPTER 30

Drug development, clinical trials, and regulatory requirements

Serge Korjian, Yazan Daaboul, and C. Michael Gibson

Contents

Summary

The drug development process as we know it today did not exist before the second half of the 20th century. Over the past several decades, regulatory agencies have been developed to monitor drug development and ensure that novel therapeutic agents are safe for human use and effective for their desired indications. The rigour and requirements with which drugs are studied and clinical trials are performed have evolved with decades of slowly expanding guidelines and regulations. After identifying a target for therapeutic intervention, drugs undergo a series of preclinical investigations in animal models. If deemed to be of potential value to humans, drugs are then tested in a series of three phases of clinical trials to evaluate their optimal dosing in humans, feasibility, generalizability, as well as their safety and efficacy. Once approved by regulatory bodies, drugs may eventually be marketed to the public. Post-marketing, drugs continue to be monitored lifelong for development of any short-term and long-term adverse events via phase IV surveillance.

The history of drug legislation and drug development

The drug development process as we know it today did not exist before the second half of the twentieth century. Although certain measures were taken by governments around the world to curtail the distribution and sale of potentially harmful substances, the earliest form of a true drug development process came about in the 1960s through legislation in the US and parts of Europe. The rigour with which drugs are studied and tested in the present day, however, is the result of decades of slowly expanding regulations, and the development of regulatory agencies to monitor drug development and ensure that novel therapeutic agents are safe for human use and effective for their desired indications.

In the past century, further expansion of regulations on drug sales were linked to pivotal patient safety events that highlighted the pitfalls of unregulated drug production,

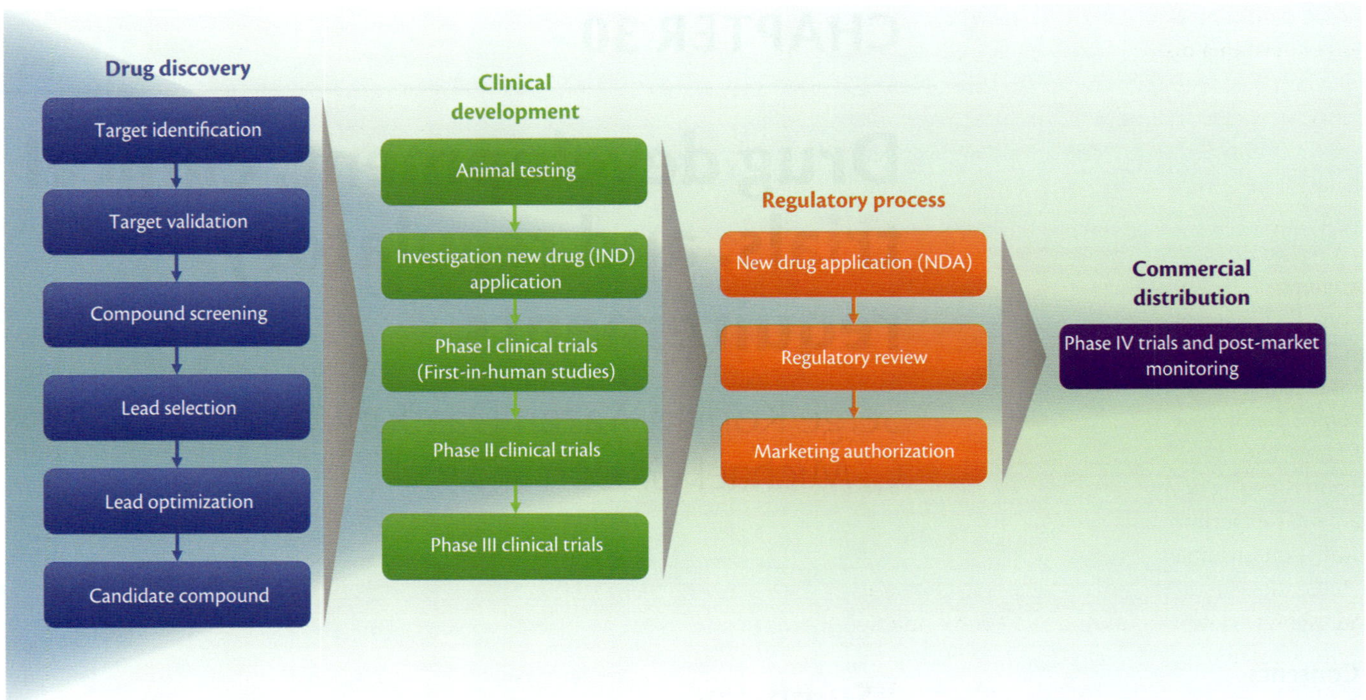

Figure 30.1 Steps of the drug development process (regulatory process based on the Food and Drug Administration (FDA) process in the US).

marketing, and distribution. The Federal Food, Drug, and Cosmetic Act of 1938 became the first legislation in the US to require evidence that a drug is safe before allowing its sale to the general public. This critical legislation was passed after a safety disaster linked to elixir sulfanilamide, where approximately 100 children died from drug-related toxicity.[1] Approximately 20 years later, thalidomide, a sleeping pill, was found to cause severe birth defects in infants in Europe. This triggered a wave of stricter drug regulations. In the US, the Kefauver–Harris Drug Amendments were passed in 1962, which now required that drug makers demonstrate that their agents are effective before sale. This set the foundation for the phased clinical trial system that is widely used in the present day. Furthermore, the Advisory Committee on Investigational Drugs was established to advise the Food and Drug Administration (FDA) on matters of drug approval and drug policy. Similarly in parts of Europe, new drug regulation laws were enacted as a result of the thalidomide scandal as well as decades of concerns around drug safety. The most significant of these laws were the Medicines Act of 1968 in the UK, and the Drug Law of 1976 in Germany.

Over the next 50 years, these laws were refined and expanded, and a more structured process for drug development was created as a direct result of these regulations (➔ Figure 30.1). In 1995, the European Medicines Agency (EMA) was established to centralize and standardize drug development and regulation across the European Union.[2] Country-specific regulatory agencies were also established around the world in the late 20th century as a result of increased scrutiny around drug safety and efficacy most notably in Germany, Japan, Canada, Australia, and China.

Drug discovery phase: from target identification to a candidate compound

Drug discovery and development is rarely a predictable endeavour and carries a very high attrition rate. Approximately one in ten compounds that show promise in preclinical testing make it to human trials in what some have termed the 'Valley of Death'.[3] These failures are due to a multitude of issues from non-reproducible primary results, safety concerns, and production difficulties, to lack of appropriate funding. Nonetheless, most novel pharmacological agents are the product of a commonly accepted pathway of early drug discovery, which we discuss in more detail.

The earliest stage of drug development involves the identification of a target for therapeutic intervention. Targets are often proteins (enzymes, receptors, antibodies, hormones), genes, or even transcribed ribonucleic acids (RNAs) that are linked to a disease process. This critical primary step is often highly time and resource intensive. Frameworks such as the one developed by the Guidelines on Target Assessment For Innovative Therapeutics (GOT-IT) working group have tried to create a structured approach to target assessment,[4] but often, the discovery of a suitable therapeutic target is not an easily mappable process.

Identifying a therapeutic target begins by having a detailed and comprehensive understanding of a disease process at the molecular level and the presence of an unmet therapeutic need. There are several desired features of a therapeutic target. A potential target should be a critical part of the disease process, preferably with an established causal relationship with the disease in models with known clinical relevance. Furthermore, a predictable expression pattern in a disease state is preferred. The therapeutic target must be safely modifiable in preclinical models. It should also be sufficiently selective to the disease process so that any modification does not alter other critical pathways, often the reason for off-target toxicities that occur during drug testing. Additionally, a good target should be 'druggable'. The term is often used to refer to a molecule that has reasonable technical feasibility to become an effective drug target. A good example of a 'druggable' target is one that is accessible to a therapeutic molecule, has a known tissue distribution, has known modulators, and can elicit a measurable biological response when modified.[5]

Once a potential therapeutic target is identified, the process of target validation proceeds. Given the vital importance of this step in the drug development process, rigorous validation of fundamental experiments is essential to avoid wasted time and resources on unsuitable targets.

Validation of a target is optimal when it is multipronged and shows comparable findings using multiple techniques. Approaches to target validation include *in vitro* testing, cell-based and *in vivo* disease models of overexpression, knock-out models, antisense oligonucleotide experiments, and comparative genomics and proteomics.

The third step in the drug discovery process is compound screening, a procedure by which suitable compounds that modulate a proposed target are tested. The approach to compound screening depends on the available knowledge surrounding a given target. If little is known about suitable modulators, then high-throughput screening (HTS) provides the most rapid and comprehensive approach to compound screening. HTS is a complex, automated, cell-based, laboratory procedure that is capable of testing the biological activity of thousands of compounds to identify potential hits that would require further investigation.[6] Given its complexity and the need for a large number of often proprietary compounds, HTS has been limited to large well-funded laboratories and pharmaceutical companies. Nonetheless, initiatives such as the Community for Open Antimicrobial Drug Discovery (CO-ADD) have allowed for open access compound sharing for HTS to help identify novel drugs, specifically antibiotics.[7] More focused compound screens can sometimes be performed when a target has previously known modulators. This approach, while less time and resource intensive, lacks the ability to identify novel therapeutic compounds. Other approaches to compound screening include structure-based virtual screening that utilizes a software to match compounds with a given target based on the three-dimensional structure of both molecules.[8]

Once a number of hits are identified, a process of refinement ensues. This process narrows down the candidates, which may be as many as hundreds, down to a select few primary agents. Initially, hits are clustered into compounds with similar structural composition or common sites of activity. Several experiments are performed to characterize the individual features of these candidates including potential toxicities (e.g. cytotoxicity to hepatocyte cell lines), absorption, tissue distribution (solubility and permeability are studied), and metabolism. In addition to understanding the basic characteristics of these hit compounds, their effective function needs to be tested. Often, a cell-based or biochemical assay is identified and carefully selected before or in parallel to the screening process for this exact purpose. Assays are dependent on the target of choice and the downstream (or sometimes upstream) biochemical and physiological effects of target modulation. These assays are preferably easily reproducible and inexpensive given the number of assays required throughout the process from compound selection to creating dose–response produce files for proposed leads. Inability to identify an appropriate testing assay can be very detrimental to the drug development process.[5,9]

As these tests are performed, clusters of compounds are eliminated, and a lead cluster is identified. Clusters may be eliminated due to off-target effects, toxicities, anticipated production issues, or poor solubility and permeability. A lead optimization process ensues whereby further testing within lead clusters identifies a small number of lead molecules that are most likely to progress to a preclinical drug candidate. These molecules are then further refined chemically to improve potency and selectivity to improve efficacy and lower any unwanted off-target effects. At this stage, one or two primary candidates can be selected, and undergo a rigorous final process of characterization in preparation for animal testing and eventual human trials. This process involves detailed pharmacokinetic and pharmacodynamic profiling, dose-response testing, toxicity profiling, as well as chemical manufacturing considerations including purity and stability, all of which are required prior to any regulatory submission.

Animal models and testing

Once a candidate molecule is identified, it requires further *in vivo* testing to evaluate its safety and efficacy. Animal models of disease used in the primary steps of the drug development process come into play once again. While several animal species may be used for preclinical drug experiments, mice are by far the most common. Mice have very favourable reproduction and maturation characteristics, low maintenance costs, and adequate genetic homology to humans, making them an excellent model for preclinical testing. Transgenesis has also allowed for manipulation of mouse genomes to create transgenic mice with either conditionally or constitutively altered expression of certain genes leading to a desired disease process.[10] These animal models can be used to test the safety and efficacy of candidate compounds.

The primary purpose of animal testing is to identify potential human toxicity. Acute toxicity testing is a short-term assessment of a single dose of the candidate being evaluated (multiple doses should evaluated in separate experiment). This helps identify a metric of toxicity defined as the median lethal dose (LD_{50}), a dose that is fatal to 50% of animals exposed. Beyond identifying an LD_{50}, acute toxicity testing can help ascertain the target organ of toxicity and help with dose selection for all further toxicity testing. Furthermore, subacute and chronic toxicity testing provide more nuanced information about multiple doses of the compound with longer durations of exposure. These experiments are guided by the acute toxicity testing results, whereby all doses studied are below the lethal threshold, but may still be potentially toxic. Valuable information about individual organ effects, teratogenicity, and carcinogenesis can be detected from these experiments.[11] *In silico* methods for toxicity testing, that is, using computational methods to analyse, simulate, and predict toxicity, have also been proposed given evidence of poor correlation between animal studies and human toxicity. These artificial intelligence models use known chemical characteristics of a compound as well as data about the physiological milieu in which they will be used to determine signals of systemic toxicity. While these methods remain in their infancy, they have garnered interest given their cost saving.

In addition to identifying toxicity, animal testing is invaluable for pharmacokinetic/pharmacodynamic modelling, dose determination, and efficacy testing in the desired disease models prior to proceeding with human testing. Data from these primary animal tests often guidance for the development of early human trials.

The initial regulatory application: Investigational New Drug applications and clinical trial applications

Regulatory bodies such as the FDA and the EMA serve to protect patient safety above all else in addition to assuring the quality of the scientific evaluation of a new compound. While they provide final market approval or rejection for a compound, they also offer invaluable independent review and guidance to maintain the integrity of the drug development process and control for financial biases and conflicts of interest. This is achieved with teams of researchers, statisticians, chemists, pharmacologists, and physicians within these regulatory authorities that review applications and conduct independent analyses of the data provided. The application and review process is long, often requiring several years after a candidate compound is identified, due to the rigour with which applications are processed and reviewed. While more abbreviated tracks for review and approval exist for rare diseases or in areas of significant unmet need, they will not be discussed here.

Any novel pharmacological compound is considered high risk for human administration, and before proceeding with first-in-human studies, involvement of local, national, and international regulatory authorities is required. Nonetheless, drug developers may contact regulatory authorities for guidance or to draw on their expertise at any point in the drug development process. The process differs by regulatory body, but the purpose of these applications remains the same. They require a detailed body of evidence from preclinical and animal studies that support transitioning the compound to human testing and eventual commercial distribution as well as a general investigational plan and the protocols for specific human studies (➔ Table 30.1).[12–15]

The FDA requires an Investigational New Drug (IND) application, which is typically submitted for compounds with promising initial animal testing before first-in-human trials; but it can be submitted at any point in the life cycle of a drug prior to testing in humans. In addition to the information discussed previously, an IND includes a detailed description of the clinical studies

Table 30.1 Requirements for regulatory submissions: Investigational New Drug applications and clinical trial applications

Requirement	Details	Purpose
Clinical protocol	Detailed investigational plan and the protocols for specific human studies	◆ Evaluate the clinical development plan and ensure that the compound will be tested in the appropriate populations and studies proposed provide needed information on safety and efficacy ◆ Ensure studies do not pose unreasonable risk of harm to human subjects, and that appropriate safety monitoring is planned. ◆ Confirm that studies follow recommended ethical practices
Chemistry, manufacturing, and controls	Chemical composition of the compound, proper identification, and detailed description of manufacturing processes and control information (placebo if applicable)	◆ Confirm that the drug is manufactured in a controlled setting with appropriate methods in a process that preserves its identity, strength, quality, purity, and potency
Pharmacology and pharmacodynamics	Details of the mechanism of action of the compound and its pharmacodynamics from *in vitro* and *in vivo* testing	◆ Understand and confirm the proposed mechanism of action and primary effects of the compound ◆ Identify any off-target effects related to interaction with endogenous molecules ◆ Identify safety concerns related to the mechanism of action of the drug
Pharmacokinetics	Pharmacokinetic profiling from *in vitro* testing and animal studies showing compound absorption, distribution, metabolism, and excretion.	◆ Confirm appropriate drug formulation and mode of administration prior to human testing ◆ Identify compound metabolites ◆ Identify safety concerns related to drug metabolism and excretion
Toxicology	Results from animal studies designed to evaluate toxicity of the compound	◆ Ensure that appropriate testing was performed and help predict any toxicity risk to humans, prior to proceeding with clinical trials ◆ Identify approximate dosing ranges

planned, including study protocols, and may be amended after initial clearance to include additional studies (under the same indication). The FDA reviews the IND application and outlines concerns or deficiencies in the application that require review and correction. Once all issues are addressed, the FDA clears the IND and clinical studies may proceed. In certain circumstances, the FDA may issue a 'clinical hold' on an IND, which is an order to delay a proposed clinical investigation or to suspend an ongoing study. While this hold may be temporary if the cause of the clinical hold can be addressed and amended, it may be permanent if it is related to concerns over patient safety. Beyond initial approval and after phase I and II clinical trials, the FDA will also provide additional input on the design of larger-scale phase III trials.

The EMA process is slightly different from that of the FDA. Applications are based on individual clinical studies and are referred to as clinical trial applications (CTAs). Prior to January 2022, clinical trial sponsors had to apply to individual ethical committees and health authorities in countries of interest to obtain approval to run clinical trials. Since new legislation known as the Clinical Trials Regulation came into effect, a single application can be submitted via an online platform known as the Clinical Trials Information System (CTIS). This was done to facilitate the conduction of multinational trials for the purpose of drug approval in the European Union. Both the IND and CTA systems require annual reports and strict safety reports of all relevant safety information.

Phase I clinical trials

Phase I clinical trials are first-in-human studies designed to assess the safety of an investigational new drug in humans. Phase I clinical trials usually enrol a small number (typically <50–60 subjects) of healthy volunteers, except in certain situations (e.g. cancer patients who have failed other therapies and have no alternative therapies available to them). Given that these studies serve as a transition from animal models to humans, they are usually higher risk and are very closely monitored. Extensive amounts of data are usually collected from subjects who volunteer to participate. Given the risk and lack of known benefit, participants are usually compensated. While strict initial monitoring, frequent follow-up visits, regular biological sampling for assays, systematic clinical examinations, and periodic questionnaires are features of most clinical trials, these are usually more extensive in phase I studies. These trials are designed to primarily understand the side effects associated with increasing doses of the agent being evaluated and thus establish a maximal tolerated dose to help guide dosing in subsequent trials. Data collected also further characterize the drug's pharmacokinetics, pharmacodynamics, mechanism of action, and toxicity in humans, which do not always correlate perfectly with testing done in animal models.

Different forms of phase I clinical trials exist, each with the purpose of understanding specific characteristics of a compound in humans. Some common study designs include single ascending dose (SAD), multiple ascending dose (MAD), and food effects trials. Trials may be developed with integrated protocols that merge aspects of these study designs to obtain the information needed without running multiple individual studies. SAD studies often enrol a small group of subjects that initially receive a single dose of the compound and if tolerated dose escalation will proceed in subsequent groups of subjects until either the maximum protocol-defined dose is reached or the maximal tolerated dose is identified, whichever occurs first. These studies can be randomized with placebo controls to compare effects of exposure to the compound being evaluated. Starting doses are often much lower than considered pharmacologically active given the risk associated with first human exposure to a novel compound and are determined using non-clinical testing in animal models. Moreover, MAD studies are designed to evaluate exposure of subjects to multiple repeated doses of a compound with defined dosing intervals to understand the safety and pharmacokinetics of multiple doses and identify the eventual dosing regimen in phase II and III clinical trials. Data obtained from the SAD trial help with the prediction of the dose and dosing intervals in the MAD trial. Food effect trials are conducted for compounds that are orally administered to understand the effect of fasting and food intake on drug absorption and bioavailability.[14,16]

Phase II clinical trials

Phase II clinical trials build upon the data obtained from phase I, to design studies that evaluate the safety and efficacy of the drug for a particular indication among patients with a certain disease or condition of interest. Phase II studies are typically larger in size than phase I, enrolling several hundred patients, and can also be randomized and placebo controlled. Phase II studies further help evaluate the safety and tolerability of a compound, while identifying early evidence of efficacy. While phase II trials heavily rely on data from SAD and MAD studies to determine optimal dosing regimens, they also serve as experiments in dose finding, further fine-tuning the dose that will eventually be used in the larger-scale phase III trial.[14]

Phase II studies can sometimes be divided into phase IIa and phase IIb studies. While this designation has many contradicting definitions in the literature, it effectively subdivides studies performed during this phase into either early or late stage. Phase IIa studies are early-stage studies conducted in a smaller group of patients. These studies can be designed with the purpose of determining safety, optimal dosing, and, less commonly, evidence of efficacy. Phase IIb studies, sometimes considered small-scale phase III studies, tend to be slightly larger in size, and designed to provide a proof of concept for a larger-scale phase III trial. Although these studies are often underpowered to truly determine efficacy, the data obtained are important to guide protocol development for a phase III trial. Similar to phase I and phase III trials, extensive data collection and follow-up are also typical. Phase II studies also provide more definitive pharmacokinetic and pharmacodynamic data among patients with a chosen disease state, which may vary from what is observed among healthy volunteers.

Phase III clinical trials

When the drug in development demonstrates safety in phase II, it may proceed into phase III. A phase III clinical trial is required to assess the product's value in clinical practice and to market it under a specific indication. In a phase III trial, the safety and efficacy of the interventional drug is compared to the current standard of care in a large number of patients who have the disease in real life (i.e. not healthy volunteers). The trial aims to demonstrate that the drug advances therapy by either improving efficacy, tolerability, safety, or a combination of all three when compared to the therapies available on the market. The investigational drug may be studied either as an alternative or as an adjunct to standard of care, and patients enrolled in the trial are usually followed up for a long period of time relative to earlier trial phases. Phase III trials continue to build the evidence to support a novel compound but further characterize its effects in a large-scale clinical setting.

A phase III clinical trial is characterized by five important features: first, it is considered pivotal, that is, it demonstrates whether a drug offers a treatment benefit to a specific population of interest and provides key knowledge regarding the therapeutic impact of the new drug when compared to standard of care. Second, a phase III trial is comparative, that is, it is designed to compare two or more therapeutic interventions, which usually include the investigational drug versus either available therapies that are considered standard(s) for care or placebo if no available therapies are present. Third, it is randomized, that is, patients enrolled in the trial are assigned to either the investigational group versus non-investigational group in a completely random manner. This randomization process is critical to minimize bias and to reduce non-measurable confounding. Fourth, the intended outcomes are predefined elaborately and unambiguously in the trial protocol prior to any patient enrolment in the trial. These outcomes should be measurable and mathematically analysable. This process permits the investigators and regulatory agencies overseeing the trial to objectively determine whether the trial succeeded or failed at meeting its intended outcomes. Finally, the trial is multisite, that is, it involves multiple sites enrolling patients simultaneously to improve the rate by which patients are enrolled, as well as to demonstrate feasibility and generalizability across different settings, countries, and ethnicities. As these sites are expected to have inherent differences, they are therefore subject to strict centralized monitoring to ensure the adequacy of data quality and adherence to study protocols and procedures.

A good phase III trial will be designed to answer a simple and measurable clinical question in an objective, reproducible, and precise manner. Phase III trial design is a key component of the trial success. In 2007, the Spirit Initiative created an international collaborative effort to standardize trial protocol items and to provide evidence-based recommendations on setting the minimum standards for protocol best practices.[17] Therefore, prior to patient enrolment, a phase III trial design undergoes rigorous protocol building that clearly describes the following: the study duration and timeline, patient population, inclusion and exclusion criteria, study groups, quality control methods, desired sample size, as well as safety and efficacy outcomes and the intended methods to statistically analyse these outcomes. Also, the protocol describes key stakeholders, the frequency and planned oversight and data monitoring process during the active trial phase, and the logistic rules and regulations for the trial. Of similar importance, the protocol document provides the legal and ethical properties of the clinical trial, including the identity and mode of action of the sponsors, regulators, and ethics boards. Therefore, the protocol must be a well-structured and accessible document prior to trial activation. While this is true for protocols of any phase trial, the large size of phase III trials, and their often exorbitant cost, warrants more extensive planning and thoughtful design. Both the EMA and FDA meet with sponsors after phase II data are obtained to provide counsel regarding the design of robust phase III clinical trials. Notably, it is not uncommon that new data emerge, either internally or externally, which would necessitate an amendment to the initial protocol. When amendments are considered scientifically sound and are approved by regulatory bodies, they are considered an acceptable pathway to change specific parts of the protocol, and therefore should not be thought of as protocol or trial failure.

As phase III trials enrol hundreds to thousands of real-life patients, they warrant independent monitoring by a Drug Safety and Monitoring Board (DSMB), which is also referred to as Data Monitoring Committee (DMC). DSMBs were first established in the 1960s to ensure the safety of subjects in clinical trials.[18] While DSMBs or DMCs are also important for smaller phase II studies, they are more often a pivotal part of the monitoring of phase III trials given their size. They usually include a small number of members, made up of trialists, clinicians, or individuals with relevant expertise, and a statistician who is deemed a non-voting member of the committee. A critical role of DSMBs is to periodically undertake risk/benefit assessment using the data available at hand during the active phase of the clinical trial and evaluate for emergence of significant serious adverse outcomes that may signal evidence of harm. Alternatively, the DSMB also evaluates for signs of early overwhelming benefit or lack or benefit, such as futility, related to the investigational drug that would require an early termination of the trial. An overwhelming signal of benefit suggests that the investigational product should no longer be withheld from patients not randomized to the investigational group, as they should ethically receive the drug. Alternatively, in the event of overwhelming evidence for lack of benefit, early stopping is important to prevent the trial from further exposing patients to futile interventions and possible harms and to minimize trial costs. While the role of the DSMB is crucial in phase III studies, it is noteworthy to mention that a DSMB remains a consultative committee, and while encouraged by regulatory agencies, its presence is not a mandatory requirement for the initiation of a phase III trial.[19]

Once the phase III trial concludes patient enrolment and follow-up, data are then analysed in an independent manner that ensures data integrity and impartiality. If the investigational drug proves both effective and safe in the phase III trial, it may then proceed to regulatory submission for formal review by the appropriate regulatory authority. Following an extensive scrutiny of the analyses and the results, the drug may then obtain approval for marketing based on the indication it receives by the regulatory agency.

Regulatory review and marketing authorization

Once the appropriate clinical studies have been conducted and robust evidence to support the safety and efficacy of a novel compound has been established, a regulatory approval process can begin with the goal of providing authorization for drug distribution and use in clinical settings. It is typical for both the FDA and the EMA to meet with sponsors prior to filing of an application to provide guidance on the legal and regulatory requirements and to avoid preventable delays in the application review. Close communication with regulatory bodies throughout the drug development process is one of the most effective ways to reduce the delays in drug approval.

The process followed by the FDA is known as the New Drug Application (NDA) and has been in place since 1938. Any drug intended for commercial sale in the US requires approval via this process. An NDA builds on the IND by adding the information gathered from human trials regarding safety, efficacy, and drug pharmacokinetics, and pharmacodynamics.[13] The purpose of the NDA is to demonstrate that the drug is safe and effective for its intended indication, that the proposed drug labelling is appropriate, and that the drug manufacturing process is appropriate and maintains the drug quality. The data are compiled into several sections, some of which are identical to the IND. These include information on the chemistry, manufacturing, and controls, nonclinical pharmacology and toxicology, human pharmacokinetics and bioavailability, and clinical data, including the results of statistical analyses of the clinical trials.[20]

Once an NDA is filed, a review team from the FDA's Center for Drug Evaluation and Research (CDER) evaluates the application and independently reviews the data provided with special focus on the study methods and statistical analyses. This rigorous review is to ensure the drug is effective and that it has no prohibitive safety concerns. The approval process is often a risk/benefit evaluation given that no drugs are completely safe. The team may also ask the sponsor for additional data during the review process. Advisory committees made up of independent experts may also be used in certain situations to help counsel the FDA prior to their decision but these committees have no authority. Once the review of a NDA is complete, it is compiled by the CDER and may either confirm the conclusions reached by a sponsor or may contradict them. If the FDA review confirms that the drug is effective and its benefit outweighs its known risks, the drug receives marketing authorization in the US. If there are issues with the NDA including concerns over safety, manufacturing, or safety, the FDA will issue a response letter to the sponsor outlining these deficiencies. The FDA may recommend corrective actions ranging from additional clinical studies to changes to drug manufacturing. After these changes are made, an application may be resubmitted; however, in certain situations, a combination of unmodifiable issues may lead to a drug permanently failing to get market approval.

The EMA is responsible for drug marketing authorizations across the European Union. Its process is very similar to that of the FDA and is known as a Marketing Authorization Application (MAA). The information required for the MAA is very similar to a NDA, with additional requirements on risk management planning and safety monitoring in case of market approval as well as planned post-market studies. The EMA also has a team of experts known as the Committee for Medicinal Products for Human Use (CHMP) that reviews these applications and is the equivalent of the CDER. The CHMP assigns a rapporteur and co-rapporteur from two different countries for the evaluation of a novel compound. These two committee members each assemble a team of experts that independently reviews the data provided in the application. To further reduce any bias and strengthen the peer review process, one or more independent reviewers from CHMP may be assigned to oversee the assessments of both teams. CHMP members and the sponsor communicate frequently during this process and any additional information needed can be provided by the sponsor. Each team will then present an independent assessment report. Once these reports are reviewed internally, a single, combined report is generated, and a decision is made by formal vote to either allow marketing authorization or outline any major objections. Any major objections by the CHMP require corrective action or it may prohibit market approval. Similar to the CDER, the CHMP may obtain external input from scientific advisory groups or ad hoc expert groups.[21]

In addition to review of the evidence, regulatory authorities will also review the drug label to ensure the proper information is provided for patients and healthcare providers and the FDA usually conducts inspections of the facilities where the drug is manufactured to ensure the facilities are compliant with regulatory requirements.

Phase IV clinical trials and post-market monitoring

Once an investigational drug is approved and now marketed to the public, it then undergoes phase IV post-marketing surveillance. Contrary to all prior phases of drug development, phase IV studies include hundreds to thousands of patients who would be receiving the drug in an uncontrolled real-world environment. During phase IV, the investigational drug undergoes continued safety surveillance through a regulated adverse event monitoring system.[22] This safety process is especially helpful as potentially fatal adverse reactions that tend to occur very rarely and may be missed in earlier trials may sometimes only be detected in the phase IV post-marketing surveillance. The safety data from phase IV studies is therefore important as signals for harm may necessitate changing the drug's prescribing information and even occasionally market withdrawal altogether.[23]

Of similar importance, data emerging from phase IV studies may demonstrate signals for new benefits, which would lead to exploring new trials for the purpose of expanding the product's indication and label. While post-marketing surveillance does not prove efficacy, which is evaluated within the controlled environment of a phase III clinical trial, it does demonstrate effectiveness, which tests the drug function at a population level including its feasibility of acquisition, its impact on organs and numerous disease states, and its interaction with concomitant drugs in real life.[22] In general, phase IV post-monitoring surveillance is expected to continue lifelong or as long as the drug remains in the market available for public consumption.

References

1. US Food and Drug Administration. Part II: 1938, Food, Drug, Cosmetic Act. Nov 2018. Available at: https://www.fda.gov/about-fda/changes-science-law-and-regulatory-authorities/part-ii-1938-food-drug-cosmetic-act
2. European Medicines Agency. History of EMA. n.d. Available at https://www.ema.europa.eu/en/about-us/history-ema
3. Seyhan AA. Lost in translation: the valley of death across preclinical and clinical divide—identification of problems and overcoming obstacles. Transl Med Comm. 2019;4:18.
4. Emmerich CH, Gamboa LM, Hofmann MCJ, et al. Improving target assessment in biomedical research: the GOT-IT recommendations. Nat Rev Drug Discov. 2021;20:64–81.
5. Hughes JP, Rees S, Kalindjian SB, Philpott KL. Principles of early drug discovery. Br J Pharmacol. 2011;162:1239–49.
6. Broach JR, Thorner J. High-throughput screening for drug discovery. Nature. 1996;384:14–16.
7. Desselle MR, Neale R, Hansford KA, et al. Institutional profile: Community for Open Antimicrobial Drug Discovery—crowdsourcing new antibiotics and antifungals. Future Sci OA. 2017;3:FSO171.
8. Lyne PD. Structure-based virtual screening: an overview. Drug Discov Today. 2002;7:1047–55.
9. Keserű GM, Makara GM. Hit discovery and hit-to-lead approaches. Drug Discov Today. 2006;11:741–8.
10. Robles AI, Varticovski L. Harnessing genetically engineered mouse models for preclinical testing. Chem Biol Interact. 2008;171: 159–64.
11. Arome D, Chinedu E. The importance of toxicity testing. J Pharm Biosci. 2013;4:146–8.
12. Chiodin D, Cox EM, Edmund AV, Kratz E, Lockwood SH. Regulatory affairs 101: introduction to investigational new drug applications and clinical trial applications. Clin Transl Sci. 2019;12: 334–42.
13. US Food and Drug Administration. New drug application (NDA). Jan 2022. Available at: https://www.fda.gov/drugs/types-applications/new-drug-application-nda
14. US Food and Drug Administration. CFR—Code of Federal Regulations Title 21. March 2023. Available at: https://www.accessdata.fda.gov/scripts/cdrh/cfdocs/cfcfr/CFRsearch.cfm?CFRPart=312
15. US Food and Drug Administration. IND applications for clinical investigations: Chemistry, Manufacturing, and Control (CMC) information. Feb 2022. Available at: https://www.fda.gov/drugs/investigational-new-drug-ind-application/ind-applications-clinical-investigations-chemistry-manufacturing-and-control-cmc-information
16. European Medicines Agency. Guideline on strategies to identify and mitigate risks for first-in-human and early clinical trials with investigational medicinal products. July 2017. Available at: https://www.ema.europa.eu/en/documents/scientific-guideline/guideline-strategies-identify-mitigate-risks-first-human-early-clinical-trials-investigational_en.pdf
17. Strengthening the credibility of clinical research. Lancet. 2010;375:1225.
18. Slutsky AS, Lavery JV. Data safety and monitoring boards. N Engl J Med. 2004;350:1143–7.
19. Bhattacharyya A, Gallo P, Crisp A, et al. The changing landscape of data monitoring committees—perspectives from regulators, members, and sponsors. Biom J. 2019;61:1232–41.
20. US Food and Drug Administration. Guidance for industry: formatting, assembling and submitting new drug and antibiotic applications. Feb 1987. Available at: https://www.fda.gov/media/71485/download
21. European Medicines Agency. Committee for Medicinal Product for Human Use: rules of procedure. Oct 2022. Available at: https://www.ema.europa.eu/en/documents/other/chmp-rules-procedure_en.pdf
22. Suvarna V. Phase IV of drug development. Perspect Clin Res. 2010;1:57–60.
23. Baber N. International conference on harmonisation of technical requirements for registration of pharmaceuticals for human use (ICH). Br J Clin Pharmacol. 1994;37:401–4.

Index

For the benefit of digital users, indexed terms that span two pages (e.g., 52–53) may, on occasion, appear on only one of those pages.

Tables, figures, and boxes are indicated by an italic *t*, *f*, and *b* following the page/paragraph number.

W